AF803245

FUNCTIONAL NEUROSCIENCE

Volume 3

NEUROMETRIC ASSESSMENT OF BRAIN DYSFUNCTION IN NEUROLOGICAL PATIENTS

NEUROMETRIC ASSESSMENT OF BRAIN DYSFUNCTION IN NEUROLOGICAL PATIENTS

THALÍA HARMONY

Routledge
Taylor & Francis Group
LONDON AND NEW YORK

First published in 1984 by Lawrence Erlbaum Associates, Inc.

This edition first published in 2022
by Routledge
2 Park Square, Milton Park, Abingdon, Oxon OX14 4RN

and by Routledge
605 Third Avenue, New York, NY 10158

Routledge is an imprint of the Taylor & Francis Group, an informa business

© 1984 Lawrence Erlbaum Associates, Inc.

All rights reserved. No part of this book may be reprinted or reproduced or utilised in any form or by any electronic, mechanical, or other means, now known or hereafter invented, including photocopying and recording, or in any information storage or retrieval system, without permission in writing from the publishers.

Trademark notice: Product or corporate names may be trademarks or registered trademarks, and are used only for identification and explanation without intent to infringe.

British Library Cataloguing in Publication Data
A catalogue record for this book is available from the British Library

ISBN: 978-0-367-75066-4 (Set)
ISBN: 978-1-003-18026-5 (Set) (ebk)
ISBN: 978-0-367-75416-7 (Volume 3) (hbk)
ISBN: 978-0-367-75421-1 (Volume 3) (pbk)
ISBN: 978-1-003-16243-8 (Volume 3) (ebk)

Publisher's Note
The publisher has gone to great lengths to ensure the quality of this reprint but points out that some imperfections in the original copies may be apparent.

Disclaimer
The publisher has made every effort to trace copyright holders and would welcome correspondence from those they have been unable to trace.

FUNCTIONAL NEUROSCIENCE VOLUME 3

NEUROMETRIC ASSESSMENT OF BRAIN DYSFUNCTION IN NEUROLOGICAL PATIENTS

THALÍA HARMONY

Escuela Nacional de
Estudios Profesionales,
Iztacala
Universidad Nacional
Autónoma de Mexico

LEA LAWRENCE ERLBAUM ASSOCIATES, PUBLISHERS
1984 Hillsdale, New Jersey London

Copyright © 1984 by Lawrence Erlbaum Associates, Inc.
All rights reserved. No part of this book may be reproduced in any form, by photostat, microform, retrieval system, or any other means, without the prior written permission of the publisher.

Lawrence Erlbaum Associates, Inc., Publishers
365 Broadway
Hillsdale, New Jersey 07642

Library of Congress Cataloging in Publication Data

Harmony, Thalía.
Neurometric assessment of brain dysfunction in neurological patients.

(Functional neuroscience; v. 3)
Bibliography: p.
Includes index.
1. Evoked potentials (Electrophysiology) 2. Electroencephalography. 3. Brain—Diseases—Diagnosis.
I. Title. II. Series.
RC386.6E86H37 1984 616.8'047547 83-16450
ISBN 0-89859-044-2

Printed in the United States of America
10 9 8 7 6 5 4 3 2 1

Note for 2022 edition

This book was written in the early 1980s and contains information up to that date. However, many new methods of analysis of the electroencephalogram (EEG) and the Event Related Potentials (ERP) of great clinical utility have been described and applied since that time; they are not described in this volume.

To Tony, Thalita, and
Antonio with love

Contents

Preface

Ten years ago, at my laboratory in the CENIC[1], E. Roy John, a group of my very young colleagues, and I, had a long talk about what the future direction for our research should be. We felt the need to carry out applied research, which would in some sense contribute to solving problems related to human welfare. The development of the neurosciences with the use of computers in the study of electrical activity of the brain had provided enough evidence to demonstrate that it was possible to move toward the application of such results. The question was whether a new methodology based on quantitative analysis of electrical brain activity, which could be sensitive enough to detect subtle brain abnormalities—not yet clinically apparent—in human beings, could be developed. In order to substantiate this possibility, it was necessary, as a first step, to demonstrate the effectiveness of the procedure in patients with well-known lesions of the nervous system. My group, at the CENIC, undertook this task. Independently, many other researchers have conducted studies in this direction. This book deals with the results obtained in this field. Dr. John, in the second volume of this series, has shown that the method is also useful in the assessment of learning-disabled children and old patients with cognitive impairment. The results obtained with these investigations have provided a tremendous amount of information about some features that are most altered in the presence of brain damage. On this basis, it is possible to jump a step forward and to search for those procedures that may be used for the early detection of brain dysfunction in asymptomatic subjects. Work on this is

[1]Centro Nacional de Investigaciones Científicas, Havana, Cuba.

now in progress; we feel optimistic of its success with the collaborative efforts of researchers in neurometrics.

I owe many people thanks; especially my friend Dr. E. Roy John for his continuous aid, ideas, criticisms, and suggestions during the last 10 years. I am also indebted to him for his dedicated labor correcting the whole manuscript of this book; to my colleagues Dr. Gloria Otero, Dr. Josefina Ricardo, and Dr. Guido Fernández for their numerous contributions to this work; to Dr. Pedro Valdés for his creative ideas in the solutions of many statistical and computational problems, for his suggestions in the writing of this book, including his writing of Chapter 7; to Dr. Alfredo Alvarez for his continuous dedication to this work; to Mr. Octavio Baez, Dr. Virgilio Rodríguez, and Mrs. Margarita Solís for programming as well as their help with much of data analysis; to Dr. Bĵorn Holmgren and Dr. Mitchel Valdés for their readings of the first drafts; to Mrs. Clara Castro, Mrs. Trinidad Virués, Mrs. Berta Castellanos, and Mr. Eduardo Eimil for their technical assistance; to Eng. Manuel Sánchez for his continuous collaboration during these years; to Mrs. Lydis Rodríguez, Mr. Juan Almira, and Mrs. Nelsa Echevarría for operating the computer; to Mrs. Silvia Pérez and Mrs. Teresa López for typewriting the manuscript; to Dr. Hansook Ahn for help in the editing of this book; to Dr. Wilfredo Torres, Dr. Juan Kourí, and Dr. Carlos Pascual for their trust and support in the realization of our work; to Eng. Luis Carrasco and Eng. Andrés Valladares for lending the computer facilities to carry out this work; to Dr. Luis Rodríguez Rivera and Dr. Guillermo Rodríguez del Pozo for lending the facilities for studying the patients, and to my husband, Dr. Antonio Fernández- Bouzas, for his continuous encouragement, help, and original suggestions, and for having patiently endured the long time I devoted to writing this book, which interfered with the pleasure of our being together. Finally, I want to express my gratitude to the Cuban people for giving me the opportunity to share in the creation of a new society, and for their example in handling many difficult tasks with love, dedication, and effort.

Thalía Harmony

1 Introduction

I. NEUROMETRICS—DEFINITION

The aim of this book is to interest clinical neuroscientists in the application of neurometrics to the evaluation of brain dysfunction in neurological patients. This methodology may produce substantial improvement in the neurological medical care of the general population.

In the last 15 years, as a result of the development of minicomputers and their application to the quantitative analysis of electrophysiological phenomena, there has been a great expansion of knowledge about the electrical activity of the brain. This activity yields a great variety of information about brain functions. Not only does the electrical activity of the brain contain valuable diagnostic information about brain lesions, but it also reveals many phenomena related to sensory, perceptual, and cognitive processes (Adey, 1974; John, 1977).

Neurometrics is a methodology, based on quantitative measurements of the brain electrical activity, for evaluating anatomical integrity, developmental maturation, and the mediation of sensory, perceptual, and cognitive processes. The goals of neurometrics are to gather accurate data sensitive to these various brain functions, to extract and quantify critical features of these data, and to classify the resulting profiles by statistical methods into clusters sharing common characteristics of brain dysfunction. Thus, neurometrics not only provides a quantitative description of brain electrical activity, but it may also indicate the diagnostic category to which an individual belongs, an application relevant for clinical purposes.

Neurometrics may be also used to discriminate among different physiological and psychophysiological processes or among different brain states. Such results provide important contributions to the knowledge of brain function, but they are not the subject of this book, which focuses on practical clinical applications and the theoretical and experimental formulations on which these are based.

II. MAJOR APPLICATIONS OF NEUROMETRICS IN CLINICAL NEUROLOGY

Many procedures are currently used for the study of neurological patients: clinical examination and complementary studies such as the electroencephalogram (EEG), laboratory examinations, X-ray studies such as angiographies, pneumoencephalograms, and Computerized Axial Tomography (CAT), gammagram, and so on. These procedures are extremely useful in diagnosing many neurological diseases, but they need skilled personnel for their performance and interpretation. In some cases, they are also very expensive and even traumatic for the patients. On the other hand, some patients have subtle functional abnormalities that are not detectable by the usual procedures. Thus, the main benefits to be expected from the application of neurometrics to the assessment of neurological patients are more sensitive, objective, efficient, and economical methods for the detection of subtle brain abnormalities. From a practical point of view, the use of neurometrics will be justified if it offers greater ease or reliability of diagnosis, reductions in costs, or requirements of special skills compared with conventional visual assessment of the EEG.

We focus on two major applications of neurometrics in clinical neurology: (1) as a mass screening procedure for the assessment of brain dysfunction or brain damage; and (2) as an aid to the specialist in obtaining a picture of the functional state of the brain, and reaching a more accurate diagnosis.

The first application is as a mass screening procedure for the assessment of brain dysfunction in those subjects who can be considered "at risk" for brain disease or damage, and in whom early detection and consequent immediate treatment will improve their prognosis. As examples, we can mention infants with pre-and perinatal risk factors; childhood diseases (38% of children with apparently uncomplicated childhood diseases show an EEG abnormality, Gibbs & Gibbs, 1964); cranial traumas; psychiatric patients and patients with headaches in whom a neurological lesion should be ruled out; chronic intoxication of workers in polluted environments; patients with peripheral signs of atherosclerosis, but asymptomatic from the neurological point of view, and so on. Appropriate preventive health programs should include the examination of these cases for early detection of brain dysfunction. Neurometrics may provide a simple, efficient, and economic way to identify within these at-risk subjects those with some sign of brain dysfunction, in order to send them directly to the appropriate specialists.

Neurometrics may be also an aid to the neurologist in a more specialized service. Neurometrics may be useful for: (1) the diagnosis of some difficult cases (e.g., multiple sclerosis patients in whom, from a clinical point of view, it is not possible to detect multiple lesions, which electrophysiological analysis may reveal); (2) studying the evolution of a case by an objective and precise procedure that permits quantitative comparisons within the same patient; (3) the evaluation of different types of treatments according to the evolution of the case; (4) the identification of different electrophysiological profiles within a group of patients with common clinical characteristics, related to different causes of similar symptoms, to selective responses to a particular treatment or to the prognosis; and (5) monitoring the brain state during anesthesia, hemodialysis, or intensive care. Neurometrics can be considered as an addition to the methods primarily sensitive to anatomical lesions (CAT, angiographies) by reflecting functional state as well as structural integrity.

At the moment great differences in the possibilities of medical care exist between countries. Perhaps those who live in countries with more developed health programs will consider that it is not necessary to seek mass screening procedures for the assessment of brain dysfunction, because this could be accomplished by the routine examinations of the at-risk population by skilled specialists. Let us assume that there are some countries that perhaps have such an abundance of specialists that they can take care of the entire at-risk population. Even they could derive a substantial benefit from mass screening to save the specialists time, so that they only need to examine those subjects who have been previously identified as suspect of having brain dysfunction or damage, eliminating the need to expend a great deal of time examining normal subjects. However, there is a world-wide general lack of sufficient specialists to permit the study of all those potential patients who may suffer from some type of neurological disease.

Let us first discuss the situation in the developed countries. Although in the period between 1960 and 1968, such countries had between 23.2 (Israel) and 7.4 (Finland) physicians per 10,000 inhabitants (Popov, 1972), the question arises whether all of them are able to detect subtle abnormalities that correspond to the first signs of a neurological disease. We suggest that, for this purpose, only neurologists, internal medicine specialists, and pediatricians are adequately prepared. Table 1.1 shows the ratio of population to available specialists of these types for several countries (in thousands). From the table, one can calculate that on the average there are about 2 neurologists, 10 internists, and 4 pediatricians, or a total of about 16 relevant specialists, per 100,000 inhabitants. Although it is well known

TABLE 1.1
Mean Ratio of Inhabitants (in thousands) Per Specialist[a]

Country	*Year*	*Neurologists*	*Internists*	*Pediatricians*
Austria	1963	26,1	9,3	19,4
Bulgaria	1963	24,4	3,4	7,3
Canada	1960	23,8	13,4	31,5
Czechoslovakia	1963	27,3	4,8	5,3
Denmark	1963	48,8	13,4	57,1
Finland	1963	29,9	17,5	36,1
France	1961	36,7	28,7	39,2
G.D.R.	1963	23,3	6,5	19,6
Hungary	1963	25,5	5,6	9,1
Israel	1963	41	5,6	7,4
Norway	1962	48,3	12,5	38,6
Poland	1963	69,1	9,2	9,4
Sweden	1963	74,5	5,0	25,8
Netherlands	1963	15,3	15,1	35,4
USA	1963	106,0	5	13,5
USSR	1968	14,4	1,9	3,2
UK	1963	311,0	25,7	119,0

[a]From Popov, 1972, table 27.

that specialists are mainly concentrated in urban areas, we assume that they are uniformly distributed throughout the country for our next consideration.

An overall estimate of the incidence of neurological diseases is 29 per 1000 inhabitants in the Soviet Union (Popov, 1972) and 38.86 in the United States (John, 1977). The overall estimate of the at-risk subjects in whom a neurological lesion should be ruled out is difficult to obtain. However, a survey of several sources estimating the incidence of head trauma (12/00, John, 1977); persistent headaches (20/00, John, 1977); perinatal trauma and newborn diseases (1.5/00, Popov, 1972); a fraction of the incidence of psychiatric illness (10/00, Lin & Standley, 1964) and of childhood disease (38% of children with childhood diseases, Gibbs & Gibbs, 1964), and the incidence of atherosclerosis (48.8/00, Popov, 1972) leads to the conclusion that somewhat more than 10% of the population is at risk of brain damage. This estimate is reinforced by the fact that the National Institute of Neurological and Communication Disorders and Strokes (NINCDS, 1973) of the United States has calculated that approximately 10% of the population of the United States may be suffering from neurological disorders. Assume that neurologists are dedicated full time to the evaluation of neurological and at-risk patients, but internists and pediatricians are only available one-fifth of their time for this purpose (this is a rough approximation based on the number of beds usually dedicated to neurological patients in a general medical service). Then, as an overall average, for each 100,000 inhabitants, there are the full-time equivalents of two neurologists, two internists, and one pediatrician.

This means that five full-time specialists must annually attend 3400 neurological cases (mean value between John's and Popov's estimates) and at least 10,000 at-risk patients, which is equal to 2680 patients/specialist/year. A careful neurological examination with a clinical history and evaluation of subtle changes takes almost one hour per specialist. Taking into account that neurological patients require much additional time for EEG and other examinations, for hospitalization, periodical examination, and so on, *it is obvious that even in the developed countries, the number of specialists who are available for studying all potential neurological patients is not adequate even if they were similarly distributed in rural and urban areas.*

A more dramatic picture of the current state of the distribution of neurologists and psychiatrists in the world is shown in Table 1.2. These results correspond to an inquiry by the Mental Health group of the World Health Organization presented in 1963. Eight countries with a total population of 20 million inhabitants had no such specialists, and 35 countries with

TABLE 1.2
Number of Neurologists and Psychiatrists for Each 100,000 Inhabitants[a]

Number of Specialists for each 100,000	*Number of Countries*	*Total Population (in millions)*
0	8	20
0,49	35	890
0,5–1,99	13	194
2,0–4,0	21	582
4,0	8	265

[a]From Popov, 1972, table 28.

a total population of 890 million inhabitants had only one specialist per 200,000 inhabitants. These numbers reveal the urgent need for medical personnel in many countries, which will take many years to acquire. In the meantime, neurometric methods for mass screening may increase the efficiency of medical care in many countries by identifying those subjects who must be studied by specialists when available, and may aid in reaching accurate diagnoses when specialists are not available. Thus, the efficiency of medical care will improve, because a general physician may take care of a portion of these cases, such as epileptics and cerebrovascular disease patients. The other cases, who need specialized examinations and treatments—for example, people with brain tumors—will be sent to specialists. Thus, the skilled personnel will be only dedicated to examining and treating such cases, leaving the remaining cases for the general physician. At the end of this book, we present a proposal for how to organize programs to attend to the population, depending on the capabilities of countries with different levels of development.

In summary, the efficiency of medical care will be improved by neurometric procedures in the following aspects:

1. Saving time of medical personnel who will study only those "suspicious" cases detected by the mass screening procedure.
2. Obtaining earlier diagnoses of the neurological diseases, which will permit immediate treatment, improving the prognosis for the patient.
3. Improving the accuracy of the diagnosis.
4. Developing preventive strategies against those factors that produce undesirable effects on the brain.
5. Providing a functional picture of the brain state of the patient, to study the evolution of the cases and the effect of treatments or remedial procedures.

III. CURRENT STATE OF NEUROMETRICS

In the development of neurometric procedures, different stages should be considered: the first, or experimental, stage and the second stage of application of the resulting methods in routine clinical practice. During the experimental stage, the aim is to select those salient features that reflect the different varieties of brain dysfunction and to develop decision rules for the classification of subjects into clusters according to electrophysiological profiles. During this stage, it is necessary to study groups of patients with definitely diagnosed lesions, to establish that the procedure is sufficiently sensitive to detect these type of lesions. For such a study, it is also necessary to obtain normative data from a population similar to the patients. Criteria for the inclusion of subjects in the referential group must be carefully defined. After the development of decision rules, it is necessary to perform replication studies to test the reliability of the procedure. In addition, the study of similar patients, but with minimal clinical evidence of cerebral lesions, is extremely important for the development of procedures sensitive to subtle brain abnormalities reflecting early stages of disease.

For the first stage, integrated teams of specialists in neurophysiology, medicine, computation, statistics, psychology and electronics are needed. After this stage, the method may be applied by a well-trained technician. Once the evaluation procedure is adequately developed, evaluation of a patient becomes rather straightforward.

To date, an enormous amount of work has been done on the quantitative evaluation of brain electrical activity, with very promising results. However, such information has not yet had much impact on clinical practice. Few neurometric procedures have been incorporated as routine examinations in the neurological services. Although several factors may delay routine clinical application of these new methods to the assessment of brain damage, one of the most important is that the development of this methodology is based on several disciplines: electrophysiology, electronic engineering, computation technology, statistical analysis, and medicine. At present, it is impossible for a single person to have sufficient knowledge in all these areas. This is why multidisciplinary teams are working in the development of such procedures. Therefore, the clinician or the electroencephalographer is confronted by a new methodology that is difficult to understand. Papers on this topic are generally written for people who work in the field. This also impedes comprehensibility for someone who does not have training in the relevant fields.

I am a physician. In my own experience, I have found it extremely difficult to understand the great variety of multidisciplinary aspects that are involved in the neurometric methodology. I have been working for many years with a multidisciplinary team, which has helped me in the study and comprehension of many different types of problems. Even with this help, it took many years before I felt capable of dealing with the variety of theoretical and technical problems involved in neurometrics. I wrote this book with the hope that it might explain and clarify these problems to other clinical neuroscientists who want to apply neurometric procedures. With this orientation, the book has been constructed in such a way that it covers the most elementary problems as well as more complex ones. At the same time, I have tried to make an up-to-date review of current quantitative electrophysiological methods and their clinical applications.

For some readers, little new information will be provided in some chapters. Nevertheless, they may be interested in particular topics in this volume. From Chapters 2 to 6, I have included data that clearly demonstrates that brain damage or dysfunction produces alterations of the EEG and of the averaged evoked responses. Chapters 7 and 8 present the mathematical bases for the statistical analysis of brain electrical activity and the development of neurometric procedures, as well as some fundamental considerations for automatic analysis. In Chapters 9 and 10, the major procedures of quantitative analysis of brain electrical activity, as well as their theoretical assumptions and practical applications, are reviewed. These analyses constitute the basis for neurometric procedures, which also take advantage of statistical theory for the establishment of decision rules to make possible the assignment of a given subject to a particular diagnostic group. Chapters 11 to 13 review the principal neurometric procedures that have been described until now, as well as their advantages and limitations.

In Chapter 14, I have summarized the more relevant electrophysiological and neurometric findings for each of the major neurological diseases, and the possible future approaches that seem to be of interest according to our actual knowledge.

In conclusion, I want to emphasize that neurometrics is not only a methodology of the future, but it is for the present as well. It is possible to take advantage of our current knowledge to achieve substantial improvement in the medical care of the general population. If neurometrics is considered as a sophisticated technique understood and used primarily for neuroscience research, it will be a long time before this knowledge begins to help people who are at risk of brain damage. Clinicians should become informed about the utility of these methods, because their participation is crucial for the utilization of what we believe is a new and valuable field of clinical neuroscience.

2 The Electroencephalogram

I. THE GENESIS OF THE ELECTROENCEPHALOGRAM (EEG)

This topic has recently been reviewed by Creutzfeldt (1974) and Thatcher and John (1977). Brain potentials arise from movements of ions across membranes, the extracellular space being the medium through which electrical currents flow and interact. One of the most striking characteristics of the EEG is the presence of rhythmic oscillations or synchronization. Many studies have demonstrated the importance of cortical–thalamic relationships in such phenomena. Synaptic potentials are a primary contribution to the genesis of the EEG, as been demonstrated by Purpura, Scharff, and McMurtry (1965) and Creutzfeldt, Kugler, Morocutti, and Sommer-Smith (1966). Investigations using microelectrodes in fiber tracts have demonstrated rather large extracellular EEG-like slow waves that make it clear that afterpotentials, or slow-wave processes closely associated with axon spikes, contribute to the EEG (Verzeano, 1972). Finally, the possibility exists that intrinsic oscillations of the membrane potential also contribute to the EEG.

In addition, it is a well-established fact that innumerable connections exist between any given neuron and any other neuron chosen nearly anywhere within the neural axis (Lorente de No, 1938). The extent and complexity of neuronal interconnectivity is responsible in part for the development of theories that maintain that neuronal population behavior is inherently statistical in nature. These theories are based on the fact that there is considerable variability in the behavior of individual neurons and that interaction of one neuron with another is so important that emergent properties appear in a population of neurons that are not discernible by observing the behavior of any individual element. Thus, in a population of neurons, there exists a certain degree of both coherence and randomness. Adey (1975) has proposed a mechanism that can exercise control of such coherence. This mechanism is supported by the fact that minute extracellular current flows can affect neuronal excitability, neural coherence, and, consequently, behavior, the frequency of the external modulating field being an important variable in the control of the EEG rhythm. In Adey's model, the macromolecular structure of the extracellular space, with numerous fixed negative charges, is believed to operate as a "sensor" and "amplifier" of weak electric fields, influencing many of the neurons in the local domain. These extracellular factors must be considered, then, as a supplemental influence modulating basic anatomic and synaptic mechanisms.

In essence, the EEG is an expression of the moment-by-moment statistical mean behavior of different populations of neurons that, in turn, is critically dependent on their functional connectivity. It is only a small step from the concept that the EEG reflects statistical features of the behavior of neuronal populations to the concept, central to the neurometric approach, that statistical analysis of the EEG will permit both the definition of normal behavior of these neuronal populations and the identification of different types of abnormality. Changes in the EEG imply changes in the coherent behavior of cells due to local effects, remote changes in input, or a combination of both, caused by physical or chemical processes.

The EEG may be recorded with electrodes attached to the scalp or with cortical or subcortical electrodes with their tips in the region selected. Special techniques have been designed for electrocorticography and deep recording. However, in this book, we refer only to data from scalp recordings, because our main purpose is to review those procedures that have been shown to be useful for the routine assessment of brain dysfunction in clinical neurology, seeking methods that can be applied for mass screening. Comparison of scalp and subdural recordings have demonstrated that only widely synchronized components of the cortical activity are observed at the scalp. Small time differences between the occurrence of similar waves in neighboring areas will reduce the amplitude of the scalp EEG. Thus, a given time difference of occurrence of waves will have a much greater canceling effect on high- than on low-frequency activity. For strictly localized activity, the attenuation from cortex to scalp can be as high as 5000:1, but for coherent activity over a wide area, it may be only 2:1 (Cooper, Winter, & Walter, 1965).

II. TECHNICAL ASPECTS OF EEG RECORDING

This topic has recently been reviewed by Broughton (1976) and MacGillivray (1974). The brain electrical activity is recorded from the scalp by electrodes connected to amplifiers and recording equipment. This electrical activity is conducted through the tissues by electrolytes. The quality of the recording, and, consequently, the degree of confidence with which it may be later measured, analyzed, and interpreted depends on all components of the electrode–amplification–recording system. What is actually recorded is the time course of the difference in voltage between two electrodes. One of these electrodes may be over an active region of the brain and the other on some relatively inactive site (referential or monopolar recording) or both electrodes may be over two different active regions (bipolar recording). Thus, it should be clear that accurate recording demands that any electrical phenomena produced by the electrodes themselves be similar and stable. Because the interface between the generator of biopotentials (the brain) and the electrode is a crucial link in the system, adequate preparation and application of electrodes is one of the most important aspects in the electrophysiological technique.

A. Electrodes

1. Electrode-Tissue Interface

The theory of electrodes is extremely complex and has been the subject of innumerable papers and texts. One of the fundamental components of all electrode systems is the electrode-electrolyte interface. The electrode may be made of a number of metals; the electrolyte may be a commercially prepared paste of gel or it may be the surrounding physiological fluid, such as is present in the subcutaneous tissue for subdermal needle electrodes. Various charge migrations are set in motion by the contact of the electrode with the electrolyte, with ionic migration from the metal into the solution and vice versa, thus creating a double layer at the phase boundary between the metal and the solution. The orientation of this double layer depends on the mutual relation of the tendency of the metals to discharge cations and osmotic pressures in the solution. If the former is stronger, the electrode is negative to the solution (the electrode loses positive charges to the solution); if the latter predominates, the electrode is positive (the electrode receives positive charges from the solution). These shifts are usually very large (on the order of mV) compared to the EEG signal (on the order of 20-100 microvolts [μV]. They can be quite different even between electrodes of similar materials and may vary from moment to moment, particularly if the surface of the electrolyte/metal interface is physically altered.

The presence of charges at the electrode surface introduces capacitative properties so that the tissue electrode interface must be considered as having both resistive and capacitative elements (i.e., a time constant, which is part of the whole recording system). From a practical point of view, this is very important, because it is meaningless to try to record slow-frequency components of the EEG activity with fine electrodes that have a smaller time constant. The total voltage between a pair of electrodes used for recording is the difference between the tissue-electrode potentials plus the ongoing physiological activity underneath each electrode. In order to observe the variable potential differences between electrodes that reflect brain activity, the larger potentials at the electrolyte-electrode interface must be held quite constant. The magnitude of the potentials actually recorded is determined by the potential drop across the amplifier inputs. If the tissue-electrode interface resistance is high, then there will be a large proportional potential drop at this point and the amplifiers will record correspondingly less of the total potential. A low electrode resistance at the electrode-tissue interface, relative to the amplifier input resistance, is therefore an important factor in achieving satisfactory EEG recordings. It is generally accepted that the electrode resistance should be less than 1/100 of the input resistance of the amplifier.

2. Polarization—The Ag/AgCl Electrode

Another characteristic of the electrode-electrolyte double layer is polarization. An electrode functioning in the limiting condition that no ions can cross the double layer is said to be a completely polarizable electrode. If the ions can move completely and freely in both directions across the double layer, it is said to be a nonpolarizable electrode. The fluctuating EEG potentials can only be measured with electrodes that are relatively nonpolarizable (or reversible electrodes). The chloriding process of silver electrodes ensures electrode reversibility. Chloriding is performed by placing the cleaned silver electrode in a solution of NaCl, the strength of which should be at least that of physiological saline (it is important to avoid evaporation and excessive concentration of saline because AgCl is slightly soluble in strong saline). The electrode is connected to the positive pole anode of a dry cell. A piece of silver is used as the cathode to complete the circuit (only silver metal should be in saline). The chloride ions in solution move to the silver electrode and form neutral silver chloride molecules that coat it. During recording, if the electrode forms the anode (relative to reference), anions from the tissue accumulate on it, especially Cl. This forms AgCl at the electrode already coated with AgCl and thus the surface quality does not change. If the electrode acts as the cathode, tissue cations react with the chloride ion of the AgCl coat releasing Ag. Again, the electrode surface remains qualitatively unchanged (Bures, Petrán, & Zachar, 1967).

Electrolyte chlorination may be a fast or a slow process. The lower the current density used (0.1 to 10 A/m²), the lower will be the final electrode resistance. The silver chloride electrode must be protected from light, drying, and friction. In use, the layer of chloride will eventually chip and break away and the electrode will produce artifacts. Rechloriding, after stripping the electrode by passing 4.5 V from the negative pole of a battery through the electrode in 5% saline until it is clean, will restore the electrode. Sodium hydroxide is produced during stripping and this saline should be discarded. The advantages of a silver/silver chloride electrode are its stability and low noise, the ease with which electrode potential can be equalized, its nonpolarizing properties, and low impedance, which ensures good quality in the recording.

3. Types of Electrodes

According to MacGillivray (1974), the general properties of electrodes suitable for routine work are:

1. *A stable electrode potential*: This means that the electrode potential should be almost constant. This process is helped by storing electrodes together in weak electrolyte solutions, and also by proper chloriding of silver electrodes.
2. *Equalized electrode potential*: Widely differing electrode potential may produce sufficient current flow between electrodes, when connected as a recording pair, to change the electrode potential itself by polarization effects. This makes the pair "noisy" and much more susceptible to movement artifacts; it also changes the inherent resistance and recording time constants. To avoid this effect, the same recommendations described in (1) are useful.
3. *Convenience of use*: Electrodes should be of simple construction and inexpensive, easy to apply, provide a stable tissue contact, and be easily removed. They should also be light in weight and strong enough to permit easy manipulation.

A variety of metals, such as gold, silver, lead, tin, solder, and stainless steel, which have in common a low chemical reactivity to electrolyte solutions, are used in routine EEG recording. From a practical point of view, the relative nonpolarizable silver/silver chloride electrode offers the best electrode properties. Electrode paste is widely needed for electrodes attached to the scalp surface. The electrolyte to skin interface is another complex system. Hair may impede good contact and the skin should be sufficiently cleaned in order to avoid a high impedance oily contact. A major objective is to achieve the lowest possible impedance from electrode to amplifier. An amplifier with input impedance not sufficiently high in relation to that of the electrode will result in distortion of the signal waveform. The resistance of a silver/silver chloride disk electrode applied to the scalp should be less than 7–10 KOhms, and all electrodes should have fairly similar resistances.

There are different types of scalp electroencephalographic electrodes. Disk electrodes of about 1 cm diameter are probably the most widely employed for routine EEG recording. They are usually cup-shaped, the concavity being filled with the electrolyte paste. Sometimes, the electrolyte paste also has adhesive characteristics (bentonite paste), or the electrode can be attached with collodion. This type of electrode gives satisfactory results for long-term recordings. It is easy to apply and remove and is comfortable for the patient.

Pad electrodes or pressure contact electrodes are held in place by a light rubber strap or head cap. The electrodes consist of a short silver rod with a knot at the contact end that is usually covered by cotton material and a small sponge. Electrodes are kept in saline and contact with the skin is made by pressure. Pad electrodes have several disadvantages (Broughton, 1976): Tension in the elastic cap sufficient to hold the electrodes in place usually produces considerable discomfort from pressure after 20 to 40 minutes; the saline may run out of the pads, increasing the electrode contact area or producing a short-circuit between electrodes, and, finally, lead wires are attached to the electrodes by crocodile clips, which may give rise to high-amplitude artifacts. However, these electrodes have been used in Europe with satisfactory results in routine records.

Needle electrodes are usually made of platinum, a platinum/iridium mixture, or stainless steel. They are 1–2 cm long and about 1 mm in diameter. The electrodes require sterilization before each recording to avoid the transmission of serum hepatitis or other infections. The needle is quickly inserted obliquely at about 30° to the surface to a depth of 5–8 mm. Their disadvantages, apart from the possibility of infection, are the risk of substantial discomfort to the patient, a greater amount of movement artifacts and, occasionally, scalp damage if the head is moved inappropriately. The use of electronic models and recordings in patients has shown that apparent EEG voltage can vary by up to 50% depending on the orientation of either one of a pair of subdermal electrodes relative to the other. It is recommended that subdermal electrodes should be placed in parallel planes, with their tips in the same direction with respect to the placement of the homologous electrodes to avoid artifactual amplitude asymmetries (Tyner & Knott, 1977).

In recent years, so-called floating electrodes have been developed for EEG. The purpose of this type of electrode is to reduce movement artifacts by recording with electrodes that are not firmly attached to the scalp. Frost (1972) designed an electrode consisting of a conical silicon–rubber sponge that sits on a flat flexible wa_er-like silicone rubber base, which contains a chlorided silver disk to which the insulated lead wire is connected. The apex of the sponge ends in a small cylindrical portion that is filled with electrolyte gel that saturates the sponge. The electrodes are attached to an elastic cap held in place by a chin strap. When the cap is ready to be used, the cylindrical portion is cut off with scissors and the cap is put on.

For some purposes, mainly for the investigation of epilepsy of possible temporal origin, the nasopharyngeal, nasoethmoid, and sphenoidal electrodes may be used.

The first of these consists of a long, moderately flexible, and insulated wire about 2 mm diameter, which is inserted through the nasal orifice until the electrode tip is near the back of the pharynx. Bach-y-Rita, Lion, Reynolds, and Ervin (1969) described a more flexible electrode formed by #20 gauge silver wire threaded through #10 gauge urethral catheter tubing. The nasopharyngeal electrodes record activity from the anteromedial temporal lobe surface, mainly the uncus. They should be sterilized and are contraindicated for sleep or induced-seizure recordings. These electrodes often produce artifacts due to swallowing, movement, respiration, and sometimes pulsation or electrocardiogram (EKG).

Nasoethmoidal and sphenoidal electrodes should be sterilized. They must be inserted under local anesthesia by medically qualified personnel. The nasoethmoid electrode (Lehtinen & Bërgstrom, 1970) is passed between the nasal septum and the conchae upwards to the lamina cribosa of the ethmoid bone. Although some breathing and pulse artifacts may appear, the electrodes are useful in recording the orbito–frontal region. They are commonly used in combination with nasopharyngeal electrodes.

The sphenoidal electrode consists of a 6 cm stainless steel needle insulated with varnish or epoxy to within 2 mm of the tip. It is inserted just below the zygoma (3–4 mm) and 2–3 cm in front of the tragus and it is passed straight in until the tip strikes bone at about 4–6 cm. A new model, which consists of a silver/silver chloride seven-stranded wire has been used with good results in long-term records up to 11 days (Ives & Gloor, 1978). The tip of the electrode lies close to the foramina ovalia and it samples activity from the inferior temporal neocortex, the hippocampus, and, to a lesser extent, the uncus (Pampiglione & Kerridge, 1956).

B. Amplification

The EEG signal is usually within 10–100 μV; thus, much amplification is necessary. The measurement of any voltage represents the difference in potential between two points. As the EEG signal is so small, interferences due to environmental electrical fields must be minimized. This problem can be solved by connecting two amplifiers together at their common or earth point and amplifying only the potential difference between the active leads, thus forming a *differential amplifier*. The problem of interference is thereby reduced, because when the two active leads have the same potential v on each with respect to the common point, the output is zero (v - v). Thus, identical inphase signals that affect the two recording points equally are "rejected." However, in practice, this rejection or "common-mode rejection" is not absolute. It is measured as the ratio of magnitude of the common mode or inphase input signal to the magnitude of the differential or out-of-phase input signal required to produce the same output voltage. The common-mode rejection ratio (CMRR) is, therefore, the differential gain divided by the common mode gain and is usually expressed in decibel form. Modern EEG amplifiers have a 50 to 60 Hz "notch" filter to remove artifacts induced by AC power lines, as well as a high CMRR, so that artifact free records can be obtained without the need for special electromagnetically shielded recording chambers that were previously required. Note that common-mode rejection results in the reduction of voltages of brain origin that occur in phase at two electrodes that are differentially amplified, yielding bipolar outputs that can be misleading (see the discussion in section D of this chapter, Bipolar Recording).

The bandpass characteristics of EEG amplifiers are defined by the low- or high-frequency limits or "cut-off" frequencies (i.e., the frequencies at which the output amplitude is 70% or 3 dB down from the actual voltage). Many amplifiers permit selection of cut-off frequencies by variable time constants (low-frequency filter) and high-frequency filters. The scalp EEG has a fundamental frequency of 10 Hz, and the signals of clinical interest are from 0.5–70 Hz or less. Another very important aspect of differential amplifiers is their input impedance. Modern amplifiers have a high-input impedance (10 Megohms). Finally, noise is generated by the electronic components of amplifiers. The quality of an amplifier also depends on the amount of internally generated noise, which should not exceed 2–3 μV.

C. Electrode Placement

Because the EEG electrode on the scalp is primarily responsive to the electrical activity of the subjacent cortex, it is obvious that the information available from an EEG examination will depend substantially on the loci selected for electrode placement. Until 1958, almost every electroencephalographer had his or her own way of placing electrodes on the head. In that year, a committee of the International Federation of Societies of Electroencephalography and Clinical Neurophysiology proposed an International System of electrode placement (the 10–20 system, Jasper, 1958). The procedure consists of the measurement of arc lengths from nasion to inion and from left preauricular point over vertex to right preauricular point. Electrodes are then placed at points 10, 20, 20, 20, 20, and 10% along each of these arcs, from which the name "10-20 system" derives. Using the points so far defined, additional arcs are positioned and electrodes are placed at similarly spaced positions along these arcs.

MacGillivray (1974) summarized the guiding principles of this system:

1. Position of the electrodes should be determined by measurement from standard landmarks on the skull. Measurements should be proportional to skull size and shape as much as possible;
2. Measurements necessary to identify the electrode position should be as simple as possible;
3. Electrodes should be spaced at equal intervals along antero–posterior and tranverse axes of the head, particularly to ensure equal interelectrode distance in bipolar chains;
4. The electrode array should be symmetrical about the sagittal plane;
5. Adequate coverage of all parts of the head should be provided with standard designated positions even though all may not be used in a given examination;
6. It should be reasonably easy to apply and retain electrodes at the site specified;
7. Designation of positions should be in terms of brain areas (frontal, temporal, etc.);
8. Anatomical studies should be carried out to determine the cortical areas most likely to be found beneath each of the standard electrode positions in the average subject.

MacGillivray (1974) emphasized that although the report of the committee gave the cerebral/electrode relations, it was not clearly explained how these were obtained.

In conclusion, this system enables one to place electrodes over corresponding brain regions in patients with heads of various sizes and shapes. It is useful because it provides standard and comparable recordings between different laboratories, but it does not necessarily place electrodes where anatomic considerations might suggest optimal information. Therefore, in some special cases, more electrodes should be placed, depending on the specific purpose of the examination. Rémond and Torres (1964) designed the LENA system for greater spatial resolution than the 10–20 system. LENA also provides constant and reproducible interelectrode distance.

D. Recording Derivations and Montages

Two basic methods of recording exist:

1. *Referential or monopolar recording,* in which EEG voltages detected by an electrode placed over some particular brain region are compared to a distant, electrophysiologically inactive reference electrode (common reference derivation). Earlobes, mastoids, the tip of the nose, the chin, or the neck are the most commonly used reference loci. Although these regions offer a choice of reference points, they are not inactive. EEG activity arising in the temporal lobe may be recorded with ear or mastoid electrodes and activity from the base of the brain, particularly from the orbital surfaces of the frontal lobes, can be recorded from the nose and chin. When a noncephalic reference is used, a variety of artifacts that obscure the EEG may be recorded: Movements and muscle activity are more easily picked up by noncephalic references than by cranial references (Lehtonen & Koivikko, 1971). Eye, tongue, and mouth movements produce large potentials between scalp electrodes and a nose or a chin reference. The Electromiogram (EMG) is often picked up from the chin, mastoid, or neck. When there is some doubt whether the reference electrode is inactive, it is desirable to compare two reference loci directly. Linked ear lobes are most commonly used as references. The advantage of monopolar recording (provided the reference is inactive) is that it gives a good definition of waveform and good location of low-voltage or absent activity, whether local or widespread.

One suggestion for overcoming the problem of selecting a reference electrode was to artificially derive a reference point that assumes an average potential of all electrodes in use (common average reference derivation). However, this procedure has several disadvantages, such as poor localization of focal activity and poor definition of waveshapes. The average reference may be very active when there is a nonsynchronous generalized high-voltage activity, when several points on the scalp have similar activity, or when there exist moderate amplitude phase-shifted components in different areas. Under such conditions, great distortions of the EEG signal are produced by the average reference.

2. *Bipolar recording*, in which EEG voltages of two active electrodes placed over the scalp are compared. In this type of recording, similar voltage fluctuations occurring inphase at the two electrodes are excluded. This causes some disadvantages: apparently localized pseudolow-voltage or

flat records; distorted waveforms; failure to record true localized low voltage under one electrode because of the contribution to the recording from the other electrode of the pair; poor and misleading location of widespread or nonlocalized activity, and inability to distinguish between a positive event in one electrode or a negative event in the other electrode. However, the bipolar recording has the advantage of yielding precise and simple localization of transient localized activity, by the appearance of transients of different polarity (phase reversal) in two EEG channels that have a common electrode connected to different sides of the amplifiers (e.g., 1–2, 2–3).

Because both procedures have their own advantages and disadvantages, both are used in routine electroencephalography. The peculiar combinations and sequences of electrode arrays in different EEG channels at the same moment constitute a *montage*. This is dependent on the number of available amplifiers. In general, it is customary to record in such a way as to observe as much of the head as possible. The routine EEG examination consists of a systematic exploration of monopolar and bipolar recordings, oriented in both the anteroposterior and the transverse planes.

E. Artifacts and Interferences

Unwanted signals from physiological sources other than the brain are frequently observed during EEG recording. They obscure the EEG potentials and, therefore, they should be eliminated. For example, there is a large potential difference between the front and back of the eye. Movements of the eyes cause large artifacts due to changes in the anatomical location of the field of this steady potential. Blink potentials are produced by a combined effect of closure of the lids themselves and a momentary turning of the eyeball. Both eye movement and blink potentials are most evident in frontal areas, but they may be present as far back as the vertex. These artifacts appear as frontal slow waves and may be confused with activity of cerebral origin. In order to reduce them, the patient should be asked to maintain the position of the eyes as fixed as possible, or to gently press the eyelids with the fingers. In Chapter 8, a procedure is discussed for automatically eliminating artifacts from the recording.

Another very important source of artifacts, the muscle potentials, is due to recording the surface EMG from underlying muscles of the scalp. Such artifacts are commonly due to tension arising from anxiety, discomfort due to the body position, swallowing, and tremor. They appear in the recordings as a profusion of brief spike potentials, most often seen in temporal regions. Simple maneuvers, such as the gentle opening of the mouth or changes in position, may reduce the amount of such artifacts. Sometimes it is necessary to increase the high frequency attenuation of the amplifiers, taking care that the sharp and fast components or the EEG should not be affected. It should also be kept in mind that with high-frequency attenuation, persistent muscle potentials are transformed into electric activity indistinguishable from genuine beta waves.

Pulse artifacts are caused by variations in the contact resistance of an electrode in the vicinity of a pulsating artery. They appear as rhythmic low-voltage sharp waves in the EEG record. The only effective remedy is to move the electrode. The EKG may be picked up in the EEG, particularly in monopolar recordings. Changing the position of the patient sometimes reduces EKG potential. Respiration artifacts may also appear, as a very slow rhythmic activity synchronous with the respiratory cycle, most often seen during hyperventilation. Sweating of the superficial skin will provoke changes in conductivity of the skin, with slow potential changes in the EEG recording. A comfortable ambient temperature should be provided for the patient in order to eliminate this artifact.

Extreme electrical interferences due to environmental electrical fields are strongly reduced by differential amplifiers with high CMRR, or with a notch filter ("hum" eliminator). *Note that these interferences are aggravated by poor technique; the most common cause of mains interference is high electrode resistance.*

F. Activation Procedures

In order to provide an estimate of the reactivity of the EEG and to provoke epileptiform discharges, different activation procedures are used, such as hyperventilation, photic stimulation, sleep recording, and drug activation. The object of hyperventilation is to reduce blood carbon-dioxide levels, causing a moderate alkalosis and cerebral vasoconstriction. The consequent alterations in cerebral haemodynamics and overall biochemistry are often very effective in enhancing or producing abnormalities in the EEG, which may be critical to the interpretation of the record. The montage selected should survey as much of the head as possible. The technique consists of asking the patient to take deep breaths and to expel all the air from the lungs when exhaling for a period of 3 or 4 minutes. There are some contraindications to this procedure: raised intracranial pressure, severe hypertension, angina, myocardial infarction, heart block, ventricular extrasystoles. If the record obtained during rest conditions is very abnormal, then this procedure will not add much more information.

The goals of photic stimulation are to determine the presence of a following response, its symmetry, and the presence of unusual responses, such as in photosensitive epileptics. The montage should include occipital, parietal, and temporal regions. Different frequencies of stimulation are explored, usually from 1–50 Hz.

Sleep recordings often reveal abnormalities not detected in the waking state; short periods of natural sleep occurring during recording may be encouraged. Thus, a dark and quiet room free from interruptions is needed. Sometimes, sleep is induced by sedatives.

Drug activation is only used after previous recordings and with specific recommendations.

III. VISUAL ASSESSMENT OF THE EEG

According to Kellaway (1973), EEG activity may be characterized in terms of: (1) frequency of wave length; (2) voltage; (3) locus of the phenomenon observed; (4) waveform; (5) interhemispheric coherence (i.e., symmetry of voltage, frequency, and waveshape at homologous placements); (6) character of wave occurrence (random, serial, continous); (7) regulation of voltage and frequency; and (8) reactivity or changes in an EEG parameter with changes in state.

In clinical practice, it is customary to differentiate the EEG into background activity, which refers to more or less general and continuous features, in contrast to paroxysmal or focal activity (Storm van Leeuwen, Bickford, Brazier, Cobb, Dondey, Gastaut, Gloor, Henry, Hess, Knott, Kugler, Lairy, Loeb, Magnus, Oller-Daurella, Petsche, Schwab, Walter, & Widen, 1966). A primary classification of the EEG background activity is most useful, not only because this characteristic of cerebral activity is really measurable with some accuracy, but because frequency differences are of major significance. A paroxysm is a phenomenon with abrupt onset, rapid attainment of a maximum, and sudden termination. Various specific electrographic patterns or sequences have been identified.

In this section, we give a very brief review of the different rhythms and patterns and the EEG abnormalities most frequently observed in major neurological diseases. The reader should consult Gibbs and Gibbs (1951b, 1952, 1964); Hill and Parr (1963); Laget and Salbreux (1967); the *Handbook of EEG and Clinical Neurophysiology* (A. Rémond, Ed.), and other books on electroencephalography for more detailed discussions. The descriptions of typical and atypical EEG patterns that follow provide a consensus of the opinions of investigators using visual examination almost exclusively. More quantitative evaluations, such as those presented later, may indicate the need to modify some of these impressions.

A. Typical Normal Rhythms

1. Alpha Rhythm

The majority (89%) of normal awake adults have, as a fundamental characteristic, a predominance of alpha rhythm in their EEG background activity (Gibbs, Gibbs, & Lennox, 1943). This rhythm was called the "Berger rhythm" by Adrian and Matthews (1934) in recognition of Berger's discovery in 1929. The alpha rhythm is generally considered to have a frequency of 8–13 Hz, and is most prominent in posterior regions with the eyes closed, under conditions of physical relaxation and relative mental inactivity. It is attenuated or blocked by sensory and especially visual stimulation and during mental activity. The most common frequency in adult subjects is around 10 Hz. This frequency decreases with senescence (Obrist & Busse, 1965). The upper frequency limit is generally considered to be 13 Hz. Rhythms at 14 Hz, of smaller amplitude, are infrequently observed. The peak-to-peak amplitude of the alpha waves is variable. In a single record, it is often possible to see regular fluctuations in amplitude, giving an envelope with a spindle shape. Simonova, Foth, and Stein (1967) asserted that in the great majority of normal adult subjects, the peak-to-peak amplitude fluctuates from 20-60 μV, amplitudes higher than 60 μV being rare. The alpha rhythms of the two hemispheres resemble each other, and at times show good bilateral synchrony, not only of individual waves, but of their envelopes. More commonly, although the overall patterns may be similar, the waves are not perfectly synchronized and there is considerable independence of the amplitude fluctuations on the two sides. By visual estimation, the mean alpha activity of the two hemispheres is different in perhaps 30% of normal adults, and markedly so in 5 or 10%, the difference being mainly in amplitude. In a high proportion of the cases that show asymmetry, the greater amplitude is on the right side (Cobb, 1963a). This asymmetry has been related to hemispheric dominance. A persistent difference in frequency between the alpha rhythms of the two hemispheres of more than 1 Hz is generally regarded as abnormal. The side of the slower rhythm is the one more likely to be the locus of a pathological process.

The amount of alpha activity increases progressively with age until adulthood. Infants between 1 and 2½ years old present brief periods of activity within the alpha frequency. By 5 years old, a child's alpha rhythm becomes clearly discernible, its amount being almost equal to the amount of theta activity (W.G. Walter, 1950; Matousek & Petersén, 1973a). From 6 to 9 years old, the child's EEG background activity also shows great variations in its frequency, with a mixture of frequencies within the alpha range and lower, but with a progressive increase of the alpha activity with age. From 10 to 13 years old, the child's alpha rhythm is almost stabilized, with similar characteristics to those observed in the adult. The proportion of alpha activity continues to increase up to 21 years old. At this age, alpha activity constitutes 70% of the total background activity in occipito-parietal derivations (Matousek & Petersén, 1973a).

Alpha slowing and intellectual deficit are quite apparent in many elderly subjects with "organic brain syndrome" (Sheridan, Yeager, Oliver, & Simon, 1955). The degree of slowing of the alpha rhythm has been found to be quantitatively related to impaired memory function, severity of intellectual deterioration, and senile changes in affect (Obrist, 1976; Short, Musella, & Wilson, 1968).

2. *Beta Rhythm*

This rhythm was also described by Berger (second-order waves). It is also frequently observed in awake normal adults. Its topographic distribution has been greatly discussed. Jasper and Andrews (1936, 1938) described a beta rhythm from 20–30 Hz in precentral areas, and beta activity superimposed on the alpha rhythm of posterior regions. They called it "gamma" rhythm, a term that is scarcely used in current literature, referring to a more rarely observed faster rhythm (35-45 Hz). Vogel and Götze (1962) described three different types of EEGs with beta activity: (1) those with beta activity in anterior regions and alpha rhythm in occipital areas; (2) a second group with continuous beta activity exclusively in occipital or in both occipital and precentral areas and a lack of alpha waves; and (3) those that presented diffuse beta activity mixed with the alpha rhythm.

According to Kuhlo (1976a), it is justifiable to give the name beta rhythm to all the EEG activity with a frequency higher than 13 Hz (Storm van Leeuwen et al., 1966). He classified the beta rhythm in three different groups: (1) the central (fronto-central) beta rhythm, which is blocked by contralateral movements or contralateral tactile stimulation; (2) diffuse beta rhythm without specific reactivity; and (3) a posterior beta (fast alpha variant) rhythm, reactive to visual stimulation.

The incidence of this rhythm in the adult population varies according to different authors (see Table 2.1). The amplitude is between 8 to 25 μV (Jasper & Andrews, 1936), although it can reach 30 μV (Kooi, 1971). In general, it is rare to observe amplitudes higher than 30 μV in the diffuse or posterior types of beta rhythm in young adults.

According to the frequency analyses performed by Matousek and Petersén (1973a), the amount of beta activity is higher in anterior than in posterior regions. They also reported that infants from 1 year old showed a relatively high proportion of beta activity (12%) in central regions, decreasing abruptly at the age of 3 or 4 (1.1%) and increasing again progressively with age, to reach 25% at 21 years old. In fronto-temporal derivations, the amount of beta activity is relatively high in 1 year old children (19.5%), decreases to a small percentage during the early years, and later increases again to 24% of the total activity in young adults. Fast activity is not a con-

TABLE 2.1
Incidence of Different EEG Rhythms and Patterns Among Adult Subjects

Type	*Population*	*% Subjects*	*Author(s) and Year*
Central beta rhythm[a]	113 army recruits	0	Gallais et al. (1957)
Central beta rhythm	309 navy pilots	28	Picard et al. (1957)
Diffuse beta rhythm	3372 engineers	4	Vogel and Fujiya (1969)
Diffuse beta rhythm	475 military recruits	33.3	Roger and Bert (1959)
Mu rhythm[b]	113 army recruits	0	Gallais et al. (1957)
Mu rhythm	507 army recruits	34.3	Roger and Bert (1959)
Low-voltage fast EEG[c]	251 healthy adults	4.1	Cohn (1949)
Low-voltage fast EEG	1000 healthy subjects	11.6	Gibbs and Gibbs (1951b)
Slow posterior arrhythmic waves[d]	147 healthy subjects	0	Hill (1952)
Slow posterior arrhythmic waves	511 military recruits	33	Gastaut et al. (1960)

[a]Beta rhythm: frequencies higher than 13 Hz (Storm van Leeuwen et al., 1966).
[b]*Rhythme rolandique en arceau* of Gastaut et al. (1952).
[c]Characterized mostly by nonrhythmic, amorphous fast activity usually not exceeding 20μV in amplitude.
[d]Potentials lasting 0.25–0.35 sec or larger, occuring over the posterior regions of the head either singly or in bursts.

stant feature of the senescent EEG, but it varies with age and mental status. A decline in the amount of beta activity at advanced ages has also been noted in subjects studied longitudinally (Obrist, Henry & Justiss, 1966). A number of investigators have reported a relative absence of fast activity in deteriorated senile patients in whom it appears to be inversely related to the occurrence of diffuse slow activity. In contrast, fast activity in normal old subjects has been associated with superior learning ability (Obrist, 1976).

The beta activity is enhanced by the administration of several types of drugs, such as barbiturates, mesantoin, meprobamate, diazepam, librium, imipramine, amphetamine, and so on, the effects being dependent on the dosage, time of administration, and individual factors.

3. Theta Rhythm

Walter and Dovey (1944) gave the name theta rhythm to the EEG activity with a frequency between 4 and 8 Hz. It is most frequently observed in childhood, a negative correlation existing between the amount of theta activity and age. Theta rhythm of high amplitude is observed in children from 1 to 5 years old in posterior regions, and is the dominant activity in children from 4 to 6 years old in central, temporal, and occipito-parietal regions. With increasing age, the amount of theta activity progressively decreases up to adulthood. In adolescents, it is possible to observe periods of theta activity from 5-7 Hz (Matousek & Petersén, 1973a). The theta rhythm is usually augmented by closing the eyes and by emotion in children up to the age of 2 to 3 years (W.G. Walter, 1950). Some electroencephalographers consider the presence of theta activity in the awake adult abnormal. However, there are some studies that demonstrate the presence of theta rhythm in healthy subjects (Gallais, Collomb, Milletto, Cardaire, & Blanc-Garin, 1957; Picard, Navaronne, Labourer, Grousset, & Jest, 1957; Volavka, Matousek, & Roubicek, 1966).

The proportion of activity within the theta band in young adults is 13% in front-temporal derivations, 17% in central regions, and 8% in parieto-occipital derivations (Matousek & Petersén, 1973a).

4. Delta Rhythm

This title was originally given by W.G. Walter (1936) to waves slower than the alpha rhythm. It is still used for those frequencies under 4 Hz (Chatrian, Bergamini, Dandey, Klass, Lennox-Buchtal, & Petersén, 1974). It constitutes the dominant activity in all derivations during the first two years of life (Gibbs & Gibbs, 1964). After this age, it tends to disappear, first in occipital and central regions and later in frontal and temporal. The presence of sufficient delta rhythm in the awake adult to be detected by visual inspection is considered abnormal. However, using frequency analysis, the existence of waves within the delta band has been demonstrated in awake healthy adults, specially in fronto-temporal derivations (Matousek & Petersén, 1973a).

At advanced ages (over 75 years), there is a significant increase in slow activity, which is more prevalent in confused senile and atherosclerotic patients than in cases with affective or involutional psychosis (Obrist & Henry, 1958). These authors also found that diffuse slow activity in elderly patients is related to prognosis and life expectancy: The majority of elderly patients with diffuse slow activity either remained hospitalized or died within a year after the EEG, whereas patients with normal EEGs or only focal abnormalities tended to have subsequent hospital release and greater survival. In relation to senescence, frontal rhythmic delta activity, usually intermittent and bilateral, has been commonly found among elderly patients with intellectual deterioration (Schwartzova & Synek, 1969); when restricted to the anterior temporal regions, it is compatible with good social adjustment in older people (Obrist, 1976).

5. Mu Rhythm

The Rolandic rhythm *en arceau*, or mu rhythm, was first described by Gastaut, Terzian, and Gastaut (1952). It is observed in the Rolandic area proximal to the hand projection in one or both sides, with a frequency of 7–14 Hz, generally associated with a beta rhythm of double frequency. It is hardly affected by mental activity or visual stimulation, but is very reactive to spontaneous or provoked limb movements, thoughts of movement, readiness to move, or tactile stimulation. The mu rhythm is composed of arch-shaped waves with a sharp negative portion and a rounded positive one. Its amplitude varies between a few to 80 μV (Chatrian, Petersén, & Lazarte, 1959). The incidence reported in normal subjects is quite variable (see Table 2.1). Great contradictions appear in the literature with respect to the age of appearance. According to Gastaut et al. (1952), it is not found before 10 years of age, and is most common between 21 and 30 years. Canali and Carpitella (1956) reported a higher incidence between 50 to 60 years of age, whereas, Beck, Doty, and Kodi (1958) and Netchine, Harrison, Berges, and Lairy (1964) found it most frequently in childhood and adolescence.

6. Low-Voltage EEG

Low-voltage EEG is characterized by activity of amplitude not greater than 20 μV over all head regions. With frequency analysis, this activity can be shown to be composed primarily of beta, theta, and, to a lesser degree, delta waves, with or without alpha activity in posterior regions (Chatrian et al., 1974). Its incidence in awake healthy subjects as well as in neurological patients is variable (Table 2.1). It is generally accepted that this type of activity is most frequently seen in older subjects, and is quite rare before 13 years of age (Adams, 1959; Gibbs & Gibbs, 1951b; Lucioni & Penati, 1966).

In some cases, it is possible to observe the appearance of brief periods of alpha activity immediately after eye closure. Hyperventilation may have no effect or may provoke the appearance of alpha rhythm. During states of anxiety and emotional stress, it is possible to observe this type of activity. A genetic factor has also been proposed in its occurrence (Vogel, 1970).

7. Slow Posterior Activities

These activities may be observed in a proportion of adult normal subjects, and include: (1) slow posterior rhythms; and (2) slow posterior arrhythmic waves (Kuhlo, 1976b). The slow posterior waves or "slow alpha variant" rhythm are characteristic rhythms of 3.5–6 Hz, but mostly at 4–5

Hz, recorded most prominently over the posterior regions of the head. They generally alternate or are intermixed with alpha rhythms to which they are often harmonically related. Amplitude is variable, but is frequently close to 50 μV. These waves are blocked or attenuated by attention, especially visual and mental effort (Chatrian et al., 1974). The incidence varied from 0.2–2.2% in a series of apparently normal individuals (Kuhlo, 1976b). Subjects displaying a slow posterior rhythm in their EEGs varied in age from 12 years (Kuhlo, Heintel, & Vogel, 1969) to 64 years (Petersén & Sörbye, 1962). The slow alpha variant has been related with grand mal epilepsy (Goodwin, 1947) or head injury (Petersén & Sörbye, 1962; Pitot & Gastaut, 1956). According to Kuhlo (1976b), there is no adequate evidence at present that establishes any definite relationship between slow posterior rhythms and any neurological disorder.

The slow posterior arrhythmic wave pattern consists of waves of variable form, lasting 0.5–0.35 sec or longer, which occur either singly or in bursts of variable duration and usually lack consistent periodicity, which differentiates them from the slow posterior rhythm. They are asymmetric in 50% of the cases, and are frequently, but not constantly, blocked by eye opening. They were found by Aird and Gastaut (1959) in 18.4% of normal controls, aged 19–22 years, and in 6% of a series of consecutive unselected patients of all ages and conditions. The prevalence of this pattern in children, adolescents, and young adults led these authors to suggest the phrase "slow posterior waves found predominantly in youth." This pattern is very similar to the "posterior temporal slow wave focus" described by Rey, Pond, & Evans (1949) and Hill (1952) in normal individuals, and present with higher incidences among subjects with psychotic or psychopatic behavior. Subsequent investigations of normal populations, including navy pilots, revealed that appearance of these waveforms in the waking EEG records of young adults is not necessarily a sign of pathology or "abnormality" (Gastaut, Lee, & Laboureur, 1960).

8. The Lambda Waves

The lambda waves are sharp transients occurring over the occipital regions of the head in waking adults during visual exploration. They are mainly positive relative to other areas and time-locked to saccadic eye movement. Amplitude varies, but is generally below 50 μV (Chatrian et al., 1974). Their incidence varies considerably (from 2–88%) in the series reported by various investigators (Chatrian & Lairy, 1976). However, by using computer summation techniques, triggered by eye movements, no failure to demonstrate lambda waves has been reported (Chatrian, 1964; Lesèvre, 1967; Rémond, Torres, Lesèvre, & Conte, 1964).

9. The Kappa Rhythm

This rhythm consists of bursts of low-voltage waves of alpha or theta frequency, occurring over temporal areas of the scalp of normal subjects engaged in mental activity. This rhythm is most prominent just posterior to the external canthi of the eyes and is best demonstrated by bitemporal recordings between these sites. According to Chatrian (1976a), the kappa rhythm has been suspected of being an artifact of ocular origin. However, a review of the available evidence suggests that vertical oscillations of the eyeballs, such as those that characterize eye flutter, do not represent the primary source of kappa potentials. The possibility that discrete lateral oscillations of the eyeballs might play a role in the generation of these waves has not been ruled out.

10. Fourteen and Six Hz Positive Bursts

The occurrence of low-voltage 14 and 6 Hz positive spikes was first reported by Gibbs and Gibbs (1951b). This pattern consists of bursts of arch-shaped waves at 13–17 Hz and 5–7 Hz, but more commonly at 14 and/or 6 Hz, generally seen over the posterior temporal and adjacent areas of one or both sides of the head during sleep. The sharp peaks of its components are positive with respect to other regions (Chatrian et al., 1974). These discharges are more common in children than in adults. Gibbs and Gibbs (1951b) reported an incidence of 15.8% among children from 5 to 9 years old; 20.8% from 10 to 14 years old; 16.5% from 15 to 19 years old; 8.7% from 20 to 24 years old. No cases older than 40 years old showed this pattern among a normal clinical population. Wegner and Struve (1977) compared these data with their findings in 2888 psychiatric patients aged 20 and above. A significantly higher incidence in the clinical sample was observed for all ages. This pattern has been associated with behavioral disorders and has been observed in some cases of epilepsy (Gibbs & Gibbs, 1951a, 1952, 1963; Hill, 1963). Thus, the clinical significance of this pattern, if any, is controversial.

11. The EEG in Early Life

Lindsley (1936) described the EEG of a child in utero that showed only diffuse slow-voltage activity, similar to that seen in the newborn. In premature babies of about 24 weeks of gestation, Scherrer, Verley, and Garma (1970) described a discontinous and asynchronous activity, and at 28 weeks, a fast rhythm was superimposed on slow waves in both occipital regions. According to these authors, the EEG activity of the full-term newborn was very similar to the EEG activity of these very young prematures when they reached the same gestational age. However, Dreyfus-Brisac (1970) considered that the EEG of premature babies, even if they reached 40 weeks of gestational age, was more disorganized than the EEG of full-term newborns. At the end of the fifth month of gestation, the EEG was discontinuous, very irregular, asymmetric, and without differentiation between sleep and wakefulness. In the eighth month, the EEG became continuous and reactive, with differentiation between sleep and wakefulness being possible (Laget and Salbreux, 1967). Dreyfus-Brisac and Monod (1965) described that although different sleep stages could be observed in prematures of 37 weeks of gestational age, cyclic sleep organization was reached only after 40 weeks of gestational age. From birth at full term up to the age of 3 months, the EEG record tends to remain uniform and is characterized by low-voltage, irregular, arrhythmic activity that is perhaps of slightly larger amplitude and slower dominant frequency in the posterior regions. At the end of 3 or 4 months, the dominant activity is within the delta band, which is maintained up to 2 years old.

Hagne, Persson, Magnusson, and Petersén (1973) performed a follow-up study of infants from birth to 1 year of age, with examinations at 2-month intervals. Recordings from temporal, parieto-occipital, and central leads for each hemisphere were obtained. A good agreement between visual judgment of dominant frequency and frequency analysis of the waking EEGs of the infants were observed. Inter- and intraindividual variations were great, but it was possible to demonstrate an increase of dominant frequency in all regions as age increased. There were differences between the three cortical regions studied in each hemisphere. An earlier dominant peak, with higher frequency and greater amplitude, occurred centrally, the latter variables reflecting amplitude and constancy of the dominant peak. Differences between homologous regions, however, were generally small.

B. Changes of the EEG During Sleep

Several sleep stages have been described in adults. The wakefulness state is considered stage O. According to Williams, Karakan, and Hursch (1974), the criterion to distinguish this stage is at least 30 secs of continuous alpha activity in occipital regions. Stage I (drowsiness, Gibbs & Gibbs, 1951b) is characterized by a decrease of amplitude of the EEG activity, with a progressive disappearance of the alpha rhythm. For Williams et al. (1974), this stage should be differentiated only in the case of less than 30 secs of alpha activity, and no more than one sleep spindle or a K complex. This pattern of activity in stage I is observed in almost all subjects 30 to 40 years old. It is not established until 10 years of age. In senescence, slow waves in frontal regions may be observed. In those subject with a low-voltage EEG, the appearance of alpha rhythm is characteristic of this stage.

The second stage (light sleep, Gibbs & Gibbs, 1951b) is characterized in the adult by the appearance of transient activity, the vertex sharp transients or K complexes that are only observed at this stage, and by sleep spindles. The vertex sharp transients are bursts of somewhat variable appearance, usually consisting of a high-voltage diphasic slow wave frequently associated with sleep spindle (Chatrian et al., 1974). They apparently occur spontaneously or in response to sudden sensory stimuli, and are not specific for any sensory modality. This stage is not easily distinguished from wakefulness or deep sleep in infants younger than 6 months. In infants 6–18 months old, the vertex sharp transients, or biparietal humps (Gibbs & Gibbs, 1951b), begin to appear, and are very clearly observed in children after 3 years of age. The sleep spindles are bursts lasting 1–2 seconds. They consist of components with a frequency of 11–15 Hz but mostly 12–14 Hz, generally diffuse, but of higher voltage over the central regions of the head. The sleep spindles decrease in amplitude and become more localized to parietal regions after 40 years of age. In the newborn, it is possible to observe activity of 14 Hz of low voltage in parietal regions, which is considered a precursor of the sleep spindle. This pattern reaches its maximum amplitude in people from 15–20 years old, decreasing after 30 years old. Sleep spindles are absent in 20% of subjects older than 60. During the second sleep stage, the dominant background activity is within the theta band, with some delta waves. Williams et al. (1974) proposed the following criterion for the differentiation of this phase of sleep: at least 2 sleep spindles or 2 K complexes, with no more than 12 seconds of delta activity during 30 seconds.

Stage III (moderately deep sleep, Gibbs & Gibbs, 1951b) is characterized by irregular delta waves mixed with some waves within the theta band. It is possible to observe sleep spindles of 12 Hz, more diffusely generalized than the sleep spindles observed in stage II. In infants, this stage is characterized by the disappearance of sleep spindles. For Williams et al. (1974), the criterion used for the definition of this stage is the presence of delta waves during periods lasting between 13 and 30 secs.

The very deep sleep (stage IV, Gibbs & Gibbs, 1951b) is defined by dominant delta waves that become more rhythmic and symmetric with deepening sleep. In this stage, the sleep spindles are not observed. In older subjects, the delta waves are of lower amplitude than in younger adults.

The rapid eye movement (REM) or paradoxical phase of sleep is characterized by low-voltage activity, accompanied by rapid eye movements and muscular relaxation. Gradual spontaneous waking, on the other hand, approximately recapitulates the stages of going to sleep, in inverse order.

In the newborn, Parmelee, Schulz, and Disbrow (1961) have distinguished two different types of activity during sleep: quiet sleep and active sleep. Quiet sleep is characterized by periods of slow waves of large amplitude with superimposed fast activity, which alternate with periods of waves of different frequencies. This pattern is observed in the premature (tracé continu) and has been called "alternant" in full-term babies by Dreyfus-Brisac (1968) and Samson-Dollfus (1955). Goldie and VanVelzer (1965) called this stage episodic sleep activity, describing it as formed by periods of 1–3 secs of large waves up to 200 μV, with a frequency between 2 and 6 Hz, alternating with longer periods of 6–10 secs of flat activity. The average duration of this stage is approximately 13.6 minutes. Active sleep presents rapid eye movements with an EEG of low or moderate amplitude containing waves of 4–10 Hz. Its average duration is 47 minutes. A transient stage between active and quiet sleep is also shown; after the active sleep stage, eye movements become slower until they disappear. Sleep spindles are rarely observed in the newborn. They become well established at 2 or 4 months of age (Williams et al., 1974).

C. Major Abnormalities Observed in the EEG

1. Modification in Frequency and Amplitude of the EEG background activity

We have indicated that the dominant frequency observed in normal subjects depends on the age and the sleep–wakefulness state. During wakefulness, the presence of more slow activity (theta or delta) than is usually observed is a sign of abnormality. In such cases, the slow activity may have a generalized or diffuse character or it may be circumscribed to a hemisphere or even to a cortical area (slow-wave focus). According to Dutertre (1977), a distinction can be made between: (1) reactional delta—anterior bursts of usually monomorphic delta activity with maximal voltage either bifrontal or medial, related to deep (organic or functional) lesions, which may be either hemispheric or subtentorial (frontal intermittent rhythmic delta activity, Chatrian et al., 1974); and (2) lesional delta—usually polymorphic delta activity exhibiting different locations according to localized (organic or functional) brain damage. Gloor, Ball, and Schaul (1977), after studying experimental lesions in cats, described that localized delta activity appears in cortex overlying a circumscribed white-matter lesion. Less commonly, localized delta activity may result from localized thalamic lesion. Unilateral diffuse delta activity appears in the side of thalamic or hypothalamic lesions. Bilateral delta activity results from bilateral lesions of the midbrain tegmentum. In contrast, localized lesions of the cerebral cortex only caused an amplitude reduction of the background EEG activity within the area of the lesion. These results show a strong correlation between white-matter pathology and the presence of polymorphic delta activity, as well as the absence of significant delta with purely cortical lesions. These results are in accord with those previously reported by other authors (Gloor, Kalaby, & Giard, 1968; Rhee, Goldensohn, & Kini, 1975; Ulett, 1945). Cerebral edema particularly affects white matter only in those cases in which decompression is not allowed. This suggests that under these conditions, the swollen hemisphere affected by the edema produces delta activity indirectly through pressure on, or displacement of, deep midline structures in the brain stem or diencephalon (Gloor et al., 1977).

In many epileptics, the background activity is composed, either exclusively or prevalently, of slow activity (in the theta and delta bands) spread over all regions of the scalp, but generally more pronounced in the anterior regions. This slow background activity is not specifically related to any one factor. It can be attributed to: (1) the disease responsible for epilepsy—in this case, the slow activity is an expression of the cerebral disease, whether organic diffuse or metabolic, and evolves with the causal disease or; (2) the epileptic attacks—transitory slowing can be observed after a single attack, or more often, after a series of attacks. In cases of chronic epilepsy, epileptics show persistent slowing of the background activity. Such cases are refractory to therapy, and are often characterized by mental deterioration and frequent seizures (Lugaresi & Pazzaglia, 1975).

Diffuse slow activity is a nearly invariable component of metabolic coma. The degree of slowing is related to the level of unresponsiveness, regardless of etiology. According to Lundervold (1975), this nonspecificity may be quite useful. The diagnosis of metabolic coma is unlikely if the EEG rhythms are not slowed in a proportion to unresponsiveness. Thus, nonspecific slow activity can be very useful in monitoring patients whose level of consciousness may fluctuate in response to an unknown metabolic abnormality.

Depression of the amplitude of the EEG activity, whether transient or diffuse, may be related to different pathological processes difficult to identify at the scalp level. Whether diffuse or localized, these processes may involve the cortex, either directly—by compression from the outside (juxtadural collection), by an epileptic cortical focus (postictal depression), or by biochemical disorders (metabolic coma)—or indirectly, in cases such as a subcortical lesion resulting in deafferentation or a cortical suppressive seizure. Their expression may be transient (suppressive burst), occasionally repetitive (iterative silence), or persistent ("*silence relatif*", Dutertre, 1977). Depression of activity should not be confused with lack of cerebral activity expressing cerebral death (electrical inactivity).

2. Abnormal Paroxysmal Activity

The following definitions have been provided by the International Federation Society of Electroencephalography and Clinical Neurophysiology (IFSECN, Chatrian et al., 1974):

Spike: A transient, clearly distinguished from background activity, with pointed peak at conventional paper speeds (30 mm/sec) and a duration from 20 to under 70 msec. The main component is generally negative relative to other areas. The amplitude is variable. [More precise definitions are provided in Chapter 12.]

Multiple-spike complex: (Polyspike complex): A sequence of two or more spikes.

Sharp waves: A transient, clearly distinguished from background activity, with pointed peak at conventional paper speeds and a duration of 70 to 200 msec. The main component is generally negative relative to other areas. The amplitude is variable.

Spike-and-slow-wave complex: This is a pattern consisting of a spike followed by a slow wave. Similarly, *sharp-and-slow-wave complex* is a sequence of sharp and slow waves.

Multiple-spike and slow-wave complex: This is a spike-and-wave complex with more than one spike.

Paroxysmal slow waves: These are waves, clearly distinct from background activity that are characterized by a duration of more than 125 msec. They may take the form of a slow-wave complex or can be observed in the form of rhythmic bursts.

In epileptics with psychomotor seizures, the interictal EEG can show bursts of theta waves, rhythmically appearing at about 6 Hz, unilaterally or bilaterally localized to the midtemporal region, and which correspond to rhythmic bursts of spikes in the rhinencephalic structures (M.G. Chatrian, 1953). These rhythmic activities are not specific to epileptics, but have also been found in subjects with psychiatric disturbances or vegetative attacks (Dutertre, 1977). Spikes and sharp waves and other paroxysmal complexes are considered as "epileptiform discharges" and have been reported in some studies of apparently healthy subjects. According to G.E. Chatrian (1976b), the finding of focal paroxysmal patterns in neurologically normal populations should be carefully assessed in the light of the subject's past history, which may or may not reveal presumably significant pathological events.

D. EEG Characteristics of the Major Neurological Diseases

1. Intracranial Tumors

The value of electroencephalography in the diagnosis and localization of tumors has been recognized ever since Walter's great pioneering work (1936). According to Gibbs and Gibbs (1964), a slow-wave focus is the most significant finding and the most nearly characteristic abnormality of brain tumors. Marked focal slowing occurs in approximately 69% of cases with cortical tumors, but only in 33% of patients with deep tumors. Absence of focal slowing occurs in half of the latter patients, but in only 10% of the former. The accuracy of localization varies with the size and location of the tumor. Very small tumors are unlocalizable because they produce no detectable abnormality. Very large tumors are unlocalizable because they produce such great disorders that no focal abnormality can be observed. Tumors that grow very slowly may produce no detectable EEG disorders; if they grow too fast, they may produce generalized abnormalities.

Cobb (1963b) analyzed the most important EEG findings in brain tumors according to their localization. Frontal tumors are the most common cause of frontal delta rhythm. The distribution of delta rhythm may be only on the side of the lesion, or it may be bilateral. Sometimes, it is largely confined to the other side, which results in difficult interpretation. Local delta activity, when seen in a high Rolandic or parietal area, is a good guide to the position of the lesion, but tumors deep in the parietal lobe sometimes give rise to a delta focus that is parieto-temporal or even temporal in position. This is a well-known source of error in localization. Parasagittal tumors are difficult to localize, because the local delta discharge may arise so near to the midline that correct lateralization distinction from a bilateral lesion is impossible. Reduction of alpha rhythm and excessive local slow activity produced by occipital and temporal tumors tend to reflect fairly accurately the site of the tumor. According to Gibbs and Gibbs (1964), focal slowing is found in 90% of cortical tumors, in 69% of tumors of the midline and central grey structures, and in 11% of tumors of the optic chiasm, brain stem or cerebellopontine angle. Paroxysmal spike activity is observed respectively in 34, 9, and 11% of the above mentioned groups. Disordered sleep patterns are observed in 16, 44, and 6% respectively. Normal EEGs are found in 4% of cortical tumors, in 14% of tumors of midline and central grey structures, and in 57% of tumors of the third group (Gibbs & Gibbs, 1964).

2. *Cerebrovascular Diseases*

Occlusions of the cerebral vessels produce three main types of electroencephalographic abnormalities: (1) an asymmetry with depression of voltage on the damaged area; (2) the presence of a slow-wave focus; or (3) the presence of spikes. According to Gibbs and Gibbs (1964), the incidence of these findings varies if the lesion is cortical or noncortical. In cortical vascular accidents, 62% of the patients showed asymmetry, 58% slow-wave focus, and 22% spikes; the EEG was normal in approximately 8% of the cases. In noncortical vascular accidents, slow-wave foci were observed with similar incidence as EEG asymmetry (approximately 30%) and 12% of the cases showed spikes; the EEG was normal in approximately 45% of these cases. In other studies, the percentage of vascular lesions exhibiting normal EEG ranges varied from 13 to 60% (Birchfield, Wilson, & Heyman, 1959; Carmon, Lavy, & Schwartz, 1966; Harvold & Skinhoj, 1956; Lavy, Carmon, & Schwartz, 1964). Frantzen, Harvald, and Haugsted (1959) and Carmon et al. (1966) found that the incidence of diffusely disturbed EEG was highest among patients with diffuse atherosclerotic changes. Unilateral slowing or depression of cortical activity is frequently correlated with hemispheric infarction or hemorrhage (Carmon et al., 1966; Martin, 1953). The EEG findings in intracerebral hemorrhages are highly dependent on the state of consciousness (Cobb, 1963b).

Aneurysms, while small and unruptured, generally did not give rise to significant changes in the EEG. Occasionally, aneurysms may be of a size and position to constitute a mass compressing the frontal or temporal lobes. In such cases, a slow-wave focus may be observed. When the rupture of an aneurysm results in subarachnoid hemorrhage, the alpha activity may be disorganized, slowed, or abolished bilaterally, and there may be generalized theta and delta activity, but these changes probably correspond with an altered state of consciousness. After recovery from the acute incident, the EEG is generally normal (Cobb, 1963b).

A cerebral arterio–venous malformation is usually diagnosed by the occurrence of a subarachnoidal hemorrhage, thus, it is very rare to record the EEG of an uncomplicated lesion. In such cases in which the patients had headaches, the EEG has been recorded and it has been possible to observe slow-wave focus or depression of alpha activity in the site of the lesion. According to Cobb (1963b), this may be due to a tumor effect produced by the angioma or to profound disturbances of blood supply. When the arterio–venous malformations produce seizures, paroxysmal epileptogenic activity may be found.

3. Head Trauma

The value of the EEG in the management of recent head injury is, first of all, that it can reveal unsuspected damage. In closed head injuries, about 35% of the cases show abnormal EEGs (Gibbs & Gibbs, 1964). It is possible to observe a decrease of alpha activity in posterior regions and an increase in theta activity in frontal and temporal areas. In open, nonpenetrating injuries, a slow-wave focus may be found at the site of the injury. Usually, the EEG normalized gradually as clinical recovery proceeds. Paroxysmal epileptogenic activity may appear several weeks or months after head trauma. In severe head injuries with subdural hematoma, the collection of fluid acts like a tumor to produce slow activity that is localized in and around the area of compressed brain, or it may produce lower voltage activity on the side of the lesion. These findings are not particularly helpful in most cases in which a subdural hematoma is suspected, because the electroencephalographic signs may be interpreted as a result of brain trauma.

Levy, Segerberg, Schmidt, Turrell, and Roseman (1952) studied the EEG of 60 patients with recent head trauma, half of them with subdural hematoma. The records were submitted to seven different interpreters who were asked whether a subdural hematoma was or was not present. The best score was 67%, and the average little better than 50%. After removal of a subdural hematoma, there is considerable variation in the rate of EEG recovery, not always corresponding to the clinical improvement.

4. Infections

Children with supposedly uncomplicated measles, mumps, chicken pox, rubella, scarlet fever, mononucleosis, or upper respiratory infections often show abnormalities in the awake recording (38%). A follow-up study revealed that only in 1% of these patients did the slow activity persist a year later. In some cases, spiking developed, with or without clinical symptomatology (Gibbs & Gibbs, 1964).

During the acute phase of encephalitis, high-voltage slow activity is usual, sometimes with the presence of spikes. With clinical improvement, the EEG becomes normal. A normal EEG, after the acute phase of encephalitis is over, is very suggestive that the patient will be asymptomatic; less than 10% have residual symptoms. On the other hand, there is a 91% chance that a patient will have residual effects if negative spikes are present. Fourteen and six per second spikes are related to behavioral disturbances; 41% of patients whose follow-up EEG showed these patterns had behavioral disturbances (Gibbs & Gibbs, 1964).

A slow-wave focus is observed in 85% of brain abscess cases. If the abscess is of great volume, the slow waves are diffuse; the depression of the voltage amplitude may be also observed when the abscess is confined to one lobule. This is seen relatively often in occipital abscesses. Paroxysmal activity may also appear (Chiofalo, Fuentes, Rodríguez, Villavicencio, & Méndez, 1976).

5. Epilepsy

(For a recent review, see Gastaut & Tassinari, 1975.) Primary generalized epilepsies are characterized by ictal EEG discharges, which are always bilaterally synchronous and asymmetrical, and specific to each type of seizure: (1) the epileptic recruiting rhythm is progressively interrupted by episodes of silence accompanying the tonic and the clonic phases of the grand mal seizure; (2) a spike-and-wave rhythm at about 3 Hz is characteristic of petit mal absence; (3) a polyspike-and-wave rhythm accompanies massive bilateral myoclonus and; (4) a spike-and-wave or polyspike-

and-wave rhythm, or a mixture of slow waves and fast waves comprising more of less rhythmic spike-and-wave complexes, accompany the clonic and hemiclonic seizures. The interictal records during rest show normal background acttivity. When hyperpnea is induced, the EEG shows slowing of background activity and, very often, spindle-shaped bursts of theta waves followed by high-voltage delta waves. Patients who have petit mal abscences show paroxysms in 80–90% of the cases, if care is taken to have a prolonged and repeated hyperpnea. The number of subjects showing interictal epileptic paroxysm is very difficult to state precisely, because the possibility of observing much paroxysms is dependent on the number, duration, and time of the recordings being made. During a single routine EEG recording of 20–30 minutes, during wakefulness, and for which photo stimulation and hyperpnea are the only activation methods employed, the number of subjects showing paroxysms in the EEG may not exceed 50% of the cases. This varies depending on the types of seizures presented. Patients with grand mal seizures only show paroxysms in 15–20% of cases, whereas patients with isolated or grand mal associated with myoclonus show paroxysms in 50–60% of the cases, principally under the effect of stimulation.

The EEG in secondary generalized epilepsies is characterized by ictal records that are usually, but not necessarily, positive. These ictal discharges include: (1) epileptic recruiting rhythms or low-voltage activity that accompanies tonic seizures, certain atypical absences, and certain atonic seizures; (2) pseudorhythmic bursts of spikes and waves at about 2 Hz, which accompany certain atypical absences and atonic seizures; and (3) isolated slow spikes and waves that are sometimes present in massive bilateral myoclonus in infants. With the exception of grand mal seizures, which are always accompanied by ictal discharge, all the other seizures may be manifested in the record only by a desynchronization of the background rhythms.

The interictal background activity in secondary generalized epilepsies is rarely normal, posterior activity usually being slower than in normal subjects of the same age. There is often a considerable amount of diffuse theta or even a diffuse delta rhythm, at times in bilaterally synchronous and symmetrical bursts. The existence of a focus of slow activity is not unusual. Interictal epileptic paroxysms during wakefulness are far more frequent in secondary than in generalized epilepsy. In encephalopathies, such as the West syndrome, the interictal records show characteristically continuous paroxysmal discharges of very high voltage (Hypsarrythmia, Gibbs & Gibbs, 1952).

The EEG in partial epilepsies may present a normal background activity or the background rhythm may be slowed, depending on the characteristics of the lesion responsible for the disturbances of the electrogenesis. The interictal epileptic paroxysms appear as spikes, sharp waves, or spike-and-wave complexes distributed intermittently over a limited portion of the scalp and constituting what is called an epileptic focus.

Neonatal status epilepticus is characterized by quite variable and complex electrographic patterns. Monomorphic rhythmic delta waves with a frequency of 1-3 Hz and positive or negative spikes of long duration, variable amplitude, and a frequency between 2-6 Hz are often recorded. A peculiar pattern consisting of an alpha-like rhythm with a frequency between 6-10 Hz and an amplitude of 25-30 μV, lasting 10-90 seconds, can appear in the Rolandic and occipital areas. The electrographic pattern sequence is variable. Discharges may be composed of the same basic repetitive waveform or by a succession of different patterns. The site of seizure discharges is generally limited to one region of a hemisphere. Interseizure records are highly correlated with prognosis: Inactive or paroxysmal EEGs without any seizure discharge are followed by death or major sequelae in 100% of the cases; abnormal tracings other than paroxysmal and inactive, by death or major sequelae in 70% of the cases, and normal or subnormal records by unfavorable clinical outcome in only 23% of the cases. Absence of sleep organization for 2 or 3 days seems to be another unfavourable prognostic feature (Dreyfus-Brisac & Monod, 1972).

6. Prognostic Value of the Neonatal EEG in Full-Term Newborns

Monod and Dreyfus-Brisac (1972) made a review of the EEG contribution to the estimation of neurological distress during the neonatal period, especially after abnormal pregnancies or deliveries. They give information relating to the prognosis for infants born after 36 weeks of gestational age. This information has been summarized by these authors as follows:

1. In the presence of a normal neonatal EEG, a small number of children die due to cardiac malformations or other causes. No cases of severe neurological sequelae have been observed in surviving babies.
2. Transitory EEG abnormalities are less alarming than persistent EEG abnormalities.
3. A paroxysmal EEG in a comatose baby, or sometimes even in a conscious baby, is consistently of very grave prognostic significance.
4. The same is true of an inactive EEG after 24 hours of life.
5. If the EEG recorded in a comatose baby is not paroxysmal, inactive, low voltage plus theta rhythms, diffusely slow, or with focalized abnormalities, there is a good chance of normal development despite a severe neurological state.

6. Rapid normalization generally implies good prognosis.
7. The presence of multiple abnormalities implies poor prognosis.
8. The presence of multiple abnormalities is more alarming than if there were only one abnormality.

IV. CRITICAL ASPECTS OF VISUAL EEG INTERPRETATION

The routine EEG examination is a harmless procedure, and it provides useful information in the study of neurological patients, as we have discussed previously. However, it has many critical aspects that make the application of more objective procedures desirable. Among these shortcomings are:

1. *Skilled personnel are needed for the interpretation of EEG records.* It is well known that accuracy in EEG interpretation is highly related to the training and experience of the personnel. In order to make the routine EEG examination available for all patients in whom a neurological disease should be ruled out, an enormous number of skilled personnel are needed for interpretation of EEG records.

2. *There is a large subjective component in the evaluation of EEG records.* According to Volavka, Matousek, Roubicek, Feldstein, Brezinova, Prior, Scott, and Synek (1971), there is a low correlation between evaluations of the same EEG records by different electroencephalographers. Majkowski, Horyd, Kicinska, Narebski, Goscinski, and Darwaj (1971), using the evaluation of 120 EEG records by 6 independent electroencephalographers, found that no agreement was reached in regard to the evaluation of normality of abnormality in 48 cases (see Table 2.2). After this independent evaluation, the participants met in order to review the EEG records jointly. In most cases, agreement was then reached, with corrections of previous opinions. Only four cases remained in which no agreement was reached. These results clearly demonstrate the subjective component influencing visual EEG interpretation. Another example of the difficulty of visual EEG evaluation is the lack of consensus among experienced electroencephalographers about what constitutes a spike. This aspect is discussed in detail in Chapter 12, but note that even experienced electroencephalographers might be inconsistent when retested with the same EEG records (Chiappa, Brimm, Allen, Leibig, Rossiter, Stockard, Burchiel, & Bickford, 1976).

3. *Great difficulty in visual EEG interpretation is related to the definition of what is really a normal EEG.* This topic has been reviewed recently by Chatrian and Lairy (1976) for the adult EEG, and by Petersén, Eeg-

TABLE 2.2
Comparison of Discrepancies in Evaluation of 48 EEG Records[a]

P:N[b]	*Number of EEG Records*
5:1	6
1:5	10
4:2	9
4:1 + 1[c]	3
2:4	6
3:2 + 1[c]	2
3:3	7
2:3 + 1[c]	3
1:3 + 2[c]	2

[a]From Majkowski et al, 1971.
[b]*P:N* is the numerical ratio of evaluation of electroencephalographers; *P* = pathological; *N* = normal.
[c]Number of electroencephalographers believing that artifacts made impossible the evaluation of the record.

Olofsson, Hagne, andSelldén (1965), Petersén and Eeg-Olofsson (1970), Eeg-Olofsson (1971), and Papatheophilov and Turland (1976) for children and adolescents. The problem of the lack of clear limits between normality and abnormality in the evaluation of EEG records might arise from two facts:

a. Great differences are observed in the incidence of different rhythms and patterns of the EEG according to different authors (see Table 2.1); such differences illustrate the considerable range of biological variation, as well as subjective judgment. Petersén, Kaiser, and Magnusson (1973) emphasize that such great interindividual variability makes objective evaluation procedures highly desirable.

b. There exist disagreements about the consideration of some waves or patterns as normal or abnormal (i.e., 14 and 6 positive spikes, Gibbs & Gibbs, 1951a, 1963), about the presence of theta activity in the adult EEG (Knott, 1976), and about the interpretation of the effects of hyperventilation, photic stimulation, and other activation procedures (which have evolved considerably since they were first introduced in clinical practice, with great caution being exercised at present by most investigators in assessing the significance of such paroxysmal EEG changes, Chatrian, 1976b). Such criterion disparities make it inevitable that the incidence of false positives among the normal population is variable according to different authors.

4. *The level of accuracy of visual EEG interpretation as a diagnostic procedure is dependent on the type and localization of the lesion.* We mentioned previously, in the case of intracranial tumors, that from 4–57% of the

records may be normal depending on whether the lesion was cortical or was located in other brain structures. Vascular occlusions exhibited a similarly wide range of normal EEGs (from 13–60%). Epileptic patients during routine awake examinations also present different percentages of normal EEGs, depending on the type of epilepsy. In patients with grand mal, 30% of the records are normal; in psychomotor epilepsy, 50% of the records are normal; in Jacksonian or focal epilepsy, 30% of the EEGs are normal, but in petit mal epilepsy, only 10% of the recordings are normal. In head trauma cases, 65% of the EEGs are normal. These figures indicate the high incidence of false negatives in visual EEG examinations of patients with major neurological diseases.

These findings justify the following assertions:

a. The visual inspection of the EEG is of great utility in a variety of brain diseases.

b. The EEG examination is not available for the whole at-risk population even in the developed countries.

c. The high incidence of false negatives calls for a great deal of improvement.

d. The incidence of false positive EEG findings among the normal population is undesirably high. These conclusions make it clear that it is desirable to develop more precise and objective procedures to extract the huge amount of useful diagnostic information that is contained in the electrical activity of the brain and to devise automatic methods to evaluate this information, in order to provide accurate diagnoses for the great majority of persons requiring EEG examination, for whom this is presently not available.

PART I:

INTRODUCTION TO EVOKED RESPONSES AND EVENT-RELATED POTENTIALS

The distinction between the "spontaneous" or "background" EEG activity of the brain and the response evoked by environmental changes is arbitrary, because many components of the intrinsic activity are themselves "responses," either to external events outside the experimental schedule or to endogenous processes (i.e., mental events). These responses are very difficult to identify, however, because there is no sign of the event that initiated them. Thus, from a practical point of view, only those responses that can be clearly related in time to a known event are considered evoked responses (ERs). The ERs to different types of sensory stimuli represent the response of the brain to the stimulus and occur at a latency determined by the central transmission time of the sensory system that was stimulated. They consist of a transient oscillation of voltage, which often is obscured by the ongoing activity.

These oscillations can be roughly divided into three latency domains, which provide different types of information. Very early events (1.5–10 msec), which must be recorded using special procedures discussed later, reflect the transmission of afferent information through successive levels of the sensory pathway. Medium-latency events (50–200 msec) reflect the arrival of afferent information at sensory and nonsensory specific cortex, and provide insight into such aspects of brain functions as sensory acuity, arousal, and attention. Long-latency events (200–500 msec), particularly the so-called late positive components or LPC, provide insight into a variety of complex cognitive processes (such as expectancy and matching of current inputs against templates constructed from previous experience). Great emphasis has been placed on the study of LPC's in recent years, because they offer a potentially unique insight into brain mechanisms mediating cognition and "higher cortical functions." In this book, we have refrained from discussing LPC's even though they have potentially important clinical applications in patients with cognitive dysfunctions. We have elected to confine our discussion to those aspects of evoked responses for which clear clinical applications have already been demonstrated. The interested reader can find extensive discussion of current LPC research elsewhere (Callaway, Tueting, & Koslow, 1978; John, 1977).

The "readiness" or "intention" potential (Bereitschaftspotential, Kornhuber & Deecke, 1965) precedes the voluntary movements. It can appear even when the movement is never actually performed; the "idea" of movement is sufficient to evoke an identifiable potential change. The readiness potential consists of a slow negative shift that begins approximately 1 second before the onset of the contraction. This potential, together with the subsequent negative and positive waves, are considered as "motor potentials" (MPs).

The contingent responses are potential changes whose appearances are contingent on the association of signals and/or action or decision by the subject. The most obvious of these is the Contingent Negative Variation (CNV), or "expectancy wave." This is a slow increase in surface negativity during the period between a warning or conditional stimulus and an imperative or unconditional one, with which the subject is in some way "engaged" (W.G. Walter, 1964a).

Imaginary potentials or responses to an omitted stimulus that is expected have also been obtained: Simple sensory stimuli are given in a regular pattern, for example in triplets, and responses in specific and nonspecific cortex are recorded. If, after a series of such presentations, the second stimulus is occasionally omitted, the response pattern shows an "interpolated response" to the omitted stimulus (Weinberg, Walter, & Crow, 1970). These emitted potentials have quite different scalp distributions depending on whether the missed stimulus was visual or auditory (Simson, Vaughan, & Ritter, 1976).

The ERs reflect not only the functional integrity of an anatomic pathway, but also various aspects of brain function related to sensory, perceptual, and cognitive processes. To cover all the information comprehensibly in one chapter is impossible. Thus, we shall only give a general description of ERs with special emphasis on their clinical applications. For further information, the reader may consult the books of Cobb and Morocutti (1967); Bergamini and Bergamasco (1967a); Donchin and Lindsley (1969); Shagass (1972); Regan (1972); Storm van Leeuwen, Lopes da Silva, and Kamp (1975); John (1977); and Desmedt (1977a,b).

From the technical point of view, the evoked responses at the scalp are recorded with the same type of electrodes described for EEG recording, silver/silver chloride electrodes being the most convenient. For placement of the electrodes, the 10–20 system is also recommended, although there are good scientific reasons to deviate from it. However, it is desirable that the placement be described in relation to the 10–20 system (Donchin, Callaway, Cooper, Desmedt, Goff, Hillyard, & Sutton, 1977). Amplification and band width of the recording system should be adjusted according to the type of evoked responses explored, because, for example, brain stem evoked responses are recorded better with a high gain and a band width up to 3000 Hz, whereas DC recording or very long time constants are used for CNV recording.

The problems discussed in relation to monopolar or bipolar recordings of the EEG are also valid for the ERs. Location of the reference electrode is crucial in ER recording. Regan (1972) discussed the benefits of bipolar versus monopolar (referential) recordings in the case of two main sources of the ER activity, of which one is of constant spatial distribution and of greater amplitude than the other. If the field due to the weaker source is of interest, then bipolar recordings are preferable because the contribution of the stronger source will be cancelled out and precise measurement of the weaker source is possible. Special attention to avoid interferences from muscle potentials and eye movements should be provided. In particular, when slow ER components are recorded, it is convenient to record simultaneously the oculogram in one channel for good control, or to use automatic artifact rejection (see Chapter 8).

I. THE AVERAGE EVOKED RESPONSE

The ERs to sensory stimuli are of very low amplitude in human beings and are obscured by the ongoing background activity. Several procedures of estimation have been developed to study them (these are discussed in Chapter 10). One of the most widely applied procedures is averaging. This procedure consists of taking a series of n samples of the EEG fluctuations that occur as a specified stimulus is repeatedly presented. Each sample begins at the instant t_0 when the stimulus occurs and is T msec in duration. This period, T, is often called the *analysis epoch*. Each sample will contain two kinds of activity: (1) the transient oscillation, which constitutes the evoked response phase locked to the time of the stimulus onset, t_0, to which we shall refer as the "signal," $S(t)$; and (2) the ongoing background activity reflecting neuronal processes unrelated to the effects of the stimulus, to which we refer as the "noise," $N(t)$. Therefore, any single sample can be considered as a composite voltage oscillation, $V(t)$, such that:

$$V(t) = S(t) + N(t).$$

The accuracy with which $S(t)$ can be defined by a single sample depends on the ratio of signal to noise (S/N) in the sample. In practice, N is as large as S, and in order to obtain a reasonably accurate estimate of $S(t)$, it is necessary to increase the S/N. This can be done by averaging a set of samples of the EEG fluctuations, $V(t)$, time locked to the repetitive stimulus. After n presentations of the stimulus, the contribution of the signal to the average will be proportional to the number of samples, because the signal is in reproducible phase relation to the time of the stimulus onset. However, because the noise is in random phase relation to t_0, the contribution of the noise to the average will be proportional to the square root of the number of samples, or $\sqrt{n}\, N(t)/n$. Thus, after n stimulus presentations, the average evoked response can be described as:

$$V(t)/n = \frac{nS(t)}{n} + \frac{\sqrt{n}\, N(t)}{n} = S(t) + \frac{N(t)}{\sqrt{n}}.$$

Therefore, if in a single sample of the EEG fluctuation, the contribution of signal and noise was S/N, in the average of n fluctuations it will be $\sqrt{n}$ S/N. The averaging improves the S/N by an amount proportional to the square root of the number of samples obtained.

The assumptions in this model are that S(t), or the signal, is considered constant or invariant during the different samples, and that the noise N(t) has zero mean with symmetrical marginal distributions. In general, it is impossible to ensure that either condition may exist. The ERs are changing according to the state of the brain, and the distribution of the EEG also varies. Therefore, the averaged ER does not necessarily represent the "prototypic" response of the brain to a stimulus. Only some components of the sensory ERs (i.e., the early components of the auditory evoked responses and the somatosensory evoked responses) are highly stable, and averaging thus provides a good approximation of their waveform. The effect of averaging is also different for the different components of the visual (Procházka, 1971) and auditory (Vivion et al., 1977) evoked responses.

Averaged evoked responses have been extensively studied. From a practical point of view, they have shown to be of great value in the evaluation of brain dysfunction in neurology, as is described later and in Chapter 13.

Average ER computations can be implemented in small, special-purpose computers of averaged transients or in general-purpose digital computers.

The analog EEG signal is led to an analog to digital (A/D) converter, which will provide a series of m digits proportional to the analog voltage, with a defined time interval or sampling frequency. At the moment of the synchronizing signal (i.e., the stimulus), the computer begins to "sweep" and each digit will be summed in a separate register, as a function of the time, or latency, at which it was sampled. As this process is repeated n times, the value of each of m registers will be proportional to the average voltage of the ER at the specific latency corresponding to that register plus the value of the noise divided by the square root of the sample size, $\sqrt{n}$. As the sample size n is increased, the contribution of the noise to the average thus decreases. The series of values of the m registers will then be a digital representation of the averaged evoked response. In the case of detection of evoked responses that precede an action or stimulus, delay recording is required or "off-line" analysis from tape run backwards.

In the study of averaged evoked responses, it has been common usage to designate the different waves according to their peak latency. Many classifications have appeared: a sequential nomenclature without regarding the polarity of the waves; a sequential denomination taking into account the polarity, and a system that specifies each component by the polarity and the mean peak latency. The last procedure is flexible and provides simple communication between laboratories.

3 Visual Evoked Responses (VERs)

VERs can be evoked by many different types of stimuli: diffuse illumination of the retina by xenon–tube flashes; focal illumination of the retina by small spots of light located in different retinal positions; a spatially structured stimulus field such as a presentation of a pattern, slow alternation of pattern-appearance, pattern-disappearance, or pattern reversal at constant mean luminance; changes in luminance or luminance modulation; moving spots or moving bar stimuli, and stimuli with some information content, such as letters, words, figures, and so on. Depending on the types of stimuli, the characteristics of the VERs change. The physical intensity, field size, modulation depth, frequency of stimulation, regularity of the pattern, stimulus color, and so on, all produce different effects on the VERs (Regan, 1972). Because VERs also change depending on the age, the experimental conditions (i.e., dark adaptation), the internal state of alertness, and the psychological state of the subject, a wide range of variables are relevant to the study of such ERs. Therefore, the type of stimulation and the technical conditions of recording should be clearly stated in each experiment, in order to permit comparison of results from different laboratories.

In VER research, the terms "transient" and "steady state" have been used in the same sense as in system theory. A transient response is obtained when, during averaging, the time between the stimuli is so long that all effects in the response are over before a new stimulus is given. If the repetition rate is increased, the effects of the stimuli merge and components or details that were separable before eventually become indistinguishably fused into one sinusoidal response. "Steady state" means that the stimulus frequency is so high that the response to all higher harmonics that the stimulus may itself contain, or that are evoked in the system because of nonlinearities that are generally present, are attenuated to such a degree that all that remains in the response is the basic frequency of stimulation. Either transient or steady state responses can be obtained by a spatially structured or unstructured stimulus field. In order to simplify the description of VERs, we first discuss the transient VERs to an unstructured field stimulus, then the steady state VERs to an unstructured stimulus, and, last, the transient and steady state VERs to structured visual field stimulation.

I. TRANSIENT VERs TO A SPATIALLY UNSTRUCTURED STIMULUS FIELD

A. General Characteristics

These VERs may be obtained by diffuse light (i.e., flashes) illuminating the entire retina, or by small spots of light located in different retinal positions. When VERs obtained by light stimulation of the foveal or extrafoveal retina were compared, stimulation of the central fovea was overwhelmingly more effective than extrafoveal stimulation (Rietveld, 1965; Eason, Oden, & White, 1967). However, flashes are the most widely used stimuli. The VERs to flashes appear very difficult to interpret because they present a great interindividual variability, as is shown in Fig. 3.1. Although the results from different laboratories display some general agreements, the specific details of polarity and latency of components are quite variable (Kooi & Bagchi,

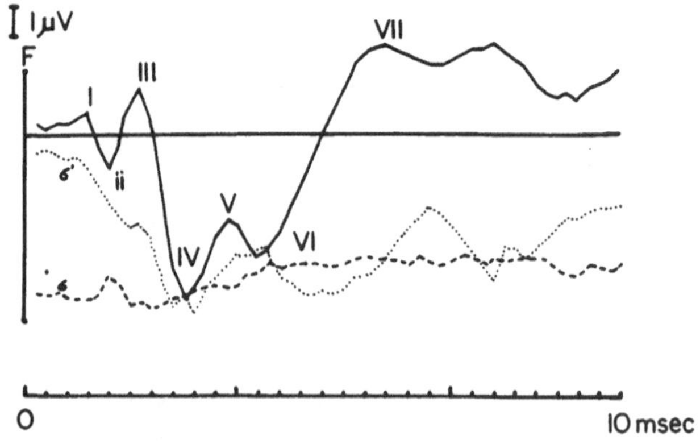

FIG. 3.1. Average VER of 1000 responses, 50 in each of 20 subjects to flash. *Dashed line*: standard deviation for the 1000 responses. *Dotted line*: standard deviation for the 20 individual average responses of subjects. (From Cigánek, 1969.)

1964a). Thus, interindividual and interlaboratory differences (Aunon & Cantor, 1977) may explain the dissimilar results obtained by several authors in trying to classify the different components according to their peak latencies. Such laboratory differences are described later in this section. Arnal, Gerin, Salmon, Ravault, Nikache and Peronnet (1972) and Valdés, Harmony, and Ricardo (1974), using two different analytical procedures, found several clusters of VERs in normal subjects. Dustman and Beck (1965a) and Lewis, Dustman, and Beck (1972) described greater similarities of the VERs between monozygotic twins than between dyzygotic twins or nonrelated children. Although VERs are more similar in children than in young adults, great interindividual variability in children from birth up to 2 years of age has also been observed (Ellingson, 1970; Ellingson, Danahy, Nelson, & Lahtrop, 1974). However, VERs to flashes seem to be highly reliable during the same period (Aunon & Cantor, 1977; Kooi & Bagchi, 1964a) with long term stability (Dustman & Beck, 1963) and, thus, with low intraindividual variability (Cigánek, 1969).

The nomenclature most commonly used (Fig. 3.1) is that of Cigánek (1961). Recording from $O_z P_z$, he described three different types of waves: the first four components (waves O to III, with mean peak latencies of 21, 39, 53, and 72 msec), which are referred to as the "early components." Wave III is the most constant. Waves IV to VII (94, 114, 134, and 190 msec) are the "late components," followed by the afterdischarge, which consists of several rhythmic waves at a frequency in the alpha range, which disappear if the eyes are opened. Cigánek also suggested that the early responses may be considered as specific responses of the visual pathways to the flash, the late components being unspecific.

VERs to flashes may be recorded on the whole scalp surface with different waveforms. Inferences concerning the intracranial location of presumptive neurogenic generators are difficult due to great interindividual variability. Amplitude maxima will correctly predict the location of a source only if it is a cortical generator whose dipole orientation is approximately perpendicular to the overlying scalp. In spite of this, there are indications that at least two distinct regions of the scalp—the occipital and vertex locations—reflect independent neuronal events: Cobb and Dawson (1960) demonstrated that the events of the first 90 msec after the flash reversed in-phase between 3 and 6 cm above the inion. Rémond and Lesèvre (1965), computing spatio-temporal maps (see Chapter 10) from equally spaced electrodes placed in the midsagittal line, found two sources: (1) the occipital region, with a negative wave at 50–80 msec latency after presentation of the stimulus and a great positive gradient between 120–140 msec; and (2) more anterior to the occipital zone, in the parieto-occipital junction, a positive wave was found with 40-45 msec latency afterdischarge. Vaughan (1969), by analysis of isopotential maps, found that both the early and late components showed a maximum overlying the occipital area, but that a later wave (200 msec) had a secondary peak in the central region. This suggests that the late components of the VERs result from two distinct generators (occipital and central), rather than from volume conduction of the occipital response.

Goff, Matsumiya, Allison, and Goff (1969), studying the amplitude distribution of the components that were more clearly discernible, found that the earliest component, at a latency of 41 msec, and the other positive wave, at 100 msec, have their maximum amplitudes in occipital regions, whereas the negative wave, at 50 msec, and waves between 150–200 msec were more pronounced at the vertex. More recently, the same group of authors (Allison, Matsumiya, Goff, & Goff, 1977) described 22 components in the VERs. Of these, six were regarded as electroretinographic, one as myogenic and the remaining as neurogenic. In the latter group, P40, N55, P60, and N70 were recorded in occipital regions. Analysis of the components in the latency range of 80–140 msec was difficult due to within- and between-subject variability, but N145 and P190 (the negativity and positivity of the vertex potential) were easily measured. Efforts at recording the activity of optic nerve and lateral geniculate nucleus by far-field recording techniques analogous to those used in recording activity of ascending pathways in the somatosensory and auditory system have not been successful (Starr, 1978).

The forementioned results have been obtained in healthy subjects, and they suggest that components between 40–100 msec may be considered as specific. However, the results obtained with the study of VERs in the presence of lesions of the visual pathway are rather controversial. The comparison of simultaneous recordings from scalp and calcarine cortex in man have shown attenuation of the first components over the scalp, with very similar waveshapes (Rayport, Vaughan, & Rosengart, 1964). Cohn (1969) described that lesions of the visual cortex produce a marked decrease in amplitude of VERs in monkeys, leaving the waveform and latencies of components little affected. Vaughan and Gross (1969), recording potentials over striate, prestriate, inferotemporal, and frontal cortex before and after brain injuries in monkeys, observed that unilateral optic tract section or unilateral striate ablation produced elimination of early wavelets in the ipsilateral striate and prestriate cortex and reduction of the entire response in ipsilateral inferotemporal cortex, concomitant with reduction in amplitude of all other components in both striate cortices and reduction in amplitude of the entire response in the contralateral prestriate cortex.

Corletto, Gentilomo, Rosadini, Rossig, and Zattoni (1967), comparing the VERs recorded at the scalp and in the cortex in man, found that they were very similar, but after removal of the occipital pole, only components between 45–120 msec were severely affected. Also in man, Vaughan and

Katzman (1964) described that lesions of the retina and optic nerve produce severe VER changes, with absent response when the affected eye was stimulated, and interhemispheric asymmetries of the VERs when lesions were located in the chiasma or in the geniculocalcarine tract. Perhaps of greater interest are observations by Jonkman (1967), Bergamini and Bergamasco (1967b), Oosterhuis, Ponsen, Jonkman, and Magnus (1969), Fernández, Otero, Ricardo, and Harmony (1970), Ricardo (1974), and many other authors, of great alteration of VERs in patients, including some with lesions outside the visual pathways, in whom no clinically demonstrable visual defects were present. These results demonstrate that VERs to flashes in man originate in both the visual specific area and in nonspecific cortex. They also suggest that details of the VER may reflect brain disease in regions outside the visual system, which interact with structures in that system.

The afterdischarge of the VERs is evoked in normal subjects during rest and with eyes closed. It has a frequency within the alpha range. A close functional relationship exists between the neural systems giving rise to the alpha activity, whether or not the systems might be physiologically identical (Barlow, 1960; Cohn, 1964; Lansing & Barlow, 1972; Lehtonen & Lehtinen, 1972; Peacock, 1970. Rémond and Lesèvre (1967) studied the variation of the VERs as a function of the phase of the alpha rhythm at the time of arrival of the stimulating flashes. They observed great differences between responses obtained triggering the flashes at maxima (source or sink): The afterdischarge was inhibited when flashes were given at the time of the maximum of an alpha source, and it was greatly increased when the flashes were triggered at the maximum of alpha sink. Dustman and Beck (1965b) reported that, with respect to a component of 57 msec of latency, the most important effect was not the phase of the alpha, but the direction of the alpha when the flash was triggered. Relations between the EEG background activity and the morphology of the VERs have also been reported by several authors (Artsenlova & Ivanitsky, 1967; Callaway & Layne, 1964; Magnus & Ponsen, 1965; Popivanov, 1974, 1977; Sato, Kitajima, Mimura, Hirota, Tagawa, & Ochi, 1971; Spilker, Kamiya, Callaway, & Yeager, 1969). These reports show that the VER waveform is highly related to the background activity. *This suggests that a possible way to reduce intra- and interindividual variability of the VER may be to synchronize the stimulus with a particular phase of the EEG activity.*

B. Changes with age and sex

VERs can be recorded even in premature infants (Hrbek, Karlberg, & Olsson, 1973, Fig. 3.2). This indicates that the presence of a VER does not

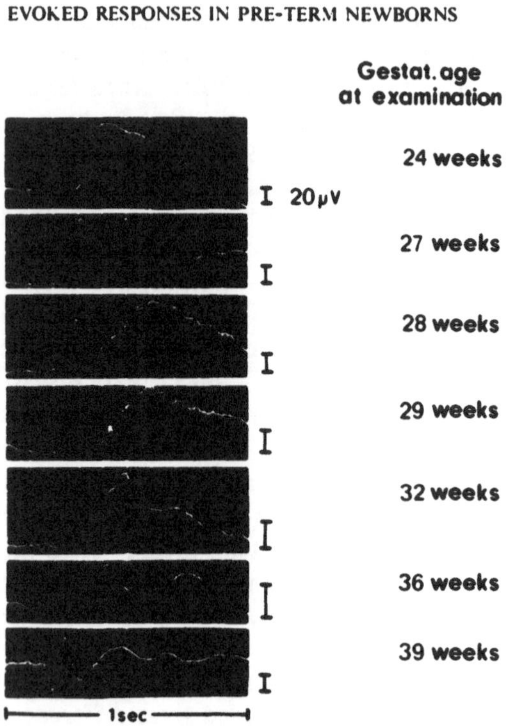

FIG. 3.2. Development of VERs in preterm newborns. (From Hrbek et al., 1973.)

necessarily imply useful visual information (Umezaki and Morrell, 1970). In premature infants, the VERs are restricted to the occipital region and spread gradually during the first months. The peak latencies decrease and the afterdischarge may develop in the third month after birth (Hrbek & Mares, 1964). Hrbek, Vitová, and Mares (1966) classified the maturation of the VERs as follows: (1) the fetal response; (2) the neonatal response, which in the second and third months changes to (3) a transient type of VER, which has some features of (4) the mature VER, into which it is gradually converted between the ages of 1 or 2 years. Similar findings have been reported by Ferris, Davis, Dorsen, and Hackett (1967), Creutzfeldt and Kuhnt (1967), Alferova (1970), Blom, Barth, and Visier (1976), and Laget, Flores-Guevara, D'Allest, Ostre, Raimbault, and Mariani (1977). Dustman and Beck (1966) and Dustman, Schenkenberg, Lewis, and Beck (1977), in a study of a group of subjects from 1 month to 81 years, found that the amplitude of occipital responses during a 250 msec time epoch is maximal at 5 to 6 years, with a decline in amplitude at 7 years of age and a subsequent rise again at 13–14 years. At the age of 16, amplitude stabilizes until the fourth decade; older subjects showed increased latencies and attenuation of late and potentiation of early components. There is a slight interhemispheric amplitude asymmetry in all age groups in central regions. VERs recorded from C4 are larger than those from C3.

Sex differences in VERs have also been reported. Higher amplitudes and shorter latencies of the different components in females than in males have been observed during adolescence and adulthood (Buchsbaum, Henkin, & Christiansen, 1974; Rodin, Grisell, Gudobba, & Zachary, 1965; Schenkenberg, Dustman, & Beck, 1971; Shagass, Schwartz, & Straumanis, 1966). During childhood, the VERs of males are reliably larger than those of females (Dustman et al., 1977).

C. Changes with the characteristics of the stimulus

There is a consensus of opinion (Wicke, Donchin, & Lindsley, 1964; see Regan, 1972; Shagass, 1972; and Cigánek, 1975, for a review) that increasing the intensity of stimulation (energy or brightness) produces VERs of greater amplitude, shorter latency, and, eventually, greater complexity (Fig. 3.3). With still higher intensities, the amplitudes do not increase further (saturation) or may even decrease. Within a certain range, the VER amplitude luminance function, when plotted in log-linear coordinates, suggests a Weber-Fechner type of logarithmic relationship between stimulus magnitude and VER amplitude, or a power law relationship, when it is plotted in log-log coordinates (Kress, 1975).

VERs may be recorded not only at the onset of the stimulus (*on* response), but at the offset or removal of stimulation (*off* responses). These responses seem to be similar in waveshape, but *off* responses are of smaller amplitude. Amplitudes of *off* responses at different luminance levels show the same behavior as *on* responses (Dinges & Tepas, 1976).

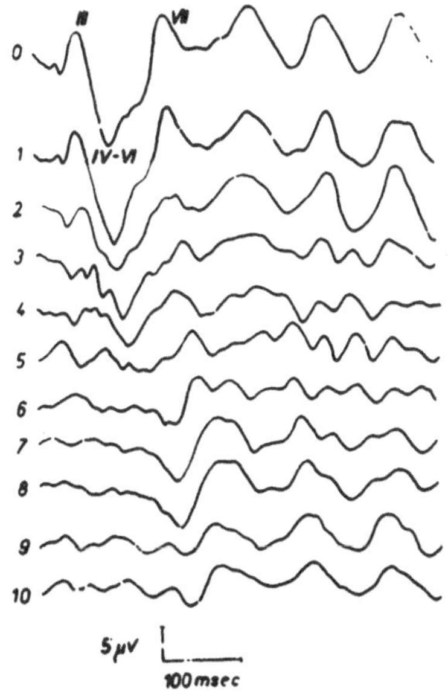

FIG. 3.3. Series of average VERs, from top to bottom progressively decreasing intensity. (From Cigánek, 1975.)

Stimulation with lights of different colors produces distinguishably different VERs (Cigánek & Ingvar, 1969; Clynes, 1969; Dobson, 1976; Grigorieva, 1977; John, 1977, Shipley, Jones, & Fry, 1965). In this context, Regan (1972) points out that before discussing the effects of stimulus color on VERs, an essential requirement is to demonstrate that the effects are indeed specific to stimulus color, and are not in reality either luminance effects or photopic-scotopic phenomena masquerading as color correlates.

D. Clinical applications

Different procedures have been used for the evaluation of VER abnormalities in the presence of brain dysfunction:

1. Various components have been identified and peak latencies and amplitudes compared between a group of healthy people and patients with brain dysfunction. This procedure has several disadvantages. In addition to the great interindividual variability of VERs, brain lesions often produce bizarre waveforms, making it very difficult to decide whether the waves observed correspond to similar waves in healthy people. It is difficult to define "abnormal" waveshapes by visual inspection, especially during the first 250 msec.

2. To circumvent the great interindividual variability, comparisons between left and right homologous VERs have also been carried out, using one hemisphere as reference for the other. Normally, VERs from homologous derivations show good waveshape symmetry. Jonkman (1967) made a systematic study in a large sample of neurological patients, measuring the peak latency difference and the peak amplitude difference for each component. He found that this comparison was very difficult to do because great waveform asymmetries appeared. Ricardo (1974) also conducted a large study with about 200 neurological patients. She reached the conclusion that these measures were difficult to make in a high percentage of cases, due to the great waveform asymmetries (Fig. 3.4). Although it was often difficult to identify the side that was abnormal, both of these authors found that waveshape asymmetry was usually much greater in patients than in normal subjects.

3. Other quantitative approaches have been used; these are discussed in Chapter 13. In this section, only those results obtained with the first two procedures are described. We shall see that even with the previously mentioned shortcomings, the results show conclusively that VERs to flashes are severely affected in the presence of many types of brain damage or disease.

The disturbances of VERs to flashes in the presence of brain damage or disease have been extensively studied. We divide our discussion of such disturbances into two parts. First, the changes observed during lesions of

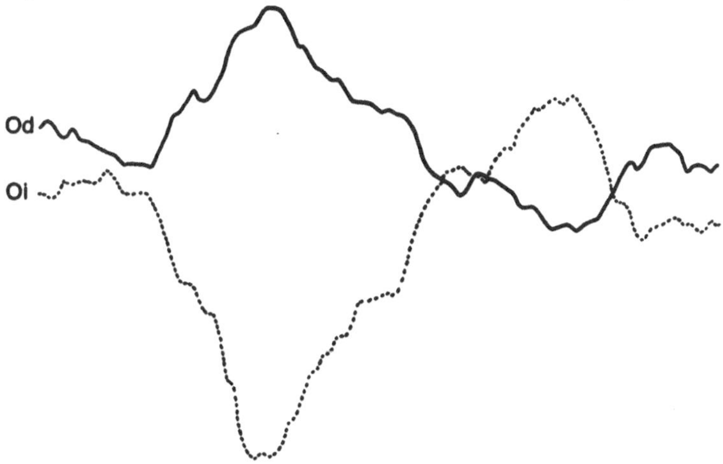

FIG. 3.4. VERs to flash recorded in left occipital (Oi) and right occipital (Od) leads in a patient with a pituitary adenoma. (From Ricardo, 1974.)

the visual pathway are examined. Subsequently, changes found in other clinical states not affecting the visual pathways are discussed.

1. Lesions of the Visual Pathway

This topic has recently been reviewed by Halliday (1975a). For the analysis of these lesions, monocular stimulation has been used.

Prechiasmal Lesions. When lesions are localized at the retina, the effects are more easily detectable in the electroretinogram (ERG) than in the VER. However, in optic atrophies and optic nerve lesions, the VERs are reduced in amplitude, whereas the ERG is normal. Table 3.1 summarizes the effects of prechiasmal lesions observed by several authors.

Chiasmal Lesions. Lehmann and Fender (1969) made a detailed analysis of a patient in whom the optic chiasm had been traumatically split some years before. They found the expected loss of the contralateral component, which has its expression in the phase reversal of the response in the contralateral hemisphere to the stimulation of each eye. This result confirms previous findings of Vaughan and Katzman (1964) and Jacobson, Hirose, and Suzuki (1968). Koshino, Kuroch, and Mogami (1977) described an increase in the amplitude and decrease of latency of the VER components after removal of hypophysial tumors. Allen and Starr (1977) describe the sudden appearance of VERs in the course of surgery in individuals with pituitary tumors who had been without vision or evoked potentials prior to the operation.

TABLE 3.1
Effects of Prechiasmal Lesions on VERs to Flashes

Reference	*Pathology*	*Results*
Ebe et al. (1964)	Retinitis pigmentosa	VERs reduced or abolished; ERG absent
	Macular atrophy	Little changes in VERs and ERG
	Optic atrophy	VERs absent; ERG normal
	Cataracts	Alterations of VERs and ERG in same cases
Vaughan and Katzman (1964)	Different retinal diseases	VERs and ERG altered
	Optic atrophy	VERs absent; ERG normal
Copenhaver and Perry (1964)	Cataracts, corneal or vitreous opacities	No relation between VER amplitude and visual acuity
	Retinal or optic nerve lesions	Relation between VER amplitude and visual acuity
	Refractive errors	Relation between VER amplitude and visual acuity
Gerin et al. (1966)	Optic nerve lesions	Reduction in VER amplitude
Ravault et al. (1966)	Optic nerve lesions	Reduction in VER amplitude
Jacobson et al. (1968)	Retinitis pigmentosa	VERs reduced in amplitude; ERG absent
	Optic atrophy	VERs reduced in amplitude; ERG normal
Rohuer et al. (1969)	Lesion of macular bundle	Loss of the early VERs to red flashes
	Trauma of the optic nerve	VERs affected according to the severity of damage
	Compressive lesions	VER changes not related to the severity of damage
	Optic neuritis	Idem
Harding (1974)	Macular lesion	Alteration of the VER component at 100 msec
Korol and Stangos (1974)	Compression of optic nerve	Absence or reduction of VERs
Novikova and Tolstova (1977)	Congenital cataracts	Decrease in amplitude and increase of latencies Same changes as in optic atrophy

Postchiasmal Lesions. Table 3.2 shows the results obtained by several authors in the presence of postchiasmal lesions of the visual pathways. The changes most frequently observed are interhemispheric asymmetries, with amplitude reduction on the side of the lesion. However, it is possible to observe the contrary. It should be emphasized that with the exception of Vaughan, Katzman, and Taylor (1963), none of the authors observed specific VER changes in the presence of hemianopia. On the contrary, many patients with cerebral lesions and without visual field impairments showed VER abnormalities of the same type as those described in hemianopic patients. Thus, abnormal VERs to flashes are not a conclusive index of lesions of the visual pathways.

VERs recorded in the early phase of occipital blindness and repeated later seem to be of prognostic value. Responses of normal shape and amplitude after monocular and binocular stimulation were followed by complete recovery of vision. Unequal and subnormal VERs obtained following monocular stimulation, and even smaller responses after binocular stimulation, accompanied permanent unilateral occipital damage resulting in homonymous hemianopia. Lack of VERs proved to be a sign preceding permanent blindness (Abraham, Melamed, & Lavy, 1975). Duchowny, Weiss, Majlessi, and Barnet (1974), in a long-term follow-up of children with cortical blindness, found that abnormalities of early components were correlated with visual ability, whereas changes in longer latency waves correlated with the level of psychomotor functions.

2. *Clinical Alterations not Affecting the Visual Pathway (see Table 3.3)*

Tumors. The most common effect on VERs in intracranial tumors has been clearly described by Jonkman (1967): asymmetries of the VERs recorded in left and right homologous areas, even though the lesions were restricted to nonspecific cortical areas or to nonsensory specific structures. These asymmetries may be observed even when the EEG is normal. No correlation was found between the side of the lesion and specific changes in amplitude or latency. The asymmetry has no relation to the type of brain tumor or the presence of intracranial hypertension. VERs were more affected when lesions of the visual pathway were present. Harmony, Fernández-Bouzas, Fernández, and Alvarez (1978b), in a follow-up study of patients with intracranial tumors that were surgically removed, described a parallel improvement of VER symmetry and clinical findings, which suggests the usefulness of VER symmetry as a procedure for the evaluation of such cases.

TABLE 3.2
Effects of Postchiasmal Lesions on VERs to Flashes

Reference	*Clinical Alteration*	*Results*
Cohn (1963)	Homonymous hemianopia	Amplitude asymmetry
Vaughan et al. (1963)	Homonymous hemianopia	Decreased amplitude of components I, II, III (Cigánek) Latency delays of I and II; interhemispheric amplitude asymmetries greater than 50%
	Cerebral lesions without visual field defects	Decreased amplitude of component II
Gastaut et al. (1963)	Homonymous hemianopia and epilepsy	Asymmetry of VERs
Kooi et al. (1965)	Homonymous hemianopia	Increased latencies on the side of the lesion Tendency to have smaller amplitude on the side of the lesion; no difference from VERs of patients with cerebral lesions without visual impairment
Crighel and Botez (1966)	Unilateral surgical excision of the occipital cortex	Absence of response on the side of the lesion in the majority of cases
Corletto et al. (1967)	Idem	Absence of components between 45 and 120 msec
Jonkman (1967)	Homonymous hemianopia	Variable effects, with frequent asymmetries; same findings as those observed in patients with cerebral lesions without visual impairment
Barnet et al. (1970)	Acute cerebral blindness	Reduction of VER amplitude related to clinical improvement
Levillain et al. (1974)	Homonymous hemianopia	Frequent asymmetries
Duchowny et al. (1974)	Cortical blindness after head trauma and meningitis	Correlations between visual acuity and changes in early components Late components related to psychomotor function

TABLE 3.2 *(continued)*

Reference	*Clinical Alteration*	*Results*
Abraham et al. (1975)	Occipital blindness	Alterations of VERs directly related to the evolution of the patient Great prognostic value
Bacsy et al. (1977)	Homonymous hemianopia	Decrease in amplitude of early VERs
Samson-Dollfus and Pouliquen (1977)	Homonymous hemianopia	Two types of asymmetries: decreased amplitude in affected hemisphere more related to vascular disorders and increased amplitude in the side of the lesion more related to expanding lesions

Cerebrovascular Disease. Oosterhuis et al. (1969) used the following criteria of normality, based on Jonkman's (1967) results: Early components are normal if there is a clear component between 60 and 100 msec, and if there is a difference of latency not greater than 5 msec or of amplitude not more than 50%, when comparing the left and right homologous VERs. The late components and the afterdischarge were considered normal if a polyphasic wave was present, with peak latency asymmetries not greater than 25 msec and amplitude differences not greater than 50%. In the analysis of the VERs in 30 patients with cerebrovascular disease, these authors reached the following conclusions: (1) the amplitude of the late components is only asymmetric in the presence of visual field defects; (2) the amplitude of the afterdischarge is directly related to the alpha amplitude; (3) when amplitude differences of the late components are greater than 50%, the smaller response is on the affected side; (4) the alteration of the early and late components is related to the severity of the illness; (5) abnormal responses were observed more often in bipolar parieto-occipital than in monopolar occipital derivations.

Creutzfeldt et al. (1966) and Ciurea and Crighel (1967) have also reported a slowing of the afterdischarge on the side of the lesion. However, Fernández et al. (1970) and Ricardo (1974) remarked that it is very difficult to identify the side of the lesion, because larger or smaller latencies or amplitudes may be detected on that side. Samson-Dollfus and Pouliquen

TABLE 3.3
Major Abnormalities Observed in VERs to Flashes in Different Clinical Alterations Not Affecting the Visual Pathway

Clinical Alteration	*A-*	*A+*	*L*	*Asym*	*Reference*
Intracranial tumors	+	+	+	+	Creutzfeldt et al. (1966); Jonkman (1967); Bergamini and Bergamasco (1967b); Schneider (1968); Crighel and Poilici (1968); Fernandez et al. (1970); Ricardo (1974)
Cerebrovascular disease	+	+	+	+	All of the above, plus Oosterhuis et al. (1969); Bohm and Droppa (1969); Samson-Dollfus and Pouliquen (1977)
Photosensitive epilepsy		+			Gastaut et al. (1963); Creutzfeldt and Kuhnt (1967); Moroccutti et al. (1966, 1968); Broughton et al. (1969); Needham et al. (1971); Brezny (1974)
Multiple Sclerosis	+		+		Feinsod and Hoyt (1975); Czopf et al. (1976)
Jacob–Creutzfeldt disease		+			Lee and Blair (1973)
Huntington disease	+				Ellenberg et al. (1978)
Alzheimer syndrome		+			Visser et al. (1976)
Chronic brain syndrome			+		Straumanis et al. (1965)
Migraine				+	Fernandez et al. (1970); MacLean et al. (1975)
Hydrocephalia				+	Ehle and Sklar (1977)
Perinatal asphyxia	+		+		Hrbek et al. (1977); Rossini et al. (1977)
Coma	+				Gerin et al. (1970); Walter and Arfel (1972)
Hysteria	+				Ivanitsky (1969)
Mongolism			+		Bigum et al. (1970)
Myxedema			+		Cooper et al. (1977)
Hypothyroidism			+		Nishitani and Kooi (1968)
Hyperthyroidism		+			Takahashi and Fujitani (1970)
Renal disease			+		Hamel et al. (1976)

[a] A − and A + mean smaller and larger amplitudes; L means delayed latencies; Asym means asymmetries.

(1977) reported that in vascular disorders, there is a tendency to find the smaller VER on the side affected. Crighel, Sterman, and Marinchescu (1971) were not able to find any correlation between the waveshape of the VERs and the duration of the disease. However, VER symmetry has been demonstrated to be a useful procedure for the evaluation of treatments in stroke patients. Fig. 3.5, shows a case with quite asymmetric and abnormal VERs, which improved after EDTA treatment (Fernández-Bouzas, Harmony, Nápoles, & Szava, 1969).

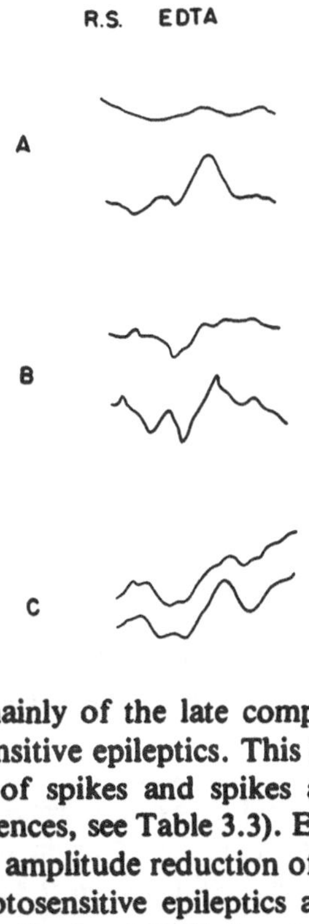

FIG. 3.5. Right and left occipital VERs in a patient with occlusion of the right parietal artery, and atherosclerosis of both internal carotid arteries. (A) The patient was in coma. (B) The patient has recovered from coma four days after EDTA treatment. (C) One month after the treatment. Calibration: 5 μV; 250 msec analysis time. (From Fernández-Bouzas et al., 1969.)

Epilepsy. An increase in amplitude, mainly of the late components of the VERs, has been described in photosensitive epileptics. This increase is dependent on the presence in the EEG of spikes and spikes and waves elicited by the photic stimulation (for references, see Table 3.3). Ebe, Meier-Ewert, and Broughton (1969) described an amplitude reduction of late components and of the afterdischarge in photosensitive epileptics after treatment with diazepam. No changes in the amplitude of VERs in other types of epileptics have been found (Aoki, 1969; Broughton, Meier-Ewert, & Ebe, 1967; Lücking, Creutzfeldt, & Heinemann, 1970). Great variability in the amplitude, waveform, and latencies of different waves of the VER have been described by Lücking (1969). This author did not find any typical alterations of VERs that could be related to the different types and etiologies of epilepsy. Later, Lücking et al. (1970) showed great differences in shapes of VERs compared to the responses of a normal control group. VERs similar to a spike and wave have been described by Morocutti, Sommer-Smith, and Creutzfeldt (1966) and Dimov, Brefeith, Menini, and

Naquet (1974). Amplitude and peak latency asymmetries have been reported by Jonkman (1967), Fernández et al. (1970), and Ricardo (1974).

Other conditions. VERs are also affected in a great variety of other clinical abnormalities (Tabel 3.3). Hrbek, Karlberg, Kjellmer, Olsson, and Riha (1977) found abnormalities of VERs in 85% of 57 neonates and infants who had been treated for perinatal asphyxia. The most frequent alterations were: the presence of a slow negative wave, larger latencies, flat responses, and a distinct decrease of VER amplitude with increasing stimulation frequency from 0.1-1 Hz (Fig. 3.6). Differences between dis-

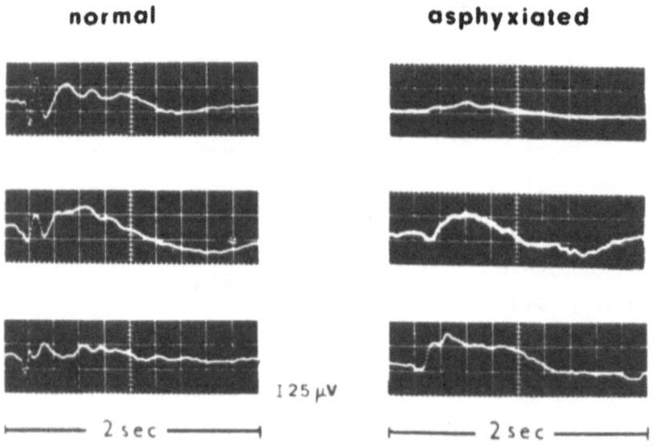

FIG. 3.6. VERs in three normal and three severely asphyxiated newborn infants. (From Hrbek et al., 1977.)

abled and normal readers are reported in the early components of VERs recorded over the left superior and inferior parietal areas, with a decrease in the number of components in the learning disabled children (Symann-Lovett, Gascon, Matsumiya, & Lombroso, 1977). Alterations of VERs in the left parietal area in children with learning disorders (Conners, 1971) and in disabled adult readers (Preston, Guthrie, Kirsch, Gertman, & Childs, 1977) seem to be a repeated finding. Njiokiktjien, Visser, and Rijke (1977), comparing the VERs of a normal group of children and another group with learning disorders, found an increase of amplitude and latency of waves II and III (93 and 144 msec) in the latter group.

Changes During Treatment. It is also a usual observation that clinical improvement is paralleled by VER improvement (Rappaport, Hall, Hopkins, Belleza, Berrol, & Reynolds, 1977). Such is the case during recovery from coma (Bergamasco, Bergamini, Mombelli, & Mutani, 1966), treatment of suprarenal insufficiency with steroids (Ojemann & Henkin, 1967); during hypothyroidism (Nishitani & Kooi, 1968) and renal disease treatments (Hamel, Bourne, Ward, & Teschan, 1976); and successful kidney transplant (Hamel, Bourne, Ward, & Teschan, 1978; Lewis, Dustman, & Beck, 1978). What is much more remarkable is the possibility of using VERs for the selection of optimal treatment according to the type of VER abnormality. In a study of 62 hyperkinetic children receiving placebo, thioridazine or d-amphetamine, an increase in latency and decrease in amplitude was found during thioridazine treatment; d-amphetamine increased latencies and amplitudes. Regression and correlation analysis of clinical symptomatology with the VER variables showed that the shorter the pretreatment latencies and the higher the amplitudes, the more disturbed was the child. Short latencies and smaller amplitudes in the pretreatment period were predictors of good therapeutic outcome with subsequent thioridazine treatment, whereas short latencies and high amplitudes were indicative of such with d-amphetamine. During therapy, the greater the drug-induced augmentation of latencies, the greater the clinical improvement (Saletu, Saletu, Simeon, Viamontes, & Itil, 1975). The mentioned results in hyperkinetic children have not been confirmed by Hall, Griffin, Mayer, Hopkins, and Rappaport (1976). R. Halliday, Rosenthal, Naylor, and Callaway (1976) have demonstrated that some VER parameters are useful predictors of clinical improvement in hyperactive children treated with methylphenidate: Children showing good response displayed large differences in VERs between a task requiring active attention and one requiring passive observing, and the amplitude of N140 and P190 component during active attention increased with Ritalin in the responders. In depressed patients, treatment with amphetamine produces different changes in VER amplitude in different groups of subjects. Buchsbaum, Van Kammen, and Murphy (1977) reported that patients who had larger P100 amplitude also tended to have larger increases in activation ratings and reduction in depression ratings. The results previously summarized must be considered as preliminary, because many complex issues are involved in such studies. However, whether or not the specific conclusions are replicated, these studies constitute a generic demonstration that in populations of patients with similar clinical characteristics, it may be possible to find clusters of subjects who share a common VER profile. The response to specific drugs seems to be directly related to particular VER profiles. *Thus, VERs may be useful not only as a diagnostic tool, but also for the evaluation and selection of the treatment.*

Some of the neurometric procedures presented in Chapter 13 also utilize flash stimuli. Results with those procedures are not to be discussed in this chapter.

II. VISUAL EXCITABILITY CYCLE

The excitability cycle of a sensory system can be investigated by applying a pair of stimuli at varying intervals and recording the ERs to the first and second stimulus (Gastaut, Gastaut, Roger, Corriol, & Naquet, 1951). The excitability cycle depends on the duration of the relative refractory period of the neurons involved in the response to the first stimulus. It is expressed as the ration between the amplitude of the ER to the second stimulus and the amplitude of the ER to the first stimulus. If it equals 0, the system is no longer excitable (absolute refractoriness). If it is smaller than 1, the system has a reduced excitability (subnormal), and if it is larger than 1, the system is more excitable (supernormal period). When it equals 1, the system has the same excitability in basal conditions.

The excitability cycle of the visual system has an absolute refractory period lasting up to 40 msec after the flash, and a period of supernormal excitability between 80 and 120 msec after the flash. From 120–150 msec after the first flash, there is a period of subnormal excitability; the return to normal excitability is observed around 200 msec (Bergamasco, 1966; Cigánek, 1964; Schwartz & Shagass, 1964). Females have a longer recovery period than males. The excitability cycle is also rather sensitive to various influences as the degree of vigilance (Cigánek, 1964); the levels of attention (Werre & Smith, 1964); drugs (Bergamasco, 1966), and sleep (Kitasato & Hatsuda, 1966; Palestini, Pisano, Rosadini, & Rossi, 1965).

Floris, Morocutti, Amabile, Bernardi, Rizzo, and Vasconetto (1967) studied the recovery cycle in normal and schizophrenic subjects. They found remarkable differences in the amplitude recovery of Cigánek's wave III (Fig. 3.7). They have also reported similar differences in a group of patients with endogenous depression (Floris, Morocutti, Amabile, Bernardi, & Rizzo, 1969). Ishikawa (1968) described a prolongation of the supernormal period in schizophrenic patients. Shagass (1972), after the analysis of different authors' data, concluded that the available results showed a reduced recovery in psychiatric patients, with the absence of diagnostic specificity.

The visual excitability cycle in epileptic patients shows a short refractory period with great facilitation of the late components (Dimov et al., 1974; Floris et al., 1969). Similar results have been observed with cardiazol activation (Bergamasco, 1966).

III. STEADY-STATE EVOKED RESPONSES TO FLICKER STIMULATION

As has already been mentioned, when averaging VERs to repetitive flashes, or flicker, the effects of the stimuli merge and components or details that were separable in the transient response are eventually indistinguishably fused into one sinusoidal response. Before the introduction of averaging techniques, it was observed that repetitive stimulation with flashes at regular intervals produced in the EEG record a rhythmic response with the same frequency as the stimulation or its harmonics (photic driving). This response was most clearly observed in occipital regions (Adrian & Matthews, 1934; Cobb & Morton, 1969; Gastaut, 1949; Gibbs & Gibbs, 1951b;

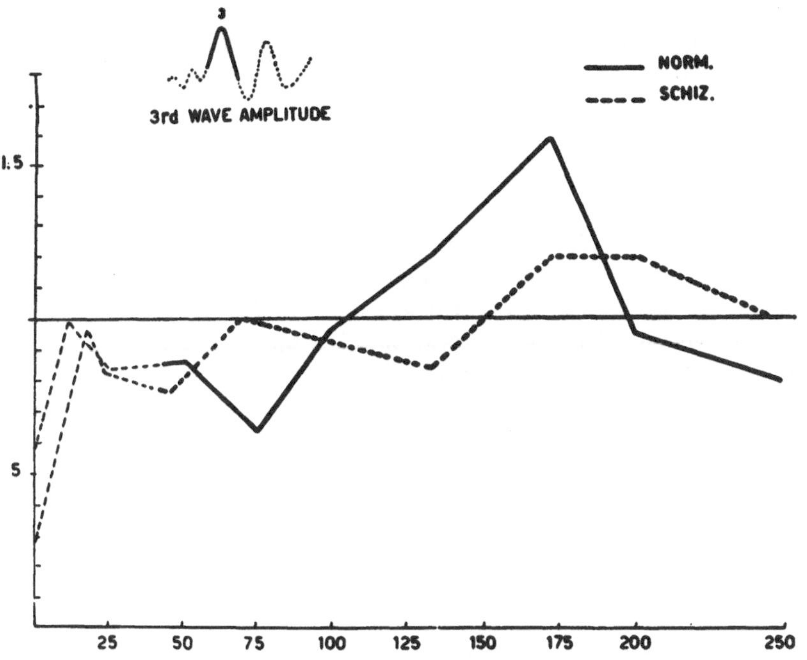

FIG. 3.7. Recovery cycle of VERs in normal and schizophrenic subjects. *Abscissa*: intervals between stimuli (in millisec). *Ordinate*: mean ratio second to first response of third wave amplitude. Note the greater recovery in normals than in schizophrenics. (From Floris et al., 1967.)

Ilyanok, 1964; W.G. Walter, Dovey, & Shipton, 1946) and was related to the spontaneous alpha and beta rhythms (Barlow, 1960; Barlow & Brazier, 1957; Mundy-Castle, 1953; Toman, 1941; Walter & Walter, 1949). Increases in the intensity of the stimulus produced an increase of the response amplitude up to a certain level, followed by a decrease (Ilyanok, 1961; Montagu, 1967). In normal subjects, a slight amplitude asymmetry of the driving response has been observed, which has been related to the hemispheric dominance (Lansing & Thomas, 1964; Masland & Goldensohn, 1967). By averaging, it is possible to record the steady-state response even when it is not observed in the EEG (Diamond, 1977; Harmony, 1975; Kitasato, 1966; Mezan, 1974; Saunders, 1976). The response is recorded better in occipital regions, but it can also be obtained from all over the scalp (Rémond & Conte, 1962; Ricardo, Harmony, Otero, & Llorente, 1974), even in frontal leads (Harmony, Fernandez, & Ricardo, 1975; Peacock & Conroy, 1974).

It has been established (Regan, 1972) that, in humans, three subsystems covering different frequency bands can contribute to the luminance ER. They have been called the low-frequency (below 13 Hz), the medium-frequency (15–25 Hz), and the high-frequency (30–60 Hz) subsystems. These subsystems can be distinguished on the basis of their topological representation as well as by their dependence on stimulus parameters. One-week-old infants are able to follow frequencies up to 3–5 Hz; at the age of 6 months, they have responses up to 12–15 Hz, and at 2 years of age, they are able to follow frequencies of 20–25 Hz (Vitová & Hrbek, 1970). The stimulation of selective quadrants of the retina has shown differences in amplitude of the steady state responses to different flicker frequencies depending on the quadrant stimulated. Flicker VERs for individual quadrants may also differ markedly between subjects and between the left and the right eye of the same object (Regan & Milner, 1978).

It has been reported that those drugs that block the adrenergic system, such as the phenothiazines, increase the driving response, whereas those that increase the adrenergic mechanisms (noradrenalin, amphetamine) produce a depression of the driving response. These results have led Vogel, Broverman, Klaiber, and Kun, (1969) and Vogel, Broverman, Klaiber, and Kobayashi (1974a, 1974b) to suggest that photic driving may reflect variations in the adrenergic system activity.

Clinical Applications

Ostow (1949) described a clear relationship between the maximal driving response to low frequencies (less than 8 Hz) and the amount of slow waves in the EEG. This may result in an asymmetric driving response in the presence of unilateral brain lesions (Brezny & Gaziova, 1964; Cantor, Young, & Wolpow, 1974; Hughes, 1960; Kooi & Thomas, 1958; Ungher, Ciurea, & Volanski, 1961), with enhanced ipsilateral responses to low frequencies in the hemisphere affected and reduced driving responses in the alpha range. Vitová (1973) has also observed a depression of driving responses in cerebral palsy and hydrocephalic infants, as well as in neurological lesions (Vitová & Faladová, 1975a). Perinatal asphyxia produced a poor driving response in neonates (Hrbek et al., 1977; see Fig. 3.8). Cigánek (1977) described abnormal driving responses to 10 and 15 Hz in epileptic patients with generalized discharges. Steady state VERs to flicker are delayed in a high proportion of multiple sclerosis (MS) patients (Richey, Kooi, & Tourtelotte, 1971); in spinal MS, this procedure can pick up patients missed by the pattern VER test (Namerow & Enns, 1972).

IV. STEADY-STATE RESPONSES TO SINE WAVE MODULATED LIGHT (SML)

Van der Tweel, Sem-Jacobsen, Kamp, Storm van Leeuwen, and Veringa (1958) introduced SML as a stimulus for evoking visual responses. The

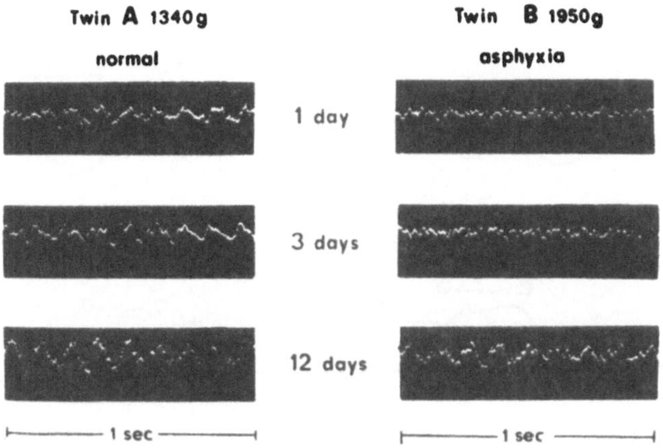

FIG. 3.8. Photic driving (8 c/sec) in preterm twins (32 weeks gestation), one normal, the other asphyxiated. Lead O_Z-P_Z. No response in Twin B at ages one and three days. (From Hrbek et al., 1977.)

amplitude of these responses is determined not only by the absolute luminance. The percentage change per cycle in stimulus luminance is often described in terms of modulation depth. Thus, the mean luminance and the percentage change can vary independently, and stimulus repetition frequency can be varied without changing the mean stimulus luminance. If the modulation depth is gradually increased, maintaining the mean luminance constant, the amplitude of the response increases until it reaches a maximum level (saturation) and may even grow smaller with higher modulation depths ("reducing," Spilker & Callaway, 1969). Saturation characteristics change depending on the intensity, the field size, the stimulus (Regan, 1968, 1977a) and the vigilance level (Spilker & Callaway, 1969). According to Regan (1968), when the stimulus repetition frequency is high, the system reaches a steady state in which it is no longer appropriate to describe the response in terms of time—that is, in terms of the latency of the components. It is better to analyze the ER in the frequency domain. A review may be found in Regan (1972). Donker (1975) studied the topography of VERs to SML. He found, as did Van der Tweel and Verduyn-Lunel (1965), that the waveform of the response was rather complex in relation to the stimulus and differed depending on stimulation frequency and localization (Fig. 3.9). The amplitude of the harmonics were largest over the occipital and smallest over the parietal scalp areas. Donker also observed considerable intraindividual variability of the amplitude of the first and second harmonics in all areas. Spekreijse and Van der Tweel (1966) have shown that the addition of noise to sine wave modulation cancels second harmonics, leaving the fundamental unchanged. In subjects trained to control

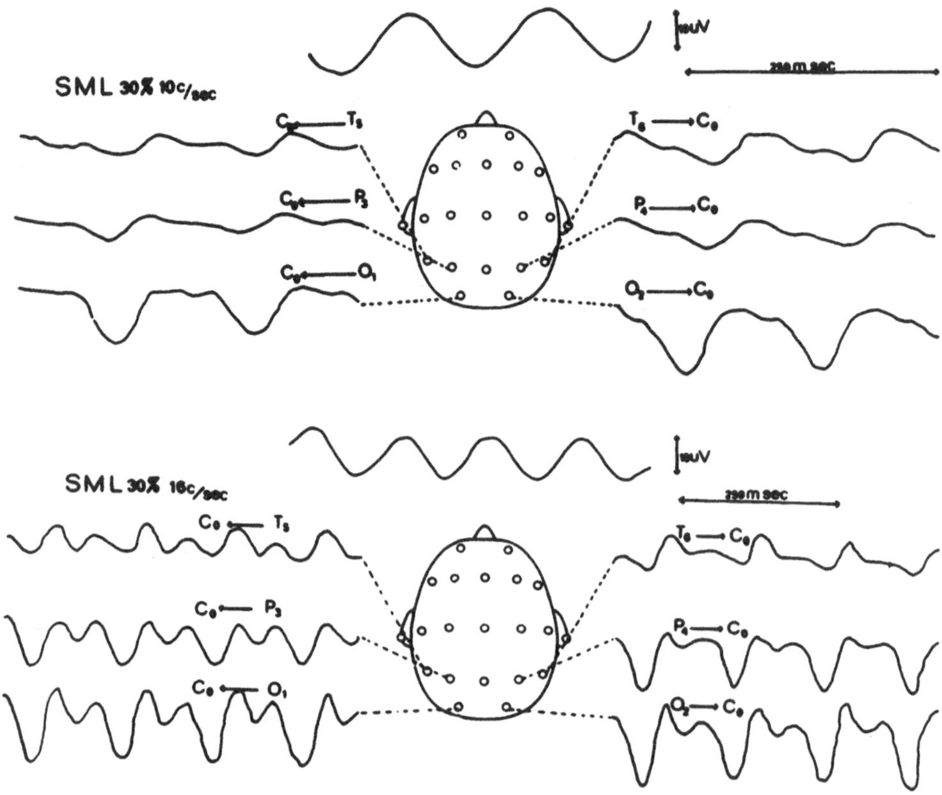

FIG. 3.9. Example of topographical distribution of average responses to SML recorded from symmetrical right and left areas. *Stimulation frequencies*: 10 and 16 Hz. *Modulation depth*: 30%. Note waveform distortion varying with stimulation frequency and localization. Analysis time 250 msec, N = 100. (From Donker, 1975.)

the alpha rhythm, Spilker et al. (1969) reported a positive relationship between the presence of alpha and the amplitude of VERs to SML, which suggests that alpha generators are influenced by SML (Townsend, Lubin, & Naitoh, 1975). However, Donker (1975) found an enhancement of interhemispheric synchronization by SML at 10 and 16 Hz, concluding that this phenomenon was not related to alpha activity.

Right-handed subjects have more symmetrical responses, the first harmonic being of higher amplitude then the second one. Left-handed subjects have greater responses over the left hemisphere, and the second harmonics are higher in low modulation depths (Pfefferbaum, 1971). The effects of adaptation of red and green color backgrounds with SML differ considerably. This yields a quantitative basis for the evaluation of VER data with respect to color vision (Van Hoek & Thijssen, 1977).

Clinical Applications

Although it has not been widely used, SML seems to be a useful procedure in the detection of brain lesions. In unilateral irritative lesions, a decrement of the response is not observed when increasing the modulation depth after the saturation level (Kamphuisen, 1969), and lower interhemispheric amplitude correlation of response to SML is observed (Donker, Njio, Storm van Leeuwen, & Wieneke, 1978). In unilateral brain lesions, Mol (1969) described great phase differences between homologous areas, as well as an abnormal delay between responses recorded in frontal and occipital regions.

V. TRANSIENT VERS TO SPATIALLY STRUCTURED STIMULUS FIELDS

A. General Characteristics

This subject has been extensively reviewed by Regan (1972). It is a general observation that transient VERs to spatially structured stimuli are much larger than those evoked by spatially unstructured stimuli, even if the light energy involved is 10,000 times lower. This suggests that these two types of VERs reflect the activities of different neuronal mechanisms. In order to change the spatial structure of the stimulus, it is possible to use a brief presentation of the pattern, to produce a slow alternation between pattern–appearance and pattern–disappearance, or to produce a pattern reversal at a constant mean luminance.

These different types of ERs have the common feature that they are greatly reduced when the retinal image is defocused. Presentation of flashed patterns produces an evoked response to changes in luminance and to pattern presentation, effects that can summate in a nonlinear manner. It is preferable, in order to record ERs to specific spatial structures, to change the spatial structure of the stimulus at constant stimulus intensity.

When VERs to a blank stimulus field are compared with VERs to a high contrast pattern field, a clear change in polarity or size of a prominent wave can be observed, with a latency of 100–150 msec in occipital regions (Harter & White, 1968; Rietveld, Tordoir, Hagenoow, Lubbers, & Spoor, 1967; Spehlman, 1965). This effect does not hold in all experimental conditions. If the checkerboard pattern is used, it depends on the check size. Allison et al. (1977) found similar topographic distribution of VERs to flashes of a localized light stimulation in the retina and to a checkerboard of larger dimensions than the one used by Rietveld et al. This might be explained by contamination of contrast-specific components of VERs to patterned stimuli by other types of VERs when the check size is increased beyond 20′(arc minute) or so (Harter & White, 1968, 1970; Padmos, Haaijman Joost, & Spekreijse, 1973).

Pattern-reversal VERs are more closely related to the ERs to pattern disappearance than to ERs to pattern appearance (Estévez & Spekreijse, 1974). The spatial distributions of potentials evoked by left- or right-half field pattern reversal or half-field pattern appearance stimuli are different (Shagass, Amadeo, & Roemer, 1976). For the first type of stimulation, four components have been described: P95, postivity contralateral and negativity ipsilateral to the field stimulated; P125, predominantly ipsilateral positivity; N165, predominantly ipsilateral negativity, and P225, predominantly positive in the midline. Pattern appearance produced an ER with three components: P125, mainly contralateral positivity; N175, mainly contralateral negativity, and P225, positive in the midline. Such difference suggest different cortical events in each type of stimulation. The waveform of the pattern-reversal VERs obtained by Shagass et al. (1976) was similar to that reported by previous authors (Eason, White, & Bartlett, 1970; Lesévre & Joseph, 1977; Lesévre & Rémond, 1972), but with longer latencies, which may be due to the luminance characteristics of the stimulus. Barret, Blumhardt, Halliday, Halliday, and Kriss (1976) also used half-field stimulation. They recorded the VERs to pattern-reversal stimuli with a transverse montage 5 cm above inion. P100 was recorded at the midline and ipsilaterally to the field stimulated, and not over the contralateral hemisphere in which, on anatomical and physiological grounds, the response is likely to originate. It was observed with a contralateral predominance only if the stimulation was confined to the macular area. A possible explanation for this unexpected result is that the cortical generators for this type of response are largely situated on the medial and posteromedial surface of the visual cortex where the neurons are transversely oriented. Thus, electrodes over the hemisphere ipsilateral to the field stimulated are optimally placed to record the response from these generator areas, whereas electrodes, over the contralateral hemisphere, are not, because they are relatively perpendicular to the axis of the generator area. The contralateral dominance of the VER to stimulus confined to the macular area may be explained because the cortical representation of the macula is at the posterior lobe and the generator neurones here could be oriented posteriorly rather than medially.

In a subsequent study, Blumhardt, Barret, Halliday, and Kriss (1978) reproduced experimentally the effect of scotomata on the ipsilateral and contralateral response to pattern reversal in one half field. They observed a linear relation of the decrement of ipsilateral P100 to the angle subtended by the central scotoma. With experimental central scotoma, a triphasic contralateral complex was demonstrated in all subjects. However, the progressive reduction of the half-field radius produces an attenuation of the contralateral response, whereas the ipsilateral P100 appeared to be relatively unaffected. They concluded that the ipsilateral P100 component was part of a response arising predominantly from that central area of the visual half field that subtended 0–8° or less, which corresponds to the visual cortex behind the calcarine sulcus. In hemispherectomized patients, Blumhardt, et al. demonstrated that although all components arise from the contralateral hemisphere to the half field stimulated, they are recorded from the opposite side of the scalp. No evidence thus supports the suggestion that callosal transfer is responsible for the ipsilateral components.

In relation to VERs produced by the appearance of a checkerboard pattern, Jeffreys (1971) reported that the responses invert their polarity when stimulation is changed from the upper to the lower half field. The longitudinal topographic distribution of the component at 80 msec was similar for stimulation of the upper and lower half fields, though with polarity reversal. The topographical distribution of the 110–120 msec peak was quite different. Jeffreys suggested that the 80 msec component was generated in the striate cortex lying within the calcarine fissure. The upper field distribution could be modeled as that due to a single dipole located in the extrastriate cortex on the under surface of the occipital lobe, and the lower field distribution as a single dipole located in the extrastriate cortex on the upper convexity of the occipital lobe. These results are similar to those obtained by Michael and Halliday (1971) with pattern reversals. Jeffreys and Axford (1972a,b) concluded that the first component is generated in the striate cortex, whereas the subsequent components are of extrastriate cortical origin.

B. Age Dependence

Spekreijse, deVries-Khoe, and van den Berg (1977) reported that 2-month-old infants have pattern-reversal VERs characterized by a single wave at 190 msec, which remains prominent until 6 months of age, but reduces its latency to 100 msec. At the age of 4 months, a negative peak at 200 msec appears. The effects of aging on VERs to pattern-reversal stimulation reveal no amplitude differences, but the first major negative and the first major positive deflections are significantly delayed with advancing age (Celesia & Daly, 1977a; Coben, 1977). These data are important for the adjustments of peak latencies according to age in clinical applications.

C. Clinical Applications

Although of relatively recent advent, VERs to structural field stimuli have found many clinical applications. They are more stable and with lower interindividual variability than VERs to diffuse light and are affected in many patients in which flash responses are normal. But, as VERs to flashes may be affected while the pattern response is normal, both types of stimuli should be used in order to detect abnormal VERs in the maximum percentage of patients.

The demonstration by Halliday, McDonald, and Mushin (1972) of a characteristic delay of the major positive component of the ER to a pattern-reversal checkerboard in retrobulbar neuritis—with this delayed response remaining beyond the normal range even during the recovery of visual acuity—opened a new field in the exploration of persisting damage of the optic nerve. In subsequent papers, Halliday et al. (1973a, 1973b, 1974a, 1974b) studied patients with MS. In all patients who had a history suggestive of optic neuritis and/or optic atrophy, the pattern-reversal VERs were delayed. Even more remarkable was the finding that in patients in whom a full opthalmological investigation did not detect any abnormality in the fields, fundi, pupils, or visual acuity, the VERs presented a significant delay. In a study of patients with progressive spastic paraplegia, it was possible to discriminate accurately those with spinal compression from MS patients by the study of pattern-reversal VERs (Halliday et al., 1974c). Similar findings in MS patients have been reported by Asselman, Chadwick, and Marsden (1975), Lowitzsch, Kuhnt, Sakmann, Maurer, Hopf, Schott, and Thäter (1976), Zeese (1976), Purves and Low (1976), Hoeppner and Lolas (1977), and many other authors. A typical recent example is shown in Fig. 3.10. The results previously mentioned have provided an extremely useful and simple procedure to detect optic nerve damage on the

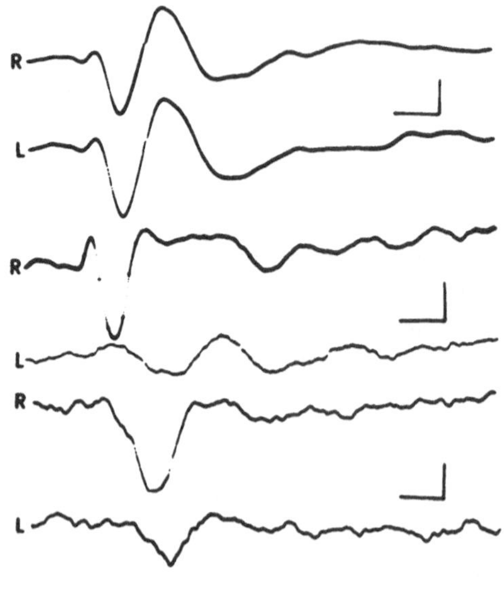

FIG. 3.10. VERs to pattern-reversal checkerboards from occipital cortex. Evoked responses to stimulation of right (R) and left (L) eyes. *Top*: bilaterally normal VERs. Positivity is downward. Calibration is 50 msec and 2.5 μV. *Center*: abnormal VER from left eye in an MS patient. Note increased duration as well as latency from left eye. *Bottom*: bilaterally abnormal VERs with both latencies prolonged in an MS patient. (From Shahrokhi et al., 1978.)

basis of the measurement of the peak latency of the major positive component. This is discussed in more detail in Chapter 13.

Delayed pattern VERs have also been observed in patients with subacute sclerosing panencephalitis (Horyd, Myga, & Kulczycki, 1977), with migraine (Rose, 1977), and in Parkinsonian cases (Bodis-Wollner & Yahr, 1977). A patient with cerebral blindness had normal pattern VERs when she saw the pattern and absent VERs when she claimed no vision (Bodis-Wollner, 1977). In monocularly deprived humans, an amplitude reduction of pattern and flash VERs has been observed in central regions when the affected eye was stimulated, but normal amplitude responses were found in occipital areas. In these patients, the VERs to a checkerboard have similar amplitude as VERs to flash (see Fig. 3.11, Glass, Crowder, Kennerdeel, & Merikangos, 1977).

Compressive lesions of the anterior visual pathways produced a wider variety of abnormalities than MS in pattern-reversal VERs (A.M. Halliday,

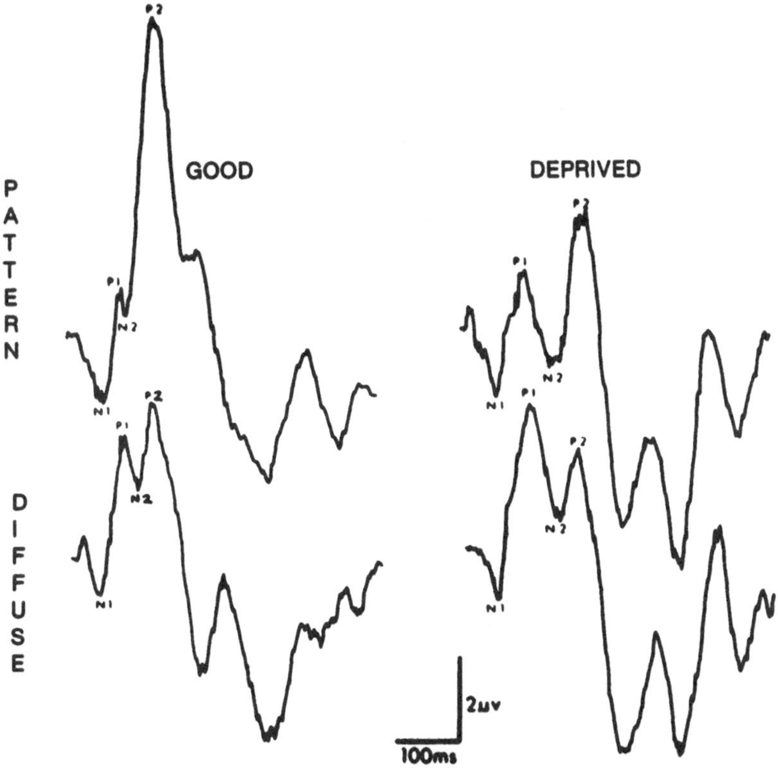

FIG. 3.11. Average of 50 VERs from occipital cortex in response to patterned and diffuse stimulation of good and deprived eyes. Flash occurs at beginning of trace with negativity down. (From Glass et al., 1977.)

Halliday, Kriss, McDonald, & Mushin, 1976). Asymmetries in the lateral distribution of the response, absence of response, or an amplitude reduction to the stimulation of the more affected side and delayed responses (but considerably faster than those observed in MS) were found in 18 out of 19 patients. According to Halliday, Barret, Blumhardt, Halliday, and Kriss (1977), in homonymous hemianopia, an "uncrossed" asymmetry of the VERs is observed: The evoked response to left- and right-eye stimulation is maximally recorded in the hemisphere contralateral to the "blind" visual field. In bitemporal hemianopia, a "crossed" asymmetry appeared: The maximal response is seen on the right side for the left eye and on the left side for the right-eye stimulation. This is in accord with their previously discussed results with half-field stimulation in normal subjects. Nevertheless, Holder (1978), using 26' checks in an 11° field, found the maximum abnormality in the VERs of the hemisphere contralateral to the field detect in all patients with chiasmal compression. This type of stimuli gives better macular stimulation than 50' checks in a 32° field used by A.M. Halliday et al. (1976), which may be one explanation for such contradictory results. As we mentioned previously, using half-field stimulation in normal subjects, Barret et al. (1976) found that if stimulation is confined to the macular area, then the VER will have a contralateral predominance. Another cause for such different results may be electrode placement. Holder used electrodes 2 cm anterior and lateral to the inion, whereas A.M. Halliday et al. recorded from electrodes 5 cm anterior and lateral to the inion.

Using a special procedure (the simultaneous stimulation method), Regan and Heron (1969) studied a patient with a hemianopic visual field defect due to occlusion of the left posterior artery. In this procedure, different retinal sites (left and right fields) are stimulated with repetitive stimulus whose repetition frequencies differ so slightly (e.g., 0.1 Hz) that they are almost simultaneous, although two separate VERs can be recorded by two parallel Fourier analyzers connected to a single electrode. Simultaneous recording had the effect that the relationship between these VERs is comparatively little affected by VER variability. Thus, the method decreases the variability and provides a "baseline", because the response to the stimulation of an abnormal part of the field can be compared with the responses evoked by the simultaneous stimulation of a "reference" area of the same eye.

Regan and Heron also studied the responses to sinusoidally modulated light (SML) to the left and right retinal half fields. The latter responses were markedly asymmetrical, although the pattern responses were very similar. VERs to patterned stimuli have contourned specific components reflecting activation of the macula, whereas VERs to SML are mainly produced by luminance changes that activate the periphery of the retina. Thus, the authors were able to conclude that it was a hemianopic field defect with macular sparing, which was later confirmed by subjective perimetry.

Another field of application of patterned VERs is the assessment of visual acuity in refraction problems. VERs to patterned stimuli are largest when the pattern is most sharply focused on the retina. Thus, the amplitude of VERs to pattern stimuli can be used to obtain an objective estimate of visual acuity. Rietveld et al. (1967) and Harter and White (1968) observed this effect for flashed pattern VERs and also demonstrated its use in refraction. According to Spekreijse, Van der Tweel, and Zuidema (1973), the negative component in the pattern-appearance VER is contour specific and therefore quite sensitive to refractive errors. Assessment of visual acuity can be done by use of different check sizes or by stepwise changes in corrective lenses. John (1977) developed a neurometric procedure based on the analysis of the statistically significant differences between VERs produced by blank and checkerboard patterns of different size (see Chapter 10, Student's Test). Assessment of refraction problems may be also done by comparing the VERs to pattern stimuli with different corrective lenses, because the maximal VER amplitude corresponds to the optimal correction (Harter & White, 1968; Novikova & Filchikova, 1977; Pastrnákova, Peregrin, & Sverak, 1975). Using pattern-reversal stimuli, Sokol (1978) estimated the development of visual acuity in infants by plotting the amplitude versus check size. He found that this plot was similar to the adult's by 6 months of age. Grall, Rigaudiere, Delthil, Legargassen, and Sourdille (1976) also described an objective procedure for assessment of visual acuity using similar concepts. According to Regan (1977a), checks whose side length is less than about 10′ to 20′ should be used in VER exploration of refraction. VER amplitude may increase when the pattern is blurred. This effect occurs in some subjects, when the check size is increased beyond 20′ or so (Regan & Richards, 1973). Regan explained this finding as follows: VERs to patterned stimuli are a mixture of a pattern-specific response and responses to local luminance changes. Each type of response has a different origin and may produce a cancellation effect in some subjects. If the check size is large, the contour-specific response will be of lower amplitude, and the response to luminance changes will predominate.

In astigmatic subjects, an asymmetry in the amplitude of VERs depending on pattern orientation is observed. Fiorentini and Maffei (1973) showed that this asymmetry persists in some subjects even after full lens correction, suggesting the existence of meridional amblyopia—that is, amblyopia restricted to a particular plane of orientation. Lombroso, Duffy, and Robb (1969) described a selective supression of VERs to patterned light in amblyopia exanopsia in a group of 22 children, who showed slight or no modification of their VERs to unstructured visual stimuli. In amblyopes, responses to small checks are more attenuated than responses to larger checks. If a plot of VER amplitude versus check size is made for the normal and for the amblyopic eye, the comparison between the shapes of these curves gives an index of the differences in acuity between both eyes (Regan, 1977a).

VI. THE STEADY-STATE PATTERN EVOKED RESPONSES

The steady-state responses to pattern reversal have dissimilar characteristics to those produced by flicker: they are restricted to low frequencies, because stimuli of frequencies greater than 30 reversals per second produce responses of very low amplitude, and they are not related to the frequency content of the EEG. The amplitude of the response to different stimulus frequencies is dependent on check size: Small checks give the largest ERs at about 5–8 Hz, whereas flicker at about 10 Hz gives the largest ERs. Large checks give sizeable VERs at both 5–8 Hz and at 10 Hz. This is consistent with the idea that VERs to large checks are a mixture of pattern and flicker responses (Regan, 1977a). The steady-state pattern responses are markedly delayed in retrobulbar neuritis patients and in some patients with the spinal form of MS (Regan, Milner, & Heron, 1976). Patients with homonymous hemianopia are characterized by a reduction of the responses in the affected hemisphere (Wildberger, Van Lith, Winjagaarde, & Mak, 1976). Recording from a blind child, with destruction of the occipital lobes except the primary projection areas, has shown preservation of VERs to diffuse light and of steady-state pattern evoked responses (Bodis-Wollner, Atkin, Raab, & Wolkstein, 1977).

VII. CONCLUSIONS

An enormous amount of work performed in the last years leads us to conclude that VERs are a valuable tool in the study of neurological patients. VERs to flashes presented a great interindividual variability that limits, but does not preclude, their use in clinical studies. The analysis of VER symmetry, which circumvent this limitation, is discussed later in this volume. VERs to flashes are affected either by lesions within or outside the visual pathway, and are extremely sensitive to a great variety of abnormal conditions. Thus, they can be used as a sensitive detector of the presence or absence of brain damage or dysfunction. VERs to different types of patterns, and in particular to pattern reversal, are highly stable and offer a unique technique for the exploration of lesions of the optic nerve, even in the absence of clinical symptomatology. Steady-state VERs are also useful for the evaluation of neurological patients. The combination of different types of stimuli makes possible the detection of a greater number of patients. This fact, as well as neurometric applications of VERs, is discussed in Chapter 13.

4 Auditory Evoked Responses (AERs)

I. INTRODUCTION

In 1938, Loomis, Harvey, and Hobart reported that a response to auditory stimulation could be observed in the raw EEG during sleep. It was composed of an initial negative component followed by a large positive wave; this response was called the "*k* complex." A year later, Davis, Davis, Loomis, Harvey, and Hobart (1939) described a diphasic negative-positive "on response" that started 50–100 msec after a tonal stimulation, followed by a much larger wave, maximal at the vertex, which was similar to the *k* complex. Since this discovery, the AERs have been intensively studied. At present, the classification of Picton, Hillyard, Krausz, and Galambos (1974) is used. These authors identified different waves in the transient AERs to click stimuli and divided them into early (0–8 msec), middle (8–50 msec), and long (50–500 msec) latency components. Recently, Picton, Woods, and Proulx (1978) reported that in response to a sustained tone burst, a negative shift can be recorded from the frontocentral scalp regions with an onset latency of approximately 150 msec. This auditory sustained potential is distinct, both in its scalp distribution and in temporal relation to the stimulus, from the transient response occurring at the onset or offset of the tone burst. It differs also from the Contingent Negative Variation (CNV) (see Chapter 6) in that it can occur in the absence of attention or during sleep.

In order to simplify the discussion of responses to auditory stimuli, early AER components and their clinical applications are discussed first, then the middle and late components, and finally the excitability cycle and the frequency following response. Clicks and tones are the stimuli most frequently used; we refer only to AERs produced by them. Semantic stimuli have also been used, but because the AERs produced by this type of stimulation have different configurations depending on the typology and characteristics of the initial consonant (S. Popov, 1977) and display different topographical distribution if nouns or verbs are used (Brown & Lehman, 1977), their study is more difficult. Thus, clinical applications using semantic stimuli have seldom been reported.

II. EARLY AER COMPONENTS OR BRAIN-STEM AUDITORY EVOKED RESPONSES (BAERs)

A. General Characteristics

Jewett, Roman, and Williston (1970), recording at the vertex and using the neck, the ear, or the chin as reference, described a consistent series of waves with peak latencies between 2 and 9 msec after click presentation. These very early auditory responses, now referred to as brain-stem auditory evoked responses (BAERs) or "fair-field" AERs, are volume conducted from regions of the brain stem. In order to observe BAERs properly, it is necessary to use high-gain $(10)^6$ low-noise amplifiers with a band pass up to 3 KHz. BAERs are computed using a high sampling rate (10–50 KHz) in response to about 2000 clicks presented at rates of 20–30 Hz and at intensities well above threshold (55–75 dB HL). The position of the electrodes most frequently used are vertex and the ear lobe or mastoid ipsilateral to the stimulated ear. The nomenclature most frequently used considers only the positive components and labels them from I to VII (see Fig. 4.1). Wave V (P6) is the component most easily identified across all subjects.

BAERs are very stable from run to run in each subject and they present a low interindividual variability both in adults and babies (Jewett & Williston, 1971; Salamy & McKean, 1976; see Fig. 4.2). Although some methodological differences exist between different laboratories, the results obtained are quite similar. Table 4.1 shows the normal peak latencies reported by several authors. Table 4.2 presents mean peak latencies, as well as the mean amplitude values and their standard deviation of the different waves to three stimulus intensities. Notice the systematic latency increase and amplitude decrease as stimulus intensity decreases. According to Rowe (1978), wave I is of low amplitude and difficult to differentiate from background noise without replications; waves II and IV are frequently absent from one or both sides; waves III and V are the most constant and reproducible peaks; waves VI and VII varied widely in waveform from one replication to another.

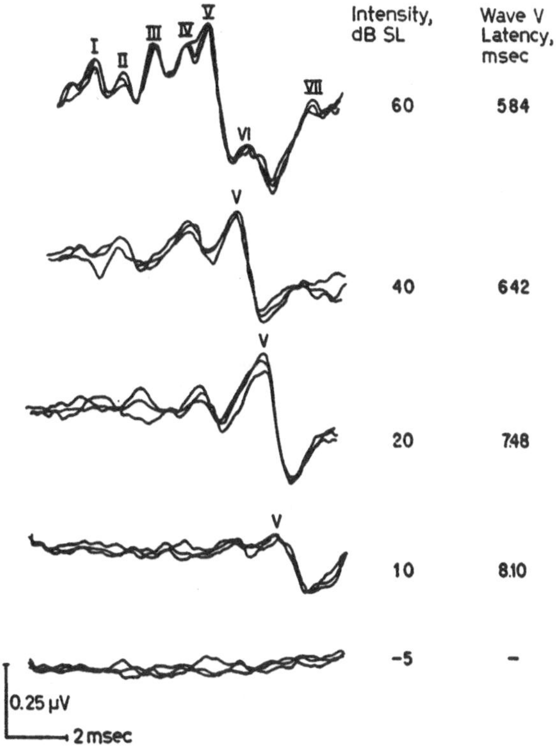

FIG. 4.1. The human BAERs to monaural clicks (30 per sec) at various intensities. Each trace sums 2000 responses; superimposed traces are replications obtained during the same recording session. Note that wave V latency increases and its amplitude decreases as signal strength weakens. (From Galambos & Hecox, 1977.)

Early work of Jewett et al. (1970) and Jewett and Williston (1971) in cats and in man clearly established that the generators of the BAERs have a neural and not a myogenic origin. The properties of wave I clearly resemble those of the neural deflections seen in the electrocochleogram recorded at the same time; wave I is smaller in such simultaneous recording, but its threshold, latency, and amplitude latency dependence on stimulus intensity are similar, indicating that the generator of wave I is the auditory nerve. The subsequent waves are considered to reflect the progressive activation of brain stem auditory structures by the acoustic message as it ascends en route to the cortex. Starr and Hamilton (1976) studied the BAERs in patients with lesions of the brain stem confirmed by autopsy and concluded that wave I reflects the activity of the VIII nerve; waves II and III reflect activity of the cochlear nuclei, trapezoid body, and superior olive, and waves IV and V reflect activity of lateral lemniscus and inferior colliculus. These conclusions agree with those reached by Buchwald and Huang (1975) and Jones, Schorn, Siu, Stockard, Rossiter, Bickford, and Sharbrough (1977) in cats, and by Stockard and Rossiter (1977) in man. The latter authors also proposed that waves VI and VII are related to thalamic activity.

In noncephalic reference recordings, waves II to VI are distributed widely over the scalp, but are most prominent at the vertex; they might also be recorded from ear, nose, and mastoid (Streletz, Katz, Hohenberger, &

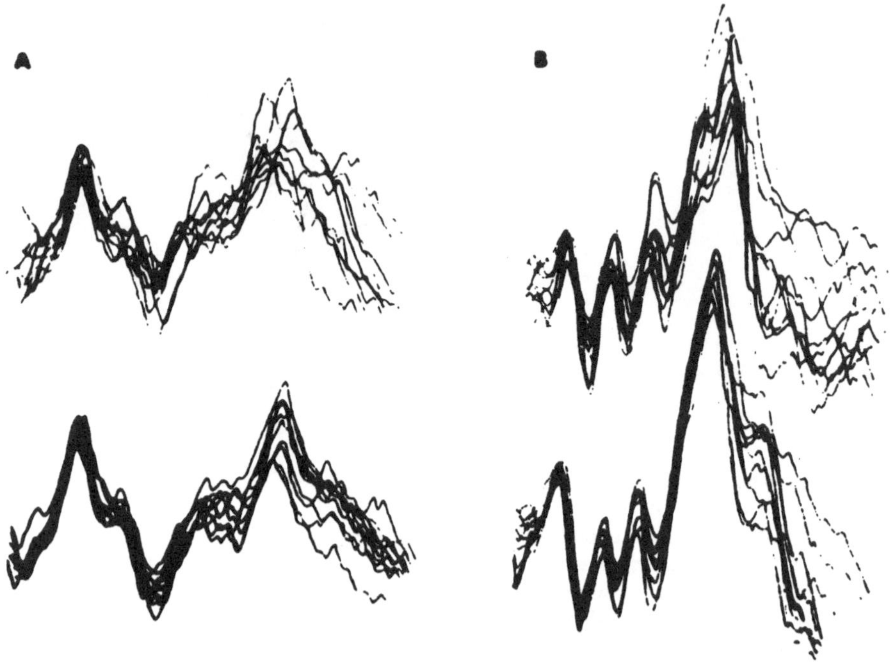

FIG. 4.2. Inter- and intrasubject variability for (A) newborns and (B) adults. Upper portion shows average BAERs for 10 different newborns (A) and adults (B). Lower portion shows 10 averages from the same newborn (A) and adult (B). (From Salamy & McKean, 1976.)

Cracco, 1977). When recording from mastoid to compare ipsilateral and contralateral BAERs (to the stimulated ear), similar properties appear. However, in contralateral recordings, the first mastoid-negative wave did not appear. Ipsilateral responses were generally greater than contralateral ones. These results agree with the notion of ipsilateral brain-stem generation of BAERs (Thornton, 1975).

BAERs are mainly produced by the activation of the basal part of the cochlea, because this portion tends to evoke better synchronized discharges than the apical part (H. Davis, 1976). According to Hecox, Squires, and Galambos (1974), the apical low-frequency fibers contribute very little to the BAER. However, Kodera, Yamane, Yamada, and Suzuki (1977), by the study of BAER thresholds to clicks and tones of different frequencies and intensities in normal and hearing impaired subjects, have shown that:

1. The thresholds of BAERs evoked by tone pips are relatively high compared to those obtained by clicks. When tone pips are used as stimuli, several cycles of the tone pips seem to contribute to provoking the BAER, which results in less synchronized discharges

TABLE 4.1
Mean Peak Latencies of Early AER Components in Normal Hearing Subjects[a]

Reference	*Stimulus Conditions*	*I*	*II*	*III*	*IV*	*V*	*VI*	*VII*
Jewett and Williston (1971)[b]	75 db/10 Hz	1.7	2.8	3.6	4.9	5.4	6.9	8.3
Picton et al. (1974)	60 db/10 Hz	1.5	2.6	3.8	5.0	5.8	7.4	8.5
W. R. Goff et al. (1977)	70 dB/8 Hz	2.5	3.6	4.5	5.7	6.4	7.9	9.9
Starr (1976)	75 dB/10 Hz	1.4	2.6	3.7	4.6	5.4	6.9	8.7
Robinson and Rudge (1977a)	75 dB/20 Hz	2.01	3.25	4.12	—	6.0	—	—
Streletz et al. (1977)	70 dB/10 Hz	1.5	2.5	3.7	4.8	5.9	7.4	—
Salamy and McKean (1976)								
(adults)	55 dB/15 Hz	1.57	2.73	3.64	4.82	5.55	6.89	—
(newborns)		2.12	3.27	4.89	5.96	7.06	—	—
(1-year-olds)		1.71	2.82	3.92	5.09	5.93	—	—
Rowe (1978)	60 dB/10 Hz	1.87	2.88	3.83	5.06	5.82	7.37	9.05
Sohmer and Student (1978) (4–10 years old)	75 dB/10 Hz	1.34	2.42	3.38	5.16	6.68	—	—

[a] Values are given in milliseconds.
[b] Estimated by W. R. Goff et al (1977a) from Jewett's figures.

than when clicks are used. This explains the smaller amplitude and higher thresholds to tone pips.

2. Wave V latency increased as the frequency of the tone pip decreased. At the stimulus intensity of 50 dB SL, the difference between wave V latency at 500 Hz and at 1000 Hz is small (0.4 msec). Near the BAER threshold (20 dB SL), the difference was 1.9 msec. These workers concluded that these results suggest that at higher intensities the BAERs evoked by 500 Hz may originate from a part of the cochlea more basal than the portion sensitive to 500 Hz. With a decrease in stimulus intensity, the more apical part of the cochlea is more selectively stimulated and presumably plays the major part in evoking the BAER, thus causing an increase in latency because of the longer travel time along the cochlear partitions.
3. Using auditory stimuli with fairly narrow frequency spectra at low frequencies, it was possible to elicit the BAER at a stimulus intensity near the subjective threshold. These responses were interpreted as "frequency-specific" BAERs.
4. In cases with sensorineural hearing loss, a high correlation was observed between subjective audiometry threshold and AER thresholds. The latter were higher by as much as 25 dB. The means

TABLE 4.2
Auditory Brain-Stem Responses (Six Normal Subjects)[a]

Latency (ms)	*75 dB*		*55 dB*		*35 dB*	
Wave I	Mean 1.4	SD[b] ±.2	Mean 1.8	SD ±.2	Mean 2.7	SD[c]
II	2.6	±.2	3.0	±.3	3.6	±.4
III	3.7	±.2	3.9	±.2	4.7	±.2
IV	4.6	±.2	5.0	±.3	5.8	±.3
IV–V	5.2	±.2	5.6	±.2	6.4	±.2
V	5.4	±.2	5.8	±.2	6.6	±.2
VI	6.9	±.3	7.5	±.2	8.4	±.2
VII	8.7	±.2	9.0	±.3	—[d]	—
Amplitude (μV)						
Wave I	.20	±.09	.09	±.04	.08	[c]
II	.16	±.06	.07	±.04	.06	±.02
III	.18	±.05	.12	±.03	.10	±.02
IV	.10	±.01	.09	±.03	.03	±.00
IV–V	.34	±.08	.25	±.09	.18	±.04
V	.25	±.04	.18	±.09	.17	±.04
VI	.12	±.07	.10	±.06	.04	±.02
VII	.09	±.03	.05	±.01	—	—

[d]: No response detected.
[c]: Responses in only one or two subjects, making the SD measure unreliable.
[b]SD: Standard Deviation.
[a] From Starr, 1976.

of the differences with 500, 1000, and 2000 Hz tone pips were approximately the same (11 dB).

B. Stimulus Dependence

BAERs are directly related to the strength of the stimulus; decreasing the intensity increases the response latency and decreases the amplitude of all the components, as is shown in Fig. 4.1 and Table 4.2 (Don, Allen, & Starr, 1977; Hecox & Galambos, 1974; Picton et al., 1974). This is extremely important for the audiometric application of BAERs. These responses have been obtained by clicks, noise bursts, and tone pips presented at regular rates up to 70 Hz. Interpeak conduction times, except possibly those involving wave II, are unaffected by a change in stimulus intensity (Rowe, 1978). Wave V latency is affected by rise time and duration of the acoustic stimulus (Hecox, Squires, & Galambos, 1976), spectrum (Kodera et al., 1977), and interstimuli interval. Increasing the click rate from 10 to 100 Hz causes a significant increase in the latency of wave V (Don et al., 1977).

However, it should be noted that Robinson and Rudge (1977b) found no significant differences in the latency and amplitude of wave V with frequencies up to 20 Hz.

C. Age Dependence

With respect to developmental changes in BAERs, Hecox and Galambos (1974) reported a progressive decline in the latency of wave V from 3 weeks to around 2 years of age. Salamy, McKean, and Buda (1975) observed a shortening of peak latency of waves I to V from birth to adulthood, and Salamy and McKean (1976), studying newborns and infants 6 weeks, 3 months, 6 months, and 1 year old, as well as normal adults, found that the adult configuration replaces the infantile response by 3–6 months. Preliminary results of these authors revealed that BAER are quite resistant to habituation following continuous stimulus presentation at any early age. Although the comparison between latencies obtained by laboratories using different stimulus intensities and/or frequencies is difficult, we can see in Table 4.1 that children from 4–10 years old have shorter latencies than adults in waves I, II, and III (Sohmer & Student, 1978). However, the peak latencies of wave IV and principally of wave V are larger in children than in adults. This result should be clarified; old subjects have longer peak latencies than young adults (Rowe, 1978).

D. Clinical Applications

1. Evoked Response Audiometry (ERA)

This term refers to the estimation of the threshold for auditory sensation by ascertaining the sound intensity required to elicit an AER. It is primarily used in those subjects who are unwilling or unable to respond to conventional audiometric tests, but are suspected of having auditory dysfunction. ERA is particularly useful in those children with suspected hearing loss who need a test requiring no cooperation—namely, very young children and those handicapped by behavioral disorders, brain damage, and mental retardation. As we see later, ERA was initially based on long latency (cortical) auditory evoked responses, but the introduction of the BAERs offers a unique opportunity to distinguish not only the sensory threshold, but the site of the lesion. That BAERs are extremely resistent to drug effects (Mendel & Hosick, 1975; Stockard, Rossiter, Jones, & Sharbrough, 1977) and that the latency of the response remains stable during different sleep stages (Mendel, 1974; Sohmer & Student, 1978) make them very suitable for

ERA, because during sedation or sleep, the threshold of the cortical AERs is elevated and their identification is less reliable than during the waking state. Brain-stem responses also offer some advantages if compared with the electrocochleogram, because it is not necessary to have an anesthetist and an otologist to place a transtympanic electrode on the promontory, and wave V is precisely related in time to the first neural wave of the electrocochleogram, with a latency difference of almost exactly 4.0 msec (Davis & Hirsh, 1977).

Hecox and Galambos (1974) described the normal relationship between signal intensity and BAER characteristics. They found that latency measures show much less intersubject and intersession variability than amplitude measures, and elected to measure wave V latency because, throughout all age groups, wave V stands out as a large, stable, and easy wave to identify. Fig. 4.3 shows the relationship between the latency of wave V and the sensation level in young adults. Galambos and Hecox (1977) found that, in patients with conductive hearing loss, wave V latency–intensity function was parallel to but displaced from the norm; the amount of this displacement of the curve to the right measures the amount of conductive hearing loss. In sensorineural hearing losses following diseases of the cochlear structures, they found so-called "recruitment," or abnormally rapid growth of loudness as the signal intensity progressively rose above threshold. Fig. 4.3 shows that at low intensity, a large discrepancy exists between the damaged ear and the normal wave V latency functions, but the curve converges upon the normal at higher signal strength. Similar findings have been obtained by Kodera et al. (1977) and Coats and Martin (1977). Sohmer, Feinmesser, Bauberger-Tell, and Edelstein (1977a) described the utility of brain-stem responses as well as cochlear and cortical evoked responses in the evaluation of nonorganic hearing loss, whereas subjective tone audiometry was not able to rule out an organic lesion. Absence of BAERs in several autistic children, indicating a profound hearing loss, has been described by Sohmer and Student (1978).

2. Lesions of the Central Nervous System

BAERs are extremely useful in the diagnosis of retrocochlear or brainstem lesions. Stockard and Rossiter (1977) recorded the BAERs in over 100 neurological patients and correlated the abnormalities of each component with postmortem or radiological localization of different brain-stem lesions. Cochlear or acoustic nerve lesions produced abnormalities of wave I. Ponto–medullary lesions produced abnormalities of wave II and all subsequent waves evoked by ipsilateral click stimulation. Hermorrhages in the caudal pontine tegmentum produced abnormally prolonged wave III and

Patient	Frequency, Hz					
	250	500	1,000	2,000	4,000	8,000
C. L.	35	40	30	35	30	40
	5	15	0	10	0	10
T. R.	25	35	40	35	45	40
	10	0	7	15	5	5
L. F.	15	30	20	25	65	65
	5	15	10	15	10	10

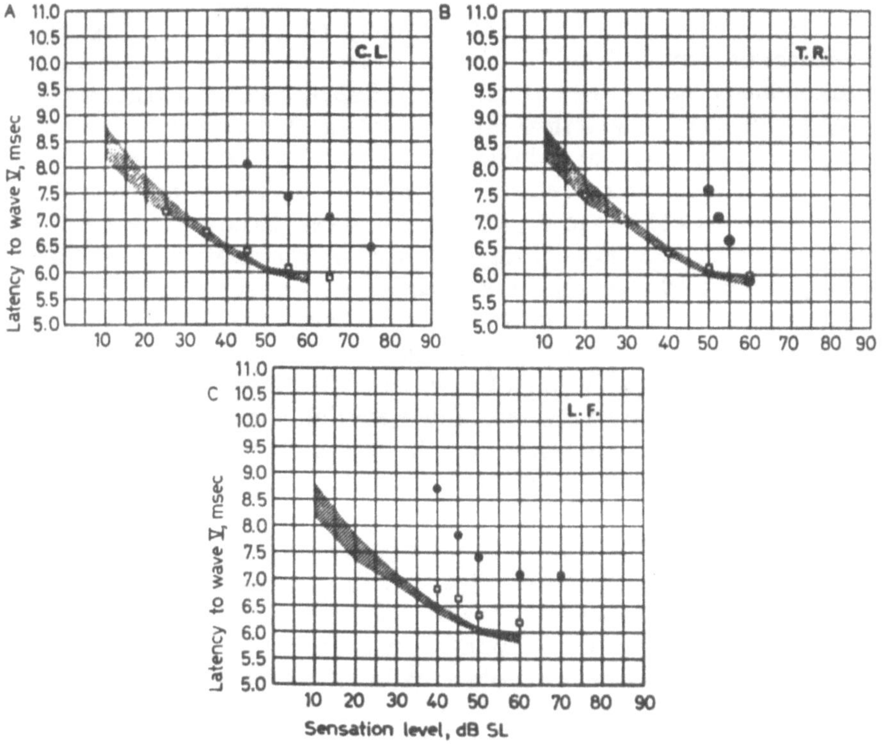

FIG. 4.3. BAER wave latency-intensity functions for three patients with predominantly unilateral hearing loss. *Hatched areas*: the normal wave V latency-intensity function. *Open circles*: wave V latencies from the "normal" ear of each patient. C.L. is a girl with monaural (solid dots) conductive loss; T.R. is an adult with flat sensorineural loss due to Menière's disease; L.F. is an adult with sensorineural loss from Menière's disease, severe above 2000 Hz. See table (top) for audiograms of each patient. (From Galambos & Hecox, 1977.)

subsequent waves. Patients with rostral pons or midbrain lesions had normal waves I, II, II, but there was a progressive delay of all waves after II. Lesions of the medial geniculate bodies caused abnormalities of the wave VI, and larger lesions of the thalamus and auditory radiation of the wave VII. They conclude that BAERs are useful in localizing and detecting certain lesions not revealed by other tests. Figs. 4.4 and 4.5 show how the abolition of one or more waves is an index of the level of the lesion. Latency delays are also very useful for the definition of lesions: In acoustic neuromas, it is possible to observe the absence of all components or a great delay in waves I and V (Daly, Roeser, Aung, & Daly, 1977; Hashimoto, Ishiyama, & Tozuka, 1977), even with normal tonal audiometry (Chiappa & Norwood, 1977). Eggermont (1977) reported that larger neuromas produced greater alterations in the responses, but that the procedure was quite sensitive, because even in tumors 0.7 mm in diameter, alterations of the brainstem responses were observed. Because interpeak conduction times are independent of stimulus intensity, these measures may be applied to patients with conductive hearing loss, simplifying the application of BAER testing in clinical neurology. The normal ranges of interpeak conduction times were computed by Rowe (1978) and they are shown in Table 4.3. Whereas waves I, III, and V are the most reliable and reproducible peaks, the conduction times from wave I to V, I to III, and III to V appear to be the most clinically useful values. A delay in I-III time would seem to indicate an abnormality in the pontine-medullary region, whereas a delay in the wave III–V portion would suggest dysfunction in the midbrain-pontine region. Delay in the wave I–V time without specific prolongation of either of its components should be considered abnormal, but without specific localizing value as to the level of the brain stem involved. Interpeak times longer than 2 SD of the normal mean have been observed in brain stem infarctions (Lynn, Gilroy, & Maulsby, 1977). Starr (1977) was able to confirm midbrain dysfunction in three patients in whom the I–V times were prolonged more than 4.4 msec. Interpeak times have been also a valuable parameter for the following up of neurological patients (Stockard, Rossiter, & Wiederholt, 1976). Fig. 4.6 shows the relation between wave I–V time and the clinical improvement in a patient believed to have central pontine myelinolisis.

Increased latencies have been observed in MS patients (Chiappa & Norwood, 1977; Robinson & Rudge 1977a, 1977b), in a case of "locked in" syndrome (Gilroy, Lynn, Ristow, & Pellerin, 1977), and in postconcussion vertigo (Rowe, 1977). According to Starr (1977), the relative amplitudes are rather consistent in normal subjects and may provide useful measures for clinical purposes. For example, the ratio of the IV–V complex to Wave I is always greater than 1.0 for signal intensities less than 60 dB SL. BAER give significant information in evaluating comatose patients. When coma is due to metabolic causes, it is very common to observe normal BAERs (Starr &

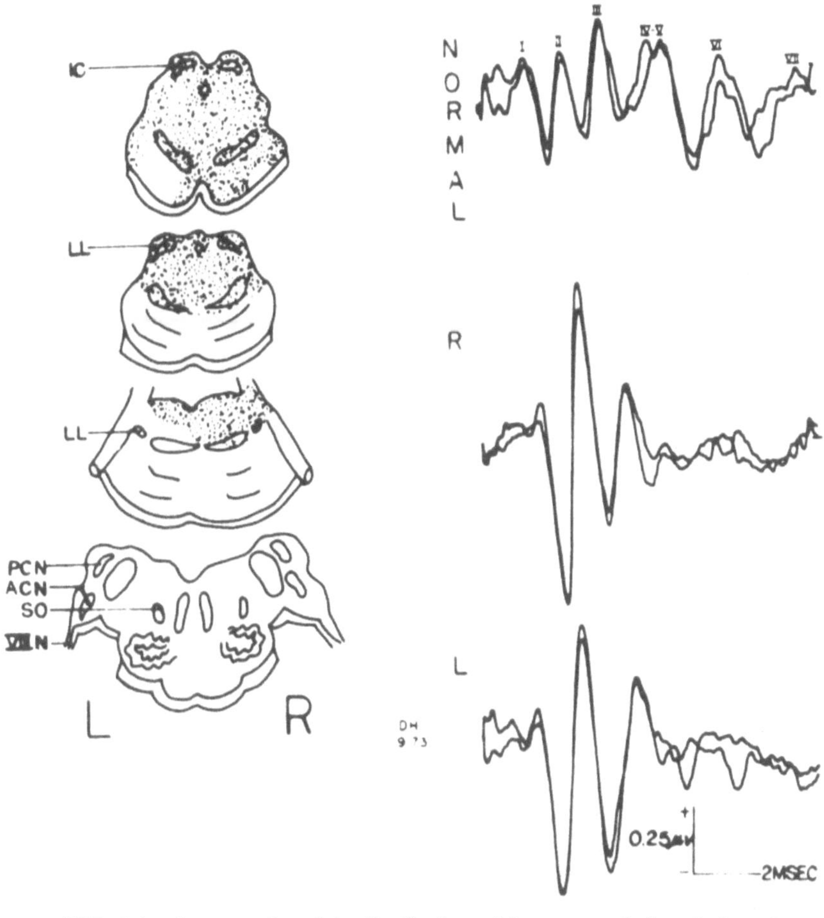

FIG. 4.4. A composite of the distribution of the neuropathology indicated by stipples (*left*) and auditory brain-stem responses from a patient with a germinoma. A normal response pattern is included for comparison. R and L refer to the side of monoaural click presentation, right (R) or left (L). This same format is used in the subsequent Fig. IC, inferior colliculus; LL, lateral lemniscus; PCN, posterior cochlear nucleus; ACN, anterior cochlear nucleus; SO, superior olivary nucleus; VIII N, VIII, cranial nerve. In this patient, waves I, II, and III seem to be intact, but the subsequent components were absent except for a small IV–V wave at prolonged latency to monaural right stimulation. Waves II and III are prolonged in latency compared to normal values, whereas wave I was of normal latency. (From Starr & Hamilton, 1976.)

Achor, 1975). Brinkman and Ebner (1977) reported a latency increase of wave V in 6 out of 20 cases of coma due to suicidal drug intoxication. In the follow-up of these patients, four recovered and wave V latency returned to normal values, whereas in the other two, the BAERs disappeared and the

NEUROLOGICAL LESIONS AND BRAINSTEM RESPONSES

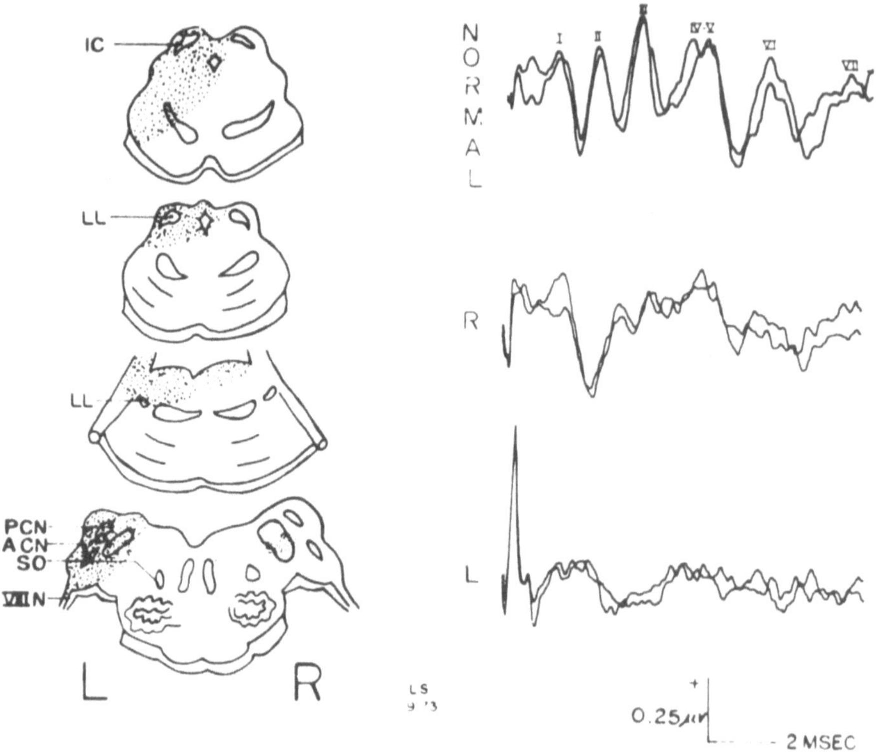

FIG. 4.5. A composite of the distribution of the neuropathology indicated by stipples (*left*) and auditory brain-stem responses from a patient with a tuberous sclerosis with gemistocytic astrocytoma involving the left midbrain and brain stem. Responses to left (L) monaural clicks at 65 db HL showed only a wave I without any other components. Responses to the clicks in the right (R) ear showed all components to be present, but the amplitude of the IV–V complex was approximately one-half of the amplitude of wave I. In normal individuals, the ratio of the amplitudes of the IV–V complex to wave I at 65 db HL is usually greater than 1.0 (mean ratio: 1.60). (From Starr & Hamilton, 1976.)

patients died. In 27 patients fulfilling the criteria of brain death, the BAERs were either absent or consisted only of wave I that, when present, was of normal amplitude but prolonged in latency. Four patients that were followed up for several days from a state of coma with evidence of preserved brain-stem and cerebral functions to a clinical state compatible with brain death had initially intact BAERs and then showed a decrease in amplitude and a prolongation of latency of waves II–V until, finally, wave I was alone (Starr, 1976). Delayed latencies of BAERs and longer brain-stem transmis-

TABLE 4.3[a]
Interpeak Conduction Time Normal Range for Young Subjects[b]

60 dB/10/sec	I-III′	III-V	I-V″	I-II″	II-III	II-V″	V-VI	V-VII
95%	2.23	2.30	4.30	1.38	1.58	3.31	2.22	3.98
99%	2.34	2.44	4.46	1.55	1.81	3.49	2.51	4.29
60 dB/30/sec								
95%	2.43	2.36	4.46	1.52	1.54	3.58	2.32	3.97
99%	2.58	2.51	4.64	1.70	1.76	3.87	2.60	4.29

[b]For old subjects, add 0.3 msec (′) or 0.2 msec (″). The times are in msecs and represent the upper limits of one-tailed confidence intervals. Times above these limits are longer than 95 and 99% of the normal population respectively. Interaural differences should be within 0.5 msec.
[a] From Rowe, 1978.

sion time (I–V time) have been reported in minimal brain dysfunction and mentally retarded children, which suggests the existence of an organic or functional brain lesion in these children, at least in the brain-stem regions concerned with auditory function (Sohmer & Student, 1978).

III. MIDDLE AND LONG LATENCY COMPONENTS OF THE AER

A. General Characteristics

Streletz et al. (1977), using a balanced noncephalic (sterno-vertebral) reference and recording in the sagittal and coronal planes, described the following middle components of the AER: a negative-positive potential with peak latencies of 8–12 msec (N9) and 10–14 msec (P11). This potential was followed by a larger negative-positive potential with peak latencies of 16–22 msec (N17) and 26–36 msec (P33). These potentials were greatest in amplitude at fronto-central locations, and were followed by a small negative potential with a peak latency of 32–42 msec (N37). With the onset of light sleep, these potentials were attenuated and the last negative wave was sometimes not observed. N17 and P33 were characterized by progressive increase in peak latency from front to back in the sagittal plane, and were more evident during sleep. That they are observed in relaxed subjects, as well as during sleep, made these authors suggest that their origin is cerebral rather than muscular. N9 and P11 have characteristics similar to

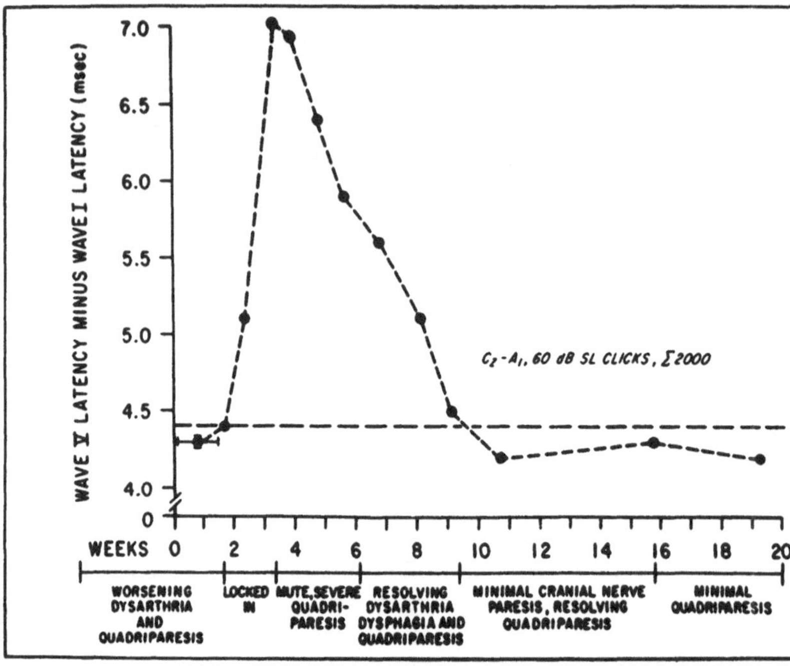

FIG. 4.6. Clinical correlates of wave V latency minus wave I latency changes in a patient believed to have central positive myelinolisis and followed up during 20 weeks. Values from eight separate recording sessions in the first 10 days of testing (*horizontal bracket*) are pooled in the first value, which has the standard deviation indicated by vertical brackets. Horizontal dashed line indicates upper limit of normal wave V minus wave I latency. C_zA_1 indicates vertex to left mastoid bipolar recording. (From Stockard et al., 1976.)

the early latency components and may also represent far-field potentials arising in subcortical structures.

Ever since Bickford, Jacobson, and Cody (1964) showed that myogenic responses could be evoked in the 8–50 msec time domain, and that these responses were heightened by the presence of cervical muscular tension and could be abolished by curare, there has been a controversy about the origin of middle auditory components. Goff, Allison, Lyons, Fisher, and Conte (1977) believe that N15 is a myogenic potential, probably originating from the postauricular musculature. This suggestion was also supported by Vaughan and Ritter (1970) and Picton et al. (1974).

W. R. Goff et al. (1977) proposed that P25, N40, and P50 may be mixtures of neurogenic and myogenic activity. P25 and P50 must be at least partially neurogenic, because these authors showed that they could be recorded from the cortical surface or depth. Neither P25 or P50 may be the primary cortical positivity, because they are suppresed by barbiturate anesthesia. These conclusions are supported by the fact that Horwitz, Larson, and Sances (1966) and Harker, Hosick, Voots, and Mendel (1977) have also recorded middle auditory components during succinylcholine paralysis in human subjects. The latter authors suggested that perhaps Bickford et al. (1964) failed to record a nonmyogenic response after curare because only 150 click stimuli were presented and summated. Summation of the response from many more stimuli is usually necessary before the smaller amplitude nonmyogenic responses become separable from the ongoing myogenic activity. Thus, paradoxically, it has been possible to record the responses generated in the brain stem from the scalp, but it has not been possible to identify unequivocally the primary cortical response generated in Heschl's gyrus.

In relation to the long latency components of the AERs, Streletz et al. (1977) described a positive potential, peaking at 45–65 msec (P51), followed by a negative–positive potential, which peaks at 70–100 msec (N83) and 140–180 msec (P149), and a negative potential with peak latency at 240–300 msec (N254). These potentials were maximal at or slightly anterior to the vertex and were recorded with lesser amplitude from the nose and mastoid, but not from the ear lobe. Because these authors found, using the noncephalic reference, that no component changed in polarity either in the sagittal or coronal planes (Fig. 4.7), they suggested that these potentials arise in widespread areas of central cortex, rather than in primary auditory cortical areas, and that they may be mediated by a nonspecific afferent projection system. These conclusions agree with those of Kooi, Tipton, and Marshall (1971) and Picton et al. (1974).

In contrast, Vaughan and Ritter (1970) proposed a dipole source, reversing polarity at the level of the Sylvian fissure, to account for the topographical distribution of the AERs on the scalp. This was also supported by their findings in the monkey (Vaughan, Arezzo, & Pickoff, 1974). Peronnet, Michel, Echallier, and Girod (1974) used a coronal montage referred to the nose, and demonstrated that: (1) there was a statistically significant interhemispheric difference in AERs to tones, with dominance of the right side; (2) there was a clear polarity reversal of the responses at the level of the Sylvian fissure in normal subjects (Fig. 4.8); and (3) the polarity reversal of the response only appears on the healthy cortex in patients with lesions involving the auditory area (Fig. 4.9). Later, Michel and Peronnet (1974) and Peronnet and Michel (1977) showed that there was a consistent predominance of the contralateral response to the stimulation of each ear, which was also in agreement with an origin of these components in the region of the auditory cortex.

These contradictory results are very difficult to understand. Middle and long latency components can be recorded from nose and mastoid when using a noncephalic reference; thus, coronal–nose recordings are actually

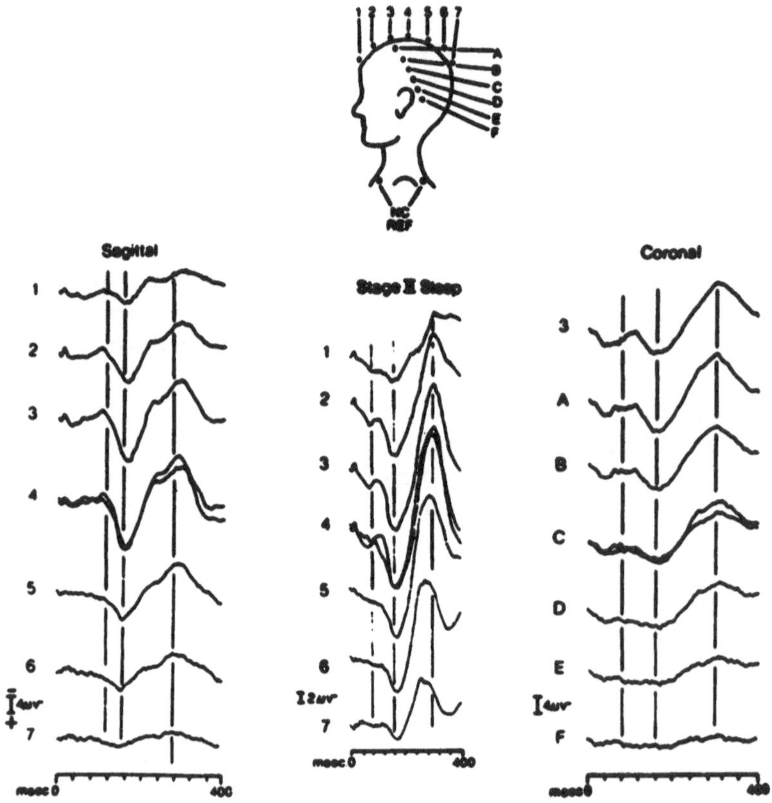

FIG. 4.7. Distribution of long-latency AERs in noncephalic reference recordings. The negative-positive potential with peak latencies of 100 and 160 msec is maximal around the vertex (leads 3 and 4) in sagittal and coronal arrays. During light sleep, the negative potential peaking at 300 msec increases in amplitude and shows progressive decreases in peak latency from anterior to posterior recording locations. (From Streletz et al., 1977.)

bipolar. If the response in temporal regions is smaller than the response at the nose, although the vertex response is larger, temporal-nose responses may appear of inverse polarity to the response recorded in the vertex-nose derivation. However, the failure to observe polarity reversal over damaged auditory cortex cannot be reconciled with this explanation, and constitutes strong argument that there is a true polarity reversal in the temporal region. Kooi et al. (1971), using a balanced noncephalic reference, noted that responses recorded from T_3 and T_4 differed from the classic vertex response in that they contained another negative intermediate wave. Based on this finding, Wolpaw and Penry (1975) studied the so-called "temporal" component of the AERs, which is formed by a positive peak (P110) and a negative peak (N150). According to these authors, neither the interpreta-

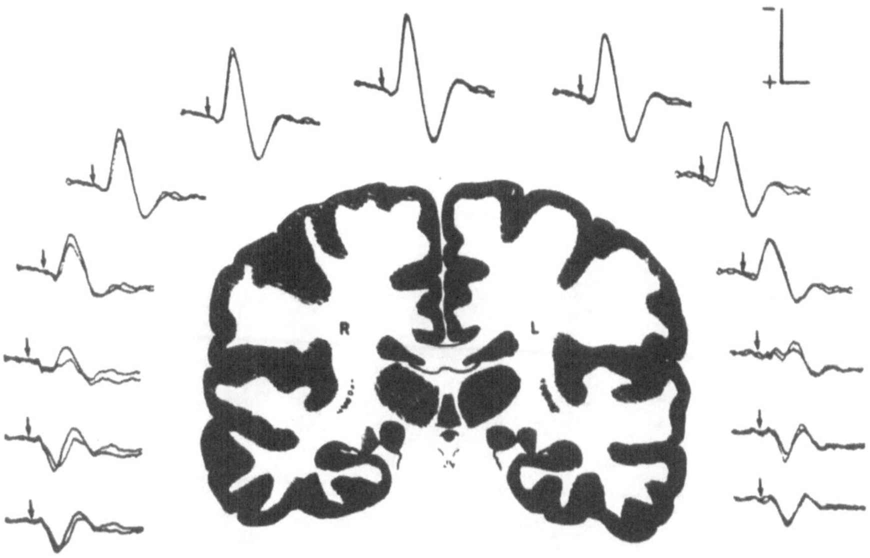

FIG. 4.8. Superaverage AERs from 26 normal hearing adult subjects, along a coronal chain referred to the nose, from the right mastoid to the left one. Stimuli are 70 dB, 1000 Hz pure tones. *Full lines*: AERs to left-ear stimulation. *Dotted lines*: AERs to right-ear stimulation. The stimulus is indicated by an arrow. Calibration: 10 μV, 100 msec. (From Peronnet & Michel, 1977.)

tions of Kooi et al. (1971) nor Vaughan and Ritter (1970) might explain their results, but the data of Peronnet et al. (1974) were more consistent with their hypothesis of a temporal complex. Wolpaw and Penry argued that what the latter authors interpreted as inverted temporal potentials were a result of different latencies in vertex and temporal regions, which clearly suggests an independent temporal component. According to Wolpaw and Penry, the vertex potential has a widespread distribution over cortex, whereas the temporal complex is probably a product of secondary auditory cortex.

N100 and P180 are the most prominent components of the whole AER. They are also the earliest potentials to be reliably modified by changes in a subject's attentive state (Picton & Hillyard, 1974). This provides a useful tool for the study of attention mechanisms (Schwent, Hillyard, & Galambos, 1976a, 1976b). Long latency components are more stable when the stimulus is triggered by a particular phase of the alpha activity (Tatsuno, Marsoner, & Wageneder, 1970), which suggests a functional relationship between the genesis of the alpha rhythm and of the AERs. Genetic effects are also present in the amplitude and waveshape of AERs, because monozygotic twins have more similar AERs than dyzygotic twins (Buchsbaum, 1974; Rust, 1975).

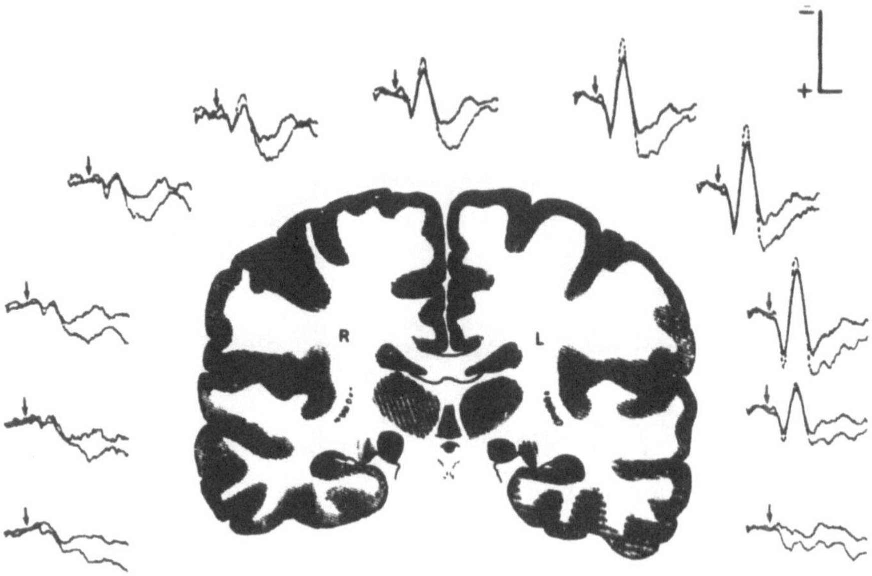

FIG. 4.9. Topographical recording of the AERs of a patient who showed a complete extinction of the left ear messages to the dichotic listening test. He presented a left regressive hemiplegia related to a Sylvian artery thrombosis with a partial revascularization by the anterior artery of the Sylvian territory. *Full lines*: AERs to left-ear stimulation. *Dotted lines*: AERs to right-ear stimulation. Calibration: 10 μV, 100 msec. It is possible to observe the absence or great amplitude reduction of AERs recorded over the right hemisphere. (From Peronnet & Michel, 1977.)

B. Age Effect On AERs

Maturational changes of the AERs have been investigated quite a bit (Barnet & Goodwin, 1965; Davis & Onishi, 1969; Lenard, Von Bernuth, & Hutt, 1969; Ohlrich & Barnet, 1972). Weitzman, Graziani, and Duhamel (1967) and Weitzman and Graziani (1968) observed that in infants of 25–28 weeks estimated gestational age, there was a diffuse scalp response, with a negative wave at 200–270 msec, followed by a large positive wave at 700–900 msec of latency. As maturation progressed, the latencies of all components decreased; by 34–37 weeks gestational age, the pattern approached that seen in full-term infants and differences between active and quiet sleep were recognizable. According to Goldstein, McRandle, and Smith (1974), the middle components are similar in newborns and in adults, P29 and N36 being more constant in latency than P18 and N21. The long latency components in the newborn varied according to the sleep state. P106 is also very stable in latency. Ellingson et al. (1974) considered that the most stable component in the human newborns was P250. They remarked that AERs are more mature than VERs at the moment of birth. At 1, 4, and 8 months of age, middle components have similar waveshapes (Mendel, Adkinson, & Harker, 1977). Crevoisier, Peronnet, Girod, Challet, and Reval (1976), recording in children aged 2–15 years in coronal montage, found that the long latency components have a lateral predominance of the response that gradually reduces in children up to 8 years old.

Children aged 2–5 years have similar waveshapes of their AERs in REM and stage 2 sleep, although in REM sleep, smaller latencies and higher amplitudes are found. Correlation between the age of the subject and the latency and amplitude of each wave showed a high positive value for P350 latency and a high negative value for the amplitude of the long latency components, exceeding 300 msec in latency in stage 2 sleep (Tanguay, Lee, & Ornitz, 1973). Similar findings were previously reported by Barnet and Lodge (1967) from the early postnatal period to 14 months of age. AERs in awake newborns are very similar to those recorded during REM sleep (Ellingson et al., 1974). According to Susuki and Taguchi (1968), AER waveshape is similar in children and adults during sleep. Barnet, Ohlrich, Weiss, and Shanks (1975) found that latencies decrease with the logarithm of age, whereas amplitude increases with age, with the exception of N100–P160, which decreases from 15 days to 3 years of life in sleeping children. The maturation of AERs was characterized by a relative increase in the long latency components, the most striking change being the development of P600. Tables 4.4 and 4.5 show the developmental changes in AER characteristics.

Recently, Ohlrich, Barnet, Weiss, and Shanks (1978) made a longitudinal study of the AERs in children from birth to 3 years old. They found an increase in amplitude and a decrease in latency, most changes occurring during the first year of life. Goodin, Squires, Henderson, and Starr (1978) recorded the AERs in normal subjects from 6–76 years old. They found a striking change in the topographic distribution of AER components: Children have a predominant parietal distribution that changes to centro–frontal dominance later on, in adults. According to these authors, aging produces an increase in latency and a decrease of amplitude in long latency components. However, Dustman et al. (1977) did not observe any change peculiar to senescence.

C. Effects of Stimulus Characteristics on Middle and Long Latency Components

On increasing the length of interstimulus intervals, a large increase in the amplitude of the long latency components (Roth, Krainz, Ford,

TABLE 4.4[a]
Number of Subjects, Mean Latencies, and Standard Deviations of the AER Components for Children from 0.5 to 36 Months of Age[b]

Age groups (months)	N_0			P_1			N_1			P_2			N_2			P_{3A}			P_{3B}		
	n	$\bar{x}$	SD	n	$\bar{x}$	SD	n	$\bar{x}$	SD	n	$\bar{x}$	SD	n	$\bar{x}$	SD	n	$\bar{x}$	SD	n	$\bar{x}$	SD
.5	3	39	12	5	72	4	6	97	17	10	217	26	10	522	109	5	654	27	8	783	101
1	1	20	—	8	65	24	9	104	34	10	214	38	10	545	139	1	474	—	10	814	105
1.5	4	34	14	6	59	14	9	95	29	10	201	33	10	395	74	3	457	69	9	655	118
2	5	27	10	5	64	32	6	101	19	10	229	55	10	488	70	2	705	204	9	775	184
3	5	43	12	7	72	19	9	114	34	10	219	33	10	459	55	6	671	49	6	794	133
6	6	29	9	9	99	27	9	139	31	10	199	28	10	442	42	8	677	97	3	686	47
9	4	39	4	8	66	26	9	91	24	10	176	23	10	394	57	4	618	139	8	713	102
12	3	33	7	9	65	11	9	109	21	10	182	31	10	380	42	7	566	106	5	663	43
15	7	36	6	8	66	16	10	105	45	10	158	36	10	356	60	5	590	167	6	726	59
18	6	28	6	8	57	19	9	88	27	10	167	20	10	353	72	6	572	103	6	685	119
24	5	37	3	6	76	19	7	91	26	10	151	22	10	323	59	9	456	99	7	690	149
30	4	36	8	8	77	19	9	113	32	10	154	24	10	314	65	9	531	112	4	671	30
36	7	30	11	8	67	27	8	100	200	10	153	21	10	325	74	9	568	116	2	648	51
Control 2 months[c]	5	27	7	8	62	17	8	96	26	10	194	34	10	503	91	6	664	99	7	838	132

[a]From Barnet et al., 1975.
[b]Values are given in msec.
[c]Analysis of the subject population and procedures revealed several variables that were not distributed uniformly across age—namely, rearing status, race, and equipment used for data collection. To test for possible effects of these variables on results, a control group of 10 white, 2-month-old, home-reared subjects was also included.

TABLE 4.5[a]

Number of Subjects, Mean Amplitudes, and Standard Deviations of the AER Components for Children from 0.5 to 36 Months of Age[b]

Age group (months)	N_0P_1			P_1N_1			N_1P_2			P_2N_2			N_2P_{3A}			N_2P_{3B}		
	n	$\bar{x}$	SD	n	$\bar{x}$	SD	n	$\bar{x}$	SD	n	$\bar{x}$	SD	n	$\bar{x}$	SD	n	$\bar{x}$	SD
.5	2	2.4	1.8	5	1.9	2.9	7	14.5	6.5	10	22.9	9.2	3	17.1	3.6	8	8.9	6.4
1	1	1.8	—	8	1.6	1.1	9	12.7	7.8	10	25.4	14.3	1	8.3	—	10	15.4	8.5
1.5	4	2.6	.8	6	2.9	2.5	9	17.7	13.9	10	26.8	23.3	3	17.0	12.6	9	17.1	10.3
2	4	1.9	1.1	5	.7	1.1	6	12.5	5.8	10	34.7	16.1	2	37.6	35.1	9	16.8	7.5
3	4	4.2	2.3	7	1.2	1.5	9	12.6	5.6	10	39.1	18.8	6	45.6	26.3	6	28.0	10.3
6	6	6.1	2.9	9	2.9	1.8	9	5.6	2.8	10	29.9	9.1	8	47.4	17.5	3	38.3	15.9
9	4	8.4	1.0	8	2.9	3.7	9	10.9	5.6	10	33.3	10.8	4	44.2	37.2	8	28.8	11.0
12	3	3.0	2.7	9	4.1	1.6	9	5.8	2.9	10	28.0	12.7	7	35.1	23.0	5	29.3	5.3
15	5	5.4	1.6	8	5.7	5.3	10	5.0	4.2	10	36.8	24.8	5	58.7	53.0	6	37.6	23.1
18	5	4.5	3.7	8	2.8	2.3	9	9.5	5.0	10	32.4	13.9	6	42.2	11.7	6	33.9	20.1
24	3	12.4	1.8	7	2.1	1.8	7	10.3	7.7	10	40.9	14.8	9	30.6	19.3	7	49.2	23.8
30	4	7.8	3.1	8	6.1	4.5	9	5.7	4.4	10	36.6	17.0	9	48.6	38.7	4	25.9	11.0
36	6	6.0	3.1	8	5.0	4.4	8	6.5	5.5	10	39.7	12.7	9	52.4	21.6	2	29.8	7.7
Control																		
2 m[c]	4	6.6	6.8	8	2.9	2.4	8	17.0	7.3	10	34.8	13.3	6	27.9	9.5	7	27.7	11.6

[a]From Barnet et al., 1975.

[b]Values are given in μV.

[c]Analysis of the subject population and procedures revealed several variables that were not distributed uniformily across age—namely, rearing status, race, and equipment used for data collection. To test for possible effects of these variables on results, a control group of 10 white, 2-month-old, home-reared subjects was also included.

Tinklenberg, Rothbart, and Kopell, 1976), as well as a reduction of latency (Surwillo, 1977a), is observed. The relation between stimulus intensity and amplitude of the long latency components of the AERs over vertex has been used as a procedure for the assessment of auditory pathway integrity and acuity (Evoked Response Audiometry). Once the threshold stimuli produced a response, progressive increase in the stimulus intensity was accompanied by continuous increase in the amplitude of the response (Davis & Zerlin, 1966; Gerin, Pernier, and Peronnet, 1972), following a linear relationship (Tepas, Boxerman, and Anch, 1972).

Increasing the intensity of clicks causes no latency changes, whereas a decrease in latency is observed with louder tones (Rapin, Schimmel, Tourk, Krasnegor, and Pollak, 1966). The latency of middle components to high-frequency tones is shorter in comparison to the responses produced by low-frequency tones (Thornton, Mendel, and Anderson, 1977). Arlinger (1976) developed a mathematical model of the relation between stimulus intensity and latency of N100, based on the assumption of an exponential relationship when using a tone pulse. The method offers a way of threshold extrapolation with rather good accuracy. AERs to the onset and cessation of pure tone stimuli are very similar in waveform, but the *on* response is generally larger than the *off* response. The curves of the fitted linear families have different slopes for the *on* and *off* responses (Schweitzer and Tepas, 1974). Frequency modulated auditory stimuli result in average vertex potentials similar to the usual AERs (Kohn, Lifshitz, and Litchfield, 1978).

D. Clinical Applications of Middle and Long Latency Components

1. Evoked Responses Audiometry

Long latency components of the AER recorded over vertex have been widely used as measures for the estimation of the threshold for auditory sensation (for a review, see Reneaw and Hnatiow, 1975). It has been well established that careful cortical audiometry provides results corresponding satisfactorily with those obtained by pure tone audiometry (Davis, Hirsh, Shelnutt, and Bowers, 1967; Morgan, Gerin, and Charachon, 1970; Rapin and Bergman, 1969; Suzuki and Taguchi, 1965; Van der Sandt, 1969). The usual difference between the two types of measures is around 10 dB, with cortical audiometry thresholds consistently higher. The components that are used for the detection of the response are P50, N100, P180, and N250. Note that the latency of these components is variable with age and brain state, and sometimes the identification of a particular component in an individual patient may be quite difficult. Rapin and Schimmel (1977) found that the chief liability of this procedure was not the failure to detect AERs, but false positive interpretation of records as showing a response when in fact no AER was present. This is the most serious error for a child, who can be denied corrective hearing amplification and proper education as a result. Therefore, special care should be taken on recording and interpreting long latency components in ERA. An automatized procedure has been described by John (1977). However, it should be emphasized (Rapin and Graziani, 1967) that the detection of clear AERs establishes the functional integrity of the afferent auditory pathway, but it is not a demonstration that the auditory input is being behaviorally utilized.

Using high repetition rates (12–30 Hz) of auditory stimulation, a sinusoidal waveshape of the AER is observed (as in VERs). The amplitude of these sinusoidal components, averaged over several thousand signals, is linearly related to the logarithm of intensity of the sound. Although the same results were obtained by clicks and pure tones, the latter produced smaller ERs and therefore a longer time averaging was needed to obtain reliable results. However, using click stimulation at repetition rates of 12–16 Hz, reliable large vertex ERs were obtained. With a 10-minute test, yielding 4 or 5 points, it was possible to establish the patient's threshold within ± 5 dB. These results, obtained by Campbell, Atkinson, Francis, and Green (1977) with a very rapid and simple procedure, are very promising for the assessment of the auditory afferent pathway.

2. *Brain Lesions*

Shimizu (1968) described lower amplitude and greater latency values of the components of the AERs in unilateral lesions of the VIII nerve (unilateral stimuli). Morrell (1974), in a patient with left hemispherectomy, demonstrated that although very small AERs were recorded on the injured side, they were the result of volume conduction (unilateral stimuli). Michel and Peronnet (1974) and Peronnet et al. (1974) described alteration in waveform and amplitude of AERs to unilateral pure tones in patients with lesions of the auditory cortical area (Fig. 4.9). These responses had a normal waveshape and coronal distribution when other cortical areas were damaged. In sections of the corpus callosum, the AERs were highly asymmetric, but with a normal waveform and topographic distribution, whereas in the agenesis of the corpus callosum, the AERs were symmetric. Barat, Paty, and Arné (1974) studied the AERs to binaural stimulation in a group of aphasic patients; they observed a decrease in the amplitude of the responses in those subjects with sensory aphasia. In the group of motor aphasics, amplitudes comparable to those of the control group were observed. In a case of auditory agnosia, great variability in the latencies of the AERs and amplitude reduction have been observed (Sheuler and Ulrich, 1977). Cant, Gronwell, and Burges (1974) observed waveform alterations of the AERs after closed head injuries; the degree of abnormality and the period needed for the restoration of a normal waveshape were related to the severity of the trauma. In patients with temporal epilepsy, changes of the AERs to clicks have been related to the degree of alteration of the EEG. When only localized spike activity was observed, without generalized EEG discharges, the response had higher amplitude and lower latency values. When the EEG alterations were generalized, there was a general reduction of amplitude of the AERs (Polujanova, Vasilieva, and Kamaskaja, 1977). Popov, Ovtcharova, Raitchev, and Tzicalova (1977) studied patients during different stages of recovery from aphasia using tones, meaningful and nonsense words with similar acoustic parameters and equal duration. They observed amplitude decreases and latency increases of AERs over the damaged hemisphere. Szirtes, Rothenberger, and Jürgens (1977) studied the AER to verbal stimuli in normal, aphasic, and right hemisphere damaged subjects. Amplitude of N100 was reduced in both types of patients, the changes being greater in the left side lesioned (aphasic) cases.

Recordings of early, middle, and long latency components in the same subject provide an opportunity to identify a hearing-impaired patient, and also permit additional statements about the nature and location of the disease process. Galambos and Hecox (1977) beautifully demonstrated this statement. Fig. 4.10 shows the BAERs and the cortical AERs in a patient with a diagnosis of mucopolysaccharidosis type III, who appeared either to be clinically deaf or to have a severe hearing impairment. The patient's BAERs were normal, but no cortical AERs were observed. With such information, the clinician has a rational basis for a therapeutic intervention.

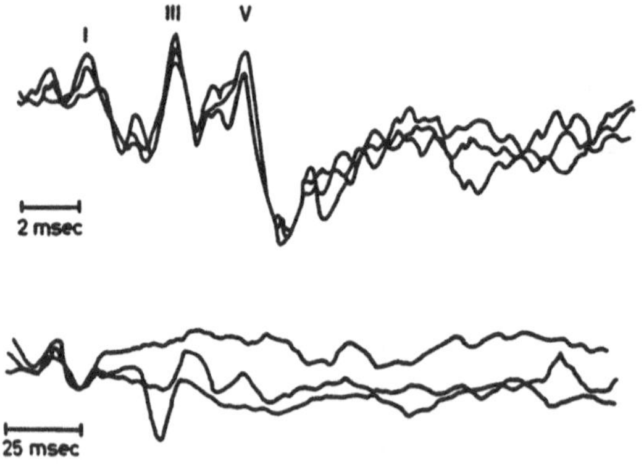

FIG.4.10. Normal brain-stem auditory evoked responses (*top*) and absent cortical auditory evoked responses (*bottom*) in a patient suffering from San Filippo's disease. Clinically, the patient appeared to have a profound hearing loss. Each superimposed tracing was obtained in response to a 60 dB SL monaural click, with positivity to the vertex upwards in all recordings. (From Galambos & Hecox, 1977.)

All the forementioned results clearly demonstrated that long latency components are greatly affected in the presence of central lesions of the auditory pathway.

3. Psychiatric and Behavioral Disorders and Other Diseases Affecting the Nervous System Barnet and Lodge (1967) described greater amplitudes of AERs in developmentally retarded children. When studying the effects of habituation on the amplitude of AERs, a lack of evoked response decrement has been found in neonates and mongoloid children (Barnet and Ohlrich, 1971). In normal children, larger left hemispheric responses are observed, whereas in children with marasmus, these differences did not appear (Barnet, Weiss, Sotillo, Ohlrich, Shkurovich, and Cravioto, 1978). In autistic children, the amplitude of the AERs increased during REM sleep, whereas in normal children, this was not observed (Ornitz, Ritvo, Panman, Lee, Carr, and Walter, 1968).

Children with poor ability to concentrate showed larger latencies of P250 and reduced amplitudes compared with children of the same age who had good ability to concentrate (Grünewald, Grünewald-Zuberbier, and Netz, 1978). Satterfield and Braley (1977) demonstrated that differences in amplitude of the different AER components between normal and hyperkinetic children are age dependent. P100–N120 was smaller at the age of 6–7 years and greater at the age of 10–12 years in hyperactive children than in normals, whereas P160–N250 was greater in the younger hyperactive and smaller at 10–12 years in hyperactive children compared with the normal group (see Fig. 4.11A and B).

Schizophrenic patients showed high variability of the AERs (Callaway, Jones, and Donchin, 1970). Lifshitz and Gradijan (1974) have shown that the amplitude reduction of the components of the AERs between 0.25 and 0.5 seconds in latency is a useful procedure for differentiation of schizophrenic from other groups. It has also been reported that schizophrenic and nonschizophrenic mental patients can be distinguished by greater differences between the AERs to tones of 600 and 1000 Hz in schizophrenic patients than in other subjects (Jones, Blacker, Callaway, and Layne, 1965). Marcus and Zuercher (1977) studied a group of adult schizoautistic patients, a group of chronic undifferentiated schizophrenics, and a group of chronic paranoid schizophrenics. The vertex responses were smaller in all three groups compared with normals. The schizophrenics also showed a smaller number of AER components, and N100 was of augmented amplitude in schizoautistics. Shagass, Straumanis, Roemer, and Amadeo (1977) also described lower amplitudes of the AERs in schizophrenic patients than in healthy subjects; the differences were more apparent from 80–150 msec after the click in vertex, frontal, central and temporal leads. Saletu, Saletu, and Itil (1973) studied the effect of psychotropic drug treatments on the amplitude of the AER components. Low amplitude of N140–P200 was associated with high ratings on behavioral items involving hallucinations, delusions, and cognitive disorientation. Even more noteworthy was the observation that during a placebo period, therapy-responsive patients exhibited shorter latencies and higher amplitudes for peaks P55 and N69 than therapy-resistent patients (Saletu, Itil, and Saletu, 1971).

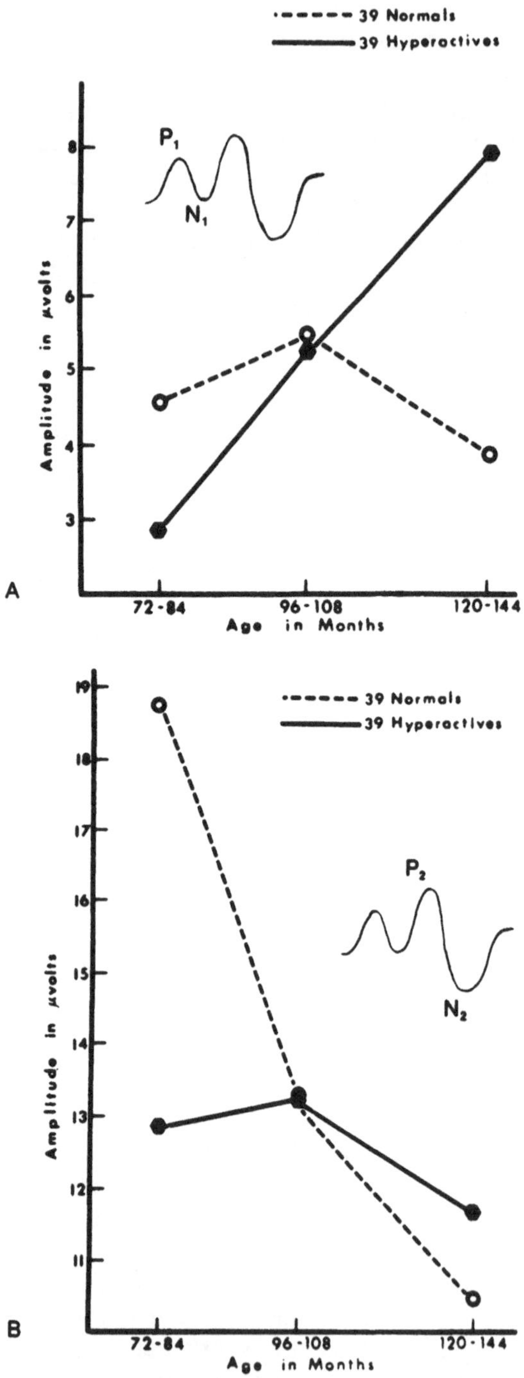

FIG. 4.11. (A) Differential effect of age on the P1–N1 component of the AER in normal and hyperactive children (from Satterfield & Braley, 1977). (B) Differential effect of age on the P2–N2 component of the AER in normal and hyperactive children (from Satterfield & Braley, 1977).

IV. EXCITABILITY CYCLE OF AERS

The auditory recovery function has not been as extensively studied as the visual or somatosensory. Ornitz, Tangway, Forsythe, de la Peña, and Ghahremani (1974) studied it in 23 normal children, from 22 to 67 months of age, during sleep. Using paired clicks, they found a clear response with interstimulus intervals greater than 40 msec and a reduction of amplitude at intervals of 250 msec. Facilitation was found with intervals ranging from 80–160 msec. The recovery cycle in autistic children has no differences from that reported in normal children (Ornitz, Forsythe, Tangway, Ritvo, de la Pena, and Ghahremani, 1974). Robinson and Rudge (1977a) studied the early BAER components to paired clicks, 5 msec apart, in normal subjects and in MS patients. The latencies of waves II to V were significantly greater than those obtained to a single click. In 15 out of 24 MS patients, a delayed wave V was observed when compared with that of normal subjects. These results were related to the fact that demyelinated fibers fail to conduct trains of pairs of impulses as well as normal fibers.

V. THE FREQUENCY-FOLLOWING RESPONSE (FFR)

If a short tone burst is repeatedly delivered via earphones to a human subject, an electrical response at the stimulus frequency with a latency of about 6 msec can be recorded at the vertex after computer averaging (Moushegian, Rupert, and Stillman, 1973). The response consists of a series of waves spaced at approximately the same interval as the stimulus frequency (i.e., 2 msec when a tone of 500 Hz is used), with an overall duration approximately equal to that of the acoustic stimulus. In general, the response is above the baseline and it resembles a sinusoid component superimposed upon a pedestal-like, slow wave response (Fig. 4.12). The FFR was be elicited by continuous tones or by tone bursts, and it is observable over a range of frequencies from 70 Hz to greater than 1.5 KH. The threshold for the continuous stimulus is lower than for the burst stimulus (Galambos and Hecox, 1977; Glaser, Suter, Dasheiff, and Goldberg, 1976).

Human FFR is generated in the brain stem (Marsh, Brown, and Smith, 1974, 1975; Moushegian et al., 1973; Smith, Marsh, and Brown, 1975). Comparison with the brain stem responses indicates that the FFR corresponds with early waves IV and V (Glaser et al., 1976). Sohmer, Pratt, and Kinarti (1977b), in control subjects and in patients with lesions of the upper brain stem, demonstrated that FFR to tone burst begins with a cochlea microphonic potential. After about 6 msec, a neural FFR is generated at the inferior colliculus and appears superimposed upon the initial response. Occasionally, an additional late FFR generated in the

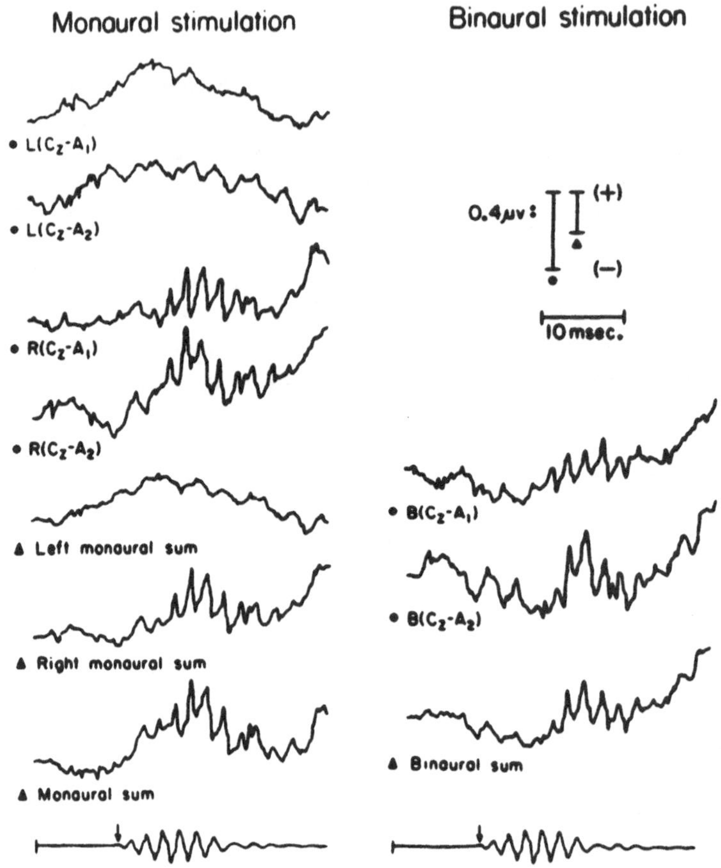

FIG. 4.12. Frequency following averaged evoked responses obtained from one subject with profound left-ear hearing loss, and normal right-ear hearing. L: monaural stimulus presentation to the left ear. R: right monaural stimulation. B: binaural stimulation. Left monaural sum is the sum of the evoked responses recorded in C_zA_1 and C_zA_2 to left monaural stimulation, and right monaural sum is the sum of the evoked responses in both leads to right monaural stimulation. Monaural sum is the sum of the evoked responses in both leads to monaural stimulation. Similarly, binaural sum indicates the sum of the evoked responses in both leads to binaural stimulation. No response to left monaural stimulation is observed, whereas a normal response to right monaural stimulation is obtained. The FFR recorded from C_zA_2 was larger in magnitude than that recorded from C_zA_1. (From Daly et al., 1976.)

postauricular muscle after about 10 msec is also superimposed to the previous responses. The microphonic component is observed to the onset phase of a monaural tone burst; reversal of the stimulus onset phase causes reversal of the microphonic response. Thus, in the averaged response in which an equal number of stimuli of both onset phases are combined, the sinusoidal microphonic component is canceled out, leaving only the neural component. The FFR is easily observed only at fairly high levels of stimulation. If the averaged recorded waveform is subjected to frequency analysis, it is possible to detect FFR at low levels of stimulation. At these low levels, it has been possible to demonstrate that the FFR is a brain stem response to the stimulation of the apical part of the cochlea. Thus, the procedure may be used to assess the integrity of the low frequency channels in audition (de Baer, Machiels, & Kruidenier, 1977). Recently, Stillman, Crow, & Moushegian (1978), using tones of frequencies lower than 350 Hz, have reported two main components, FFR1 and FFR2, with 1.7 msec latency difference, suggesting two brain-stem sources for these responses. With tones of higher frequency, FFR2 is obscured by the presence of FFR1.

Monaural stimulation of either ear evoked larger responses from the ipsilateral electrode derivation than from the contralateral electrode. Binaural stimulation evoked responses of equal amplitude in both sides, each larger than either the ipsilateral or contralateral monaural response, but slightly smaller than the sum of the ipsilateral and contralateral monaural responses (Daly, Roeser, & Moushegian, 1976; Gerken, Moushegian, Stillman, & Rupert, 1975). These results indicate that FFR arises from at least two separate symmetric neural sources, each activated by one ear. FFR can be obtained in normal adults and in children as young as 9 weeks of age (Marsh et al., 1975).

The FFR has been studied in hearing-impaired subjects. In unilateral hearing loss, monaural stimulation produces a flat response (Daly et al., 1976; Moushegian, 1977). Fig. 4.12 shows the FFR of a patient with pronounced left-ear hearing loss. Using a forehead reference and an active electrode on the mastoid, Yamada, Yamane, & Kodera (1977) studied the simultaneous recordings of the brain stem response and the FFR taken under three conditions: (1) the connection of the two electrodes to the two inputs of the amplifier was kept constant and the phase of the tone bursts was alternated on successive stimuli over 2000 presentations, which resulted in BAER recordings and FFR canceled out by the successive phase reversal; (2) the inputs from the electrodes and the phase of the tone burst were kept constant over 2000 presentations, with simultaneous BAER and FFR recordings; and (3) during the first 1000 stimuli, the forehead electrode was connected to input 2 and the mastoid electrode to input 1 of the differential amplifier and the initial phase of the tone burst was negative. During the second 1000 stimulus presentations, the electrode inputs were reversed and the initial phase of the tone burst was positive. This procedure canceled the contribution of the BAERs, leaving FFR alone.

This technique allows a detailed study of patients with hearing loss, because it makes available the actual frequency response characteristics of the auditory pathway. As previously described, patients with lesions of the upper brain stem have no FFR.

VI. SUMMARY

It is beyond question that AERs are very useful in the evaluation of the functional and anatomical integrity of the auditory pathway. The early components, or brain-stem auditory evoked responses (BAERs), have been related to the activation of the auditory nerve (Wave I), cochlear nuclei (Wave II), superior olivary complex (Wave III), lateral lemniscus and inferior colliculus (Waves IV and V). Generators of waves VI and VII have not yet been defined, although it has been proposed that they may have a thalamic origin. BAERs have been used to study conductive and sensorineural hearing loss, as well as in the assessment of brain-stem lesions in patients suspected of tumors or degenerative diseases. They have also been used to define the functional integrity of the brain stem auditory pathways in comatose patients.

Middle latency components (8–50 msec) are supposed to be mixtures of neurogenic and myogenic activity. At present, it has not been possible to identify unequivocally the primary cortical response generated in Heschl's gyrus. Many contradictory results appear in literature concerning the origin of long latency components (50–500 msec). Some authors considered that they are mediated by a nonspecific afferent projection system, whereas others have proposed that long latency components arise in the region of the auditory cortex. Evidence presented in patients with lesions involving the auditory area constitutes a strong argument in favor of the latter hypothesis. The main clinical application of middle and long latency AER components has been in the assessment of auditory thresholds (Evoked Response Audiometry), but they seem to be also very useful in the study of patients with brain lesions that affect the auditory area, in cranial traumas, and in psychiatric and behavioral disorders.

From this chapter, it might be concluded that recording of early, middle, and long latency components in the same patient not only provides an opportunity to identify a hearing-impaired patient, but also permits additional statements about the nature and location of the patient's disease process. Some neurometric approaches based on the study of AERs are presented in Chapter 13.

5 Somatosensory Evoked Responses (SSERs)

Somatosensory evoked responses may be evoked by percutaneous electrical stimulation of the peripheral nerves, fingers, or toes, by mechanical stimulation, by thermal stimulation, or by nociceptive stimulation. Different types of nerve fibers are activated depending on the stimulus, producing different types of evoked responses. The responses may be recorded at the scalp or over the spinal cord. In this chapter, we first discuss the SSERs recorded at the scalp by different types of stimuli; later on, we discuss the spinal evoked responses.

I. SSERs TO NONPAINFUL ELECTRICAL NERVE STIMULATION

A. General Characteristics

At the scalp, the percutaneous electrical stimulation of peripheral nerves produces an ER with very constant early components and variable late components (Debecker & Desmedt, 1964; Goff, Rosner, & Allison, 1962; A.M. Halliday, 1975b; Madkour & Abdel Hamid, 1967). The early responses are due to impulses conducted in peripheral fibers at over 15 m/sec (Dawson, 1956; Desmedt, Franken, Borenstein, Debecker, Lambert, & Manil, 1966). The afferent volley travels by the dorsal column pathway and the medial lemniscus (Giblin, 1964; Halliday & Wakefield, 1963), relaying in the ventro-posterior nucleus of the thalamus (Domino, Matsuoka, Waltz, &

Cooper, 1965; Pagni, 1967) and reaching the cerebral cortex. On unilateral stimulation of peripheral nerves, the early response is mainly recorded over the contralateral Rolandic area.

For recording the very early potentials, a large sample is needed. It is also necessary to take special precautions with the reference electrode. Wiederholt and Kritchevsky (1977) recommend that the knee or the dorsum of the hand opposite to the one stimulated be used as reference, because Cracco and Cracco (1976) demonstrated that the first two waves are very similar at the vertex, nose, and ear when using this reference. Because of the resulting cancellation effect, the waves are not well defined in vertex-ear derivations (Fig. 5.1). By unilateral stimulation of the median nerve, the first component has its latency at 9–10 msec with positive polarity at the scalp (P9) and negative over the clavicle. It is considered a far-field reflection of activity in the brachial plexus. The second potential has a mean peak latency at 11–12 msec, being positive (P11) over the fifth cervical level and negative below; it is related to the activation of the dorsal column or the postsynaptic activation of the dorsal nuclei (Cracco & Cracco, 1976; Hume & Cant, 1978; Jones & Small, 1977; Wiederholt & Kritschevsky, 1977). The third component is positive in the scalp and negative in the cervical region and has a peak latency of 13–14 msec (P14); this, according to Nakanishi, Shimada, Sakuta, & Toyokura (1978), is the result of the activity of the afferent pathways from the medulla to the thalamus, reflecting the activity of the medial lemnisal system in the brain stem.

The early cortical activity (presynaptic) is represented by N19 or N20. It has been called the initial negative wave and may be recorded in the posterior part of the contralateral hemisphere from the Rolandic area backwards (Calmes & Cracco, 1971; Giblin, 1964; W. R. Goff et al., 1962). The component is followed by a positive–negative–positive complex up to 30 msec (Halliday, 1975b). N20 and P30 show a clear polarity inversion across the central sulcus (Broughton, 1969; Goff, Matsumiya, Allison, & Goff, 1977).

Another component that has been found by several authors is P45. It can be recorded over a wide area, but it is still predominantly contralateral and has its maximal amplitude in the parietal region (Giblin, 1964; G. D. Goff et al., 1977; W. R. Goff et al., 1962). Long latency components show more variability, both in amplitude and latency, than early components. P100 is extremely large at the forehead and is detectable at nearly all scalp locations. According to G. D. Goff et al. (1977), it has two possible origins: a posterior neuronal source and a frontal myogenic source. N140 and P190 constitute the vertex potential. The N260–P300–N360–P420–N460 sequence of components is presumed to be neurogenic with some similarity to the occipital alpha rhythm (G. D. Goff et al., 1977). Very similar shapes of SSERs have been recorded from the scalp and from the dura (Broughton, 1969;

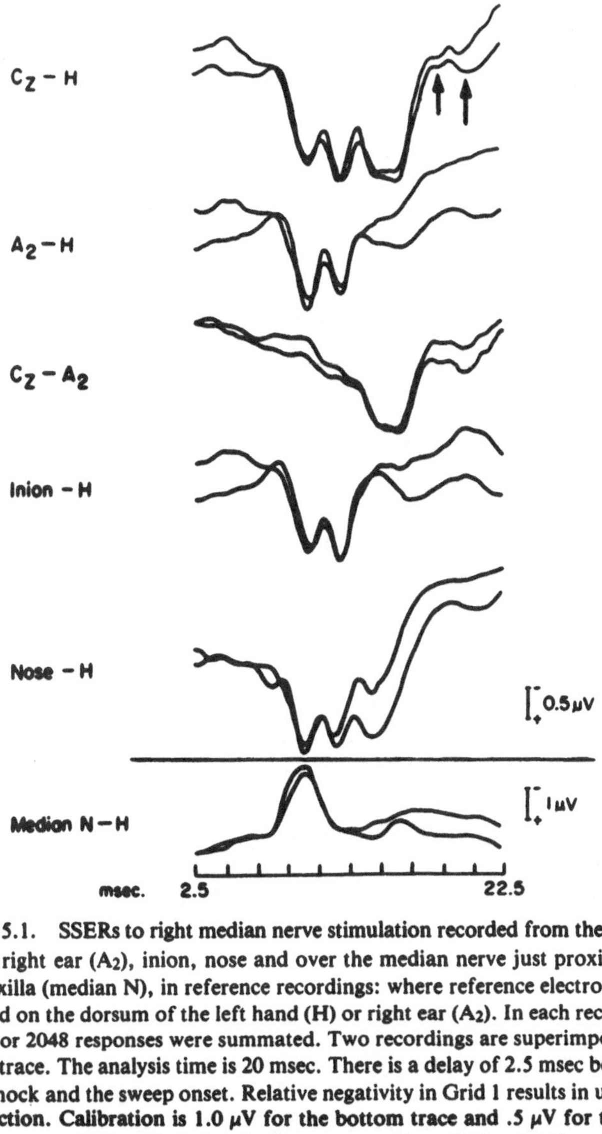

FIG. 5.1. SSERs to right median nerve stimulation recorded from the vertex (C_z), right ear (A_2), inion, nose and over the median nerve just proximal to the axilla (median N), in reference recordings: where reference electrode was placed on the dorsum of the left hand (H) or right ear (A_2). In each recording 1024 or 2048 responses were summated. Two recordings are superimposed in each trace. The analysis time is 20 msec. There is a delay of 2.5 msec between the shock and the sweep onset. Relative negativity in Grid 1 results in upward deflection. Calibration is 1.0 μV for the bottom trace and .5 μV for the top five traces, as indicated. In hand reference recordings, P10 and P12 are clearly seen at the vertex, ear, nose, and inion. whereas in vertex–ear derivation these components are not observed. The latency of onset of the first positive potential recorded from the scalp, nose, and ear is similar to that of the negative potential recorded over the stimulated median nerve 2 cm proximal to the axilla (*bottom trace*). (From Cracco & Cracco, 1976.)

Domino et al., 1965; Kelly, Goldring, & O'Leary, 1965; Stohr & Goldring, 1969). Asymmetries of the late components related to handedness and side of stimulus delivery have been suggested: To right stimulation, right-handed subjects have greater responses in C_4 than in C_3, whereas to left stimulation, the left handed have greater responses in the left side (Barret, Halliday, & Halliday, 1977). N118 and P180 increased their amplitude during movement (Lee & White, 1974).

The stimulation of the peripheral nerves of the legs elicits a similar set of potentials, though they are somewhat delayed because of the additional length of the ascending pathway (Desmedt, 1971).

In relation to the sources of the ipsilateral responses, it seems that the early waves, which are recorded only when the contralateral area is adequately functioning, are produced by ipsilateral cortical generators activated by the contralateral area via the corpus callosum (Liberson, 1966; Tamura, 1972; Williamson, Goff, & Allison 1970). Regarding the late components, some contradictory results have been obtained. Williamson et al. (1970) found that unilateral cerebral lesions, which disrupted primary somatic pathways at or above the thalamic level and were characterized by reduced or absent early contralateral components, also showed alteration of the late components in both hemispheres. This is contradictory to the results obtained by Yamada, Kimura, Young, & Powers (1978), who described essentially normal ipsilateral late components despite absent or markedly depressed contralateral responses. Evidence that ipsilateral long latency components are not strictly dependent on the contralateral response has also been provided in hemispherectomized patients (Hazemann, Oliver, & Fishgold, 1969; Matsumiya, Gennarelli, & Lombroso, 1971). These long latency components have also been described in patients with agenesis of the corpus callosum, which suggests the existence of an independent ipsilateral cortical generator of these components. In tumors of the rostral and caudal portions of the corpus callosum, the ipsilateral SSERs are normal, but when the whole corpus callosum is affected, lower amplitudes of the long latency ipsilateral components are observed (Taghavy, 1977). Possibly, both an ipsilateral cortical generator and callosal transmission of the contralateral response contribute to the long latency ipsilateral components.

Velasco, Velasco, Maldonado, & Machado (1975) and Velasco & Velasco (1975) studied the differential effect of thalamic and subthalamic lesions on early and late components of the SSERs, concluding that the first components correspond to the various proprioceptive impulses that travel by the lemniscal pathway to the thalamus and cortex, and that the late components (P180) correspond to a parallel activation of a nonspecific, polysynaptic, extralemniscal reticulo–thalamo–cortical pathway. This hypothesis is supported by the results of Pagni (1967) and Fukushima, Mayanagi, & Bonchard (1976). The latter authors recorded the SSERs to peripheral nerve stimulation in various thalamic structures. In the specific relay nucleus, the SSERs were recorded only contralaterally and were characterized by a positive deflection with a peak latency of 17.5 msec (occurring 1–2 msec before initial negative cortical component), whereas in the association and unspecific thalamic nuclei, ipsilateral and contralateral SSERs had similar characteristics, with early and late positive-negative complexes. These results strongly suggest that the ipsilateral components recorded in the absence of the contralateral primary cortical area are mediated by the nonspecific diffuse projection system.

B. Age Dependence

Maturational changes of the SSERs have been described (Hrbek, Karlberg, & Olsson, 1973; see Fig. 5.2). In preterm newborn infants below 30 weeks gestational age, the major or single component is a very slow negative wave, most distinct in the corresponding projection area. During further development, this component decreases and faster components appear. At 29 weeks of gestation, constant primary components are observed, the relationship between latency and gestational age being linear after 30 weeks of gestation. Vertex components increased during development (Hrbek et al., 1973). The duration of the early negative component decreases progressively with age, and its latencies to onset and to peak also follow a consistent pattern when the body length is taken into account; at the age of 8 years, the adult pattern is approached (Desmedt, Brunko, & Debecker, 1976). Lüders (1970) Tamura, Lüders, & Kuroiwa (1972) studied the effect of aging on the SSERs of adult normal subjects from 19–70 years old. They observed a slight increase of peak latencies in older subjects. Amplitude changes follow a

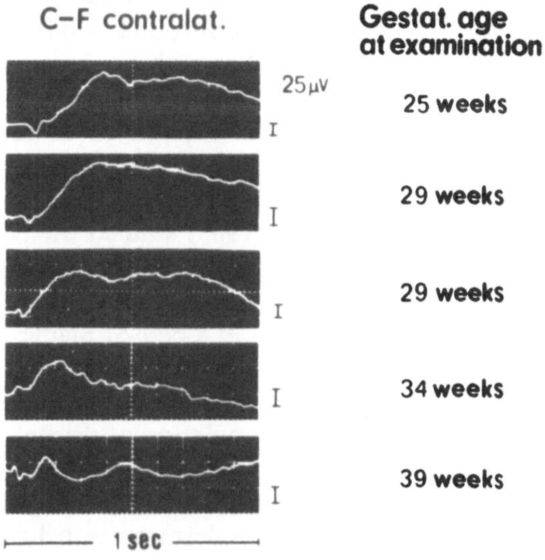

FIG. 5.2. Development of SSERs at different conceptional ages recorded over centro-frontal contralateral cortex. (From Hrbek et al., 1973.)

U-shaped curve, decreasing between 30 and 45 years of age and increasing afterwards.

C. Clinical Applications

1. Peripheral Nerve Lesions

Increased latencies, longer duration of the components, and amplitude reduction may be observed (Bergamini, Bergamasco, Fra, Gandiglio, Mombelli, & Mutani, 1965; Desmedt et al., 1966; Giblin, 1964; Kondo, 1977) with a clear relation between the severity of the sensory loss and the degree of alteration. Halliday (1967) emphasized that amplitude, latency, and waveform are independently affected and that these independent changes may reflect the relative amount of conduction delay and temporal dispersion of the sensory volley. In the Carpal tunnel syndrome, the volley may remain well synchronized but is delayed by the lesions, whereas in polyneuritic lesions, there is a desynchronization of the volley (Halliday, 1975c).

2. Spinal Lesions

Halliday and Wakefield (1963) clearly demonstrated that delayed and/or reduced amplitude of SSERs were observed only in patients with impairment of joint position sense. Similar findings were also reported by Giblin (1964), Bergamini, Bergamasco, Fra, Gandiglio, Mombelli, & Mutani, (1966a) and Kondo (1977). No abnormalities in the SSERs to electrical nerve stimulation have been found in patients with alterations of pain and temperature sensations but with preserved joint position sense, nor in patients after spinal tractotomy (Larson et al., 1966a). Lesions of the dorsal column produced similar alterations of the SSERs as those observed in peripheral neuropathy, with persistence of abnormal SSERs after clinical recovery (Halliday & Wakefield, 1963). Namerow (1968) and Baker, Larson, Sances, & White (1968) studied the SSERs in patients with MS and reported a great incidence of abnormal responses in those patients with impairment of joint position sense and vibration sensibility. Independence of the spinal sensory fibers in a pair of Siamese twins joined by lumbo-sacral spinal column fusion was demonstrated by recording the SSERs to popliteal nerve stimulation of each twin (Bergamini et al., 1966a).

SSERs to electrical stimulation of dermal segments have proved useful in the detection of lesions of the dorsal column. By this method, SSERs of lower amplitude, increased latency, or absence of response may be observed in the stimulation of the dermatome below the spinal compression, even when the patients do not yet have sensory impairment (Baust & Jörg, 1974, 1977). Kondo (1977) reported that by stimulation of the median, ulnar, femoral, and peroneal nerves, it is possible to detect the level of the spinal-cord lesion. However, Katz, Blackburn, Perot, & Lam (1978) described that in spinal transection below C7, the SSERs to median or radial nerve stimulation were affected in the latency range from 40–60 msec, suggesting that SSERs are not solely determined by the activation of the fibers entering the spinal cord and the relay nuclei, but also reflect more complex interactions within the central nervous system. SSERs have also been utilized to monitor spinal-cord function in the operating room in individuals undergoing laminectomy for removal of spinal-cord tumors or on individuals undergoing correction of spinal-column curvature (Allen & Starr, 1977). As we see later in this chapter, the evoked spinal-cord responses also seem to be a valuable procedure for the study of spinal lesions.

3. *Brain-Stem and Thalamic Lesions*

In vascular lesions with a Wallenberg or Weber syndrome, no significant abnormalities of the SSERs are observed. But, in patients with a locked-in syndrome, the SSERs are depressed, with prolonged latencies (Noel & Desmedt, 1975; see Fig. 5.3). Nakanishi et al. (1978) described the absence of N15 to median nerve stimulation in patients with brain-stem lesions, whereas it was present in patients with thalamic lesions. Lesions of the VL thalamic nucleus produced no alterations of the early components of the SSERs (Domino et al., 1965), but a decrease in amplitude of P180 (Velasco et al., 1975). When the VPL thalamic nucleus was affected, the earlier cortical components N19 and P24 were particularly altered, although all components were reduced if the lesion was large (Domino et al., 1965). Patients

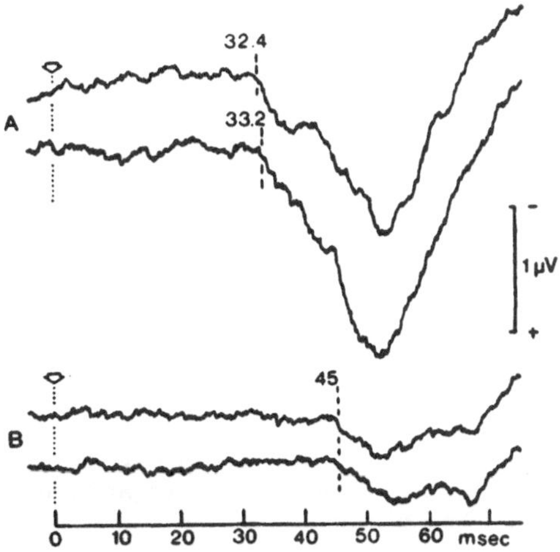

FIG. 5.3. SSERs to electrical stimulation of the right (A) and left (B) median nerves at the wrist in a patient with a "locked-in" syndrome. Two separate trials on the same day show the consistency of the potential. (From Noel & Desmedt, 1975.)

with a cerebrovascular accident and thalamic syndrome had a reduced voltage and increased latency of the SSER in the affected side (Fig. 5.4).

4. Cerebral Lesions

In relation to cerebral lesions, A. M. Halliday (1975c) remarks that the main differences, when compared with lesions of the afferent pathway, are the absence of latency changes and the incidence of cases in which abnormal SSERs and impaired position sense could not be correlated. Liberson (1966) studied 17 patients in which a right hemiplegia and aphasia appeared 4 months before the study. He observed a striking relation between the degree of alteration of the SSER and the severity of the aphasia, although responses to flash and click stimulation recorded in the same derivations were not affected. Larson, Sances, and Baker (1966b) also studied patients with strokes in which the alteration of the SSERs were not related to sensory loss. They followed the cases over 1–10 months, observing that the alterations of the SSER remained even in the presence of clinical improvement. Branston and Symon (1974) described a linear relationship between the rate of depression of the SSERs and residual blood flow in baboons. Kaplan (1978) found decreased amplitude of the SSERs over the affected hemisphere in patients with strokes.

Kato, Lüders, Miyoshi, & Kuroiwa (1970) observed alterations of the SSERs in 29 out of 69 cases with brain lesions. The abnormal response was

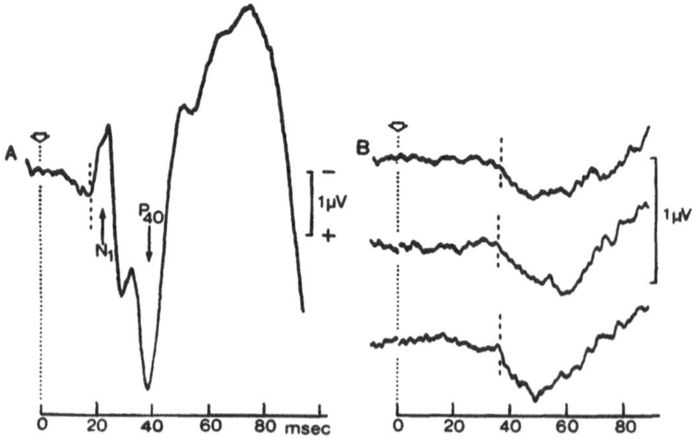

FIG. 5.4. SSERs evoked by electrical stimulation (arrow) of the right (A) and left (B) median nerves at the wrist, in a patient with a right thalamic lesion. Three separate trials performed in the same day are shown in (B). The vertical interrupted lines indicate the onset latency of the cerebral potentials. N1 early surface negative component is present in (A) but not in (B). (From Noel & Desmedt, 1975.)

highly correlated with injuries of the somatosensory pathway. Components P14 and N18 were abnormal only when an impairment of position sense was present. The other components were more generally affected by lesions of the parietal lobe, which is in agreement with previous findings of Laget, Mano, & Houdart (1967). Williamson et al. (1970) studied patients with infarctions in the territory of the middle cerebral artery or unilateral infiltrating neoplasms. They observed a good correlation between the SSER and the clinical sensory loss. Kuroiwa, Kato, & Umezaki (1968), in a study of agnostic syndromes, observed that SSERs were greatly depressed in Gerstman's syndrome as well as in patients with hemy-palesthesia, being normal in visuospatial agnosia. A decrease in amplitude of P180 has been observed in cerebrovascular lesions (Velasco, Velasco, Lombardo, & Lombardo, 1977), and in Parkinsonian patients with akinesia (Velasco & Velasco, 1975). Shibasaki, Yamashita, & Tsuji (1977a) developed diagnostic criteria based on SSER measurements that seem to be very powerful in the detection of cerebral lesions. These are discussed in Chapter 13.

The first studies in epileptics were reported by Dawson (1947a, 1947b). He found higher amplitudes of the SSERs in a patient with myoclonic epilepsy. Similar observations have been reported by A. M. Halliday (1965, 1967); Lüders, Miyoshi, & Kuroiwa (1972); Foit & Cigánek (1975), and Hirose & Hishikawa (1977) in the same type of patients, and by Broughton et al. (1967) and Vitová and Faladová (1975b) in photosensitive epileptics. However, no differences in amplitude have been reported between normal subjects and centrencephalic epileptics (Bacia & Reid, 1965). Injection of diazepam produces reduction of amplitude of VERs and SSERs in photosensitive epileptics (Broughton, Meier-Ewert, & Ebe, 1966). In Jacksonian epilepsy, the SSERs may be of higher amplitude (Fig. 5.5) or absent on the side of the tumor (Fig. 5.6), as has been shown by Düsseldorf (1975). In a group of patients with different types of myoclonus, Shibasaki, Tamashita, & Kuroiwa (1977b) studied the SSERs and the Motor Potentials. In the Ramsay Hunt syndrome, they found an increase of amplitude of SSERs, with the absence of the readiness potentials. In myoclonic epileptics, only an increase of amplitude of the SSER was observed, whereas no abnormalities were found in essential myoclonus. Similar findings were previously described by Halliday & Halliday (1970).

In all infants and children with motor disabilities due to various causes (anoxia at birth, preterm birth, and gran mal states), differences between the SSERs recorded from the two hemispheres were observed. Abnormalities were recorded in the contralateral hemisphere to the side of the body affected (Laget, Salbreux, Raimbault, D'Allest, & Mariani, 1976). In full-term and preterm newborn infants who were treated for perinatal asphyxia, 65 percent had a low amplitude of the SSER and absence of the primary initial components (see Fig. 5.7, Hrbek et al., 1977).

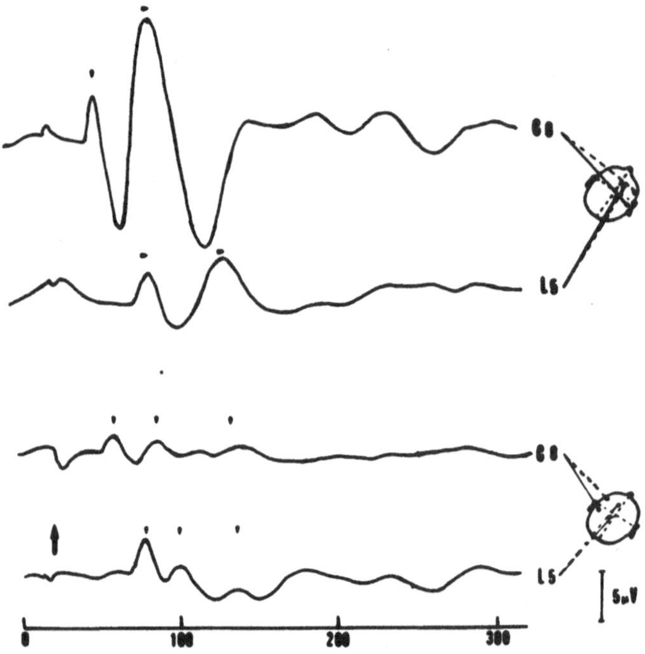

FIG. 5.5. SSERs to left (*top*) and right (*bottom*) median nerve stimulation in a patient with Jacksonian attacks on the left side. A right centro-parietal solitary metastasis was found. The EEG and carotid arteriography were normal. The scintigraphy showed a discrete parietal-median accumulation. (From Düsseldorf, 1975.)

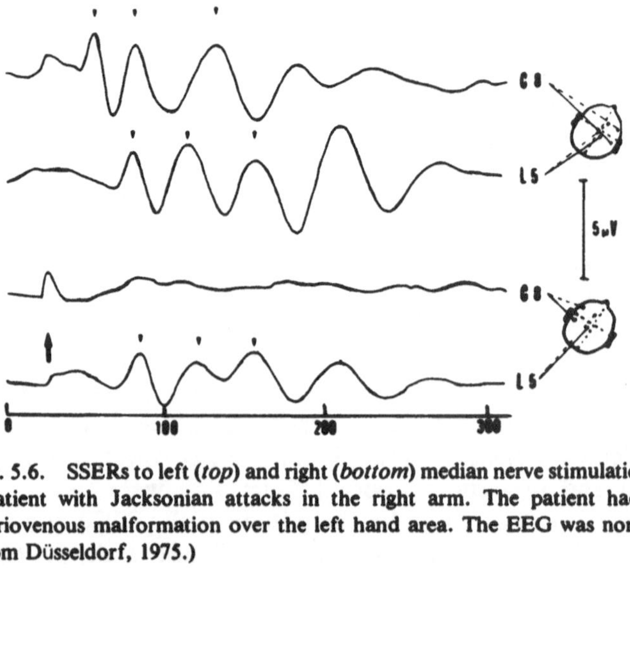

FIG. 5.6. SSERs to left (*top*) and right (*bottom*) median nerve stimulation in a patient with Jacksonian attacks in the right arm. The patient had an arteriovenous malformation over the left hand area. The EEG was normal. (From Düsseldorf, 1975.)

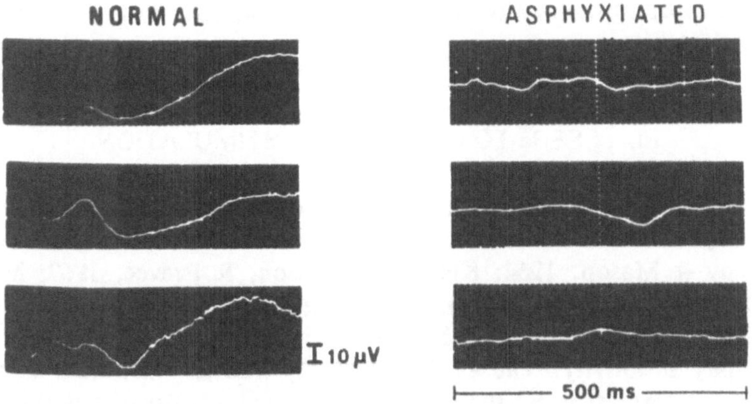

FIG. 5.7. SSERs recorded in contralateral CF leads to stimulation of the median nerves in three normal and three severely asphyxiated newborn infants. (From Hrbek et al., 1977.)

Abnormal SSERs have been also reported in hepatolenticular degeneration (Lüders, Kato, & Kuroiwa, 1969; Samland, Przuntek, & Dommasch, 1976), in hyperthyroidism (Takahashi & Fujitani, 1970), and in renal insufficiency (Lewis et al., 1978). In a group of schizophrenic patients, Shagass et al. (1977) observed reduced amplitude of the components, after 100 msec, in the VERs, AERs, and SSERs. Increased negativity of the N60 component of the SSER was observed in chronic paranoids when compared with other patient subtypes. Saletu, Saletu, Itil, & Simeon (1975) also reported decreased amplitudes of long latency components in schizophrenic children.

II. SSER EXCITABILITY CYCLE

The stimulation of the peripheral nerves with a pair of electrical stimuli separated by different intervals produces changes in the second response that are related to the excitability of the system, and are described by the ratio of the amplitudes of the responses. The excitability cycle has an initial return to full responsiveness by 20 msec, followed by a phase of reduced responsiveness and then by a second phase of full recovery or supernormal excitability, peaking at 120 msec, followed by a return to normal excitability around 200 msec. Psychiatric patients with personality disorders, psychiatric depression, or schizophrenia have similar depressed recovery curves, particularly in the early phase up to 20 msec. A clear relationship has been demonstrated between the degree of abnormality of the recovery response and the clinical improvement of psychotic depressed subjects (for a review, see Shagass, 1972). In epileptic patients, the SSER excitability cycle shows a short refractory period, which also happens with the visual excitability cycle.

III. SSERs TO MECHANICAL STIMULATION

Following mechanical taps to the fingers, the SSERs are similar to those obtained by electrical stimulation, but they have slightly longer latencies (Halliday & Mason, 1964; Kjellman, Larsson, & Prevec, 1967; Meijes, 1969). Larsson & Prevec (1970), by tapping the thenar eminence, obtained latencies of 33 and 55 msec for the two positive waves and 42 msec for the intermediary negativity. The earlier positivity had its maximum over the primary sensory area, but the later positivity had a wider distribution with its maximum generally at vertex. Latencies of the early positivity vary systematically with the part of the body stimulated, as in the case of the response to electrical stimulation, but the later positivity does not have the same consistent dependence on the stimulating site. SSERs to tendon taps are also similar to those evoked by electrical stimulation, those produced by stimulation of the lower extremities being simpler and of longer latency than those evoked by stimulation of the upper extremities (Gantchev & Yankov, 1974; Hrbkova, 1969). Evoked responses accompanying monosynaptic reflex to mechanical stimulation of muscles and tendons were studied in newborn babies by Hrbek, Hrbkova, & Lenard (1968, 1969). An example is shown in Fig. 5.8. The responses were more clearly seen in the contralateral Rolandic area, latencies becoming shorter during the neonatal period. These responses were dependent on the behavioral state. In regular sleep, the late components were larger, whereas in REM sleep, they became smaller and the early components achieved greater prominence.

Clinical applications of SSERs to mechanical stimulation seem to be as reliable as those produced by electrical stimulation. Hrbkova (1969) described an amplitude increase of these responses in the place of the epileptogenic focus, as well as a depression of the responses in unilateral brain lesions. Prevec & Butinar (1977) also found the absence of some components and increased latencies in MS patients. An extremely interesting result was obtained by DeMarco & Tassinari (1977) in the study of SSERs to a single Achilles tendon percussion in 8000 unselected children: 105 of these children had an extremely high amplitude response. In this group, 22 were already epileptic, and in 15 children of the remaining 83 that were followed up for several years, clinical signs of epilepsy appeared later.

SSERs to tendon taps have been related to a proprioceptive origin. However, in patients with dissociated sensory losses due to lesions of the spinal cord, mechanical stimulation with taps, pinpricks, and touch stimuli produced SSERs that had features different from those obtained by elec-

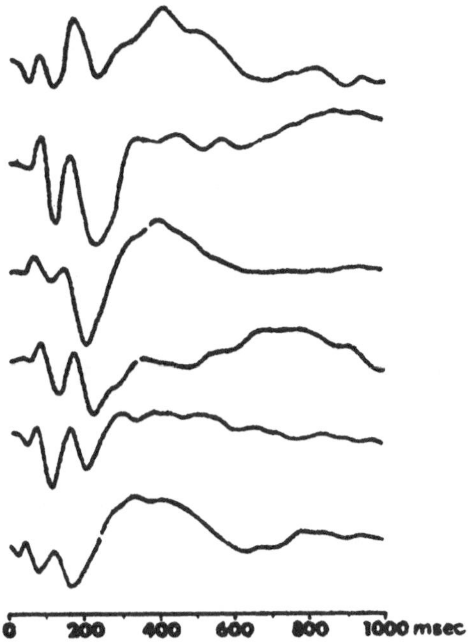

FIG. 5.8. Responses to tapping the biceps tendon in six different children. The first five (from top downward) are newborns; the lowest is from a 5-week-old infant. Contralateral CF leads. Irregular sleep. 50 responses were averaged. (From Hrbek et al., 1968.)

trical stimulation. Nakanishi, Shimada, and Toyokura (1974) studied 33 young, healthy adults and 61 patients with neurological disorders. Alterations of the SSERs to mechanical stimulation were observed in seven out of eight patients with impaired pain–temperature and tactile sensations but preserved joint position sense. In a patient with such a dissociated sensory loss, the SSERs were elicited by electrical stimulation, but no response was obtained by mechanical stimulation of the affected side. Conversely, in a patient with loss of joint position sense and preserved touch and position sensations, cortical evoked potentials were produced by pinprick stimulation, but not by electrical stimulation. *Such findings suggest that the afferent impulses responsible for the SSERs to mechanical stimulation of the fingers travel by the ventrolateral tracts.* More information is needed to support this statement, but if it is true, both types of stimuli would be complementary in the study of the integrity of the somatic sensory pathways.

IV. SSERs TO PAINFUL STIMULATION

Chatrian, Canfield, Knauss, & Lettich (1975) described the SSERs to electrical stimulation of the tooth pulp, which produced a subjective sensation of sharp pain. They found clearly evoked responses over the scalp with two concurrent sequences of events, one maximal in midline areas and the other over lower postcentral regions, thus demonstrating electrophysiologically the existence of a representation of tooth pain sensation in the somatosensory cortex of man. The midline events have their sources in parasagittal locations anterior to the central sulcus, which may represent activation of the anterior part of the cingulate gyrus. These ERs represent the first objective, measurable, nonverbally mediated sign of central events associated with the perception of acute experimental pain in man.

Drechsler, Wickboldt, Neuhanser, & Miltner (1977) recorded the SSERs to the electrical stimulation of the V nerve in a group of volunteers and in a group of patients with trigeminal neuralgia before and after thermocoagulation of the ganglion Gasseri. In healthy subjects, they found the following components: N5, P9, N13, P23, N34, P44, N100, N180. The first wave was related to the ganglion response. Before the intervention, the patients showed increased latencies of N5, P9, and N13, and decreased amplitudes of all the components. After intervention, N5 and P9 disappeared and amplitudes and latencies of P13 to N100 were normalized. Component N180 was not observed before or after intervention. ERs to noxious thermal stimuli induced by brief pulses of laser-emitted radiant heat were composed of a late negative–positive component (130–160 msec), which correlated in latency with the stimulus intensity and in amplitude with subjective sensation. This response was larger at the vertex (Carmon, Mor, & Goldberg, 1976).

V. SPINAL-CORD EVOKED RESPONSES (SCERs)

A. General Characteristics

The first waves of the SSERs to electrical stimulation recorded at the scalp are the reflection of the activation of peripheral nerves, dorsal roots, dorsal column, and postsynaptic activation of dorsal nuclei. These components may be recorded in the spinal cord, using intrathecal electrodes (Ertekin, 1976) or electrodes introduced in the epidural space (Shimoji, Higashi, & Kano, 1971), or directly situated on the skin surface over the spine (Cracco, 1973). With intrathecal recordings from lower cervical and lower thoracic intervertebral levels to the stimulation of the median, ulnar, and posterior tibial nerves, Ertekin (1976) showed that the evoked responses varied in shape and size depending on the position of the electrode. Behind the cord dorsum and around the midline, the segmental evoked response was composed of fast, sharp early, and slow late components. This was called a CD potential and its first component was related to the activity of the ascending dorsal funiculus fibers. When the tip of the intrathecal electrode was lateral to the midline within the vertebral canal, a triphasic compound response of very high amplitude, related to activity of the spinal roots, was observed. If the electrode tip portion was close to the posterior horn of the spinal gray matter, a very small triphasic spike and two later components were related to the pre- and postsynaptic activity of the horizontally oriented fibers within the segmental gray matter of the posterior horn. Ertekin (1978) made a comparison of the human SCERs recorded by the intrathecal, epidural, and surface recordings. The early sharp component of triphasic shape and short duration was observed in the three recordings, but with an amplitude in the subdural of one-third, and in the cutaneous recordings of one-tenth, of that observed in the intrathecal responses.

With electrodes introduced into the posterior epidural space and recording in the same or adjacent spinal segment from which the stimulated nerves originated, Shimoji, Matsuki, & Shimizu (1977) found an initial positive spike (P1) and subsequent slow negative (N1)–positive (P2) potentials in cervical and lower thoracic regions. This response was clearly elicited by the stimulation of the common peroneal nerve, but was not elicited by even a strong stimulation of the fifth toe. SSERs over the scalp were clearly demonstrated to both types of stimulus. These results are contradictory to those of Matthews, Beauchamp, and Small (1974) and Kopec & Edelwejn (1978), who recorded clear spinal responses with surface electrodes to the stimulation of the fingers. A series of negative-going peaks recorded on the surface, to the electrical stimulation of the median nerve, have been described by Matthews et al. (1974), S. J. Jones (1977), and Small & Jones (1977). The latter authors designated the series of negative-going peaks recorded over the cervical spinal cord to median nerve stimulation as N9, N11, N13, and N14.

Table 5.1 shows the mean latency values and their standard deviations and the latency range of the different components of the simultaneous evoked responses to median nerve stimulation at the scalp in C_3 and C_4 (10-20 system) and over the spinal cord at C2 and C7 levels using F_z as reference. Hume & Cant (1978) found that peak latency of N20 at the scalp and N14 from the neck have a positive correlation with arm length and height. However, the difference in latency between these components was independent of arm length and can be used to measure conduction velocity in the central somatosensory pathway in man. Cracco & Cracco (1976) provided evidence that suggests that uncontaminated SCERs to median nerve stimulation are difficult to record from the surface in cervical leads when the reference electrode is placed on the scalp, nose, or ear, because these sites will record the far-field potentials whose latencies are similar to those of cervical spinal responses (Fig. 5.9).

Following the stimulation of the posterior tibial nerve at the ankle, the surface evoked responses varied in form depending on the position of the active and reference electrodes. Using T6 as reference, at the L4 and S1

TABLE 5.1[a]
Latencies of Evoked Responses to Median Nerve Stimulation[b]

A. *At the scalp* (C_3 and C_4 vs F_z)

Peak	*X*	*SD*	*Range*
P15	15.4	1.0	13.4–18.2
N20	19.4	1.1	17.2–22.0
P20	22.2	1.0	20.2–24.4
N25	24.1	1.6	21.5–28.0
P25	26.9	1.5	25.1–31.5
N35	33.6	2.4	26.8–40.5
P45	43.6	3.9	35.8–54.2
N55	54.9	2.6	49.9–59.1

B. *At the spinal level*

	C2			C7		
Peak	*X*	*SD*	*Range*	*X*	*SD*	*Range*
N10	9.5	.7	8.1–11.3	9.4	.6	7.8–10.3
P10	10.5	.7	9.1–12.0	10.6	.6	10.6–11.1
N12	—	—	—	11.7	.7	10.5–12.9
P12	—	—	—	12.3	.7	10.6–13.4
N14	13.8	.9	12.0–15.6	13.7	.8	11.7–15.4
P20	18.2	1.0	16.0–20.0	18.1	1.1	16.3–20.4
N20	19.5	1.2	19.6–22.1	19.6	1.3	17.0–22.1
P25	23.7	2.6	19.8–31.5	24.1	3.2	18.5–31.5

[a] From Hume and Cant (1978).
[b] Values are given in milliseconds.

levels, the response presents two peaks: a dominant early negative wave with approximately 11 msec of latency and a subsequent wave with 15 msec of latency. The first component has characteristics that suggest that it represents neural activity ascending in the dorsal roots of the cauda equina. The second main negative deflection may represent the dromic and antidromic discharges in the ventral roots (a reflexly elicited volley), with a possible contribution from slow fibers in the dorsal roots (Delbeke, McComas, & Kopec, 1978; Dimitrijevic, Larssen, Lehmkuhl, & Sherwood, 1978). Jones & Small (1978) recorded the SCERs from C2 to L4 using various references (midfrontal, sacrum, contralateral ankle). They observed a negative-going potential (N23) of maximum amplitude from T12 to L2 and a progressive reduction in amplitude caudally and rostrally. The lumbar potential had a latency of 31 msec between C2 and T3 and of 40 msec at the

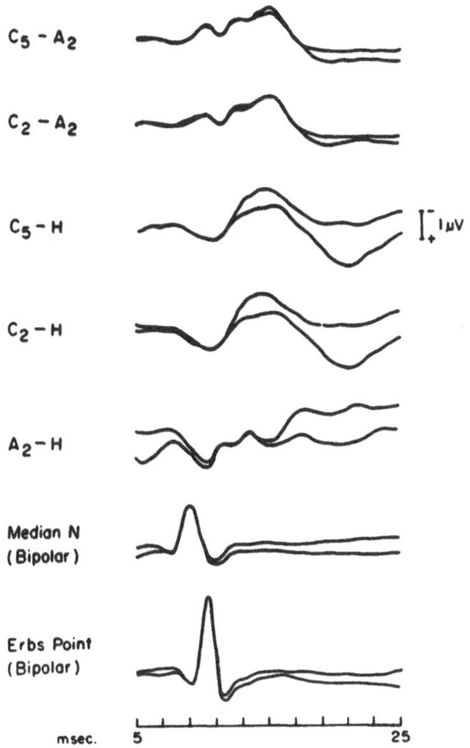

FIG. 5.9. Right median nerve evoked potentials recorded over the fifth and second cervical spines in ear and hand (H) dorsum reference recordings. Each recording summated 1024 or 2048 responses. Two recordings are superimposed in each trace. In hand-reference recordings, the cervical response consists of an initially positive triphasic potential. In cervical–ear leads, it consists of small upward deflection that is bilobed. The first upward deflection is similar in latency to the first positive potential recorded from the ear and cervical spine in hand-reference leads. The initial portion of the second upward deflection recorded in cervical–ear leads is similar in latency to the second positive potential recorded from the ear in the hand-reference lead. The entire second upward deflection is similar in latency to the negative potential recorded in cervical–hand leads. The latency of onset of the first positive potential recorded from the ear is similar to that of the negative potential recorded over the stimulated median nerve just proximal to the axilla (*second trace for bottom*) and less than that of the negative potential recorded over the brachial plexus (*bottom trace*). (From Cracco & Cracco, 1976.)

scalp. The negative potential recorded in cervical regions was very consistent with midfrontal reference, but was less well seen with other references. This suggests that it may be due to a positive component appearing at the midfrontal region, with a possible additional negative potential recorded over cervical spine. Based on the study of other mammals, Delbeke et al. (1978) interpreted the different waves observed in the major negative component at T12 as follows: The first notch may correspond with the dorsal column (DC) activation, the next one (N_{1a} from Austin & McCouch, 1955) may be due to activity in the termination of sensory fibers within the dorsal horn, and the remainder of the major negative component may be related to the depolarization of internuncial neurons and relay cells within the dorsal horn. A long positive wave following this major negative component (P2 of

Shimoji et al., 1977) may correspond to the primary afferent depolarization (Eccles, Kostyuk, & Schmidt, 1962) responsible for presynaptic inhibition.

The forementioned results demonstrate that with surface recording, it is possible to obtain technically satisfactory SCERs. Because this recording method is harmless, its advantages in comparison with intrathecal and epidural recordings are obvious.

B. Clinical Applications

SCERs seem to be very useful in the study of spinal-cord lesions. Shimoji, Kano, Morioka, & Ikezono (1973), using the epidural recording technique, reported an absence of responses to ulnar and posterior tibial nerves at C2 level in a quadriplegic patient. Using the same procedure, Caccia, Ubialli, & Andreussi (1976) studied a group of patients with radicular lesions and with spinal-cord lesions, comparing the potential from the healthy side with that from the impaired limb in the cases of unilateral root lesions. They concluded that the amplitude of the SCERs was the only parameter significantly changed on the side of the radicular impairment at both the cervical and thoracic levels, whereas the propagation velocity of the response of the still excitable fibers (probably cutaneous) was never found to change significantly. In massive lesions of the spinal cord (acute transverse myelitis), the SCERs were absent above the lesion, whereas in cases with extrinsic compression of the spinal cord (Pott's disease), the SCERs recorded above were present but of markedly lower amplitude. Ertekin (1977) described absent responses or responses with decreased amplitude and longer latencies in patients with lesions of the first sensory neuron or when the posterior funiculus was involved. No changes were observed in the SCERs in lesions of the anterior horns and/or motor roots. Frankel, El-Negamy, & Sedgwick (1978) found, in complete lesions of the lumbar cord, the absence of the major negative component after stimulation of the posterior tibial nerve, and no response in cauda equina lesions. In MS patients, Small, Beauchamp, & Matthews (1977) reported increased latencies and the absence of any potential in the SCERs to median nerve stimulation in 40 percent of patients with purely ocular manifestations and in 89 percent of the severely disabled MS patients, for an overall accuracy of 75 percent. In those cases with no clinical signs of sensory loss in the upper limb, 70 percent had abnormal SCERs. Similar results have been described by McInnes (1978).

VI. SUMMARY

SSERs evoked by percutaneous electrical stimulation of the peripheral nerves, fingers, or toes, have shown to be very useful in the evaluation of the functional and anatomical integrity of the afferent lemniscal pathway, even when the patients do not yet have sensory impairment. The early waves may be recorded at the scalp (far-field potentials) or over the spinal cord. The first recordable neural activity reflects the activation of the peripheral afferent fibers. Subsequent waves have been related to the activation of dorsal column, dorsal nuclei, thalamus, thalamo–cortical radiations, and primary somatosensory cortex. Long latency components show more variability and arise both from the primary somatosensory and association areas.

There is a clear relation between SSER alterations and vibration and position sense impairment in those patients with lesions of the afferent pathway. However, patients with cerebral lesions may have abnormal SSERs, even without sensory impairment.

Some evidence suggests that mechanical stimulation to the fingers produces SSERs that reflect the activation of the ventrolateral spinothalamic tract. If this is so, both types of stimuli would be complementary in the evaluation of the integrity of the somatic sensory pathway.

It has been demonstrated that with surface recordings, it is possible to obtain technically satisfactory recordings of the spinal-cord evoked responses. Detailed analysis of these responses produced by stimulation of different peripheral nerves has demonstrated that they are very useful in the assessment of spinal-cord lesions that affect the afferent sensory pathway.

In Chapter 13, some neurometric procedures based on the analysis of the SSERs are discussed.

6 Other Event-Related Potentials

I. CONTINGENT NEGATIVE VARIATION (CNV)

A. General Characteristics

Using the following paradigm—first, a conditional signal (S1), such as a click, a constant delay of 1 second or more, and then a second or imperative stimulus (S2), such as a series of repetitive flashes to which the subject responded by pressing a button—W.G. Walter, Cooper, Aldridge, McCallum and Winter (1964) demonstrated a slow negative potential in the interstimulus interval (see Fig. 6.1). This potential was called the Contingent Negative Variation (CNV). It was related to the psychological state of "expectancy" and therefore has sometimes been designated as "E wave" (Cohen & Walter, 1966). J. Cohen (1969), with a mastoid reference, found that its maximal amplitude was usually seen at the vertex. Weinberg and Papakostopoulos (1975), using a pattern-recognition procedure and with elimination of electro-oculogram artifacts, studied the CNV of different brain areas to determine whether they have the same characteristics. The results showed that the frontal CNV was different in form and smaller than the response recorded at the vertex, central, and parietal regions. This seemed to suggest that these differences reflected different functions of the cerebral sites with respect to the information that has to be processed. Several recent studies have also provided evidence that two distinct negative shifts contribute to the classical CNV. These components can be clearly distinguished when the S1-S2 interval is prolonged (Rohrbaugh, Syndulko, &

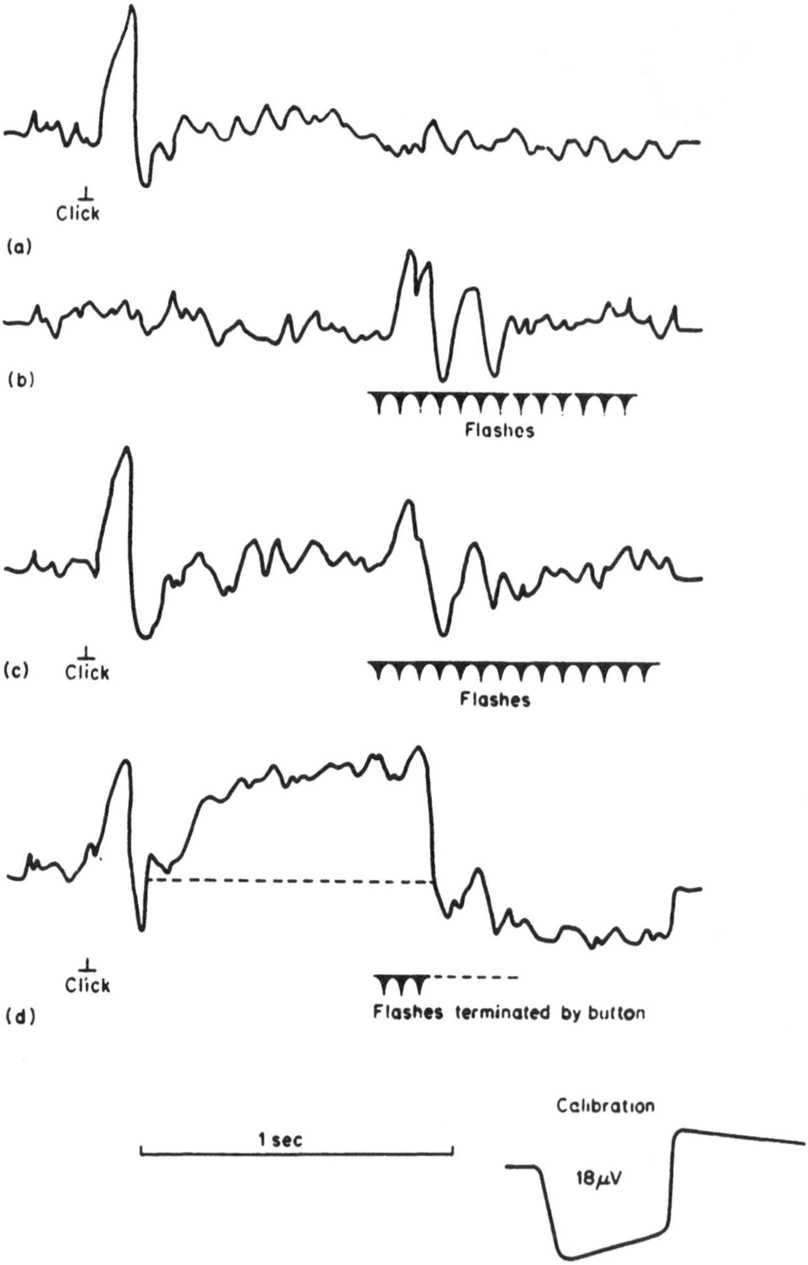

FIG. 6.1. Average of response to 12 presentations. (a) Vertex response to click alone. (b) Response to a series of flashes. (c) Response to click followed by flashes. and (d) CNV appears as slow negative wave following the click before subject presses button to stop flashes. (From Walter et al., 1964.)

Lindsley, 1976; Simson, Vaughan, & Ritter, 1977). The early component has been associated to an orienting response to S1 (Gaillard & Perdok, 1977). It reaches its peak at 400-700 msec after S1 and is maximal in the posterior frontal region with auditory stimuli; it has a parieto-occipital and a central foci after visual S1 stimulation, which suggests its generation in primary and secondary areas (Simson et al., 1977). The later component, considered either to reflect expectancy for S2 or preparation for the motor response (the readiness potential), has a predominantly central distribution, with probably generators in motor and premotor cortex.

There is a general consensus on two important aspects:

1. The CNV may be generated independently of a motor action. Cohen and Walter (1966) found CNV in a situation in which subjects expected a projected picture as the S2 with no overt response on the part of the subject, or when the subjects responded to S2 with a word that they freely associated to a word presented as S1. It does not matter whether the subject says the word aloud or merely thinks of it as an ideational response.

2. The CNV is not a single phenomenon, but a composite potential from different intracranial sources, whose distribution varies as a function of task variables and sensory modality of stimulation. Thus, tasks that permit the establishment of a preparatory motor set are characterized by shifts arising from Rolandic cortex, or "readiness potential" (Grunewald, Grunewald-Zuberbier, Netz, Sander, & Homberg, 1977; Otto & Leifer, 1973; Syndulko & Lindsley, 1977; Vaughan, 1969, 1975).

Usually, the CNV ends with the second stimulus, but in some subjects it can remain for a short period after the imperative stimulus, or drop out for about .1 sec and then resume a marked negativity, returning only gradually to a baseline within 1 or 2 seconds (Bostem, Rousseau, Degossely, & Dongier, 1967). According to Gauthier and Gottesmann (1976), the post-imperative part of the CNV may be significantly prolonged when two types of interferences are applied at the same time between S1 and S2. Hillyard (1969) observed the same phenomenon when the subject had made a correct rejection task. CNV has been related to psychological events identified as expectancy, decision (W.G. Walter, 1964b; Weinberg, Michalewski, & Koopman, 1976), motivation (Irwin, Knott, McAdam, & Rebert, 1966; McAdam, & Seales, 1969), volition (McAdam, Irwin, Rebert, & Knott, 1966), conation (Low, Borda, Frost, & Kellaway, 1966), and arousal or the physiological state of excitability (McAdam, 1969).

CNV is rather constant in normal subjects, not only from trial to trial, but from year to year. It is not fully developed until 20 years of age. Although CNV waves have been observed in very young children, these were transitory. In most children before the age of 7 to 8 years, large secondary waves that do not seem dependent on stimulus association or voluntary participation have been observed; thus, only after the age of 7 does typical

CNV begin to appear (Shagass, 1972). The amplitude of CNV partly depends on changes in parameters of stimulation, accurate perception of the stimuli, interval between the two stimuli, probability of association of both stimuli, changes in responses, individual differences, and changes in some physiological functions (J. Cohen, 1969; Low, Coats, Rettig, & McSherry, 1967; Naitoh, Johnson, & Lubin, 1971; W.G. Walter, 1965, 1975). CNV amplitude increases with a high attention level, whereas during different levels of arousal, its amplitude shows an inverse U-shape (Timsit-Berthier, Gerono, & Rousseau, 1977).

B. Clinical Applications

CNV was studied in organic cerebral diseases by McCallum and Cummins (1973). It was of lower amplitude over the cortical area corresponding to the localized lesion; the more diffuse the lesion, the more widespread was the CNV abnormality. If a localized lesion produced a diffuse clinical effect such as behavioral dysfunction, the CNV was suppressed diffusely. Lower amplitudes have also been observed in senile patients (O'Connor, 1977) and in serious mental deficits (Bergamasco, Benna, Covacich, & Gilli, 1977). Reduction of CNV on the affected side in 80% of patients with vascular diseases has been described (J. Cohen, 1975). No clear and constant asymmetries in form and amplitude of the CNV were observed in relation to the side or extent of frontal lobe lesions (Zappoli, Papini, Briani, Benvenutti, & Pasquinelli, 1975). Low and Purves (1975) reported that no CNV were recorded in patients with lesions invading or distorting the thalamus on either side. No significant changes of CNV amplitude have been found in chronic hepatic encephalopathy (Jones, Binnie, Bown, Lloyd, & Watson, 1976). Amplitude of CNV was smaller in subjects with traumatic head injuries (Rizzo, Amabile, Caporali, Spadero, Zanasi, & Morocutti, 1978).

Zimmermann and Knott (1974) compared the CNV to verbal responses in normal speakers and in stutterers. Similar vertex responses were found in both groups. However, normal subjects have a clear left dominance of the CNV in frontal regions that was not observed in stutterers.

CNV responses have been widely applied in psychiatric patients. The most striking changes, with virtually no CNV, were obtained by W.G. Walter (1970) in patients considered to have an antisocial type of psychopathic disturbance. Anxious patients, as well as schizophrenic patients, showed small CNV amplitude, but variability was greater in the latter group. The schizophrenic patients maintained a CNV reduction even during treatment and clinical improvement (Abraham & McCallum, 1977; Abraham, McCallum, Docherty, Fox, & Newton, 1974). McCallum and Walter (1968) described a significant reduction of the amplitude of CNV with distraction in patients with high anxiety.

Timsit, Koninckx, Dargent, Fontaine, and Dougier (1969) observed a great prolongation in the duration of the CNV after the imperative stimulus in the great majority of psychiatric and in one-third of neurotic patients. Reduced CNV amplitude has also been described in hyperkinetic children (Ward, 1976). Children with no ability to concentrate also have a reduced CNVs (Grunewald-Zuberbier, Grunewald, Netz, & Klenkler-Wehler, 1977).

CNV has also been used to design an objective test of the threshold of perception of a simple acoustic stimulus. A tone of adjusted intensity is delivered as S1, and a light as S2. A CNV is generated between both stimuli if the subject perceives the tone, but if not, the CNV does not appear (see Fig. 6.2). Prevec, Lokar, and Cernelc (1974) described that acoustic stimuli near threshold frequently produced a CNV of higher amplitude than those following stronger stimuli. They claimed that the essential advantage of CNV audiometry over ERA is that it was possible to determine the threshold of subjective perception of an acoustic stimulus. However, CNV audiometry cannot be used in small children or infants, because CNV is not reliable at that age. Brix (1975) used the CNV as a proof of concept

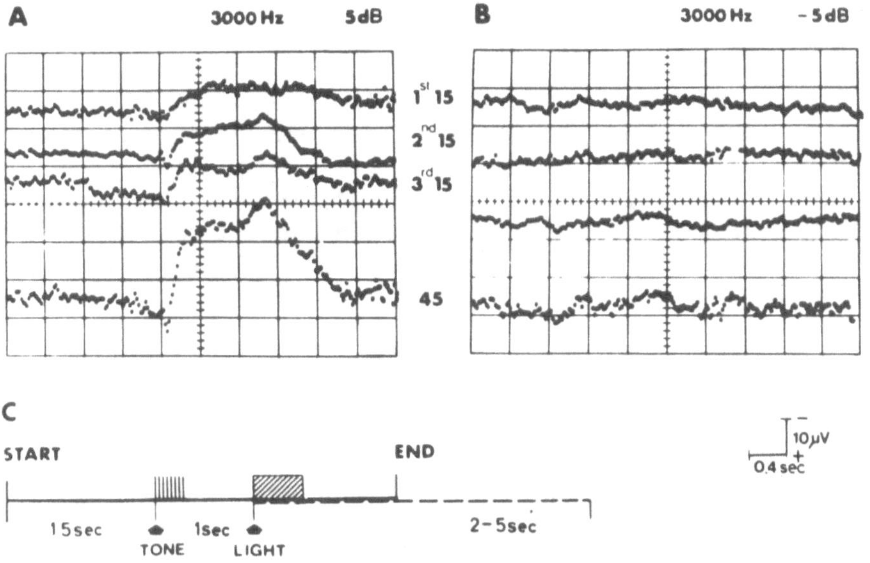

FIG. 6.2. (A) The CNV generated when an acoustical stimulus of 3000 Hz and 5 dB was perceived. The *upper three traces* represent summated consecutive series of 15 responses whereas the *bottom trace* was obtained by summation of all 45 responses. (B) The acoustical stimulus of 3000 Hz and minus 5 dB was not perceived and the CNV was not generated. The traces were obtained as in A. (C) The sequence of analysis and stimuli used to record the CNV. (From Prevec et al., 1974.)

discrimination in aphasic patients. The second imperative stimulus is made dependent on the concept of the word that is given as S1 (objective speech audiometry).

II. THE MOTOR POTENTIALS

A. General Characteristics

Scalp potentials that occur before and immediately following the onset of motor activity have been investigated by recording the EEG in one track of a multitrack recorder, recording a signal synchronous with the onset of muscle activity on another track, and averaging backward and forward off-line. Using this method, Kornhuber and Deecke (1964, 1965), Vaughan, Costa, Gilden, and Schimmel (1965), and Gilden, Vaughan, and Costa (1966) described the cortical potentials antecedent to the onset of movements, or motor potentials (MPs). Similar MPs have also been found to precede phonation (Ertl & Schafer, 1967; Schafer, 1967) and voluntary eye movements (Barlow & Ciganek, 1969; Becker, Hoenne, Iwase, & Kornhuber, 1972).

Although MPs vary substantially from person to person and in different movements executed by the same subject, the following distinct components, associated with movements of the extremities, tongue, and face, can be generally defined: (1) a slow negative shift that begins approximately 1 second before the onset of contraction. This is the readiness potential (Bereitschaftspotential or RP) of Kornhuber and Deecke (1965) or N1 wave; (2) the premotion positivity (P1), a small sharp potential that begins 50 to 150 msec before the onset of movement; (3) a sharp longer negative deflection or motor potential (N2); and (4) a final large positive wave (P2), which usually begins shortly after the onset of contraction, but which may sometimes precede it (Deecke, Scheid, & Kornhuber, 1968), and which is included in the term "motor potential."

Direct recording on the cortical areas has clarified the origin of these waves. N1 or RP is recorded in contralateral precentral and central areas; N2 is predominantly contralateral in precentral cortex, related to the specific area of the muscles involved; P2 is also predominantly contralateral to the movement in pre- and postcentral gyrus (Arezzo & Vaughan, 1975; Groll-Knapp, Ganglberger, & Maider, 1977; Papakostopoulos, Cooper, & Crow, 1975). A marked positive shift in the frontopolar and prefrontal cortical region and in the nucleus medialis thalami has also been reported (Groll-Knapp et al., 1977). An analysis of the time relationships of the voluntary movement and slow potentials led these authors to suggest that decision and design of movement is started in the thalamic-prefrontal system. From there, a motor RP is initiated in premotor cortex and subcortical structures.

Kutas and Donchin (1977) observed that, in right-handed subjects, N1 was larger over the hemisphere contralateral to the responding hand. In left-handed subjects, there was clear contralateral dominance with the right-hand movements and very little dominance when responding with the left. The mean time interval between the onset of the RP and the onset of motor activity is shorter for activation of the right hand than for the activation of the left hand (Baba, Asano, Nakamura, & Orimoto, 1976/77). The RP amplitude is larger in healthy right-handed men (Papakostopoulos, 1978). During sustained contraction, a prolonged positive shift has been observed at central and postcentral recording sites (Otto & Benignus, 1974). The P1 component is discernible in the majority of cases, dominant on the cerebral hemisphere ipsilateral to the contracting muscles; with bilateral simultaneous movements, P1 is not observed in any subject. Based on these results, Shibasaki and Kato (1975) proposed that P1 is related to an inhibition of imitative movement of the opposite hand (mirror movement).

In the previous section, the relationship between the CNV and the RP was discussed. It was stated that during the CNV paradigm, all tasks that require the establishment of a preparatory motor set were characterized by an RP, as part of the CNV. The phasic potentials (positive and negative) that follow the RP were interpreted by Gilden et al. (1966) as the corticospinal discharge immediately preceding the motor contraction, based on the fact that the interval between these cortical potentials and the muscular activity varies depending on the length of the neural pathway between the brain and the contracting muscles. A different interpretation of the N2 component has been made by Papakostopoulos et al. (1975). They considered this component as a signal of reafferent activity resulting from a movement. Shibasaki and Kato (1975) also considered that N2 might not reflect activation of the corticospinal pathway, because, in most cases, N2 has its onset after the start of muscle contraction. However, Vaughan (1975) emphasizes that the functional significance of the late components need to be elucidated, because it is questionable whether they represent a kinesthetic feedback generated by muscular contraction because deafferentation of the extremities failed to alter the MP configuration in monkeys.

B. Clinical Applications

Shibasaki (1975) and Shibasaki and Kuroiwa (1977) have made an important contribution to the application of MPs to the study of neurological patients. In 80% of the cases with unilateral cerebral lesions of various etiologies, abnormal MPs were found. The most common observation was a decrease in amplitude of N1 on the affected hemisphere (see Fig. 6.3), although the absence of this component in the injured side, or an increase in amplitude on the affected side, were found in a small group of patients. The MP abnormalities were observed in patients with or without hand weakness, and with or without pyramidal signs.

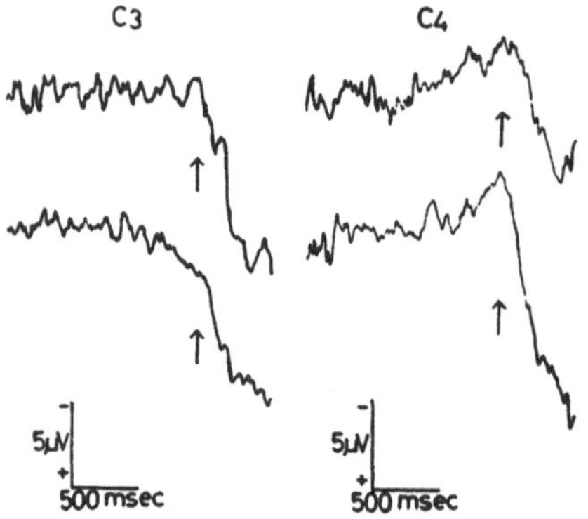

FIG. 6.3. Average cortical potentials (averaging of 200 samples) associated with right fist clenching (*upper tracings*) and with left fist clenching (*lower tracings*) in a 64-year-old woman with glioblastoma in the hand sensory-motor area of the left hemisphere. There is no negative component recognizable on the left central region (C_3). Arrows indicate the start of muscle contraction. (From Shibasaki, 1975.)

Shibasaki and Kuroiwa (1977) also observed the absence or depression of the RP in 62% of patients with central hemispheric lesions, in 90% of Parkinsonian patients, and in 58% of patients with cerebellar ataxia. In cases of cerebellar ataxia without myoclonus, the RP was normal. In cases of midbrain cerebrovascular lesions, 75% of the patients showed depression of the RP. The RP may be absent in midbrain or thalamic lesions. In a case with ataxia and right midbrain cerebrovascular accident, the RP was not obtained with movement of the right hand, whereas it was normal during left-hand movement. These authors also observed that the RP is not observed during the first 10 days immediately after thalamotomy, but in the next 6 months, it is completely recovered. Infarcts of sensory thalamus did not affect the RP, whereas more widespread thalamic tumors produced disorganized RP. Baba et al. (1976/77) also reported that after stereotactic thalamotomy, the RP remains without great changes, but that in a patient with a vascular lesion and a thalamic syndrome, the RP was absent on the affected side. Another interesting result is that MPs are also affected in psychiatric patients without motor dysfunction (Delaunoy, Gerono, & Rousseau, 1977).

The forementioned results opened a new field of exploration for the application of the MP, which is the electrophysiological representation of one of the efferent cerebral functions.

III. SUMMARY

In previous chapters, we have directed our discussion to those components of the sensory evoked responses that are directly related to the physical characteristics of the stimulus (exogenous components). By contrast, there are event-related components that may be related only partially to the physical characteristics of the stimulus, being more dependent on the subject's prior experience, intentions, and decisions (endogenous components). Although exogenous components are elicited by stimuli, this does not imply that the information processing associated with the stimuli is identical for all presentations of a given stimulus. We have seen changes in the morphology of exogenous components caused by changes in the state of the subject. Thus, the processing associated with these components also depends on events internal to the nervous system. The defining characteristic of the exogenous components is that they are always elicited by external stimuli. Whereas some endogenous components may reflect further processing of the stimulus input, others do not, but rather are related to the use made of stimulus information. Long latency events (N200, P300), CNV, and the Readiness Potential (RP) may be considered as endogenous components. The CNV is not a single phenomenon, but a composite potential from different intracranial sources, which has been related to several psychological events identified as expectancy, decision, volition, conation, attention. It has been found to be of lower amplitude in patients with cerebral lesions, but it has been more widely studied in psychiatric patients. CNV has been also used in the assessment of subjective perception of auditory stimuli (evoked response audiometry) and as a proof of concept discrimination in aphasic patients (objective speech audiometry). The RP appears prior to self-paced voluntary responses, and it is considered the first component of the motor potentials (MPs). In the CNV paradigm, all tasks that require the establishment of a preparatory motor set are characterized by an RP as part of the CNV. RP abnormalities have been observed in patients with unilateral cerebral lesions of various etiologies. Exploration of motor potentials in neurological patients has opened a new field of application in clinical neurophysiology.

The study of the endogenous components offers the opportunity for the exploration of more complex mechanisms mediating cognition and "higher cortical functions." Great emphasis has been placed on their study in recent years, and many aspects must still be clarified. Nevertheless, we believe that in the near future, endogeneous components will provide important information for clinical purposes.

PART II:

QUANTITATIVE ANALYSIS OF BRAIN ELECTRICAL ACTIVITY

7 Statistical Bases

by Pedro Valdés

I. INTRODUCTION

This chapter presents a survey of statistical methods relevant to neurometric evaluation of brain function. A practical approach to the classification and use of different techniques is discussed without any pretense to theoretical completeness or rigorous presentation. Rather, an attempt is made to place in perspective the bewildering number of different methods by emphasizing the main questions that must be asked, the basic assumptions that the data must meet in order for various methods to be used legitimately, and the price of violating these assumptions.

It is impossible to collect or interpret data without a set of hypotheses, whether explicitly defined or, more commonly, unconsciously accepted. It has been repeatedly stated by philosophers of science that reality can only be coped with by simplifying it enough to grasp it theoretically and manipulate it experimentally. It may be worthwhile, at this point, to emphasize that no question can be meaningfully asked, no hypothesis tested that does not rest implicitly on some sort of a model, or schema, which describes the possible relationships between events or features associated with certain events. It is essential to try to make such models as explicit as possible, because the definition of what will constitute an acceptable answer to the question asked depends very much on the characteristics of the model.

Statistical data analysis techniques are based on certain assumptions. Unless the fit is acceptably good between the features of a theoretical model and the assumptions or requirements of a particular data analysis procedure, the answer to the question being asked may well be untrustworthy, misleading, or just wrong. This is particularly dangerous these days, because standard statistical computer program packages invite the unwary to use the most available or fashionable methods in the field irrespective of their appropriateness.

Statistics may be viewed as the application of the scientific method to situations in which chance is not negligible. By chance, we do not suggest that the relationships to be studied are subject to capricious influences. We mean that any subset of measurements that we obtain must be regarded as selected more or less fortuitously from a much larger set of possible measurements that might have been made. A problem immediately arises: How typical of the larger set can we assume the subset to be? Alternatively, how similar to the first measures would we expect measures from a second subset to be? The variability between measures from successive subsets represents the chance or stochastic elements of the measurements or the sample selection process.

Therefore, the stochastic elements must be explicitly incorporated into the theoretical model. Ideally, each piece of scientific work would require its own specific probability model and a statistical treatment optimal for that model. From this, and from the questions asked, the analytic procedures follows.

There are mainly three reasons why this strategy is not usually adopted. In the first place, many models and questions constantly recur in different situations, such as how to estimate a certain fixed physical constant corrupted by noise. These frequently posed questions and answers make up a considerable body of the statistical literature. Statistics tends to focus upon these stereotyped problems, rather than teaching how to formulate a plausible answer to an uncommon problem. In the second place, the methods and language of statistics are rather esoteric. They are intended for the specialist who is usually not a laboratory worker. This leads the nonspecialist in the laboratory to try to solve a problem by using certain time-tried and respectable methods as an economy of effort, with the clear danger of uncritical acceptance of possibly incorrect methods by the mathematically unsophisticated.

The third reason why investigators do not develop their own methods is that all too often, clearly defined hypotheses or models are not at hand. What one really wants to do is to examine a sample of data in the hope that it will suggest some hypothesis. One turns to statistics to help examine the data. Statisticians are increasingly being called upon to serve as data analysts. This has resulted in important new contributions on how to handle data (Tukey, 1978). However, it is the laboratory worker who has the most thorough scientific understanding of the data and undue reliance on the statistician to carry out what may constitute the crucial theoretical activity may be unwise.

The heart of neurometrics is the statistical treatment of quantitative parameters of brain electrical activity. The value of these measurements in a particular individual must be related to a known or estimated population distribution of such measures in a way which permits objective classification of that individual for some practical diagnostic purpose, with the greatest possible accuracy. Therefore, though the *user* of neurometrics may accept the results on the basis of their performance, those that want an insight into the basis of neurometrics should have at least an intuitive idea of the statistics employed. Those that *produce* neurometrical procedures must have a deeper knowledge about statistical methodology and frequent access to competent advice.

Thus, in order to be able to select a correct statistical treatment of one's data, it is important to clearly establish the questions one wants answered, the type of theoretical-stochastic (probabilistic) models one is willing or forced to accept (Fig. 7.1). If one attends to these three aspects—questions,

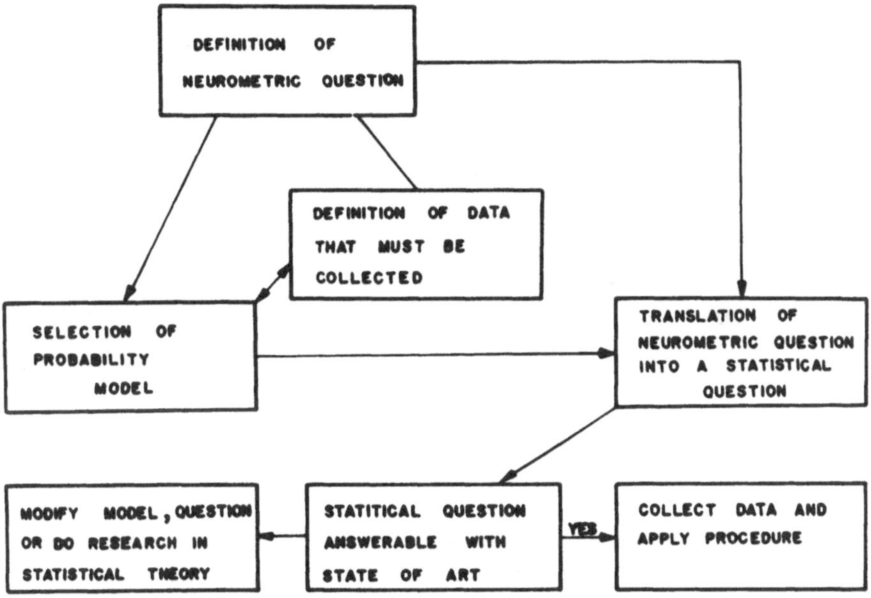

FIG. 7.1. *Sequence of steps involved in applying statistical methods to a neurometrical problem.* The question to be asked must first be defined. Then, an appropriate probability model must be selected. The data to be collected will depend on the model selected or, alternatively, the availability of certain data may determine the type of model chosen. This two-way type of interaction is indicated by a double-headed arrow here. The probability model selected permits a statistical formulation of the neurometric question that may be of a standard type or not. If not standard, the questions or model must be adjusted or new methods developed. When an adequate procedure is identified, data are collected and the statistical procedure applied.

type of data, and models—then certain methods are usually indicated. We shall attempt to review these methods ordered according to their suitability for different types of questions or data.

Before attempting this review of the most common statistical procedures, we want to stress, even at the risk of being repetitious, that statistics is not a branch of science amenable to recipes. If the standard methods do not seem well devised for a particular problem, then the adequate solution must be sought. Because this often involves difficult or even unsolved theoretical issues, a practical solution is to carry out simulations on digital computers. This approach, which is not described in detail here (see, however, Enstein, Ralston, & Wilf, 1977), is also based on the use of a mathematical model for the expected results.

The stochastic elements are supplied by the computer program. One can, therefore, carry out a large number of simulated "experiments" and study the permissible distribution of results.

A. Statistical Questions

For our purposes, we roughly group statistical questions into the following four divisions:

1. A *sample* of data is the set of items that happened to be observed from a larger, unobserved *population*. If one could know the relative likelihood of the constitutive items of the population, then the degree of typicity of a given sample would be clear and there would be no doubt about what inference to make. This is not the situation in reality. A probability model must be accepted as reflecting the distribution of items in the population. This has decisive consequences, because it strongly influences the statistical procedures to be employed in analyzing the sample. A first question is then the *determination of the acceptable probability model*. In the absence of theoretical reasons for choosing a particular probability model, an examination of the sample itself may be of use. For this purpose, *tests of goodness of fit* are used to ascertain the acceptability of proposed probability models. A different situation arises when the general form of the distribution is known and only the value of certain constants must be determined. In this case, these parameters must be *estimated*.

2. It is often of interest to assess or test the existence of certain relationships among features of the data—the existence of linear relationships among features, the grouping of values into clusters, the presence of extreme values of features, and so on. Such questions are about the *structure of the data*. Recently, many graphic and informal methods have been developed for this purpose, as well as more formal procedures (Everitt, 1978).

3. Samples are often obtained in different situations. The changes from one situation to another are either controlled by the investigator (experimental data) or only observed by him or her (survey data). In either case, it is of interest to know whether measures are altered from one situation to another. *Sample comparison techniques* come into use to answer such questions.

4. In other situations, one wants to use the available information to make predictions about an observed individual. Such is the case in giving a presumed diagnosis of a disease. Predictive Methods like *Regression* and *discriminant analysis* have been devised for such purposes.

B. Types of Measurements

Most types of data can be represented in a variety of ways and the particular representation that is selected—rank order, absolute value, percentage, and so on—is best treated with a different type of statistics. Some common types of data are:

1. *Categorical data*, for which only membership in a certain class can be specified.
2. *Ordinal data*, among which an ordering relation such as "better" or "higher" can be established.
3. *Numerical data*, on which the usual arithmetical operations can be performed. Most important are data that can be measured as *real numbers* (numbers that can be represented along a linear scale usually by a decimal value). In some applications, such as frequency analysis, where amplitude and phase information must be coded in a single number, *complex numbers* are used (numbers that must be represented as points on a two-dimensional plane, one dimension of which is a real number and the other that is referred to as *imaginary*).

In neurometrics, the usual measurements are numerical, though other types are sometimes used in the analysis of samples. Examples of different types of measurements are: presence or absence of an EEG spike (categorical); "normal," "slightly distorted," and "abnormal" waveform in evoked-response studies (ordinal); coefficient of a Fourier transform (complex number). Throughout this volume, we plan to define measurements when they are introduced.

The classification of measurements is further complicated by the number of different measurements (variables) obtained from a single observation. If there is only one variable, then *univariate* probability models and statistical techniques are to be used. This constitutes the usual content of traditional statistical courses. However, in practice, it is much more common to make more than one observation per experimental unit. For example, weight, height, and age may be obtained for a sample of subjects, and the evoked response is usually portrayed as a sequence of digitized values sampled at different time points, and soon. In all these cases, the result of an observation on an experimental unit is not just a number, but an ordered array of numbers. Such ordered arrays of numbers are called *vectors* and the type of statistical technique developed for vector-valued observations is called *multivariate. (See Table 7.1).*

TABLE 7.1
Summary of Concepts Related to the Type of Observation Process

	TYPE OF MEASUREMENT		
Usual Statistical Concepts	Single Measurement on an Observation	Multiple Measurements on Observations	Multiple Observations of same Quantity at Different Time Instants
Type of probability model	Univariate probability model	Multivariate probability model	Stochastic process
Unit observation	Observation	Observation	Realization of stochastic process or *time series*
Collection of unit observations	Sample	Sample of vectors	Collection of time series
Type of statistical procedure	Univariate statistics	Multivariate	Time-series analysis

At this point, it is important to discuss the way to represent univariate and multivariate data. This will help us to formulate many of our problems geometrically and, therefore, to have an intuitive understanding of what is being asked, something that is usually obscured by formulas. Any single measurement can be represented as a point along a scaled line that has an origin (Fig. 7.2).

If two measurements are made on an experimental unit—say amplitude and latency of a peak in an evoked response—then one can represent this on a plane, the position of the observation being fixed by its two *coordinates* (a_1 and a_2, a_1 being the first measurement and a_2 the second). A few important points follow. In the first place, instead of a single number, we are now dealing with an ordered pair of numbers, a vector. This vector, because it has two components, is *two-dimensional* and each component can be taken as the projection along the axes x_1, x_2 of a two-dimensional plot, in a plane

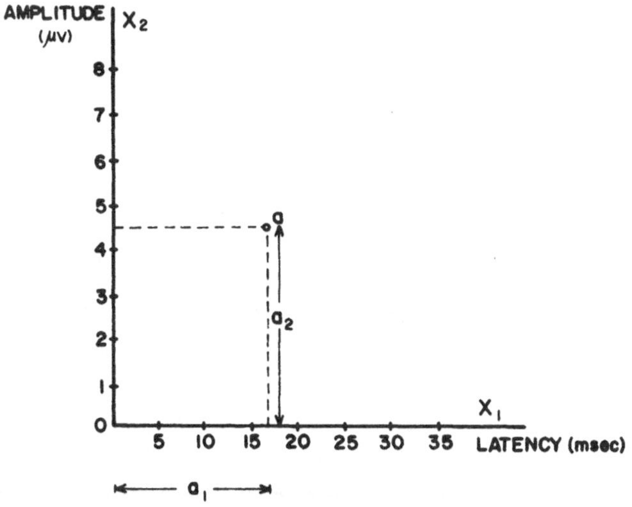

FIG. 7.2. Representation of two simultaneous measurements as components of a vector. As an example, the amplitude and latency of an evoked response peak are portrayed as a point a on the plane defined by all possible values for the latency and amplitude. The latency in msec of the peak determines its abscissa a_1, or horizontal displacement, and the amplitude (in μV) of the peak its ordinate, a_2, or vertical displacement. Thus, two features are extracted from the evoked response, latency and amplitude, each a real number representable along a linear scale. The combined information latency-amplitude is representable as a point or vector a with two components (a_1, a_2) along the X_1 (latency), X_2 (amplitude) axes. The set of all (x_1, x_2) vectors is a two-dimensional space.

(Fig. 7.2). If *three* measurements have to be worked with simultaneously, the obvious extension of the forementioned procedure is to represent the observation as an ordered triple (a_1, a_2, a_3) or *three-dimensional* vector. Its graphical representation must be in three-dimensional space (Fig. 7.3).

The extension of these ideas to more than three variables is immediate. If p (when p is an integer) variables are measured on an experimental unit, then the observed measurements can be ordered in a *p-dimensional* vector. We shall denote such vectors (a_1, a_3, . . .a_p) by boldface letters, in this case $\vec{\mathbf{x}}$. Once again, we may take the different numbers in a as the coordinates (or projections on the axes) of a *p-dimensional hyperspace*. Though such spaces cannot be visualized as two- or three-dimensional spaces can, another type of representation is possible. If the values of the successive components a_1, a_2 . . are plotted as functions of the integers 1, 2. . . (Fig. 7.4 A and B), a graph is obtained that permits the vector to be portrayed.

In many cases, the number of variables (components) is very high, but there is a great degree of dependence between successive components. This is usually the situation when a certain quantity is measured as successive in-

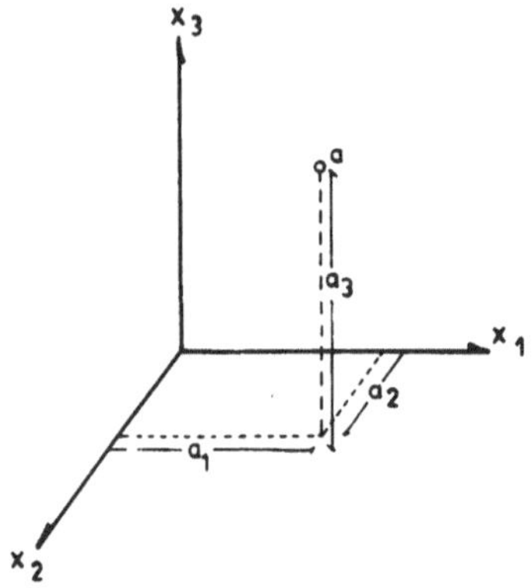

FIG. 7.3. *Representation of three measurements as components of a vector.* If a third value is added to the values measured in Fig. 7.2, then a three-dimensional representation is necessary. Point *a* has now three components: a_1, a_2, and a_3. This vector representation of observations may be carried over to more than three dimensions, though other types of pictorial representations are then necessary (see Fig. 7.4).

stants of time. For example, an EEG sampled at equidistant time points (see Fig. 8.1) or an evoked response are instances of this type of vector. These special types of vectors are called *time series* (though the successive components need not be values obtained at different time instants, electrical activity at different cortical depths being an example). Special methods, known as *Time Series Analysis*, are used for this type of observation.

In order to deal with the complexity of reality, vector-type observations are needed, and the concepts of hyperspace, time series, and many others are added to the already difficult vocabulary of statistics. Nonetheless, these concepts ultimately simplify reasoning about multiple observations. For reference, a survey of important hyperspace concepts is presented in section II of this chapter.

As a summary, measurements can be single (in which case they may be categorical, ordinal, or numerical), or multiple, in which case they are represented as vectors (ordered arrays) of single measurements. Table 7.1 summarizes the concepts presented.

C. Probability Models

A certain type of probability model, for reasons discussed later, known as the *Gaussian* or normal probability distribution (defined later), holds a very prominent place in statistical theory and practice. Methods that assume this distribution are among those called *parametric*. (More precisely, the name parametric should be applied to methods that assume a certain general type of probability model, completely specified except for the values of certain numerical parameters). This is to distinguish them from other types of methods that do not assume a very specific type of probability model and, therefore, are called *nonparametric*.

The advantage of parametric methods is that their properties have been very thoroughly ascertained. As a result, questions about the accuracy of estimation and prediction can be answered with relative precision, provided that restrictive assumptions are satisfied. Nonparametric methods have the

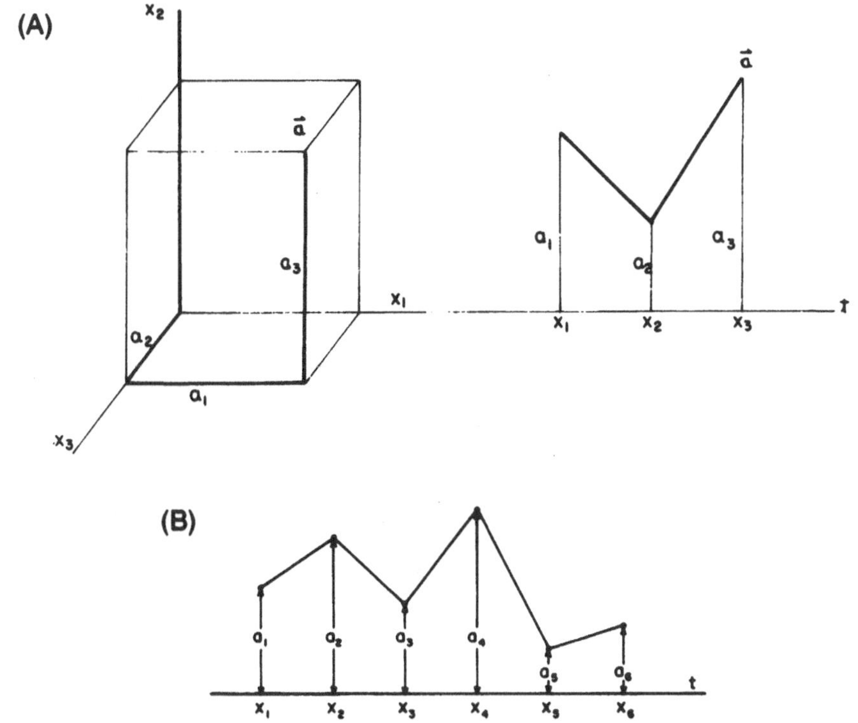

FIG. 7.4. Two equivalent ways to represent a three-dimensional observation, as a *vector* (as in Fig. 7.3) on the left, or as a *time series,* on the right. In the time-series representation, the values (a_1, a_2, a_3) are not plotted as coordinates along different axes (as in the vector representation), but as different ordinates along a common abscissa. The time-series representation is usually used when the components are more than three, they are measured in the same units, and they represent samples of the same quantity obtained at different time instants, in which case the values of the abscissa (t in this graph) is the time at which the sampling was performed. (B) *Time series with more than three components.* In this case, a graphical vector-type representation as in (A) is not even possible, but the time-series representation is still useful. The set of all possible time series is a hyperspace.

advantage that these assumptions can be relaxed, which is particularly advantageous with small samples or unknown population distributions. The price one pays for this generality is that questions can only be answered generically, rather than in precise detail. One particularly unpleasant consequence of using nonparametric methods is the loss of *power* (defined as the probability of detecting differences when they exist).

Table 7.2 gives examples of well-known statistical methods appropriate to certain types of measurement and statistical questions.

A *neurometric* procedure must extract a quantitative feature of brain electrical activity and relate it to a known or estimated population distribution of such measures in such a way as to permit an objective decision to be

TABLE 7.2
Choosing One of the Well-Known Statistical Methods

	TYPE OF MEASUREMENT		
Statistical Questions	One Variable (Univariate)	Many Variables General	(Multivariate) Time Series
How to evaluate the probability model?	Chi-squared (χ^2) Test for goodness of fit One sample Kolmogorov-Smirnov test	Multivariate Normality tests	Test for Stationarity
How to examine the structure?	Histograms	Scatter plots Regression Factor analysis Cluster analysis	Fitting of autoregressive models Spectral analysis
How to assess the effects of change?	t test Analysis of variance (ANOVA)	T^2 test Multivariate analysis of variances (MANOVA)	ANOVA for time series
How to make predictions?	Confidence intervals	Regression Discriminant analysis	Regression for time series

[a] The definition of the statistical question and the type of measurement often suggests the type of well-known methods available that might be useful. To illustrate this point, some well-known methods are presented here, classified according to the question and the type of measurement. The actual method used depends on many considerations, among which the appropriate type of probability model is prominent.

made about observed individuals for some practical purpose. For example, it is known that the evoked potentials from symmetrical (homologous) derivations display high waveshape and amplitude symmetry in healthy individuals (see Chapter 3). The demonstration that a given patient, at risk of some brain disease, displays evoked potentials with statistically significant asymmetry constitutes a positive clinical finding based on a neurometric procedure. On the other hand, although it might be of scientific interest to compute and display the bispectrum from young adults or to plot the chronotopogram (see Chapter 9), such measurements cannot be considered neurometric until they are quantitatively compared to a data base and until some correlates of departure from normative values have been identified. The ready availability of data-processing techniques has resulted in a proliferation of quantitative electro physiological findings of which only a fraction are currently of neurometric utility.

The importance of following the logic expressed in Fig. 7.5 cannot be overemphasized. An adequate probability model should be selected for two reasons. If the model does not accurately reflect the characteristics of the process under study, misleading or even erroneous results may be obtained. Even when the model fits the data, the parameters measured may not reflect relevant information for neurometric purposes. Careful consideration should be given before selecting parameters for study, since there is ample evidence that inclusion of noisy and redundant information can cause difficulties in interpretations and even vitiate an analysis.

The second step, the study of the structure of the data, is important in revealing natural groupings of the data and interrelationships between variables. This step can be decisive in the selection of diagnostic groups, in the redefinition of parameters and in the selection of statistical methods to be used in subsequent steps. In the third step, statistically meaningful differences are sought for parameters in different groups.

It is of no use to try to predict on the basis of chance differences. Insignificant differences require reexamination of definition of groups, measurement procedures, and selection of variables. Significant differences provide a justification for trying prediction. The final step is the selection and implementation of a predictive procedure. A successful outcome validates a neurometric procedure; inadequate accuracy leads to the reevaluation of the model and reexamination of the structure of data.

General introductions to statistical theory can be found in Lindgren (1962). The area of non-parametric in multivariate statistics is covered by Puri and Sen (1970), and of parametric methods by Morrison (1976). Time series analysis is developed in Anderson (1970), Brillinger (1975), and Hannan (1970).

We shall now review some of the methods available for answering the four types of questions, taking into due consideration the probability model.

II. VECTORS AND MATRICES

Vectors and matrices provide a convenient shorthand for expressions used in the analysis of multiple observations and some basic concepts shall therefore be presented in order to facilitate further discussions. In the first section of this chapter we mentioned that an ordered array of numbers (be they real or complex) is called a *vector*. The length of the array is the *dimensionality* of the vector and the constitutive numbers, the *components* of the vector, these being numbered according to their order. Vectors are denoted by an arrow above a lower case letter e.g. $\vec{a}$. The components of a vector are usually represented with the same letter and a subscript denoting the position of the component in the vector: a_i being the i-th component of vector $\vec{a}$. It is also convenient to recall that for vectors with a dimensionality lower than 3 a pictorial representation is straightforward, but that for more than 3 dimensions a different sort of graph is needed (Fig. 7.5). However,

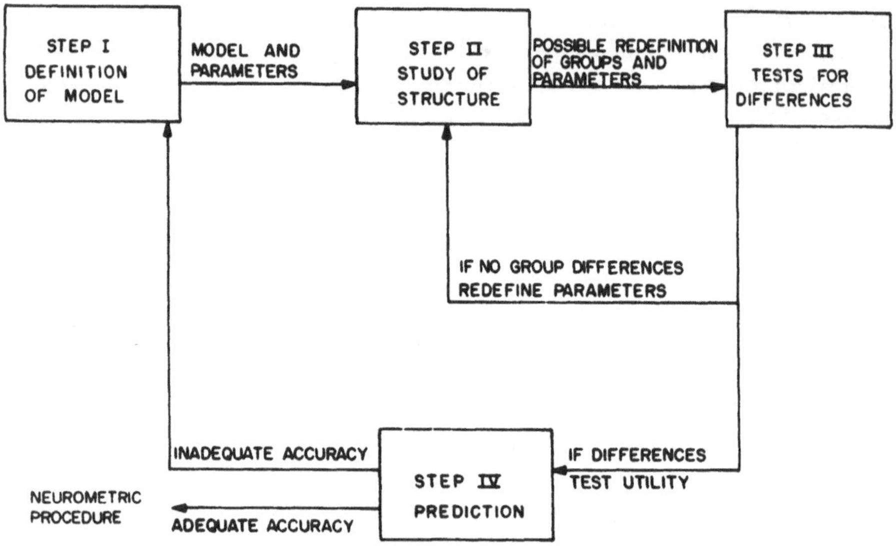

FIG. 7.5. *Sequence of steps in the application of statistical methodology for the construction of a neurometric procedure.* A model, of variable complexity, that establishes certain numerical parameters of brain electrical activity must be defined. The aim is to find parameters that vary for different groups (normals, patients, etc.). In the second step, the structure of the data collected is studied in the hope of sharpening the definition of groups and parameters. The demonstration of the existence of differences between values of parameters in the different groups is the objective of Step III. If these differences exist, then in Step IV, a procedure for the prediction of the group to which an observed individual belongs is developed. If accurate this becomes a neurometric procedure.

the formulas defining operations with vectors are the same no matter what the dimensionality, this being one of the advantages of vectorial notation.

As well known a convenient way to assess the general tendency of a group of data is to compute their average. For univariate data, a_i this is done by simply adding the values and dividing by the number of values (say N). This can be expressed in a formula as:

(Eq 7.1)
$$\bar{a} = \frac{1}{N} \sum_{i=1}^{N} a_i$$

In this formula the Greek symbol Σ stands for "summation," the subscripts $i = 1$ below the Σ and N above indicating that the values a_i from $i = 1$ to N must be summed. The bar above the a on the left signifies "average."

In the multivariate case, a useful summary of the data is also given by the mean of each variable. A convenient way to introduce this concept is by defining the *sum of two vectors*. This is no more than the sum of corresponding components of the two vectors considered. For example:

(Eq 7.2) $$\begin{bmatrix} 1 \\ 0.5 \end{bmatrix} + \begin{bmatrix} 2 \\ 3 \end{bmatrix} = \begin{bmatrix} 3 \\ 3.5 \end{bmatrix}; \vec{x} + \vec{y} = \vec{z}$$

In this case Eq. 7.2 is shorthand for the fact that two vectors, $\vec{x}$ with components 1 and 0.5, and $\vec{y}$ with components 2 and 3 sum to form another vector $\vec{z}$ with components (3, 3.5). Note that vectors must have the same dimensionality in order to be summed. In Fig. 7.6, this same sum is represented both in vector and time series representation.

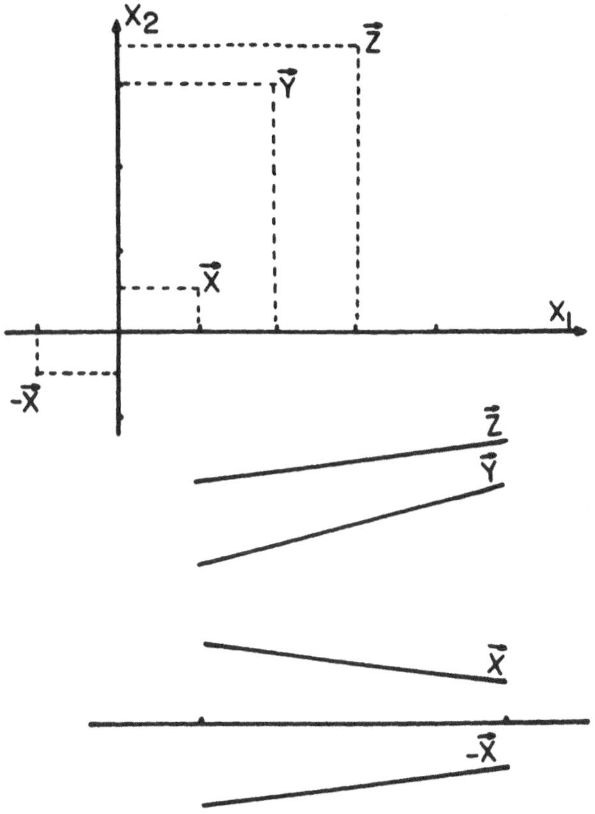

FIG. 7.6. *Vector sum*. This Fig. illustrates the concept of vector summation, for example, in which the two-dimensional vectors $\vec{X}^T = (1, .5)$ and $\vec{Y}^T = (2, 3)$ are summed to obtain the vector $\vec{Z}^T = (3, 3.5)$. *Top, vector representation. Bottom, time-series representation. The superscript* ^{T} indicates that vectors are really column vectors and not row vectors (see text). $-\vec{X}$ is the result of multiplying the vector $\vec{X}$ by -1 (see text).

The summation of vectors formally has the same properties as ordinary numbers. Thus the extension to the summation of N vectors is evident. We can therefore define the *average* or *mean* vector a a sample of N vectors $\mathbf{a}_i$ as:

(Eq. 7.3a)
$$\vec{\bar{a}} = \frac{1}{N}\sum_{i=1}^{N} \vec{a}_i$$

It might be useful to illustrate a typical application of these conventions to the management of electrophysiological data. Imagine that, in response to some specified stimulus, a series of X single evoked potentials is recorded from each of 6 head regions on each of a group of Y patients. The single evoked potential can be described as a time series, the successive components of the vector being the voltage sampled at successive increments of time after the stimulus. We can denote such an evoked potential as $\vec{e}_{ij}$, where the subscript $\mathbf{i}$ indicates the number of the evoked potential in the series of N events and the subscript $\mathbf{j}$ refers to the head region from which it was recorded.

Previous chapters have discussed the Average Evoked Response, which is just the average of the $\vec{e}_{ij}$ component by component. Thus, for any region $\mathbf{j}$, the average evoked response $\vec{e}_j$ is the mean vector:

(Eq. 7.3b)
$$\vec{\bar{e}}_j = \frac{1}{N}\sum_{i=1}^{N} \vec{\bar{e}}_{ij}$$

Now suppose that 6 head regions for which $\vec{\bar{e}}_j$ is available in each patient are comprised of 3 symmetrically located pairs of regions. In Chapter 13, the diagnostic utility of the asymmetry of the averaged evoked responses from homologous regions is discussed. One way to represent the asymmetry is to compute the difference wave obtained by subtracting corresponding components of the average evoked responses, $\vec{\bar{e}}_j$, recorded from the two symmetrically located electrode derivations of an homologous pair. The operations of vector subtraction are defined below in Eq. 7.4. Another estimate of symmetry can be obtained by the computation of the correlation coefficient defined below in Eq. 7.9.

Let us define the bilateral asymmetry as the vector $\vec{r}_{jk}$, where $\mathbf{j}$ indicates to which of the 3 regions the subscript refers and $\mathbf{k}$ identifies a particular patient. The average or mean asymmetry across the 3 homologous pairs of regions in patient $\mathbf{k}$ is given by the mean vector:

Eq. 7.3c)
$$\vec{r}_k = \frac{1}{3}\sum_{j=1}^{3} \vec{r}_{jk}$$

Further, the average value of mean asymmetry in the group of Y patients is given by the mean vector:

(Eq. 7.3d)
$$\vec{\bar{r}} = \frac{1}{Y}\sum_{k=1}^{Y} \vec{\bar{r}}_k$$

Very simple procedures, consisting of computations of vector sums, mean vector and vector differences, have allowed us to obtain a quantitative description of the average evoked response, the asymmetry in average evoked response between homologous regions, the overall asymmetry between large portions of the two hemispheres in each patient, and the average asymmetry within a group of patients. These iterated simple operations could put us in a position where it might be feasible to construct a neurometric procedure. For example, if one knew the distribution of $\vec{\bar{r}}$, one might utilize the difference between $\vec{\bar{r}}$ and $\vec{\bar{r}}_k$ to estimate the probability that patient k displayed an abnormal interhemispheric asymmetry. It is instructive to depict an actual average of a small number of three dimensional $\vec{\bar{r}}_k$ vectors. Inspection of Fig. 7.7 illustrate that this sample forms a swarm in 3-space (this type of graph is called a scatter plot) and that the average $\vec{\bar{r}}$ is the center of gravity of the swarm.

The multiplication of a vector by a number is simply obtained by multiplying each component by the number. This represents a change of scale of the graph, for example in Fig. 7.6, a multiplication of $\vec{x}$ by 2 would maintained its general orientation in the graph at the top or its waveshape in the graph on the bottom but with a magnification in "size" (to be defined more precisely later). In particular a multiplication of a vector by -1 reflects it with respect to the origin ($-\vec{x}$ in Fig. 7.6). The difference of two vectors is then defined as follows $\vec{x} - \vec{y} = (-1)\vec{y} + \vec{x}$. Important types of difference vectors are obtained by subtracting the mean vector of a sample

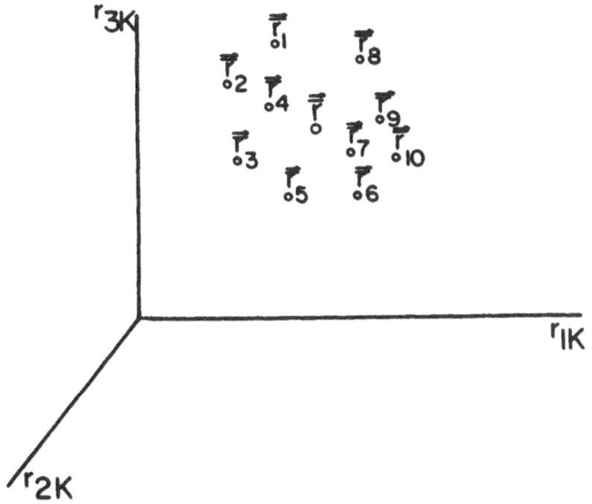

FIG. 7.7 Vector average of six neurometric vectors $\vec{r}_i$. The vector average, $\vec{\bar{r}}_i$, is the center of gravity of the swarm of $\vec{r}_i$, thus indicating the central tendency of the cloud of points.

from each member of the sample. This operation is a critical step in many neurometric procedures:

(Eq. 7.4) $$\Delta\vec{\mathbf{r}}_k = \vec{\mathbf{r}}_k - \vec{\mathbf{r}}$$

In equation 7.4, $\Delta\vec{\mathbf{r}}_k$ denotes the difference vector of individual k with respect to the mean. In neurometric applications, this difference vector is important since (if the mean of the normal population is used in the difference) it reflects the profile of deviations from normality for a given individual. With appropriate scaling, the *probability* that a particular difference vector belongs to a normal individual can be estimated. This is the Z vector, discussed in Chapter 11, but introduced later in this section.

Multiplication of vectors can be of many types. We shall only define one type (scalar multiplication). It gives as a result, not another vector, but a number. In order to define this type of multiplication we must distinguish between *row vectors* like $\vec{\mathbf{x}} = (x_1, x_2, x_3)$, and *column vectors* such as

$$\begin{bmatrix} x_1 \\ x_2 \\ x_3 \end{bmatrix}$$

Introducing the transposition operation will permit us to denote column vectors. The transposition of a vector is the operation of changing a row vector into a column vector (preserving the order of the components) or vice-versa. It will be denoted by superscripting the vector to be transposed by a t. Thus $\vec{\mathbf{x}}^t$ is the transpose of $\vec{\mathbf{x}}$. (It is easily seen that $\vec{\mathbf{x}}^{tt} = \vec{\mathbf{x}}$). Therefore all vectors with a t superscript will be column vectors. With this in mind we may define the product of two p-dimensional vectors $\vec{\mathbf{x}}$ and $\vec{\mathbf{y}}^t$ as:

(Eq. 7.5) $$\|\vec{\mathbf{x}}\ \vec{\mathbf{y}}\| = \vec{\mathbf{x}}\ \vec{\mathbf{y}}^t = \sum_{i=1}^{p} x_i y_i$$

This expression is the sum of the component-wise products of the two vectors. In Fig. 7.8 we illustrate this in the special case when we multiply a vector by itself. This defines the length-squared, or $|\vec{\mathbf{x}}|^2$. In 1, 2 or 3 dimensions the *square root* of $|\vec{\mathbf{x}}|^2$, i.e. $|\vec{\mathbf{x}}|$, is the ordinary length of the vector $\vec{\mathbf{x}}$ or in other words the *distance* of $\vec{\mathbf{x}}$ from the origin 0. For more than 3 dimensions $|\vec{\mathbf{x}}|$ can be thought of as a *hyperlength* or length in hyperspace. In the case of evoked responses, it can be given an interesting interpretation. It is the energy (rather a multiple) of the $\vec{\mathbf{e}}_i$. In the case of the neurometric vector of differences from the population mean, $\Delta\vec{\mathbf{r}}_k$, it represents an overall measure of abnormality. It is formed by finding the square root of the sum of the squared neurometric deviations for each measure. Usually, the individual deviations are first normalized by transforming them into

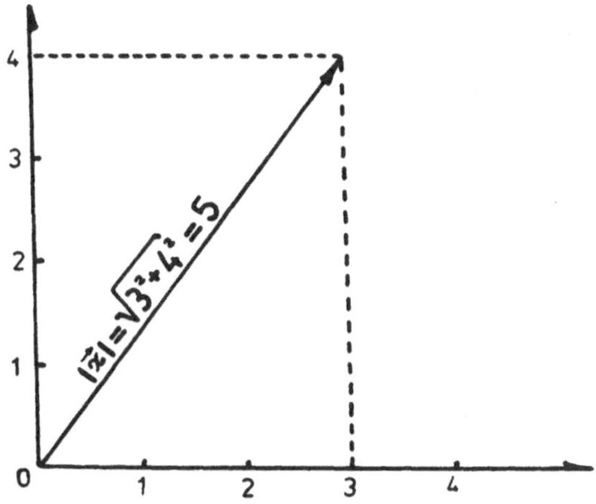

FIG. 7.8. The *length* of a vector $\bar{x}$ is defined as the square root of the product of $\bar{x}$ by itself, denoted by $|\bar{x}|$. In this FIG. for 2-space, the concept is illustrated in the case of a vector with components 3 and 4, the length being 5. The length represents a sort of root-sum of squares measure of difference from the origin. In the case of neurometric parameters, this length is the overall measure of deviance from normality if the space is centered at the mean of normals.

standard deviation units (Z-transform, see next section), defining the probability that each deviation represents an abnormal finding.

We have used the word "*distance*," which has an obvious connotation in ordinary space. The vector notation will permit us to define (Euclidean) distance for hyperspace as:

(Eq. 7.6)
$$d(\vec{x},\vec{y}) = \sqrt[n]{(\bar{x} - \bar{y}) (\bar{x} - \bar{y})'}$$
$$= \sqrt{\sum_{i=1}^{p} (x_i - y_i)^2}$$

Thus, the distance is also a sort of root sum of squares measure of difference between two vectors. It is of great utility in neurometrics, and statistics in general, to make precise the notion of similarity of two observations. It is usual in statistics to define those observations as similar if the distance between them is small. This opens up interesting possibilities, such as the ability to define mathematically what a "subgroup" or cluster is, but this will be discussed later.

The concept of distance has been so useful that generalizations of it have been made, to which we shall refer as they turn up, only one sample sufficing for the time being. Suppose that N observations x_i have been made. We already have a measure of central tendency, the mean $\bar{x}$. But we can also use a measure of *dispersion* around the mean. From elementary statistics courses this is known as the (sample) standard deviation:

(Eq. 7.7)
$$s_x = \sqrt{\frac{\sum_{i=1}^{N}(x_i - \bar{x})^2}{N-1}}$$

The point is that if we order the observations into a vector (N-dimensional) $\vec{x}$, and subtract the mean $\bar{x}$ from each component then the standard deviation of the sample is the length $|\vec{x}|$ divided by $1/\sqrt{N-1}$. Thus, the standard deviation is a sort of scaled length.

To continue with the uses of vector multiplications, suppose two variables have been measured on N subjects, let us call the values for variable $\vec{x}$, x_i and those for variable $\vec{y}$, y_i. Let us proceed as above, subtracting from each component of the $\vec{x}$ vector (formed by aligning the N observations into an array) the mean $\bar{x}$, and $\bar{y}$ from the corresponding components of $\vec{y}$. What happens can be visualized by looking at the case where $N = 5$ in the representations, as in Fig. 7.9. In 7.9a the components of $\vec{x}$ and $\vec{y}$ tend to vary together, in 7.9b they vary in opposite directions, and in 9c they do not vary together at all. The result of forming the vector product $(x\,y')$ is clear; in a) it will be positive, in b) negative and near 0 in c). This prompts us to use the vector product of the observation vectors for two variables as a measure of relationship or covariation between the two variables. As a matter of fact this is the definition (plus a scale factor $1/N-1$) of the *covariance* of variables x and y:

$$S_{xy} = (\vec{x}\,\vec{y}') / (N-1) \qquad \text{(Eq. 7.8)}$$

If we previously scale each variable-vector to unit length, then Eq. 7.8 turns into the definition of the *correlation coefficient* between variables x and y:

$$r_{xy} = \vec{x}\,\vec{y}' / |\vec{x}|\,|\vec{y}| \qquad \text{(Eq. 7.9)}$$

r_{xy} is a dimensionless quantity between 1 and -1 for perfect covariation

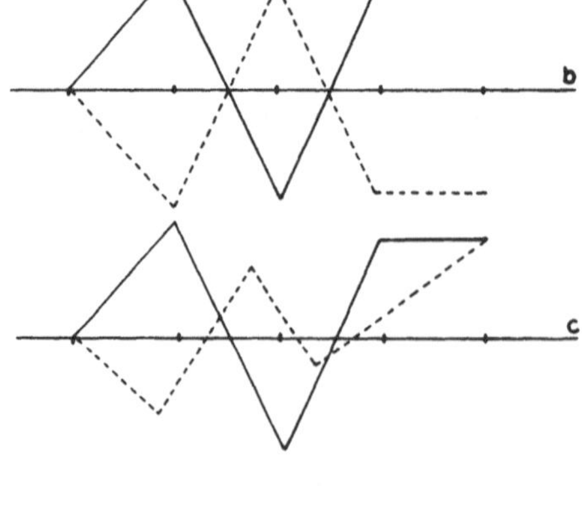

FIG. 7.9. *Time-series representation of the two vectors* $\vec{x}$ (—) and $\vec{y}$ (----) formed by five observations of variable x and y. The ith component of $\vec{x}$ corresponds to that of $\vec{y}$. The means $\bar{x}$ and $\bar{y}$ have been subtracted from each vector (this corresponds to an elimination of the DC shift for each vector). In (a), the two variables covary; in (b), they covary inversely; in (c), they do not covary.

and inverse covariation, respectively. If x and y do not covary, then r_{xy} should be near 0.

Suppose we wish to represent a set of N evoked responses simultaneously. We would then have N p-dimensional vectors. Such data may also be ordered as tabular arrays. In the case of the $\vec{\mathbf{e}}_i$ we get a table with p columns and N rows. Such tables are called *matrices*. They are generalizations of vectors.

Examples of matrices are:

$$\begin{bmatrix} 1 & 3 & -11 \\ 0 & 5 & 0 \end{bmatrix} \quad \begin{bmatrix} 10 & 7 & 2 \\ 3 & 5 & 0 \\ 1 & 2 & 8 \end{bmatrix} \quad \begin{bmatrix} 10 \\ 10 \end{bmatrix}$$

Matrices are denoted by boldface uppercase letters. They can be considered as vectors with vector components. For example:

$$\begin{bmatrix} 1 & 3 & -11 \\ 0 & 5 & 0 \end{bmatrix} = \begin{bmatrix} \vec{\mathbf{a}} \\ \vec{\mathbf{b}} \end{bmatrix} \text{ with}$$
$$\vec{\mathbf{a}} = (1 \quad 3 \quad -11) \text{ and}$$
$$\vec{\mathbf{b}} = (0 \quad 5 \quad 0)$$

Matrices are classified according to the number of columns and rows. A matrix can have any number of rows or of columns. An *$r \times c$ matrix* is a matrix with r rows and c columns. Above are a 2×3, 3×3, and a 2×1 matrix. Special important cases of matrices are vectors, as can easily be seen; Row vectors are $1 \times p$ matrices and column vectors are $p \times 1$ matrices. Another special class of matrices are *square matrices*; these have the same number of columns as rows.

The components of a matrix are identified by a double suffix indicating the row and column that it occupies. Thus, a_{ij} is the number in the ith row and jth column. Matrix operations are readily defined as follows: The addition and subtraction of matrices is done component-wise as in vectors. It is, therefore, obvious how to define an average matrix. Matrix multiplication is a bit more complicated. It is defined for those matrices **A**, **B** in which the number of columns of **A** is equal to the number of rows of **B**. Suppose that **A** is an $r \times c$ matrix and that **B** is a $c \times s$ matrix. Represent them as if **A** were formed by r, c-dimensional row vectors $\vec{\mathbf{a}}_i$ and **B** as s, c-dimensional column vectors $\vec{\mathbf{b}}_j$. Then, the matrix product of A and B is defined as the matrix **C** with elements $c_{ij} = \vec{\mathbf{a}}_i \, \vec{\mathbf{b}}_j$. This is best seen with an example, Fig. 7.10.

The multiplication of a matrix by itself permits the definition of *powers* of a matrix. The square of a matrix **A** is $\mathbf{AA} = \mathbf{A}^2$, the cube $\mathbf{AAA} = \mathbf{A}^3$, and so on. The *square root* of a matrix **A** is the matrix that squared gives **A**. $\mathbf{B} = \mathbf{A}^{1/2}$ if $\mathbf{BB} = \mathbf{A}$.

$$\begin{matrix} \vec{a}_1 \\ \vec{a}_2 \end{matrix} \begin{bmatrix} 1 & 3 & -11 \\ \hdashline 0 & 5 & 0 \end{bmatrix} \begin{bmatrix} \vec{b}_1^T & \vec{b}_2^T & \vec{b}_3^T \\ 10 & 7 & 2 \\ 3 & 9 & 0 \\ 1 & 2 & 8 \end{bmatrix} =$$

$$\text{A (2×3)} \qquad \text{B (3×3)}$$

$$= \begin{bmatrix} |\vec{a}_1\ \vec{b}_1^T| & |\vec{a}_1\ \vec{b}_2^T| & |\vec{a}_1\ \vec{b}_3^T| \\ |\vec{a}_2\ \vec{b}_1^T| & |\vec{a}_2\ \vec{b}_2^T| & |\vec{a}_2\ \vec{b}_3^T| \end{bmatrix} =$$

$$\text{C (2×3)}$$

$$= \begin{bmatrix} 1\times10+3\times3-11\times1 & 1\times7+3\times9-11\times2 & 1\times2+3\times0-11\times8 \\ 0\times10+5\times3+0\times1 & 0\times7+5\times9-0\times2 & 0\times2+5\times0+0\times8 \end{bmatrix} =$$

$$= \begin{bmatrix} 9 & 12 & 86 \\ 1 & 45 & 0 \end{bmatrix}$$

FIG. 7.10. *Matrix Multiplication.* The 2 x 3 matrix **A** is multiplied by the 3 x 3 matrix **B** to give the 3 x 3 matrix **C**. **A** is subdivided into two rows of three-dimensional row vectors $\vec{a}_i$, and **B** is subdivided into three rows of three-dimensional column vectors $\vec{b}_j^t$. The elements of **C** are formed according to the rule for vector multiplication: the element $c_{ij} = |\vec{a}_i \vec{b}_j^T|$.

Besides serving as a condensed representation of data from different vectors, matrices are useful to represent ways of transforming vector observations. If we have a vector observation and we wish to form another vector observation obtained from the first by summing any combination of components multiplied by weights, then we can find an appropriate matrix to do the job. For example, if I want to divide every component of the neurometric vector r_k by a weight, say the standard deviation of each variable then this can be done by multiplying with the matrix:

$$\begin{bmatrix} 1/S_1 & 0 \ldots\ldots\ldots\ldots\ldots & 0 \\ 0 & 1/S_2 \ldots\ldots\ldots\ldots & 0 \\ 0 & 0 \ldots\ldots\ldots\ldots\ldots & 1/S_p \end{bmatrix}$$

The effect on a neurometric vector r_k of first subtracting the normal population mean for each dimension and then dividing each difference value by the corresponding standard deviation is to construct a vector $\vec{z}_k$. Each component of $\vec{z}_k$ is scaled in standard deviation units. This provides a common metric for all components of $\vec{z}_k$ or dimensions of the hyperspace, no matter what the physical dimensions of the initial variables. In this manner, components as different as energy, frequency, phase,symmetry, etc. can be compressed in terms of *probability of occurrence in a normal population*. Thus, vectors transformed in this fashion yield a highly condensed description of the relationship of a set of neurometric measures obtained in a particular individual to the distribution of those measures in the normative data base. This is the *Z*-vector define by John et al. (1977) that is further discussed in Chapter 11. The length of the vector represents the overall probability that patient *k* belongs to the a normal population.

The type of scaling operation just defined may be generalized. When dealing with univariate measurements scaling is the *division* of all observed values by some appropriate constant (which obviously cannot be zero). The corresponding scaling operation would be an analogue to *division* defined for matrices. This operation may be defined in terms of multiplication as follows:

The *identity matrix* **I** of order n is the n × n square matrix which has l's in the diagonal and O's elsewhere. Its most important property is that when multiplying a vector it does not modify the vector in any way: $\vec{\mathbf{X}}\mathbf{I} = \vec{\mathbf{X}}$. **I** constitutes a generalization of the number 1. The inverse of a number x is that number y such that xy = 1 we may define the *inverse of a n by n matrix* **A** as that matrix $\mathbf{A}^{-1}$ such that $\mathbf{A}\,\mathbf{A}^{-1} = \mathbf{I}$. Not all matrices have inverses. There is a set of n × n matrices which are *non invertible or singular*, corresponding, with respect to matrix inversion, to the role played by zero for numerical division.

There is a way of associating a number to each square matrix, that serves as a criteria of invertibility (besides having other use in statistics). This number, called the *determinant* of the matrix, is zero when the matrix is non invertible and different from zero otherwise. We will not go into the details of how to compute the determinant in this chapter. Rather the formulae for 2 × 2 and 3 × 3 matrices are presented. $|\mathbf{A}|$ is the symbol for the determinant of matrix **A**.

$$\begin{bmatrix} a & b \\ c & d \end{bmatrix} = ad - bc$$

$$\begin{bmatrix} a & b & c \\ d & e & f \\ g & h & i \end{bmatrix} = \begin{matrix} aei + dhc + gbf \\ -gec - hfa - dbi \end{matrix}$$

III. PROBABILITY MODELS

A. Sample Spaces, Random Functions, and Probability Distributions

In any scientific endeavor, when a measurement is undertaken (be it of the univariate, vector, or time-series type), there is a degree of uncertainty associated with it. This might be due to the impossibility of controlling all determining factors or to inherent variability. Whatever the cause, the final result is that it is not possible to make precise statements about the exact value a measurement will have. This unpredictability is not always present in the same degree. In some situations, it is so negligible that it is ignored altogether and one talks of deterministic experiments or models, the classical examples being those of some parts of physical science. In the biological and behavioral sciences, however, the situation is quite different. No two patients are exactly the same, signs and symptoms are associated with certain diseases, but only loosely, and so forth. The important point, nonetheless, is that, "nondeterministic" is not the same as "unlawful." Symptoms are not tightly coupled with diseases, but there are regularities (physicians act upon them). A drug that is effective against a given disease might not cure all cases, but it does a great proportion. As was pointed out in section I of this chapter, specific *probability models* reflect the stochastic or chance elements, of reality and serve as a foundation for rational inference and decisions.

It, therefore, seems important to discuss the different types of probability models for use in neurometrics, how to apply them to the data, and how to test for their adequacy.

In order to fix ideas and relate theoretical constructs to reality, we employ throughout this section the following example of a chance experiment: In Part I, the concept of an evoked response was introduced. As discussed there in greater detail, when a brief, intense stimuli is presented to the sensory organs of a subject, a chain of highly coherent neural events is elicited. This produces potential differences that are superimposed (or combined, depending on how one views the physiology of ERs) on the ongoing EEG, which reflects, in turn, the unending and event-unrelated transactions of the CNS. Let us consider the presentation of a single stimulus (Fig. 7.11). The result is a voltage-time function $e(t)$, which is a time series. If the voltage values at time instants t_1, t_2, and t_3 are assembled into an array, we have a vector or multivariate observation $\vec{e}$. Any single component of $\vec{e}$, say $e(t_2)$, is a numerical measurement.

Any one of these measurements may vary from one stimulus presentation to another. Probability theory permits a description of this variability as subject to laws. Statistical theory uses this information to make inferences or decisions. The first step is to define the *sample space*. This is the set of all possible outcomes of a chance experiment—in our example, the collection of all possible variations of neural responses to the same stimulus that could produce different ERs. The fact that only a minimal fraction of such possible "brain responses" will be actually observed is immaterial and does not affect the utility of the model. We can not assign equal plausibility to all brain responses, nor does experience suggest this. The simultaneous discharge of *all* the neurons in the brain, for example, with the resultant "giant ER" is something that we do not expect. We are thus led to consider different *events*, or members of the sample space and to assign weights to their relative plausibility or possibility of occurrence. These are the *probabilities* assigned to the events in the sample space. Thus, if we consider the event "the whole nervous system goes bang," we assign probability 0 to it. On the other hand, the event "some neuron responds to the stimulus" is almost absolutely certain and to it, we assign a probability of 1. All values

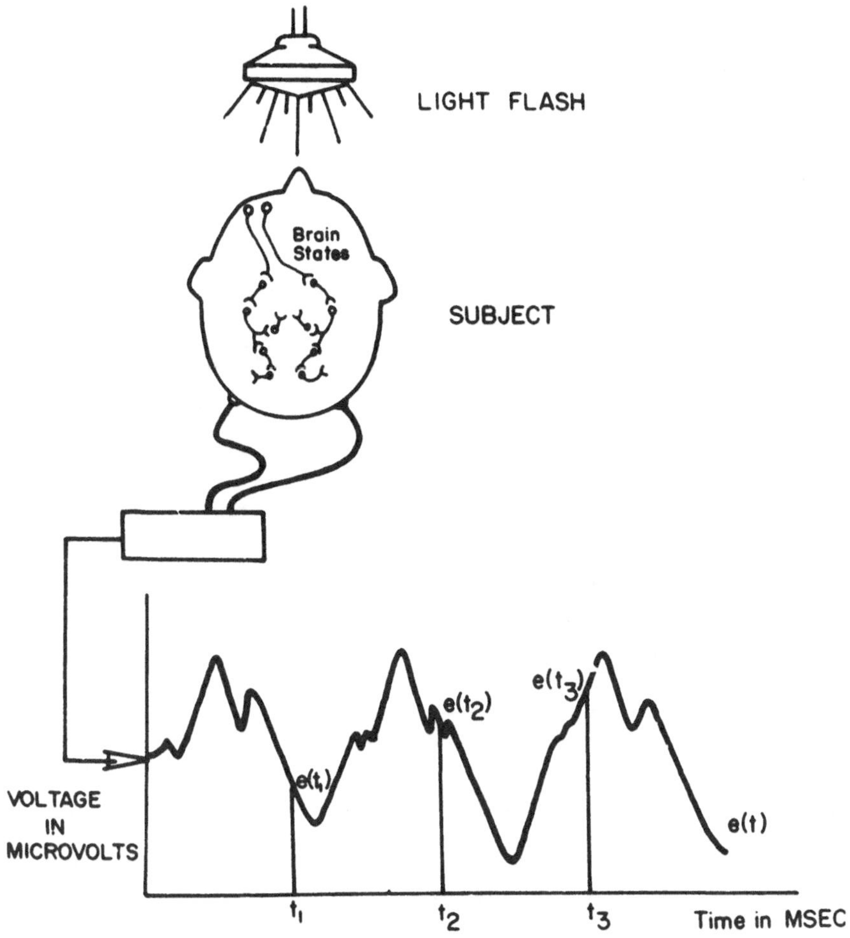

FIG. 7.11. *Evoked response as result of a chance experiment.* The presentation of the stimulus produces a chain of brain states that can be indirectly monitored by measuring the voltage difference between two electrodes on the scalp as a function of time. The resulting voltage–time function can be considered as a *time series* $e(t)$ or, assembling voltage values at time t_1, t_2, and t_3 into a vector $\vec{e} = [e(t_1), e(t_2), e(t_3)]$ as a multivariate observation or, if only the voltage at one time instant is considered, as a numberical univariate measurement.

of probability, therefore, go from 0 (impossible event) to 1 (certain event).

Let us now consider specific measures of brain responses (what we really work with), the ERs. Each brain state has its own particular electrical signature, the ER associated with it. (Possibly, many brain states have the same ER, so the correspondence is not necessarily one to one). The probabilities of the different possible brain states determine the probability of different types of ERs. We must change focus from a sample space of "brain responses'' to that of functions (or vectors or numbers). The probabilities assigned in the original sample space induce an assignment of probabilities in the sample space of all possible functions. The act of measurement moves us into the world of functions, vectors, or numbers, and these are mathematically tractable.

All this might seem a mere technicality. Usually one starts off as if the original sample space were the set of all possible ERs. The point is that what we are really interested in is brain states. A different way of measuring brain responses, by measurements of blood flow for example, would give us a very different set of functions and associated probabilities. We can define different measure spaces on the *same original sample space*. The rule that relates a given set of brain states to certain functions is known as a *random function* (or *random vector, or random variable* depending on the type of measurement). Fig. 7.12 schematizes the concepts discussed, assuming a very limited number of possible brain states for the sake of illustration.

To express things more formally, a probabilistic model starts by defining the *sample space* Ω as the set of all possible outcomes (elementary events) of a chance experiment. Subsets of the sample space (for example, all brain responses of a certain type) are *compound events* (or simply *events*). Probabilities are assigned to events in the sample space, 0 to the event that has no member (the 'empty' event, or is impossible) and 1 to the sure event (the whole sample space). Mappings that associate numbers, vectors, or functions with subsets of the sample space are known as *random variables, random vectors*, or *random functions* respectively. These random quantities and the probabilities that are induced by the sample space are the subject matter of probability theory.

There are two usual ways to specify the assignment of probabilities to random quantities. If the random quantities vary discretely, then to each value of the random quantity a probability value is directly associated. This is a discrete probability distribution. The probability assignments in Fig. 7.12 are of this type. Discrete probability distributions can be portrayed as shown in the inset of Fig. 7.12b.

When random quantities vary continuously, technical problems arise in assigning probabilities to every possible event. In order to give an idea of this, let us consider the simple event ''the evoked response at time i is *exactly* 4 μV,'' and the (compound) event ''the evoked response at time i is between 3.5-4.5 μV.'' The first event is highly improbable. In fact, due to measurement error and other random factors, it is highly unlikely that the observed value could be any exact number. In probability theory, this is recognized by assigning probability 0 to any *point* of a continuous random quantity. On the other hand, the compound event just mentioned has a nonzero probability. A distribution function in the spirit of the discrete probability assignment in the previous paragraph would be of no use, because the value for each x would be 0.

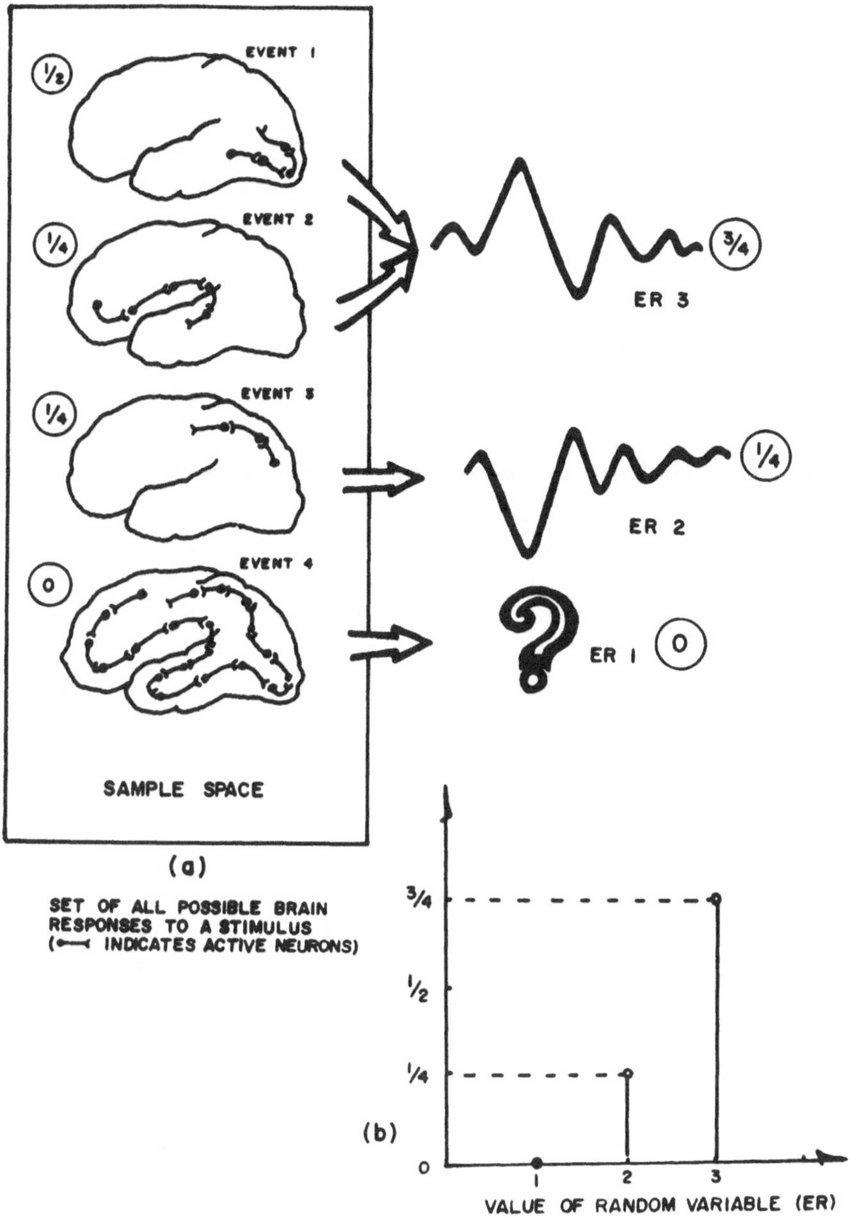

FIG. 7.12. *Sample space, probabilities and random functions.* a) The sample space is defined by the set of all possible outcomes (responses) of the experiment of stimulus presentation. For simplicity, our example is limited to 4 possible outcomes. Each brain state produces an evoked response (ER). The outcome (ER) of stimulus presentation in brain state 1 and 2 is assumed to be indistinguishable. Brain state 3 yields a different outcome. Brain state 4, simultaneous discharge of the whole brain, is impossible. These four brain states have different probabilities, represented by the circles at the left of the 4 schematized state diagrams. The mapping of the set of brain states into the set of outcomes is a random function which generates different probabilities for each type of ER, represented by the circles to the right of each ER.

What is then possible, in many cases, is to define a function that assumes numerical values for each value of the random quantity, that are *not* probabilities. What *is* a probability is the *area* (or volume, or hypervolume) underneath this function. Fig. 7.13 shows an example of the case of a random variable. The bell-shaped curve does not depict probability, but the shaded area is the probability that the random variable x has a value between x_1 and x_2. Such functions are called *probability densities*; their fundamental property is that when suitably integrated over a certain region, they yield probabilities. In what follows we limit our attention to densities.

The name "density" is inspired by the following geometric interpretation: If we consider the values of a random quantity as points in p-space, we can visualize them as a swarm or cloud of points. The density or concentration of points is quantified by the density function. The number or quantity of points in any particular region or hypervolume of the cloud depends on the shape of the region and the values of the density function in that region.

B. Moments

Probability distributions and densities are characterized by certain quantities known as *moments*. These summarize important properties of the probability models and, therefore, merit some attention.

As mentioned repeatedly, stochastic measurements are not totally unlawful, but rather, they tend to cluster around certain values. This vague idea is made more precise by the definition of the *first moment* of the probability distribution, or density. This is simply the *mean* or *average*. In many situations, one can consider the mean as the "real value" around which chance displaces the actual values observed. This type of thinking is embodied in the use of the Average Evoked Response as if it were "the" response of the brain to a stimuli. Explicitly, the model supposes a fixed

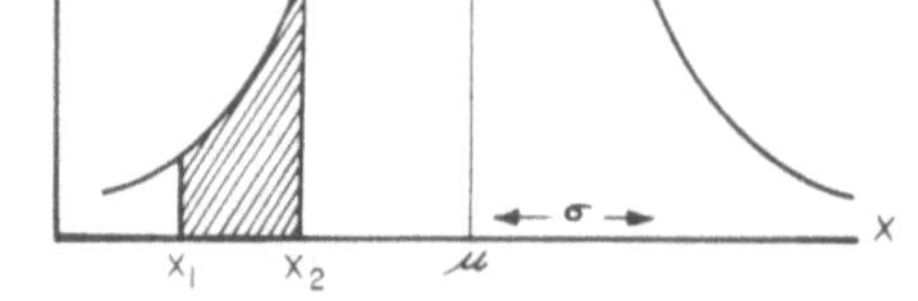

FIG. 7.13. *Example of a probability density*. The probability of a random variable falling in the interval between x_1 and x_2 is the corresponding *area* under the density function $= \int_{x_1}^{x_2} f(x)\, dx$. This particular density function is the normal or *Gaussian* density function. μ is the *mean* and σ the *standard deviation* of the distribution (see text).

response π upon which a random noise β is superimposed due to the ongoing brain activity. In formula:

(Eq. 7.10) $$e(t) = \pi(t) + \beta(t).$$

In this equation, $e(t)$ represents the time-dependent observable voltage changes in response to a stimulus, $\pi(t)$ is the fixed evoked response, and $\beta(t)$ is the "noise" due to uncontrolled factors.

If only one variable, $e(t_2)$ for example, is considered, then the values of this variable should cluster around $\pi(t_2)$. If a very large number of observations are made, the mean would be the center of gravity of the distribution. An important point is that the mean is not the only summary statistic to indicate the values around which random quantitites cluster. The *mode* (or most frequent value) and the *median* (or value for which the probability of the random variable being either greater than or less than is ½) are alternatives much used in nonparametric statistics. However, if the density is symmetric, these concepts coincide (Fig. 7.14). The formula for the mean of variable x is:

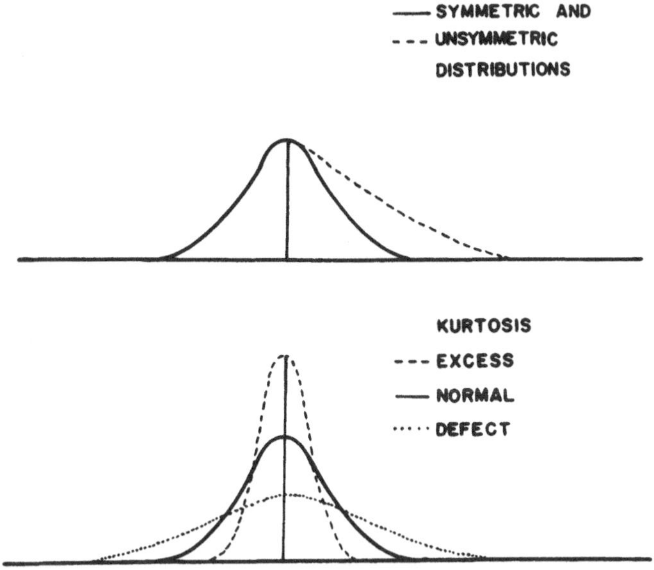

FIG. 7.14. *Moments of univariate densities.* The first moment or mean (μ) is the center of gravity of the density. The median (the value for which half the values are less and half larger) and the mode (most frequent value) are also measures of *location*. The variance, or second moment about the mean, σ_2, is a measure of *dispersion*. The standardized third moment about the mean or skewness, β_{11}, is a measure of asymmetry. When $\beta_{11} = 0$, the density is symmetric, and median, mean, and mode coincide. When $\beta_{11} = 0$, the curve is *skewed*. The standardized fourth moment about the mean is the kurtosis β_{21}. The higher the kurtosis, the more "peaked" the curve.

(Eq. 7.11) $$\mu = E(x) = \int xf(x)\,dx.$$

Eq. 7.11 expresses that the mean μ, or $E(x)$, is the average of x weighted by the density $f(x)$ [$E(\quad)$ is an operator to be interpreted as "taking the mean of whatever is in the parentheses].

When more than one observation is made, in multivariate observations, the *mean vector* is simply the mean of each component variable:

(Eq. 7.12) $$\vec{\mu} = E(\vec{\mathbf{x}}) = (\mu_1, \ldots \mu_p).$$

For example, the average evoked response is the sample analogue of a population sample mean. If one remembers Fig. 8.7, the mean vector corresponds to the center of gravity of the swarm.

The first moment is not enough in most cases. It is usually of interest to know not only the most typical or "true" value, but to take into consideration the characteristics of the random fluctuations around the mean. In geometric terms, considering once again the distribution of values specified by a probability model as a swarm of points in hyperspace, the mean vector only is a *measure of location*. It tells where the center of gravity of the swarm is, but contains no information about the size of the cloud of points, its shape, and so on. For this purpose, *higher order moments* are necessary.

Suppose that we center the swarm of points at the origin of the coordinate axes—that is, that we put the mean vector equal to 0, because we are now going to concentrate on the variability around the mean and the actual value of the mean is immaterial.

For a single variable x, the degree of spread or *dispersion* around the mean is measured by the *second moment* (around the mean) or *variance*. Its value is given by:

(Eq. 7.13) $$\sigma_x^2 = E[(x - \mu)^2] = \int (x - \mu)^2 f(x)\,dx.$$

This equation defines α_x^2, or the variance of x, as the mean value of the square of the difference between x and its mean μ.

$\sqrt{\sigma_x^2} = \sigma_x$ is the *standard deviation*.

As can be seen in Eq. 7.13, the variance is a sort of mean-square measure of departures from the mean. A physical interpretation in terms of the evoked-response example is that it is proportional to the mean amount of energy expended by the brain at time t_2 for a given type of stimuli.

When two or more totally unrelated variables are considered, then the overall size of the swarm of points is determined by the values of the variances for each variable. These variances express the degree of variability along the different axes.

When there are relationships or dependencies among the variables, the situation is somewhat more complicated. To fix ideas, consider two variables and the corresponding plot of values in 2-space. The greater the degree of correspondence between the values of each variable, the more the swarm of points clusters around a straight line (Fig. 7.15). Therefore, the *shape* of the cloud will depend not only on the variances, but also on the degree of relationships between the variables. This is measured quantitatively by the *covariances*, defined as:

$$\sigma_{12} = E\,[\,(x_1 - \mu_1)\,(x_2 - \mu_2)\,]. \qquad \text{(Eq. 7.14)}$$

The covariance is the mean value of the cross product of $x_1 - \mu_1$ and $x_2 - \mu_2$. As can be seen from Eq. 7.14, the covariance of a variable with itself is the variance ($\sigma_{11} = \sigma^2_{x1}$) and $\sigma_{12} = \sigma_{21}$—that is, the covariance of a variable x_1 with x_2 is the same as the covariance of x_2 with x_1. Covariances are 0 when x_1 and x_2 are *independent* (have no relationship) and can vary up to $\sqrt{\sigma_{11}\,\sigma_{22}}$ when a perfect *linear* relationship is present.

In the example for two variables, there are three second order moments: the variance σ_{11} and σ_{22} for variables x_1 and x_2, and the covariance between x_1 and x_2, σ_{12}. In general, the shape of the *p*-dimensional distribution is influenced by the variances and covariances between the variables. These are conveniently arranged in a *p* by *p* matrix Σ, the *variance-covariance* matrix. In this matrix Σ, any entry σ_{ij} is the covariance between variable *i* and *j*. Thus, the elements in the diagonal entries (Fig. 7.16) are the variances. If the variables are all independent, then the covariances are 0 and the matrix Σ is diagonal matrix (a matrix with only diagonal nonzero elements).

Just as was done for the mean, we can also fix the value of the variance-

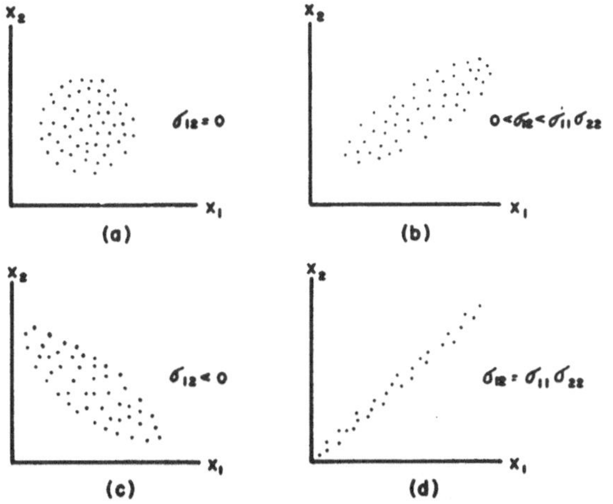

FIG. 7.15. *Covariance between the variables x_1 and x_2.* In each graph, the probability density is proportional to the density of points. In (a), the covariance of x_1 and x_2 is equal to 0. The variables are independent and they form a spherical-like swarm of points in the x_1x_2 plane. In (b), there is a moderate amount of linear dependency between x_1 and x_2 and the covariance is greater than 0 but less than its maximum value σ_{11} σ_{22}. In (c), a situation similar to (b) is present, but the relationship between x_1 correspond to lower values of x_2, and σ_{12} is negative. In (d), a perfect linear relationship exists between x_1 and x_2 and σ_{12} attains its maximum (positive) value $\sigma_{11}\,\sigma_{22}$.

covariance matrix in order to concentrate on other differences between models. If, for example, we not only subtract from the variable x, but we also divide by σ_x, we will then have a variable with 0 mean and variance 1. It is *standardized*.

For a vector $\vec{x}$, this can be done by substracting the mean and multiplying by the inverse of the square root of Σ, $\Sigma^{-½}$. In this case, we obtain a distribution with a geometric representation of a swarm of points z_i centered at the origin, spherical in shape, and with the same dispersion in any direction (Fig. 7.16). This transformation can be expressed:

(Eq. 7.15) $$\vec{z} = (\vec{x} - \vec{\mu})\Sigma^{-½}$$

($\vec{z}$ is the standardized vector, $\vec{\mu}$ and Σ the mean vector and the variance-covariance matrix, respectively).

This standardized form of expressing **x** is so important that the distance between any two points $\mathbf{z}_1$ and $\mathbf{z}_2$ in the swarm is called by a special name, the *Mahalanobis distance*.

The moments of *third* and *fourth* order (with respect to the standardized representation) are known as the *skewness* and *kurtosis* of the distribution. For a single variable x, these are denoted by β_{11} and β_{21} (Fig. 8.14). These quantities measure, respectively, the *symmetry* and peakedness of the density (Fig. 7.17). They, therefore, specify further the shape of the density. The

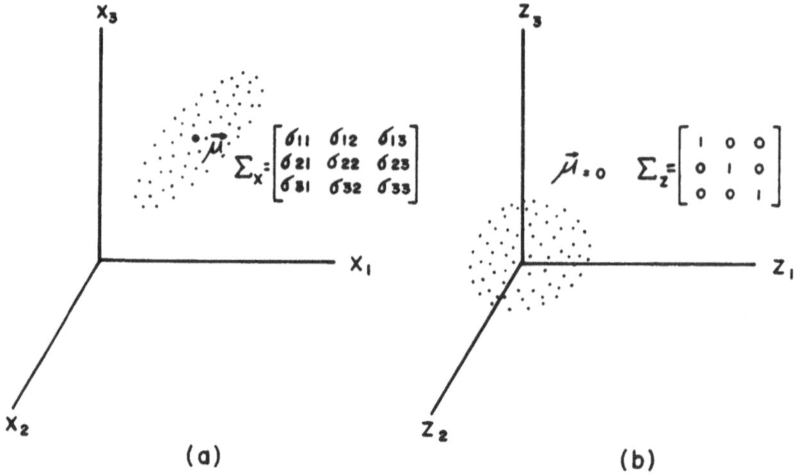

FIG. 7.16. *Standardization of a three-dimensional probability density.* In (a), the density of points before the transformation. The vector $\vec{\mu}$ indicates the *location* and the variance-covariance matrix Σ_X, the *shape* of the swarm of points. After applying the transformation $z = (x - \mu)\Sigma_X^{-½}$, where $\Sigma_X^{-½}$ is the inverse square root of Σ_X (b) a distribution is obtained that has zero mean and a spherical shape. The variance-covariance matrix Σ_Z is now the identity matrix, with 1's in the diagonal and 0 elsewhere.

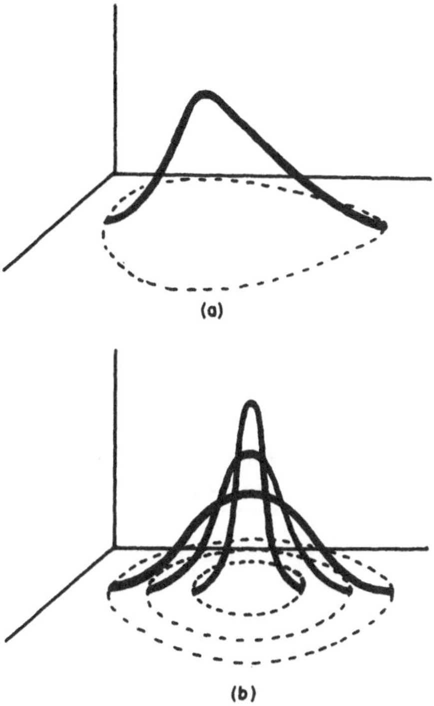

FIG. 7.17. *Multivariate skewness and kurtosis.* In (a), a skewed or asymmetric two-dimensional probability density is portrayed. As can easily be observed, the dome-shaped surface is more "stretched" to the right. In (b), three different densities are superimposed to illustrate different degrees of kurtosis for densities that have the same mean and that are symmetrical.

generalization of these measures to p dimensions is denoted by β_{1p} and β_{2p} (Fig. 8.17). We do not go into further details here.

It is possible to extend the notion of moments to higher orders than the fourth. For reasons seen later, this is not necessary for our purposes. We, therefore, now turn to the most frequent types of properties assumed for models used in neurometrics.

C. Gaussian Probability Models

A variable is said to have a *Gaussian* (or *normal*) distribution if its probability density is defined as:

$$y = \frac{e^{-\frac{1}{2}\frac{(x-\mu)^2}{\sigma}}}{\sqrt{2\pi\sigma}} \qquad \text{(Eq. 7.16)}$$

Eq. 16 represents the well-known bell-shaped curve (Fig. 7.13). In this equation, x is the value of the random value, μ the mean value and σ the standard deviation; y is the value of the probability density associated with a particular value of x.

A random vector is said to be Gaussian (or multinormal) when the density y associated with any particular vector $\vec{x}$ is:

(Eq. 7.17)
$$y = \frac{\exp[-\tfrac{1}{2}(\vec{x} - \vec{\mu})^T \Sigma^{-1} (\vec{x} - \vec{\mu})].}{(2\pi)^{1/2}\sqrt{|\Sigma|}}$$

In this equation, $\vec{\mu}$ is the mean vector and Σ the variance-covariance matrix. It is a generalization of Eq. 16 in which the random variable x is replaced by the random vector $\vec{x}$; the mean μ by the mean vector $\vec{\mu}$; the scalar value $(x - \mu)^2$ in the exponent by the scalar result of the matrix multiplication $(\vec{x} - \vec{\mu})^T \Sigma^{-1} (\vec{x} - \vec{\mu})$ (these operations were defined in section II of this chapter) and the standard deviation σ is replaced by the determinant of Σ. It also represents a bell-shaped curve for two dimensions (Fig. 7.18). In three dimensions, samples from a multinormal distribution lie within a volume that is ellipsoidal (football-shaped) in any cross section. For more than three dimensions, it is best to portray the distribution in time-series representation. The values for any particular variable have a Gaussian distribution—that is to say, they are *marginally Gaussian* (Fig. 7.19).

Gaussian-type distributions recur again and again in statistics for the following reasons:

1. The Gaussian distribution is completely specified by its moments of first and second order. The mean μ and variance σ^2 in the univariate case and the multivariate mean vector $\vec{\mu}$ and variance-covariance matrix Σ completely describe the location and shape of the Gaussian distribution.

2. Not only is the Gaussian distribution attractive because of its mathematical simplicity, but also the *central limit theorems* (Feller, 1965) explain its widespread appearance. These theorems state that if a stochastic process Z is the sum of N independent processes X_i, and if the variances of the X_i's are not large compared to that of Z, *then no matter what the distribution of the* X_i, Z tends to have a Gaussian distribution as N tends to

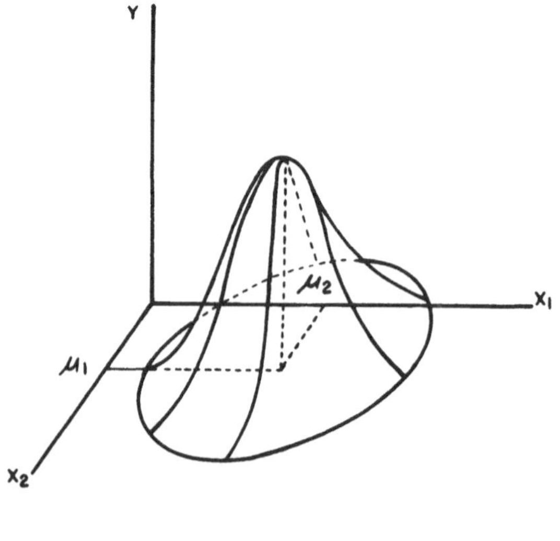

FIG. 7.18. *Two-dimensional random vector* $\vec{x}$ *with a Gaussian distribution.* The vector formed by x_1 and x_2 is distributed according to the density in the Y axes. The familiar bell-shaped curve is this density. The Gaussian density is completely specified by its mean vector (μ_1, μ_2) and covariance matrix Σ. Note that x_1 and x_2 are each Gaussian (marginal Gaussianity). The converse need not be true—marginal Gaussianity does not ensure overall Gaussianity (see text).

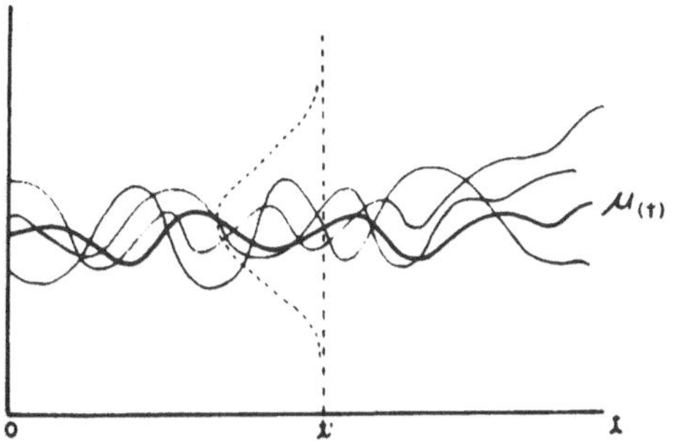

FIG. 7.19. *Gaussian time series.* The distribution at any time (t' in the figure) is univariate Gaussian. *Note that this is not enough.* The distribution of values at any set of time instants must be multivariate normal (see text). A Gaussian time series is completely specified by the mean function μ (t) and the covariance σ (t_1, t_2) between any pair of time instants.

infinity. *This means that a process that is the outcome of many weak, independent sources tends to be Gaussian.* Because many processes studies in biology can be approximately considered the outcome of many weak influences, and because many quantities considered in statistics are the weighted sum of random variables, the central limit theorem guarantees Gaussianity when the sample size is large enough.

In spite of this, all too frequently, the Gaussianity assumption is not valid. How situations of this type may occur is illustrated in Fig. 7.20. Suppose that we are obtaining evoked responses, as depicted in Fig. 7.11 and 7.12. Suppose also that the brain responses to a stimulus oscillates spontaneously between state 1 and 2 with equal probability. For each state, the electrical activity is Gaussian, so that if for two time instants t_1 and t_2, we plot separately the densities of the ERs for each brain state, we obtain the bell-shaped Gaussian surfaces (Fig. 7.20a). The combined process (called *a mixture*) is not multinormal; instead of being bell-shaped, the density has a butterfly-like shape, as seen in Fig. 7.20b. Yet, if one measures each variable $e(t_1)$ and $e(t_2)$ separately, as envisaged by projecting the combined mixture on either of the axes $e(t_i)$, they have a Gaussian distribution. The example just given illustrates the fact that univariate normality does not ensure multinormality.

The consequences of nonnormality, uni- or multivariate, are quite diverse. Some procedures are quite insensitive to certain kinds of deviations from multinormality, whereas others completely break down. In recent years, there has been considerable effort expended in the search for *robust* methods that stand up to violations of assumptions, and in the theoretical and computer-simulated evaluation of the effects of different types of nonmultinormality (see, for example, Mardia, 1970 and Olson, 1974).

If the sample is known to have been obtained from a nonnormal population, then the appropriate use of transformations, such as taking the square root of all the data, may be a remedy, either in the univariate case or in the multivariate situation (Andrews, Granadesikan & Warner, 1971). However, sometimes this is not possible and either a suitable probability model must be found, or nonparametric methods tried (Puri, 1970; Puri & Sen, 1971).

For the reasons previously stated, it is of considerable theoretical and prac-

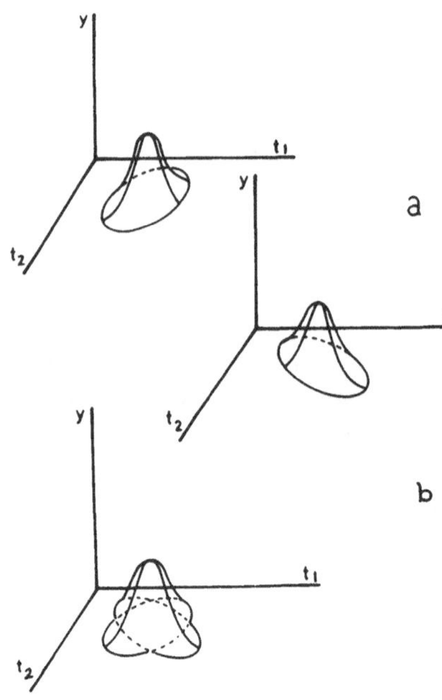

FIG. 7.20. *The combination of multinormal distributions* can generate a nonmultinormal distribution. Evoked responses to a certain stimulus are obtained while the brain oscillates spontaneously and equiprobably between two different stages, 1 and 2. If each state is considered by itself, the evoked responses obtained have a multinormal distribution, shown in (a) for only two time instants t_1 and t_2. (b) When the combined process is observed—that is, when the evoked responses are gathered irrespective of which state the brain is in, a distribution results that is *not multinormal.* This happens even though the distribution for each time instant is normal. This illustrates that a distribution may be univariate normal but not multinormal.

tical importance to be able to examine the Gaussianity of the data. For univariate samples, the problem has had a long history in statistics, and widely used methods are the Chi-squared test and the Kolmogorov-Smirnov one-sample test.

In spite of their popularity, extensive empirical computer-simulation studies, carried out by Shapiro and Wilk (1965), Shapiro, Wilk, and Chen (1968), and Lilliefords (1967), have shown these methods to perform poorly. They recommend the Shapiro and Wilk Omnibus test as the most powerful, and tests for skewness and kurtosis as second best. Because skewness and kurtosis tests generalize to multidimensional data, we explain them here.

As already pointed out, skewness and kurtosis are the third and fourth moment of the standardized distribution. These parameters reflect the degree of asymmetry and peakedness of the density. Because the Gaussian distribution is completely specified by its mean μ and variance σ^2, the values of all moments higher than the second are the same no matter what values μ and σ^2 take on. For a univariate Gaussian distribution, the skewness is 0 and the kurtosis is 3. Skewness and kurtosis tests for univariate normality are based on measuring the skewness and kurtosis for the sample and assessing the difference between the actual and theoretical values. If these differences are greater than those expected due to chance, then it is concluded that the sample does not come from a normal population. This is an example of a *test for goodness of fit*.

Multivariate normality is much more difficult to test and has received attention only in the last decade (Andrews et al., 1973; Gasser, 1975; Malkovich & Afifi, 1973; Wagle, 1968). Andrews et al. (1973) propose a graphical method that is based on the fact that the squared Mahalanobis distances d_i^2 of sample vectors from their mean are approximately Chi-squared distributed. (The Chi-squared distribution arises when variables that have normal distributions are squared and summed. This happens when a distance squared is obtained). We discuss this method in greater detail in section IV of this chapter, in connection with the detection of outliers.

Mardia (1970) generalized kurtosis and skewness measures for any number of dimensions, basing them on the concepts of Mahalanobis distances. Significance tables for both measures are available (Valdes, 1978).

When studying *time series*, it might not be possible to obtain more than one sample record. Such situations arise, for example, in the study of the spontaneous EEG when only one record is available for a given situation. This unique record is all that can be used to assess Gaussianity. Many authors have applied univariate Gaussianity tests to the sample values of such records, oblivious to the correlations between values obtained at successive time instants. The shortcomings of proceeding in this fashion and the difficulties involved in really testing Gaussianity have been pointed out by many authors (see, for example, Gasser, 1977). It appears that additional restrictions, such as stationarity, are always necessary in order to conduct tests for this assumption.

D. Stationarity, Ergodicity, and Mixing

As already stated, time series are a particular case of multivariate observations in which the variables measured are obtained at sequential time instants and therefore require special models. Time series can be sequences of discrete or continuous values, referred to either as *discrete valued* or *continuous valued*. Again, they may be observed continuously or only at discrete time instants. The former, *continuous time parameter series*, are the output from analog devices; a prime example is the EEG. *Discrete time parameter series* are encountered in digital processing of neurometric data. Time-varying potential changes, such as the EEG and evoked responses are modeled by the use of stochastic continuous time parameter series in theoretical work, and by discrete time parameter series in practical computer analysis. The underlying probability models for time series are called *stochastic processes*.

Stochastic processes can be rather intractable to mathematical analysis. If they have certain properties, then straightforward statistical procedures are appliable. Gaussianity (see the previous discussion) is one such property.

Another desirable property is that of *stationarity*. The time-series representation of stationary processes looks the same in spite of any time shift imposed on the time axis. Fig. 7.21a shows some time series that are stationary and Fig. 7.21b, shows some that are not. This is stated with more precision by saying that a stochastic process is *strictly stationary* if its probabilistic properties do not depend on time. In particular, this means that the mean function is constant, and that the covariance between two time instants t_1 and t_2 only depends on how far apart in time they are. For the sake of illustration, consider a discrete time parameter time series. At each time instant t_i, $\mu(t_i)$ must be constant. The covariance between values observed at t_i and t_j must be the same as the covariance for those observed at t_{i+k} and t_{j+k}; otherwise, these properties would be changing in time and the process would not be stationary. The covariances depend only on the difference $i-j$. This defines a peculiar type of covariance matrix, called a Toeplitz matrix. Fig. 7.22 shows a 10×10 Toeplitz matrix. As can be seen, only 10 distinct values occur, those in the first row. The rest of the matrix is obtained by reordering this row. A graph of any of the rows of this type of matrix against time is also known in the literature as an *auto-covariance function*—that is, the covariances between successive time points within the same discrete time process.

If only the mean is constant, then we speak of *first-order* stationarity. If the covariances also do not depend on time, then the process is known as *second-order stationary* or *weakly stationary*. Because the first two moments completely specify a Gaussian distribution, second-order stationary Gaussian processes are strictly stationary. It is fundamentally second-order stationarity that is assumed and tested for. This assumption introduces great simplifications into the description and analysis of time series, as is described later.

Stationarity can be assessed in two conditions: when replications of samples may be obtained (as in evoked-response studies) and when this is not possible (single EEG record). Valdes (1978) developed a test procedure for

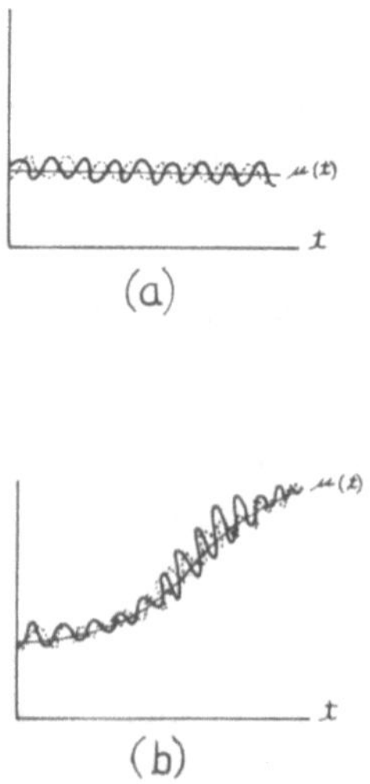

FIG. 7.21. *Stationary and nonstationary stochastic process.* In (a), two samples of a stationary stochastic process are represented. $\mu(t)$ is the mean of the stochastic process. Notice that changing the time axis by shifting the scale would not affect the appearance of the graph. In (b), there is a trend in the properties of the stochastic process; the mean $\mu(t)$ and the amplitude of oscillation change with time. The process is therefore *nonstationary*.

TOEPLITZ MATRIX

Covariance of variable i with variable j

	1	2	3	4	5	6	7	8	9	10
1	a	b	c	d	e	f	g	h	i	j
2	b	a	b	c	d	e	f	g	h	i
3	c	b	a	b	c	d	e	f	g	h
4	d	c	b	a	b	c	d	e	f	g
5	e	d	c	b	a	b	c	d	e	f
6	f	e	d	c	b	a	b	c	d	e
7	g	f	e	d	c	b	a	b	c	d
8	h	g	f	e	d	c	b	a	b	c
9	i	h	g	f	e	d	c	b	a	b
10	j	i	h	g	f	e	d	c	b	a

$\sigma_{ij} = \sigma_{|i-j|}$

FIG. 7.22. *Covariance matrix of a stationary process.* The covariances do not depend on the absolute times betwen two observations, but only on the difference between them—that is, $\sigma_{ij} = \sigma_{|i-j|}$. Thus, there are only 10 distinct values in the matrix, each row being a reordering of the previous one. This type of matrix is called a *Toeplitz matrix.*

the first case. As for the second case, in spite of many approximate and empirical methods (which usually only test first order stationarity), the only theoretically well-founded procedure available appears to be that of Priestley and Rao (1969), based on the concept of a time varying spectrum.

Another property is *ergodicity*, a term borrowed from statistical mechanics. Ergodicity means that averages formed at any time instant across all possible samples (called *ensemble averages*) are equal to averages across all the time points for a sufficiently long sample. This justifies, if the process is ergodic, the analysis of only one time series, if a sufficiently long record is available.

The *mixing* assumption specifies that the covariance of a stochastic process diminishes for the time points that are widely spaced. This corresponds to the fact that random influences usually make the predictibility of the values of a time series more and more difficult as time elapses.

The concepts presented in this section are interrelated, as can be seen in Fig. 7.23. Also included in this Fig. are statistical procedures that depend on assuming these properties.

Before turning to another point, consider briefly a very important type of stochastic process to be used subsequently. It exhibits the properties of stationarity and mixing to an extreme degree. *White noise* is defined as a

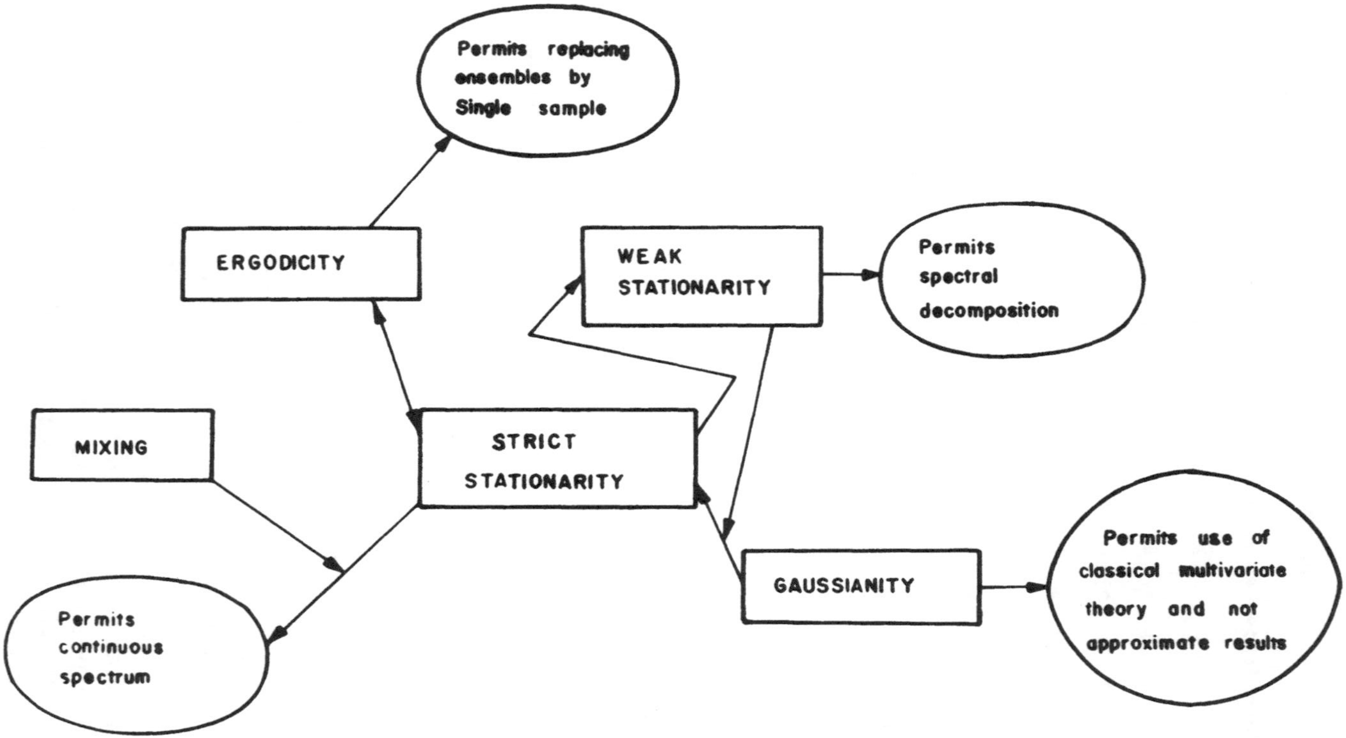

FIG. 7.23. *Relationships between the concepts of Gaussianity, stationarity, ergodicity, and mixing.* Arrows indicate that concepts may be derived from each other under specified assumptions. In ovals are statistical procedures based upon various assumptions.

stochastic process that has zero mean and for which the covariance between any two distinct time instants is zero.

IV. ANALYSIS OF THE STRUCTURE OF THE DATA

Even when a neurometric problem has been formulated, an adequate probability model selected, and the actual data collected, in the majority of cases, it is of interest to further analyze the sample obtained before ascertaining differences between clinical groups or trying to set up a diagnostic procedure. This need to further analyze the data stems from a recognition that the raw data collected is wastefully redundant as to the information that is useful for the problem at hand. Consider a typical 1-minute sample of EEG from eight channels, sampled at 100 Hz. The data in this case is 48,000 numbers! The existence of regularities in the data, be they consistent relationships among the variables or the recurrence of similar patterns for different individuals, permit summarizing descriptions that may be used to attain a minimal set of measures that are not redundant and that contain all the neurometrically relevant information.

In this part of this chapter, we review a group of statistical methods useful for what we call *analyzing the structure of the data.* The data collected is usually in the form of a *data matrix* (Fig. 7.24). This is a $N \times p$

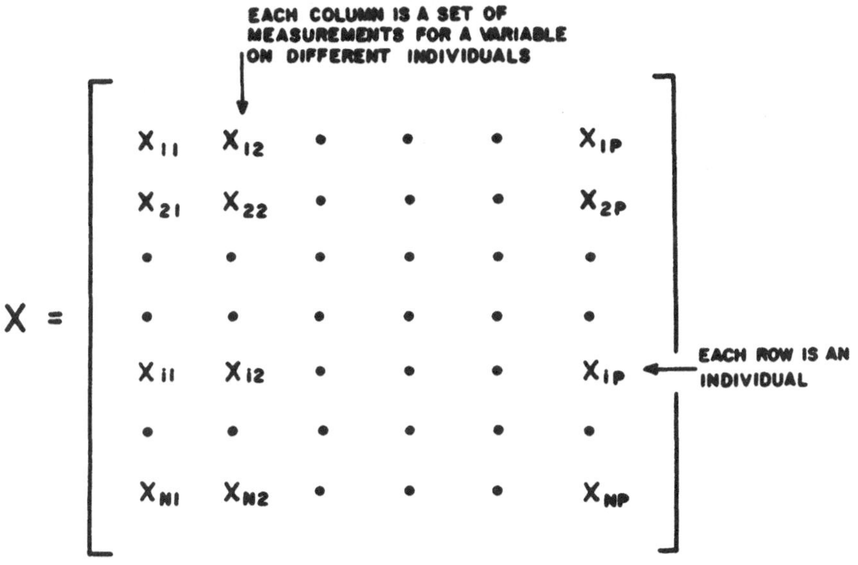

FIG. 7.24. *The data matrix.* Each row i of the data matrix X is the vector of observations for individual i, formed by p measurements x_{ij}. Methods for analyzing the structure of the data scan either the rows (individuals) or the columns (variables).

matrix **X**, in which N is the number of individuals and p the number of variables. Following the standard terminology, we refer to each row of the data matrix as the information for an *individual*, though this does not imply that each individual is a different subject (each row, for example, might be a replication of some vector measurement on the same subject.) The problem is to use the data matrix to study the structure of the data. This may be done from two points of view: studying relationships among the variables (columns fo the data matrix) or studying the relationships among the individuals (rows).

A. Relationships Among the Variables

Statistical methods for analyzing relationships among variables may be subdivided according to the nature of the variables involved and the type of relationship assumed. The types of variables may be:

1 *Actually observed variables*, which is data that can be collected. In all the Figs. of this section, these are symbolized by squares.
2. *Hypothetical or latent variables*. These cannot be observed, only inferred from the observed data. They can be considered as occult "generators." They are symbolized by circles.
3. *Standard variables*. The variables take on values of mathematical functions, such as sine, cosine, etc. They are denoted in all Figs. by triangles.

The problem is to determine whether a relationship between a set of observed variables and a set of another type of variables (observed hypothetical, or standard) exists, and to quantitatively measure the degree of relationship (Fig. 7.25). For example, if we try to determine the degree of dependence of a certain neurometric parameter on age, we are studying the relationship of two observable variables (Fig. 7.25a). If we are tyring to describe all the evoked responses from different derivations as a function of a small number of basic waveforms, then we are relating observed variables (evoked responses) with hypothetical variables (basic waveforms) (Fig. 7.25b). Finally, if we try to describe an EEG as the combination of different periodic waveforms (as is usual in spectral analysis), then we are relating the EEG record (observed variables) to the set of sine waves of different frequencies (standard variables) (Fig. 7.25c).

It is now pertinent to discuss the rather vague term "relationship" we have been using. Relationship is the tendency of the observed variables (possibly obscured by "noise") to vary in a certain fashion when another set of

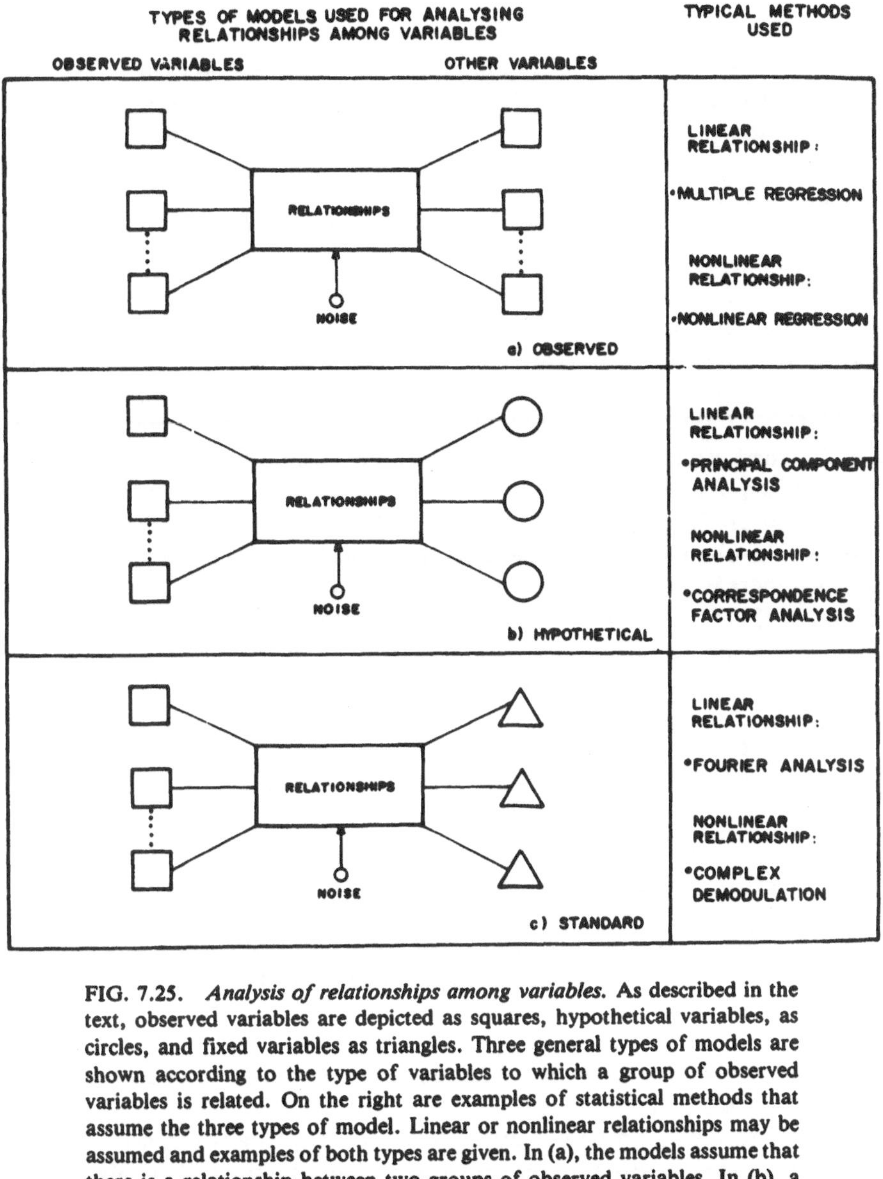

FIG. 7.25. *Analysis of relationships among variables.* As described in the text, observed variables are depicted as squares, hypothetical variables, as circles, and fixed variables as triangles. Three general types of models are shown according to the type of variables to which a group of observed variables is related. On the right are examples of statistical methods that assume the three types of model. Linear or nonlinear relationships may be assumed and examples of both types are given. In (a), the models assume that there is a relationship between two groups of observed variables. In (b), a group of observed variables is assumed to be related to unobservable hypothetical variables. In (c), the observed variables are described in terms of certain fixed mathematical functions (standard variables). In all models, the hypothetical variable "noise" obscures the functional relationship. Dotted lines connect dependent variables.

variables (observed, hypothetical, or standard) varies. By no means does this indicate the existence of *causal* relationships. The methods to be reviewed only explore the existence of phenomenological relationships. They might suggest determining mechanisms, but these must be established using experimental methods. Saying that an EEG record has 60% of activity in the alpha frequency band (8-13 Hz) is certainly helpful descriptively, but no one would imagine a sine wave generator (at least without experimental evidence) hidden among the folds of the cortex. We stress this point because many workers using the methods described in these sections claim that "they might suggest underlying physical mechanisms . . ." Although this is not impossible, the bulk of results has been of descriptive value. It seems probable that the elucidation of physiological mechanisms will come from the construction of well-designed models that will suggest the appropriate statistical analysis and not from the use of general purpose statistical methods whose generality and widespread usefulness comes from drastically simplifying assumptions.

As with probability models, the degree of specification of the type of relationship increases the precision with which inferences may be made, but enhances the possibility of not fitting the data. One may play safe and possibly lose precise information or be specific and get either a lot of or no information. To illustrate, suppose we are interested in case (a) of Fig. 7.25, the relationship between two sets of observed variables, in this case the EEG recorded at two different derivations. To measure the usual correlation between these two EEGs is to assume a *linear* relationship (Fig. 7.15). We might reject the existence of such a linear relationship if the covariance (or its scaled version, the correlation) is near 0, when in reality some other sort of relationship (such as a logarithmic relationship) is present. Recently, many papers have proposed the use of parameters derived from information theory in order to avoid this situation. What these parameters measure is the departure of the data from total independence (no statistical relationship at all). Although based on a minimum of assumptions, there is a drastic reduction of possibly very relevant information. A flexible strategy should be used, tailored to the problem; in fact, various methods should probably be tried out on the same data.

We now review the methods appropriate for studying the relationship of observed variables to other observed variables, to hypothetical variables, and to standard variables. In each case, we indicate: (1) the model; (2) other assumptions and consequences; (3) interpretation in terms of the data matrix; (4) mathematical formulation in formulas; (5) procedures for checking for fit; (6) neurometric examples and comments on use. Tables summarizing the information given are included for reference.

B. Relationships Between Two Groups of Observed Variables

1. Nonparametric Measures of Association.

These measures do not assume any particular type of relationship between observed variables or groups of observed variables. The model is based on the supposition that some sort of relationship exists between the observed variables that makes the assumption of statistical independence untenable. Well-known representatives of this type of measure are which quantify the departure from statistical independence, the *Chi-square statistics, non-parametric correlation coefficients*, and the *mutual information measure.* The first is useful for categorical data or data reduced to categorical form. The particular type of correlation coefficient discussed is the *rank-order correlation* that uses ordinal data or numerical data reduced to ordinal form. The mutual information is applicable to any kind of data, but we illustrate its use with categorical data.

We illustrate with a concrete example. Suppose two EEG records are obtained at the same time, for example from the same individual, but for two different leads. We want to measure the interrelationship between the two leads. To do this, we have two N-component vectors, $\vec{x}$ and $\vec{y}$, the two EEG records. The first components of each vector, x_1 and y_1, are the sampled voltage values for the two leads at time t_1, and in general we have N pairs (x_i, y_i). For the time being, we ignore the fact that there are intercorrelations between the successive x_i and y_i. *This is because, for the sake of illustration, we are going to apply to the EEG methods that are only valid when the samples obtained for different i are independent.* (This requirement is incorrectly ignored by some authors. The correct procedures to apply to EEGs have been developed for time series and are discussed in section IV.D of this chapter.)

Let us, furthermore, perform a drastic reduction in information. When a component x_i or y_i is positive or zero, we put a 1 in its place, when negative, a 2. Thus, for $N = 3$ the vector $\vec{x} = (2.5, .1, -3.3)$ is turned into $\vec{x} = (1, 1, 2)$. We have reduced numerical data to categorical data, simplifying, but also throwing away information. Denote by n_{11} the number of pairs (x_i y_i) in which both components are 1, by n_{12} the number of pairs in which the first components is 1 and the second 2, and so forth. We obtain a *contingency table* like that of Table 7.3. Summing a column, the first for example, we obtain n_1, the number of times the x_i are positive. If we divide by N, we obtain estimates of the *probability* of the events considered.

Thus, $\hat{P}_{ij}$ is the estimate probability of x being i and y being j simultaneously. (The hat "^" above a symbol denotes the *estimate* of the population

TABLE 7.3
Contingency Table Used to Calculate Chi-Squared Statistic and Mutual Information Measure[a]

	$x_i = 1$	$x_i = 2$	
$y_i = 1$	n_{11} $\hat{p}_{11} = n_{11}/N$	n_{21} $\hat{p}_{21} = n_{21}/N$	$n_{.1} = n_{11} + n_{21}$ $\hat{p}_{.1} = n_{.1}/N$
$y_i = 2$	n_{12} $\hat{p}_{12} = n_{12}/N$	n_{22} $\hat{p}_{22} = n_{22}/N$	$n_{.2} = n_{12} + n_{22}$ $\hat{p}_{.2} = n_{.2}/N$
	$n_{1.} = n_{11} + n_{12}$ $\hat{p}_{1.} = n_{1.}/N$	$n_{2.} = n_{21} + n_{22}$ $\hat{p}_{2.} = n_{2.}/N$	$= n_{1.} + n_{2.}$ $= n_{.1} + n_{.2}$

[a] Two EEG channels recorded at the same time (x and y) are obtained. The numerical values in the vectors x_i, y_i are substituted by a 1 if a positive or by 2 if negative. The Table has as entries n_{kl}, the number of times x_i takes on the value k ($k = 1$ or 2) *and* y_i also takes on the value 1($l = 1$ or 2). These values divided by the total number of components of x and y, N, give estimates of probabilities. For example, $\hat{p}_{11}$ is the estimated probability of x_i being positive *and* y_i being positive.

parameter). $\hat{P}_{i.}$ is the estimated probability of x being i and $\hat{P}_{.j}$ is the probability of y being j.

The *multiplication rule* for independent events (Feller, 1965) states that if x and y are independent, then:

$$\hat{P}_{ij} = \hat{P}_i \hat{P}_j \qquad \text{(Eq. 7.18)}$$

The Chi-squared statistic and the mutual information are based on Eq. 18. Applying the formulas in Table 7.4, the Chi-squared statistic for this situation is:

$$\chi^2 = (\hat{P}_{11} - \hat{P}_{1.}\hat{P}_{.1})^2 / \hat{P}_{11} + (\hat{P}_{22} - \hat{P}_{2.}\hat{P}_{.2})^2 / \hat{P}_{22} + (\hat{P}_{12} - \hat{P}_{1.}\hat{P}_{.2})^2 / \hat{P}_{12} + (\hat{P}_{21} - \hat{P}_{2.}\hat{P}_{.1}) / \hat{P}_{21} \qquad \text{(Eq. 7.19)}$$

And the *mutual information is:*

$$I(x,y) = \hat{P}_{11} \log \frac{\hat{P}_{11}}{\hat{P}_{1.}\hat{P}_{.1}} + \hat{P}_{22} \log \frac{\hat{P}_{22}}{\hat{P}_{2.}\hat{P}_{.2}} + \hat{P}_{12} \log \frac{\hat{P}_{12}}{\hat{P}_{1.}\hat{P}_{.2}} + \hat{P}_{12} \log \frac{\hat{P}_{12}}{\hat{P}_{2.}\hat{P}_{.1}} \qquad \text{(Eq. 7.20)}$$

As can be easily seen from Eq. 18, 19, and 20, both the mutual information and the Chi-squared statistic are 0 when the variables are independent. These measures increase for increasing dependence. The fancy-sounding "information theory" parameter measures the same thing as the Chi-squared statistic.

Let us continue the illustrative example. Instead of just being interested in polarity of the EEG signal, we now establish a rank ordering among the elements of the vector $\vec{x}$ and $\vec{y}$. For the $\vec{x}$ vector in Eq. 20, this rank ordering gives a vector $\vec{x} = (3, 2, 1)$. We lose less information than before, because the relative ordering of the EEG records is preserved. We may now find the differences $d_i = x_i - y_i$ and apply the formula for the rank-order correlation coefficient (Table 7.4). We have another measure for relationship between lead x and y. This measure is 0 if no relationship holds, -1 if x has the reverse ordering of y, and 1 if they have the same. Tables for assessing the significances or correlations for different values of N may be found in Siegel (1970).

These methods are applicable with a minimum of assumptions. They are equally useful for any type of data if the appropriate transformations are made. They also entail a loss of detail that might be essential.

The loss of detail is very important. For example, if it is possible to demonstrate that the two EEG vectors $\vec{x}$ and $\vec{y}$ both might have come from Gaussian populations, then applying the concept of mutual information to the multinormal density gives an expression that is essentially a logarithmic transformation of the ordinary correlation coefficient used to assess linear relationships. In this case, the use of Eq. 20 seems wasteful of mutual information.

2. Linear Relationships Among the Observed Variables: Linear Regression Models

Two groups of variables are said to be *linearly related* if they can be expressed as weighted sums of each other plus an error term. To make the discussion more precise, consider two neurometric variables x_1 and x_2. If the equation:

$$x_2 = \alpha x_1 + \beta \tag{21}$$

is valid, then the two variables are linearly related (their graph in 2-space is a straight line). In practice, neither x_1 or x_2, is precisely determined; rather, they are random quantities and Eq. 21 is substituted by:

$$x_2 = \alpha x_1 + \beta + \varepsilon \tag{22}$$

in which an error term is included to reflect the deviations from an exact linear relationship. This is known as a (simple) *linear regression model*. This model is schematized in Fig. 7.26. The method of *least squares* may be used to estimate the parameters α and β of Eq. 22. This consists of finding values

TABLE 7.4
Measures of Nonparametric Association[a]

Measure	*Formula*	*Values which the Measure Takes*	*Type of Data That May be Used*
Chi-squared statistic	$X^2 = \sum_{i=1}^{n} \sum_{j=1}^{m} \frac{(\hat{P}_{ij} - \hat{P}_{i.}\hat{P}_{.j})^2}{\hat{P}_{ij}}$	O for independence. Increases with increase in functional dependence.	Categorical
Mutual information	$I_{(x,y)} = \sum_{i=1}^{n} \sum_{j=1}^{m} \hat{P}_{ij} \log \frac{\hat{P}_{ij}}{\hat{P}_i \hat{P}_j}$	O for independence. Increases with increase in functional dependence.	Categorical, ordinal, numerical
Rank correlation	$r = 1 - \frac{6 \sum_{i=1}^{n} d_i^2}{n(n^2 - 1)}$	O for independence. Negative values up to -1 for inverse relationship. Positive values up to 1 for direct relationship.	Ordinal

[a]Measures of association used to quantify the degree of dependence between variables x and y. Suppose that x and y can each have n and m states *t* respectively. Then $\hat{P}_{ij}$ is the estimated probability of x being in state i and y in state. $\hat{P}_{i.}$ is the estimated probability of x being in state i; $\hat{P}_{.j}$ is the probability of y being in state j. These probabilities are estimated by counting the number of occurrences of each event and dividing by the total number of events. For example, $\hat{P}_{ij} = n_{ij}/N$, where N is the total number of occurrences of x and y observed and n_{ij} the number of those occurrences in which x took on state i and y took on state j. For the calculation of the rank of correlation, the observations for each variable (x and y) are rank ordered, d_i is the difference between the rank order of x_i and y_i.

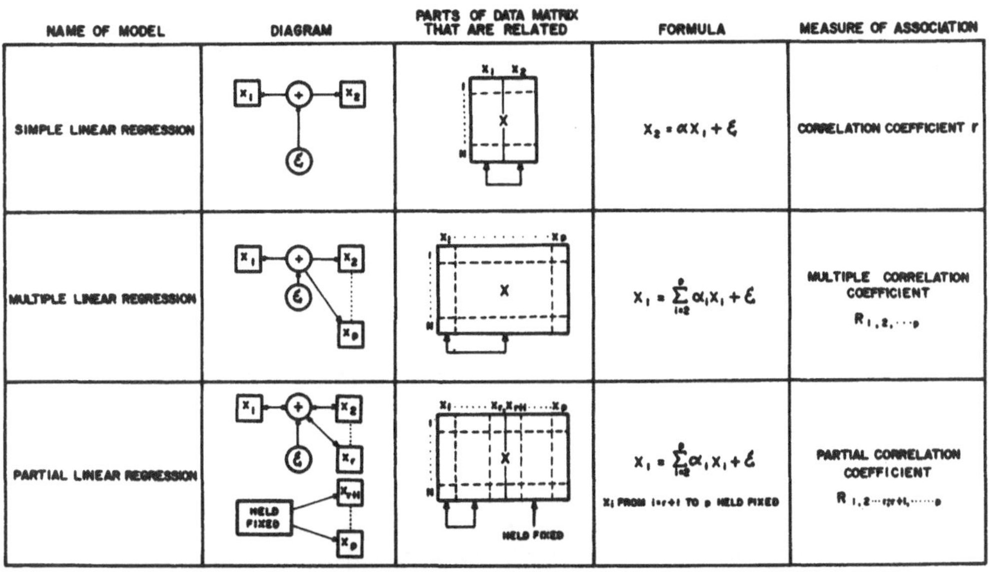

FIG. 7.26. *Linear regression models.* The x_i are the observed variables represented by squares. E is the error term (hypothetical, because it cannot be directly observed) represented by a small circle. The arrows represent linear interactions symbolized by the circle containing the + sign. N is the number of individuals in the data matrix and p the number of variables.

a and b, which substituted in Eq. 22 in place of α and β minimize the values of:

$$e_i = ax_{1i} + b - x_{2i} \tag{23}$$

In this equation, x_{1i} and x_{2i} are the values of x_1 and x_2, respectively, for individual i.

The e_i, known as the residual, are just the estimates of the noise . This procedure is quite general. Its geometric meaning is easily seen in Fig. 7.27. The points in that Fig. are the data points for pairs of value of x_1 and x_2. A functional relationship $x_2 = f(x_1)$ is postulated where $f(.)$ is a function belonging to a family of functions that depend on certain parameters θ. The method of least squares consists in varying the θ until the sum of the squares of the errors e_i (the differences between $f(x_1)$ and the data points in the vertical direction, marked by the lines labeled $e_1, e_2, \ldots, e_7$ in the Fig.) is a minimum.

If we, furthermore, assume that the noise has a Gaussian distribution, then exact tests of significance for the fit of the model may be legitimately carried out. We do not discuss these tests for goodness of fit, but, rather, consider a related concept, that of the *association coefficient* derived from the linear model. It may happen that the data do not adjust well to Eq. 22, either because the functional relationship is not linear, or because any functional

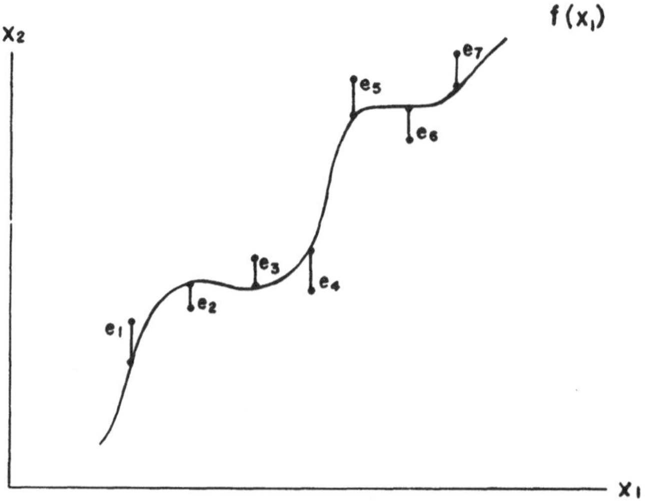

FIG. 7.27. *Fitting a functional relationship* between x_1 and x_2 by *least-squares method*. The functional relationship $x_2 = f(x_1)$ is to be fitted. The function f depends on certain parameters Θ_K. The data is represented by points, in this case 7. For any given values of Θ_K, f will have a certain form. The difference of the data points from the function may be measured by the vertical distances of the data points to the function f, in the figure represented by the vertical lines labeled e_i. These are the *residuals*. The sum of the residuals squared, E, is a measure of the goodness of fit of the functional relation. The method of least squares tried to vary the Θ_K so as to minimize E.

relationship is swamped by the excess of noise ϵ. In any case, statisticians define measures of association that quantify how much of the variation in the data is due to the functional relationship and how much is due to noise. In the example under discussion, this is measured by the *correlation coefficient*, mentioned earlier in this chapter. If the noise is so large that no linear relationship is really present, the correlation coefficient is 0.

If a perfect linear relationship is present, then the correlation coefficient is 1 in absolute value (positive or negative depending on the slope of the line; see Fig. 7.15).

Care should be exercized in interpreting the correlation coefficient because the existence of a nonlinear functional relationship may result in a zero linear correlation coefficient. This and other possibilities of misfit of the model may be detected by plotting the residuals e_i against the values of $ax_{1i} + b$. If the model is correct, then the e_i should be randomly distributed around zero. Tendencies to cluster, extreme values, and other departures from assumptions are diagnostic checks that something is wrong.

The preceding comments are applicable to all types of regression models. In Fig. 7.26, the principal types of linear regression models are presented. A brief comment on each type follows:

1. *Simple linear regression*: This model has been discussed previously.

2. *Multiple regression*: A linear relationship is postulated between an observed variable and a set of observed variables. A least-squares solution is always possible; more exact tests for degree of fit are available, if a multinormal distribution is assumed for the error vector. The measure of association is the *multiple correlation coefficient*, a simple generalization of the correlation coefficient. A geometrical representation of the multiple regression of a variable y on x_1 and x_2 can be seen in Fig. 7.28.

3. *Partial regression*: This is a variant of multiple regression in which the effects of certain variables are "partialled out." It is useful for studying the relationships of a variable (predicted variable) with others (predictor variables) independent of the effects of other variables (concomitant variables).

4. *Canonical correlations*: This model is useful in studying the linear interrelationships between two different sets of observed variables. We discuss this in a later section, after analyzing the use of hypothetical variables.

We now give some neurometric examples of the use of these concepts. The simple linear correlation coefficient may be used to assess whether any particular neurometric parameter depends on age. If this is so, the variation due to age may be "partialled out" using partial regression in order to obtain an

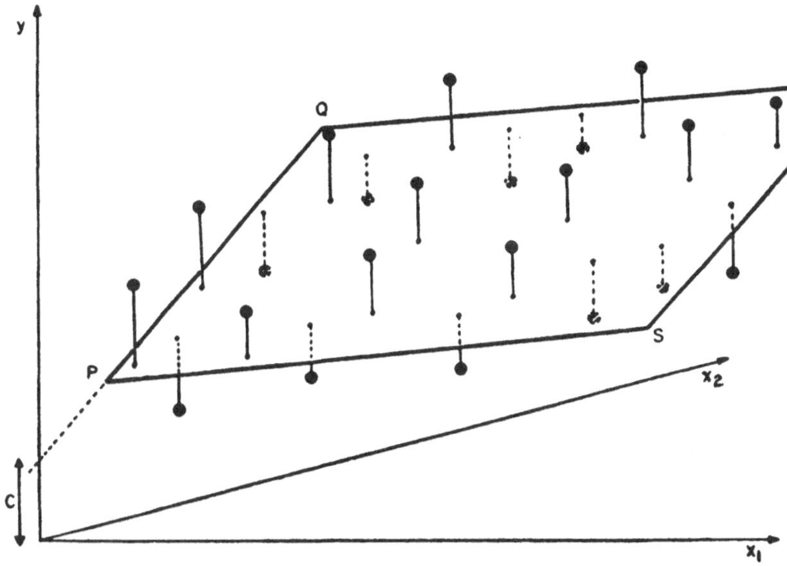

FIG. 7.28. *Multiple regression.* This is a geometrical representation of a multiple regression of the variable y upon variables x_1 and x_2. This is a generalization of Fig. 7.27. In this case, the plane *PQRS* is the least-square best fit plane. It minimizes the square of the sum of the residuals, represented here by the vertical lines projecting from the data points to the plane.

age-independent measure. Matousek and Petersén (1973b) give a particularly interesting example of the use of multiple regression (discussed in Chapter 11). They found the regression of age on a set of neurometric parameters. One can then calculate the "EEG age" of a given individual and compare it to the biological age (the age-dependent quotient).

3. Nonlinear Relationships Among the Observed Variables: Nonlinear Regression

Linear relations are the most simple and mathematically tractable type of interrelations between observed variables. This is the reason that linear models are usually tried as the first option. Even when the fit is not exceptionally good, linear regressions may serve as a first approximation, valid perhaps for certain restricted values of the observations. An example of this is multiple regression mentioned int he previous section, undertaken by Matousek and Petersén (1973b). John has prepared regressions of a large number of neurometric parameters on age. The functional relationship that is the best fit to the Matousek and Petersén normative data is not linear, but a fourth order polynomial of the form:

$$x = a_o + a_1t + a_2t^2 + a_3t^3 + a_4t^4, \qquad (24)$$

in which x is the neurometric parameter and t age in months.

This illustrates that when one needs a better fit than the one linear regression gives, it is necessary to turn to some form of nonlinear regression. We do not go into details here, but simply point out that the general observations of the previous section also apply to nonlinear regressions. Both least-squared and Gaussian-based methods of fitting the nonlinear equations are available. They are much more time consuming than in the linear situation. In nonlinear regressions, as in linear regression, examination of the residuals is very valuable.

4. Step-Wise Regression Methods

These are not really a new type of regression model, but rather a computational procedure for selecting a minimal amount of observed variables (called independent variables) necessary to explain a given observed variable (called a dependent variable). Theoretically, one could fit the regression models of this action using all possible subsets of independent variables. For example, if the dependent variable y is to be regressed upon x_1 and x_2, then the regression of y upon x_1 alone, upon x_2 alone, and upon both x_1 and x_2 are carried out. The minimal best-fitting regression equation is then chosen. This procedure is feasible only for small numbers of variables because the number of possible subsets of p independent variables is 2^p. Efficient methods for examining all possible subsets are described in Enslein (1977).

When the number of varibles is so great that not even the efficient methods for testing all 2^p regressions are feasible, then *step-wise regression methods* are used. A typical step-wise regression procedure is as follows:

1. Select that independent variable (say x_1) that best explains the dependent variable y.
2. Partial out the effect of the selected variable x_1 from the remaining $p - 1$ independent variables, $x_2, \ldots, x_p$.
3. Look for the variable among the remaining independent variables that, together with x_1, best explains the dependent variable y.
4. Repeat step 2 as long as acceptable accuracy is achieved.

Step-wise methods are among the most popular programs used and are available in many statistical computer program packages. In spite of this widespread use, many prominent statisticians have pointed out that it is an empirical method. Its properties are not well understood. Also, there are concrete examples in which it gives biased results. These considerations should prompt the user to view the output from this type of program as a heuristic aid, rather than as statistically conclusive results.

C. Relationships Between Observed Variables and Hypothetical Variables

The next group of models for the analysis of structure involving interrelationships among variables have the peculiarity that the observed variables are related to *hypothetical variables* also called *latent variables*, factors, or components (Fig. 7.25). The general idea is that a certain minimal amount of unobservable "primary variables" combine and interplay to produce a host of observable variables. If these primary variables could be estimated, they would contain all the information on the observed variables without any redundancy. It was precisely in this setting that the psychometrics, forerunners of this methodology called their attempts at extracting underlying "intelligence factors" *factor analysis*. Since then, the subject has freed itself from any specific content and has become a part of standard multivariate techniques.

These methods have a clear advantage in compressing data. Instead of working with a data matrix with 100 variables, for example, it is often possible to have a new data matrix with only 10 variables and essentially the same information. The interpretation of the hypothetical variables, however, is a tricky business. There is a certain indeterminacy in the solutions: If a certain set of hypothetical variables "explain" the data matrix well, then there are infinitely many sets of hypothetical variables that do just as well. The constraction of mathematical criteria for selecting *the* solution has involved a large number of statisticians (see Morrison, 1976), but all the criteria seem to have an artificial character. The practice of naming factors and interpreting them is rather ad hoc. It thus seems that the principal value of these methods is of parsimonious description, to a much lesser extent, suggestion of hypotheses, and almost never, the suggestion of actual "generators" of the data structure.

As with the interrelationships between observable variables, we consider nonparametric, linear, and nonlinear types of relationships of observed with hypothetical variables.

1. Nonparametric Latent Structure Methods

The most widely used nonparametric method for uncovering latent structure is *correspondence factor analysis.* This method can be used with any type of data. The relationships among the observed variables are summarized in a sort of nonparametric correlation matrix, which is a table of the Chi-squared statistic of nonparametric dependence between all pairs of observed variables. From this matrix, the method constructs a two- or three-dimensional plot of the correspondence factors. The variables are portrayed on these plots as points and the distance between two variables reflects their degree of association. These plots are especially useful because the individuals may also be plotted together with the variables. (This is discussed in connection with the analysis of structure for individuals in section F of this chapter). This method has been used successfully by Arnal, Gerin, Salmon, Nakache, Maynard, Peronnet, and Hugonnier (1971) in describing visual evoked potentials in normal and amblyopic subjects.

2. Linear Latent Structure Methods

The two principal types of models are *principal component analysis* and *factor analysis* (Fig. 7.29). They both perform a linear transformation of the data matrix in order to obtain a new data matrix with fewer variables. In other words, if the original data is representable in p-dimensional hyperspace, then these methods linearly transform the data (they form weighted sums of the columns of the data matrix) in order to represent them in an r-dimensional hyperspace (r is usually substantially less than p).

What *principal component analysis* does can be seen graphically in Fig. 7.30. In the Fig., the method is illustrated with an example consisting of a set of data collected for three variables, x_1, x_2, and x_3. These data form a swarm

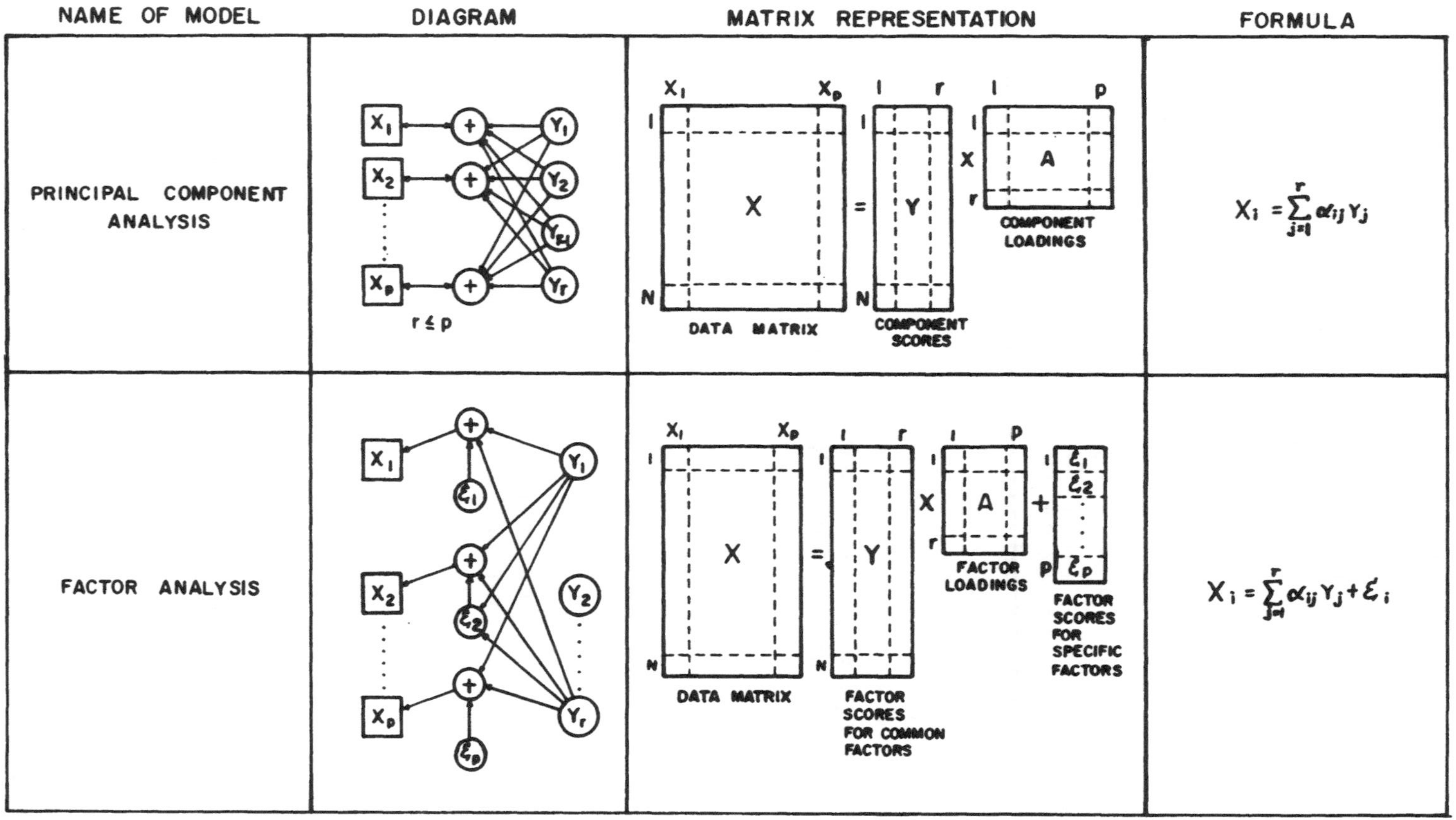

FIG. 7.29. *Linear latent structure models.* The x_i are *observed variables,* represented by squares. The $\mathbf{Y}_i$ are hypothetical variables, the *common factors,* represented by circles. The ζ_i are also hypothetical variables represented by squares, the *specific factors.* The presence of specific factors is what characterizes *factor analysis* as distinct from *principal component analysis.* Circles containing plus signs and the arrows stand for linear interactions.

of points that is elongated and points along a certain direction. The swarm is highly concentrated along a longitudinal axis that points up and to the right, indicating a high degree of covariance between the different variables. The principal component transformation (with coefficients a_{ij}) forms weighted sums of the data matrix. These weighted sums can be considered as a new reference system (Fig. 7.30)—that is, as new variables y_1, y_2, and y_3. These new variables have the property that most of the variation of the swarm of points lies along y_1, most of the remaining variation along y_2, and what is left along y_3. If we were to discard any of the three variables y_i, we would certainly start with the third, and perhaps even the second, because most of the variation is along y_1, y_1 is called the *first principal component*, y_2 the *second principal component*, and so on. An important property of the principal components is that they are statistically independent. They, thus, permit a description of the data with the minimum number of variables that are uncorrelated. These ideas carry over to more than three variables (Harman, 1960).

Principal component analysis is usually carried out after putting the mean of the swarm of points at the origin (this was done in Fig. 7.30). All the information necessary to calculate the coefficients a_{ij} for the transformation is contained in the variance-covariance matrix. The coefficients a_{ij} are called the principal *component loadings*. The values of the individuals for the principal components are the principal *component scores*.

If the original variables x_i are not in the same units, then they are usually scaled to unit variance. This is equivalent to working with the correlation matrix instead of the covariance matrix. In terms of Fig. 7.30, this means not only putting the mean of the swarm at the origin, but also giving the elongated swarm a ball-like shape before the transformation. Principal components obtained from correlation matrices are *not* equivalents to those obtained from covariance matrices.

Factor analysis is a slightly different model. It specifies two different types of new variables. *Specific factors* explain variations that are uniquely characteristic of each original variable x_i.The *common factors* explain the variation of the data that is common. Thus, factor analysis may be considered a sort of principal component analysis after the specific factors have been removed. More precisely, this is a type of factor analysis known as *principal factor analysis*.

Principal component analysis is a special case of factor analysis in which the specific factors are considered to be zero. This distinction should be clear, because what usually is called factor analysis in program packages and publications is really principal component analysis.

Factor analysis concentrates interest on the common factors. As for principal components, the coefficients linearly relating the original variables x_i to the factors are called *loadings*. The values of the common factors for each individual are called *scores*.

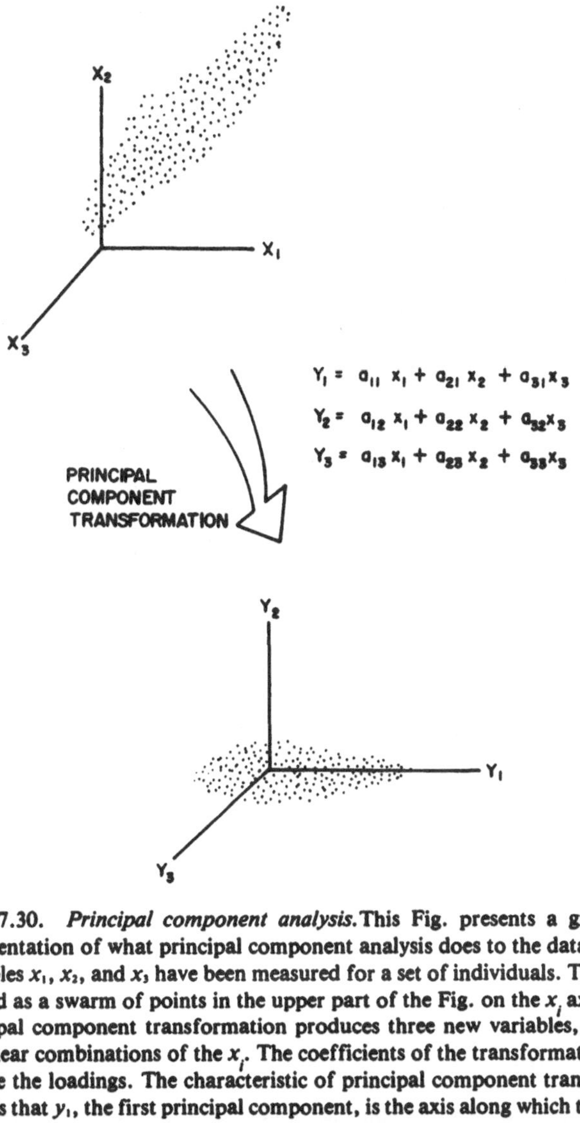

FIG. 7.30. *Principal component analysis.* This Fig. presents a graphical representation of what principal component analysis does to the data. Three variables x_1, x_2, and x_3 have been measured for a set of individuals. These are plotted as a swarm of points in the upper part of the Fig. on the x_i axes. The principal component transformation produces three new variables, y_i, that are linear combinations of the x_i. The coefficients of the transformation, the a_{ij}, are the loadings. The characteristic of principal component transformations is that y_1, the first principal component, is the axis along which the principal direction of variation of the swarm of points lies. The second principal component, y_2, accounts for most of the remaining variability. y_3 has very little variability left. The projection of the individuals on the y_i axes (that is, their values for the new variables) are the scores.

Both principal components and factor analysis produce sets of new variables that are highly parsimonious descriptions of the original data matrix, but these new variables are difficult to interpret. In the hope of clearing up the relations between the new variables and the original ones, statisticians have developed further transformations called *rotations*. One of the most popular is the *Varimax rotation* of Kaiser (Morrison, 1976). What this transformation does is shown graphically in Fig. 7.31. Here, we plot a set of "old" variables x_i in terms of the "new" factors. The principal component solution is given in Fig. 7.31a. As can be seen, the first principal component y_1 is close to all the x_i and y_2 is not. This is precisely the characteristic of principal components. There are two groups of x_i variables, however, and performing a rotation on y_1 and y_2 can bring each of them near to one of these groups and far from the other, as in Fig. 7.31b. This (the statisticians say) might facilitate the interpretation of these variables, the *varimax axes*.

Under certain conditions, varimax scores (designed as the values of the varimax variables for each individual) tend to be more stable from one sample to the other. Principal component analyses, followed by varimax rotation, has been used in the description of evoked responses (John, Ruchkin, &

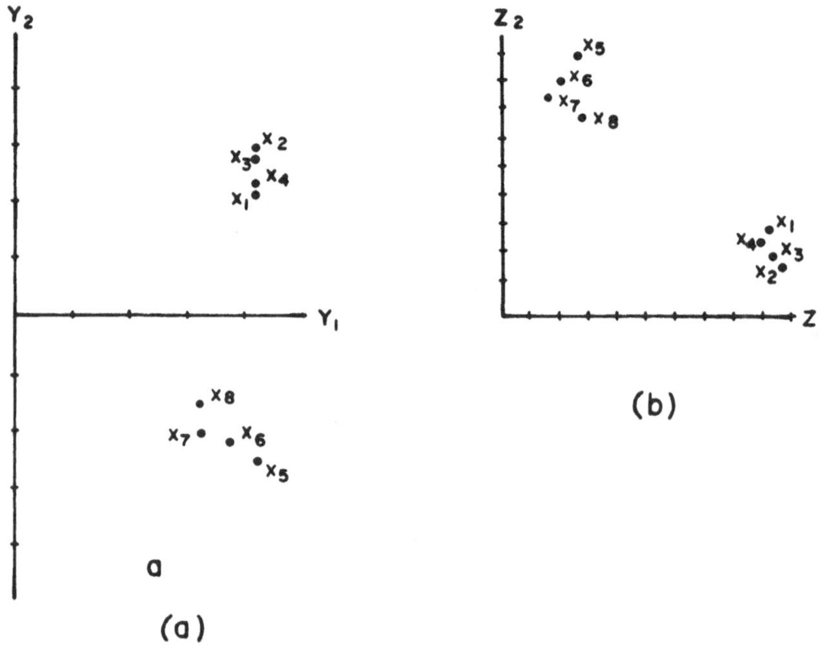

FIG. 7.31. *Varimax rotation.* The varimax rotation is a transformation of principal components or factors to enhance their interpretability. This Fig. gives an example in which eight original variables x_i have been analyzed by principal components. Two principal components were found to explain most of the variation of the sample. However, the interpretation of these principal components is very difficult. a) If the variables are plotted as functions of the two principal components, y_1 and y_2, it can be observed that two groups of variables exist. b) A Varimax rotation is an analytical procedure to rotate the axes y_i until each axis is as near to a cluster of variables and as far away from others as possible. This rotation gives a new set of axes, z_1 and z_2, that (hopefully) might be easier to interpret.

Villegas, 1964; Kavanagh, Darcey, & Fender, 1976; Valdés, unpublished results).

There are two other models that merit discussion here. These are *canonical correlation* and *canonical coordinates analysis*. *Canonical correlation analysis* (Fig. 7.32) is the generalization of the linear regression models. As can be remembered, in these analyses, *one* observed variable was compared to a set of observed variables. When *two sets* of observed variables are to be compared, a single linear relationship is not enough and *canonical variates* are introduced. Suppose that we want to compare p variables x_i with r variables y_i (these are all observed variables). To do so, we form a hypothetical variable ζ_1 that is a linear combination of the x_i and another hypothetical variable n_1 that is a linear combination of the y_i. We do this in a way that ξ_1 and η_1 have the highest possible correlation. These are the *first canonical variates* and their correlation is the *first canonical correlation*. We then form two new hypothetical variates ξ_1 and η_2 with the highest possible correlation that are independent statistically from ξ_1 and η_1. These are the *second canonical variates* and their correlation is the *second canonical correlation*. This is continued until we have partitioned the total correlation between the x_i and y_i into the canonical correlations. Canonical correlation analysis is of use in studying the dependence relationships (of linear type) between two sets of variables. It has not been used very much in neurometrics.

Canonical coordinate analysis (the use of the word "canonical" for different things is confusing, but standard statistical jargon) or, as it is sometimes called, *discriminant factor analysis*, does not compare sets of variables, but different groups of individuals for which the same variables have been measured. Suppose we have k different groups, with unequal mean vectors but with the same covariance matrix. This can be imagined as a set of k swarms in p-dimensional hyperspace. These swarms have the same shape, but they are displaced with respect to each other (Fig. 7.33a). Imagine now that we standardize (section IIB of this chapter) these swarms—that is, we turn them into spherical clouds of points with unit variances along any direction (Fig. 7.33b). We then do a sort of principal component analysis and project these clouds onto a space of much smaller dimension (Fig. 7.33c). The axes of the new space are the *canonical coordinates* (or canonical functions). The advantage of this representation is that we have all the information about differences between the groups in standardized and condensed form. The use of the canonical functions for prediction are studied in section V of this chapter.

In neurometric applications, the data matrix is sometimes transposed: Rows are changed to columns and what was an individual becomes a variable. For example, in doing principal component analysis of evoked responses, Donchin (1966) considers each evoked response as an individual and the samples value of the evoked response at a particular time instant as a variable.

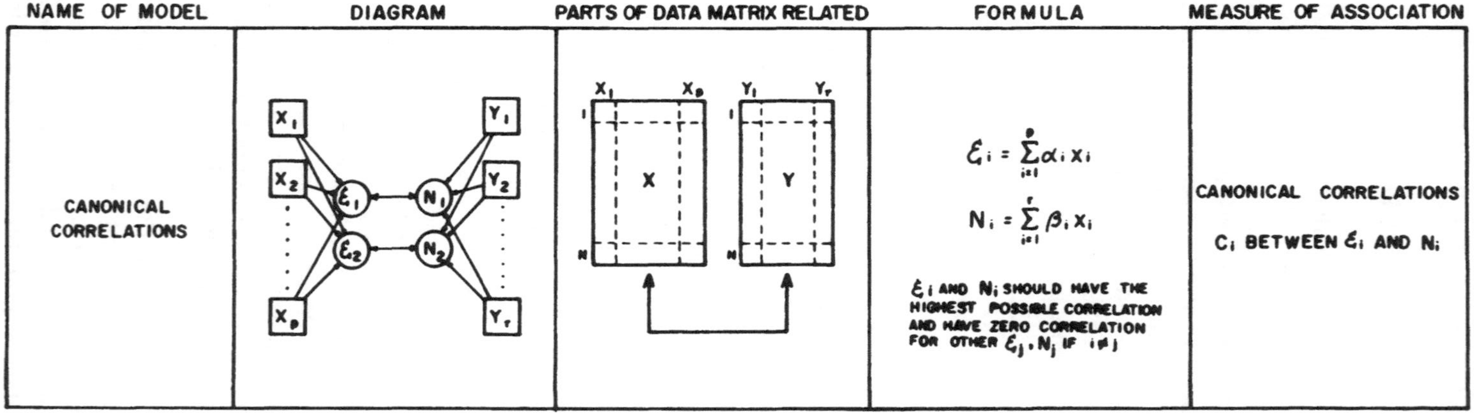

FIG. 7.32. *Canonical correlations.* The x_i and y_i are observed variables, represented by squares. The ζ_i and N_i are hypothetical variables, represented by circles. The arrows represent linear combinations. The ζ_i and N_i are the canonical variates, selected in such a way as to have the highest possible correlations and zero correlation for other ζ_j and N_j if $j \neq i$. The correlation between ζ_i and N_i is the ith canonical correlation, indicated by the double-headed arrows.

This is precisely the terminology that has been used in this chapter up to now (Fig. 7.24). John et al. (1964) perform their analysis the other way around: Each evoked response is treated as a variable and each time instant as an individual. This latter procedure overlooks the fact that individuals must be independent samples and this certainly is not true for successive values of a time series. Time-series methods have been developed for this purpose (see section IVE of this chapter). Nonetheless, for descriptive purposes, the analysis may be carried out as if the evoked responses were variables.

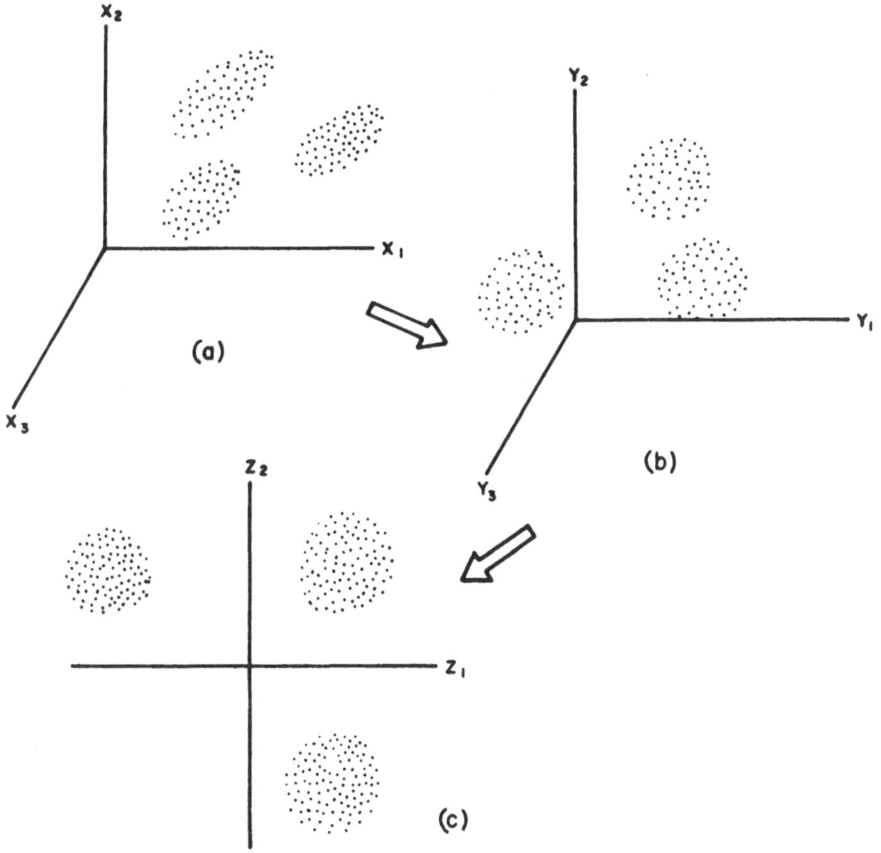

FIG. 7.33. *Canonical functions or discriminant factor analysis.* In (a) is represented the result of measuring three variables x_1, x_2, and x_3 for three different samples, one from each of three different groups. The individuals are represented as points, the sample for a group is a swarm of points. The three swarms are identical in shape, but have different means (in other words, they have the same covariance matrix). In (b), the z transformation is performed to transform the swarms into spherical clouds of points. This is done by standardizing the variables x_i. In (c), the canonical coordinates or functions have been extracted. These are linear combinations of the original x_i such that the most parsimonious description of the differences between groups is obtained.

Because the methods presented in this section use the covariance or correlation matrix obtained from the data as a basic, they present the same limitations as the correlation coefficient for describing interrelationships between waveform of brain electrical activity. Because the correlation coefficient is a sort of average of cross products of observed values, fast activity and transients tend to be lost in the overall slower components. Once again, special time-series methods must be used to deal with this. An excellent discussion of the use and shortcomings of latent structure methods in evoked-response studies may be found in John, Ruchkin, and Vidal (1978).

3. Nonlinear Latent Structure Methods

An obvious generalization of the process of forming hypothetical variables by linear combinations of the observed variables is to relax the condition of linearity. The hypothetical variables would now be nonlinear transformations of the original variables. This is a topic that has not been developed very much, though such extensions of factor analysis and discriminant factor analysis have been described.

D. Relationships of a Set of Observed Variables with Fixed Mathematical Functions or "Standard Variables"

Loosely speaking, the models treated up to now can be conceived heuristically as some sort of device that, given some input, performs a transformation that is subject to noise, resulting in the observed variables. The transformation could be linear or not, giving rise to linear models or nonlinear models. Regression models have (in this imprecise analogy) observed variables as input. The latent structure methods of the previous section had hypothetical variables as input. An obvious extension is to use some family of standard mathematical functions as input—that is, to express the observed variables as some sort of transformation of what we call "standard variables."

This sort of representation is most useful when the observed variables are all measured in the same scale; in fact, the principal use of this type of model is for the description of time series, discussed in the next section. We discuss this type of representation primarily to prepare for the study of time series.

Many different families of mathematical functions may be used to represent observed variables. The most well known are the sine and cosine functions. These are used in the Fourier frequence domain description of time series. However, any family of functions with certain properties may be used, depending on the particular application. For instance, Dumermuth, Gasser, Hecker, Herdan, and Lange (1976) present an example of an EEG record expressed as the combination of square pulses (the Walsh transform). In this analysis, the concept of "sequency" substitutes for that of frequency.

Sine waves, and the sets of square pulses (used in Walsh transforms) look the same no matter what time segment is considered—that is, they are stationary functions. The type of observed variables that may be modeled by this sort of function are therefore also stationary.

When transient effects are present, then modifications of stationary functions may be necessary. Amplitude modulated sine waves are an example. John et al. (1978) comment on the use of a nonstationary square wave family of functions in the study of ERs, the Haar Transform.

E. Time-Series Models

The methods for studying the structure of the data considered up to now are general-purpose univariate and multivariate statistical procedures. We now consider in more detail the problem of observations made on physical quantities during a certain period of time. These measurements may be considered the output of a system, physical or biological, and therefore any two successive measurements will have some sort of specific relationship. This poses special problems for statistical inference and originates specialized mathematical techniques for coping with them.

Let us repeat some definitions given in preceding sections. A graph of some physical quantity plotted against time, supposed to be just one of potentially many such graphs selected at random, is a *time series*. The underlying probability model is a *stochastic process*, and the particular time series considered is a *sample function* or *realization* of the stochastic process. There is some sort of probability measure associated with each time series. For a given stochastic process, some graphs are more probable than others. Typical examples of time series are an EEG record or a single trial-evoked response from a single derivation. These are *univariate time series* because only one measurement is available for each instant of time. The measurement of multiple parameters simultaneously, as when recording a multichannel EEG, results in a set of graphs; to each time instant corresponds a set of measurements. These are *multiple time series* or *multivariate time series*.

The two examples of time series given, the EEG and evoked responses, illustrate some further distinctions to be made. The EEG can potentially be recorded for as long as we wish, the duration of an evoked response is bounded by its onset—the stimulus—and a not-very-well-defined end point that is either another stimulus or the complete recovery of the "background" activity. This illustrates that time series can be defined for *all* t (where t is a time instant) or only for an *interval* of time ($0 < t < T$). Another difference between the EEG and the evoked response is that evoked responses that are "equivalent" for a given purpose may be obtained by simply repeating the stimulus (while trying to maintain the subject in the same conditions), whereas in EEG studies, only one record is usually available for examination. In the first case, we may obtain *multiple replications* of the time series, whereas in the second, we have only *one replication*.

Time series may have values for every time instant (*continuous time parameter*), as when obtained by analog devices, or may be an ordered series of measurements at certain discrete time points (*discrete time parameter*), which is the usual case in digital signal processing.

Transforming a time series is termed *filtering* it. The mathematical transformation itself is a *filter*. For example, consider a p-dimensional vector. In the terminology of this section, it is a univariate, discrete time parameter, time series, which takes integer values from 1 to p. Multiplying by a matrix (section II of this chapter) is to linearly transform it. This will now be called *linear filtering* and the matrix is the linear filter.

1. Special Problems Posed by Time Series

First consider the evoked-response situation. Suppose we are recording from r derivations, that we obtain N replications of the single-trial evoked responses. Each single-trial evoked response consists of p voltage values arranged in a vector. This is the case of an r-component multiple time series, with discrete time parameter, measured at p time instants. Table 7.5 illustrates the situation. How is this data to be analyzed? We outline some incorrect and widely used procedures:

1. Consider each derivation as if it were a variable. Treat the values obtained at different time instants as if they were independent. This means taking each row as a vector (Fig. 7.34a) having pN individual components. The usual multivariate procedures are then applied as outlined in previous sections. An example of this type of operation is the factor analysis carried out by John et al. (1964) in which each evoked response is considered a variable and the time instants are individuals. Another example, this time for a single time series, is the analysis of Gaussianity by different authors (Elul, 1969; Gasser, 1975) in which a single EEG record is considered as a variable and the sampled values as individuals. *These analyses overlook the fact that substantial and patterned correlations exist between the successive time instants of a time series.*
2. Take each single-trial evoked response as a p-vector and perform a separate analysis for each of the r derivations (Fig. 7.34b). This procedure is more acceptable, but has the drawback that there exist interactions between derivations that would make some sort of a joint analysis desirable.
3. Form a vector with pr components, aligning the single-trial evoked

TABLE 7.5
Data Matrix Collected in a Multivariate Time-Series Experiment[a]

	1st Replication Time Instant			*Nth Replication Time Instant*		
	1	2	p	1	2	p
Derivation 1	$x_{11}(t_1)$	$x_{11}(t_2)$...	$x_{11}(t_p)$	$x_{1N}(t_1)$	$x_{1N}(t_2)$...	$x_{1N}(t_p)$
Derivation 2	$x_{21}(t_1)$	$x_{21}(t_2)$...	$x_{21}(t_p)$	$x_{2N}(t_1)$	$x_{2N}(t_2)$...	$x_{2N}(t_p)$
....	....	....	....	....	....	....
....	....	....	....	....	....	....
....	....	....	....	....	....	....
Derivation R	$x_{R1}(t_1)$	$x_{R1}(t_2)$...	$x_{R1}(t_p)$	$x_{RN}(t_1)$	$x_{RN}(t_2)$...	$x_{RN}(t_p)$

[a]This is the data matrix obtained in a multivariate time-series experiment, when the time parameter is discrete and replications are available. R is the number of time series; p is the number of time instants t_i for which the R time series are measured. N is the number of replications. In the Table, $x_{ij}(t_k)$ is a single measurement, obtained from the j replication, for the ith time series at time instant k. For each replication, each row is a p vector denoted by x_{ij}. For each replication, the multiple time series is the matrix X_j. (i denotes the time series and j the replication).

responses from a single replication into a single vector (Fig. 7.34c). Then apply multivariate statistical methods to the pr-dimensional sample. This method is much preferable to 1 and 2 because all joint spatio-temporal information for a single presentation of a stimulus is combined into a single vector and each vector is an independent sample (one for each stimulus). This legitimizes the application of usual statistical methods. It does have the inconvenience of requiring the analysis of vectors of high dimensionality. It is well known that at least more replications must be obtained than variables. This might make the whole problem practically unmanageable.

There are two further considerations that indicate that although possible (especially using variant 3 from the preceding list), the straightforward application of standard multivariate methods to time series is not quite adequate.

The first consideration stems from the fact that standard multivariate methods are designed for any type of variables, which do not even have to be measured in the same scale, or even to measure similar things. In time series, by contrast, the different components of the time-series vectors are the *same measurement performed at different time instants*—that is, the same quantity is measured in the same scale, presumably produced by an underlying

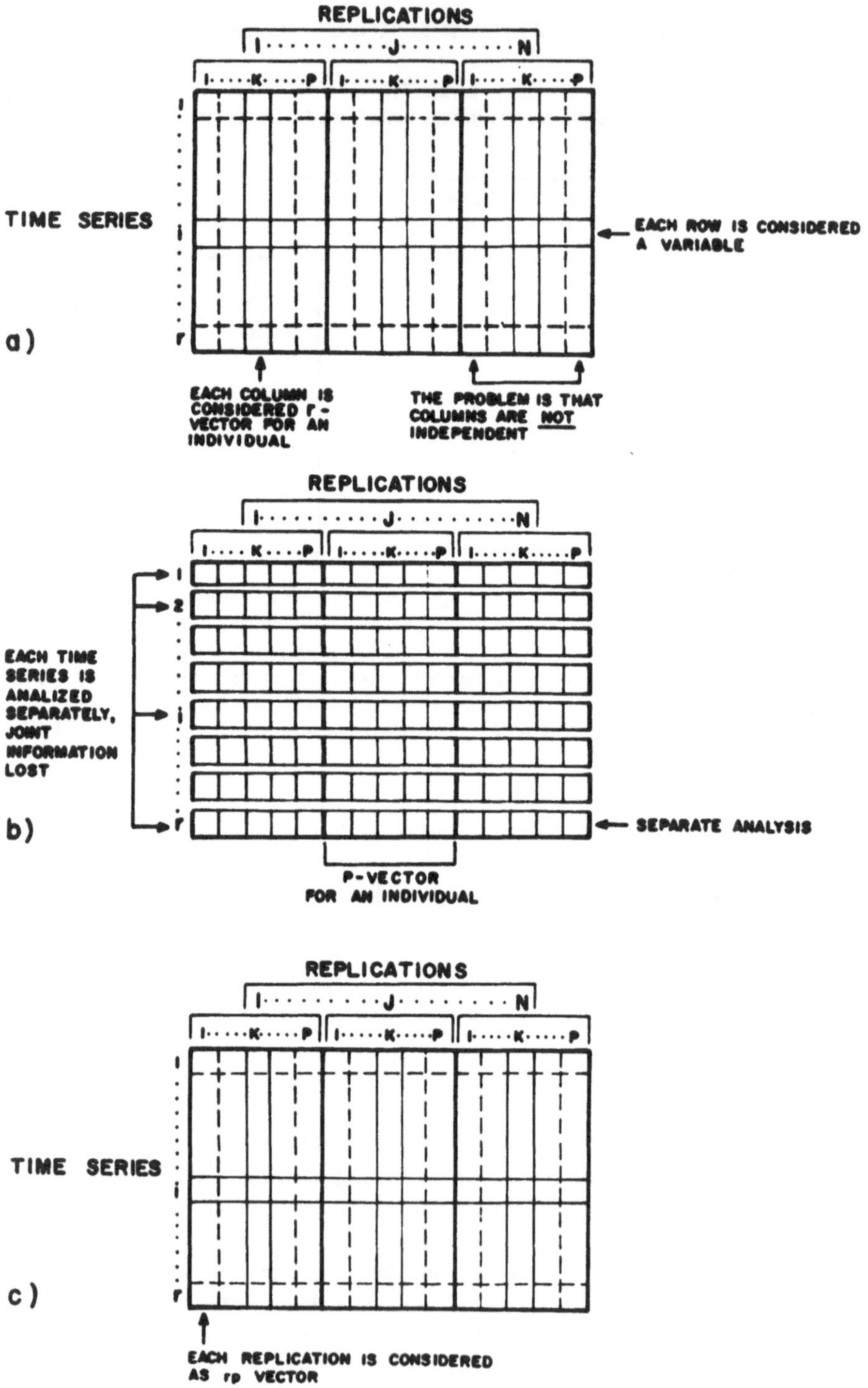
REPLICATIONS
1 . . . . J . . . . N
1 . . . . K . . . . P
TIME SERIES
EACH ROW IS CONSIDERED A VARIABLE
a)
EACH COLUMN IS CONSIDERED r-VECTOR FOR AN INDIVIDUAL
THE PROBLEM IS THAT COLUMNS ARE NOT INDEPENDENT
REPLICATIONS
EACH TIME SERIES IS ANALIZED SEPARATELY, JOINT INFORMATION LOST
b)
SEPARATE ANALYSIS
P-VECTOR FOR AN INDIVIDUAL
REPLICATIONS
TIME SERIES
c)
EACH REPLICATION IS CONSIDERED AS rp VECTOR

FIG. 7.34

physical or biological mechanism that is apt to introduce certain relationships among the successively measured variables. The explicit introduction of specifications of these interrelationships permits considerable simplifications, as is described later.

The second difficulty is illustrated by an example. Suppose we are interested in uncovering the underlying latent components of the evoked responses obtained from a single derivation. One way of doing this is to apply *principal component analysis* (section IV C.2 of this chapter) (Arnal et al., 1972; John et al., 1964; Kavanagh et al., 1976; Valdés, unpublished). Everything is adequate if a situation such as that shown in Fig. 7.35a corresponds to reality. The observed evoked responses are simply the sum of basic waveforms, each amplified by a certain constant. But, if we have a single waveform that shifts in time (Fig. 7.35b), then principal component analysis will identify different basic waveshapes when there is really only one. Standard multivariate methods cannot handle such time shifts. In a two-dimensional representation of data, if both two dimensions correspond to time, then it is conceivable that something happening in t_1 might be retarded and therefore appear at t_2. But, if the two dimensions are dissimilar, for example, height and weight, this jump from one dimension to another is meaningless.

What has been discussed up to now argues for the need for special methods to deal with time series. This is even more evident when the data available is just one replication, as is common with the EEG. From the point of view of standard multivariate methods, this is like having only one sample to work with. Introducing certain assumptions offers a solution, and gives a practical meaning to the rather esoteric concepts of *ergodicity* and *stationarity* discussed in section III of the chapter. The assumption of *ergodicity* assures us that statistics computed for a sufficiently long sample of a single time series will behave similarly as to statistics computed at one time instant for a very large sample of different time series. In addition, *stationarity*, or the invariance of statistical properties with shifts in the time axis, permits the introduction of very simple models that we now review.

Time-series descriptions are divided into two large groups: linear and nonlinear. Each is further subdivided accordingly if the data are described in the original *time domain* or if some sort of relationship with standard variables is carried out (section IV.D of this chapter). The most frequent way

---

FIG. 7.34. *(Opposite page) Different ways of analyzing a multiple-time series experiment.* r is the number of time series; N is the number of replications; p is the number of time instants sampled. In (a), each column (instant) is considered an r-vector, giving pN individuals. In (b), each row (variable) is considered separately, which results in r separate analysis of Np-vectors. In (c), each replication is considered an rp-vector, there now being N individuals (see text for discussion).

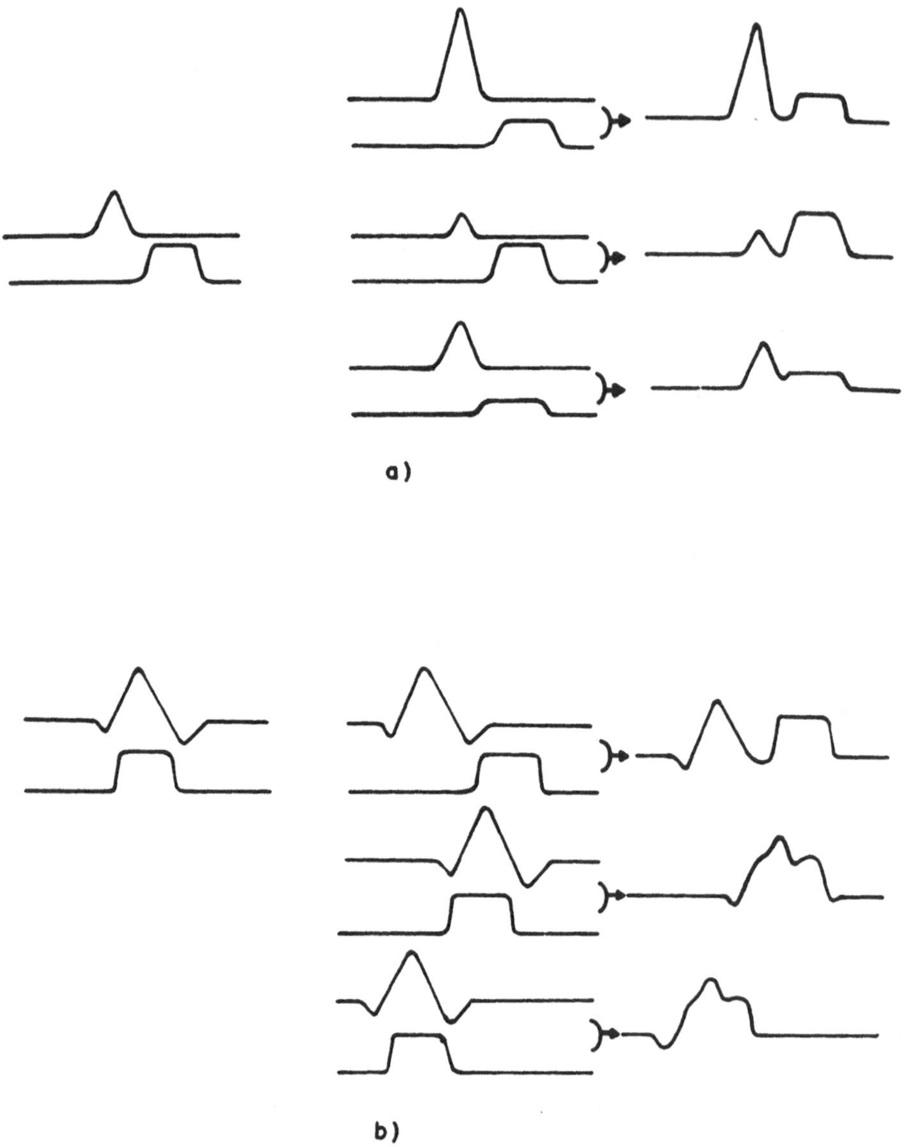

a)

b)

FIG. 7.35. *Difficulties of principal component analysis with time-shifting waveforms.* In (a), the ideal situation from principal component analysis is presented. Two basic waveforms (on the left), in fixed 'phase' relations but in different linear combinations (on the middle) produce a set of waveforms (on the right). Principal component analysis will have no difficulties in recovering the original two basic waveforms. In (b), however, the basic waveforms shift in time and relative to one another. A principal component analysis will identify many more basic waveforms than actually present.

to represent time series is as transformations of sinusoidal waveforms. This is *frequency domain representation.*

A summary of the different ways to analyze the structure of time series is presented in Table 7.6.

2. Linear Stationary Time-Series Models: Frequency Domain

The simplest models suppose that the observed time series is the result of linearly combining stationary processes. This representation is adequate for

TABLE 7.6
Different types of Descriptions of Time Series[a]

Type of Model		*Descriptive Domain* *Frequency*	*Time*
Linear models	Stationary	Spectral analysis	Moving Average (MA) Model Autoregressivve (AR) Model Autoregressive Moving Average (ARMA) Model
	Nonstationary	Time-varying spectrum	Autoregressive Integrated Moving Average (ARIMA) Model AR, MA, and ARMA Models with time-varying coefficients Kalman filtering Karhunen-Loeve Expansion
Nonlinear models		Complex demodulation Polyspectra (bispectrum, trispectrum) Cepstrum	Decomposition in terms of Wiener kernels

[a] The table is divided according to the domain of description of the time series (frequency domain or time domain) and according to the type of model that is chosen. Linear models suppose that time series are the outcome of linear combinations of certain events that can be either stationary (time invariant with respect to statistical properties) or nonstationary. Nonlinear models assume relationships more complicated than the linear. In each entry, some examples are given of descriptions developed for each type of model and domain. There is an equivalence between frequency and time domain descriptions. The methods are discussed in the text.

selected segments of the EEG and as a first, approximate solution in other cases.

Consider the following heuristic model (which should not be viewed as an actual model of neural machinery). We have a bank of sinusoidal wave generators. Each generator g_i produces a sinusoidal wave with fixed frequency f_i (in Hz). The amplitude of the generator may be adjusted to a value a_i. The phase shift ϕ_i of the waveform may also be modified. The outputs of all g_i are summed. This produces, for fixed f_i, g_i, and ϕ_i, a deterministic waveform $Y(t)$. This way of representing waveforms, in terms of sums of sinusoidal waveshapes, is termed Fourier analysis. The situation is schematized in Fig. 7.36a. This may be formalized by the following equation:

$$Y(t) = \Sigma\, a_i \sin(f_i t + \phi_i) \tag{25}$$

This equation expressed that $Y(t)$ is a linear combination of sinusoidal waveshapes. It is well known that the types of functions representable in this way include all of those that might be a result of a real experiment. For example, if the f_i are all integer multiples of each other, the function is periodic; if not, it is aperiodic. In some applications, the number of generators might have to be infinite, the frequencies arbitrarily close to each other, and the summation Σ, replaced by an integral, giving what is known as the integral Fourier transform. This will not change the general interpretation of the heuristic example under discussion.

Let us look at another way of specifying the function $Y(t)$ in terms of its frequency components. In Fig. 7.36b, we look inside each generator g_i. The output of frequency f_i, amplitude a_i, and phase shift ϕ_i can be obtained as the sum of a sine wave generator and a cosine wave generator, with outputs amplified by s_i and c_i respectively. These combine in the way shown in Fig. 7.36c to produce the amplitude a_i and phase ϕ_i. The interesting point is that, except for the frequency f_i, the output of the generator g_i is completely specified by a point in 2-space. We have mentioned that magnitudes that are representable in a plane are called *complex numbers*. They permit the codification of amplitude and phase information into a single number. The appearance of complex numbers in time-series analysis corresponds to the unique problem of treating phase information, unknown in standard statistics. The complex number $Z_i = (C_i, S_i)$ is the complex coefficient for frequency f_i.

We have already mentioned that for fixed z_i the $Y(t)$ is a fixed deterministic signal. But, consider now the following experiment: Obtain a series of different $Y(t)$, changing the values of z_i in a random fashion after each trial. In this case, we are dealing with a stochastic process, and the individual $Y(t)$s are time series. The stochastic process is determined completely by the type of probability distribution of the z_i, so specifying the distributions describes the stochastic process in the *frequency domain* (in terms of frequency components) instead of in the time domain.

Before continuing this discussion, we must digress and define some terms for the description of random complex quantitites. A complex number may be viewed as a two-dimensional vector. A *univariate complex density* is a multivariate bidimensional density in the complex plane. If a complex variable has an associated density that is bivariate normal, with the real and imaginary (first and second components) parts statistically independent, and

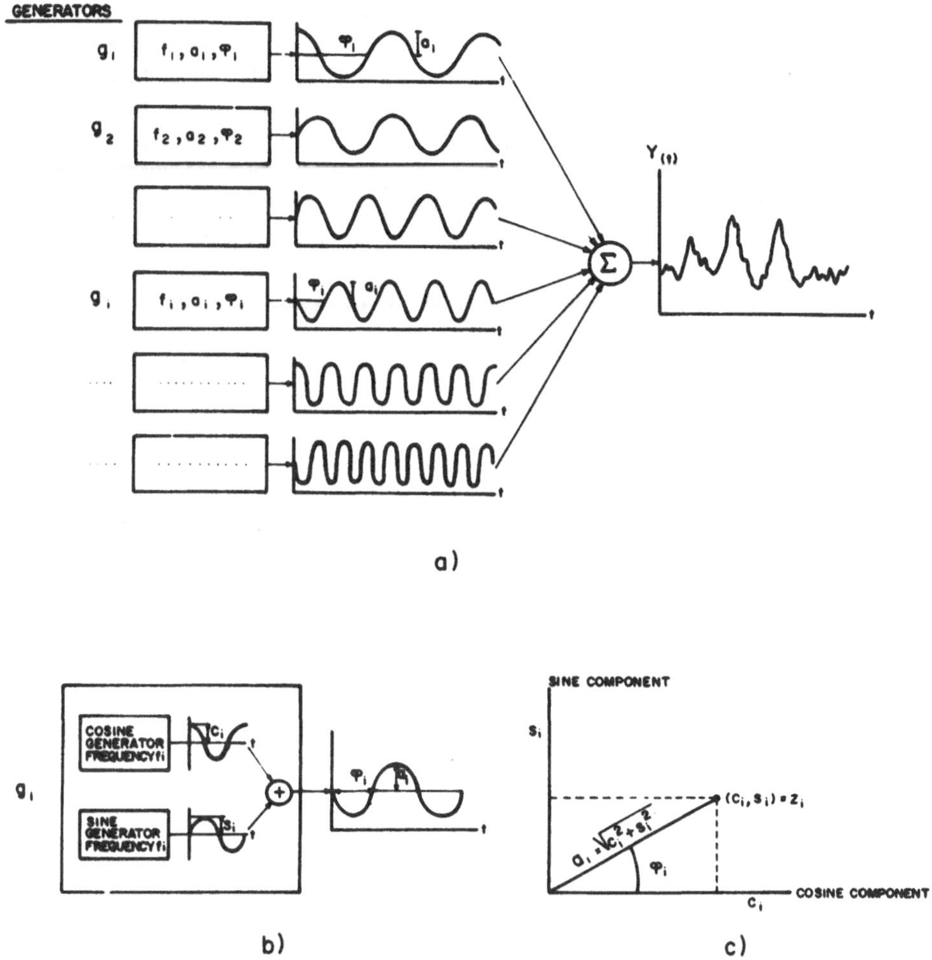

FIG. 7.36. *Heuristic representation of frequency domain in treatment of time series.* In (a), a time series $Y(t)$ is shown as the summation of outputs of a bank of generators g_i that output sinusoidal waves with frequency f_i, amplitude a_i, and phase Φ. In (b), the generator g_i is shown as the sum of a sine wave generator with amplitude s_i and a cosine generator with amplitude c_i (frequency f_i, fixed). The dependence of a_i on c_i and s_i is shown in (c). This illustrates that the information of phase can be combined with that of amplitude into a single *complex number* $z_i = (c_i, s_i)$. If the z_i are random, then the $Y(t)$ are realizations from a stochastic process described in the frequency domain by the mean and variances of the z_i.

if the variance for each component is equal to $\sigma^2/2$, then the complex variable has a univariate complex normal density with mean equal to the pair (μ_1, μ_2), in which μ_1 is the mean for the real part and μ_2 the mean for the imaginary, and variance σ^2. This is shown in Fig. 7.37.

The model most frequently used in time-series analysis is that shown in Fig. 7.36, with the z_i having a complex univariate distribution with 0 mean and variance $S(f_i)$. The function $S(f_i)$ is the *power spectrum* of the stationary process. In clinical applications, the variance for different frequencies is often summed to yield the classical *frequency bands* (alpha, beta, theta, and so on).

Description in terms of the power spectrum is analogous to giving the variances in a multivariate statistical problem, with the advantage of being able to ignore the covariances because the contributions at different frequencies are statistically independent. *Thus, one of the prime problems of time-series analysis, the intercorrelations within a time series, is solved.* One may now proceed to carry out separate univariate analysis for each frequency. The price paid is to use a more complicated statistical framework, that of *complex statistics.*

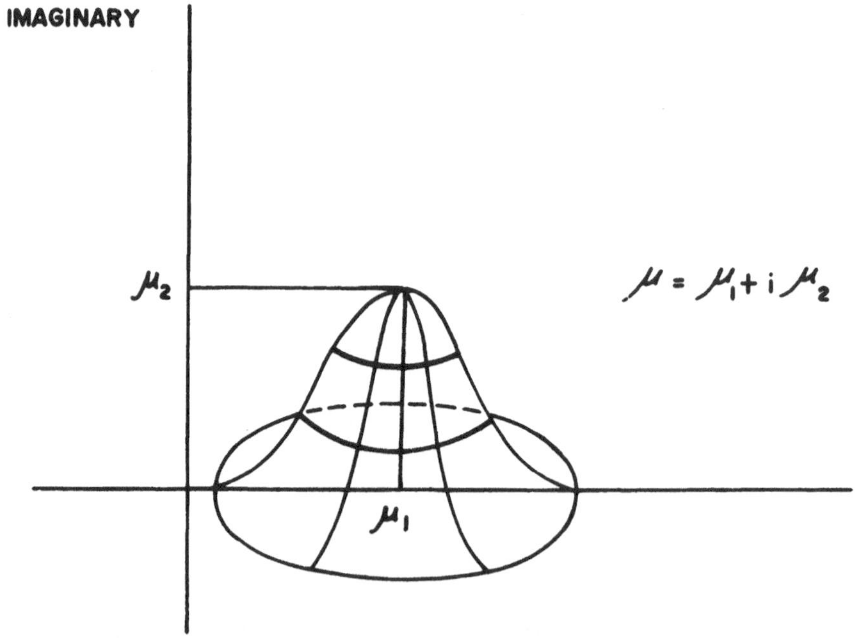

FIG. 7.37. *Complex univariate normal variable.* The complex variable z has a gaussian distribution if each component, real (z_1) and imaginary (z_2), has a univariate normal density and if the vector (z_1, z_2) has a bivariate Gaussian density with zero covariance between z_1 and z_2. The variance of the two components should also be equal, say $\sigma^2/2$. The mean of the density is the complex number formed by the mean of the real and imaginary parts. The variance is two times the variance of its components—in this case σ^2.

In practice, one does not know the values of $S(f_i)$. The task of Fourier analysis is to estimate these quantities from an observed time series. The practical problems involved in doing this are discussed in the next section. In the meantime, we consider the possibilities of the frequency domain representation from a theoretical point of view.

One of the advantages of the frequency domain description is the elegant and simple representation of linear filters (contrasted with the situation in the time domain description). The effect of a linear filter on any time series is completely specified by stating its effects on each separate frequency component—that is, by specifying the changes it will produce in amplitude and phase. The effects of the filter on the amplitudes of each component is multiplicative and known as the *gain* of the filter for that frequency. The effect on the phase is additive and is known as the *phase response* of the filter. The gain $G(f_i)$ and the phase $F(f_i)$ functions of the filter describe its effects. The effect on the function $Y(t)$ is, from Eq. 25:

$$Z(t) = \Sigma\, G(f_i)A_i \sin\,[f_i t + \phi_i + F(f_i)], \tag{26}$$

in which $Z(t)$ is the transformed filtered time series.

The effect of applying a filter to a stochastic process is to multiply the spectrum $S(f_i)$ by $G^2(f_i)$. This generates an interesting interpretation of stochastic processes.

We have previously mentioned that the simplest type of stochastic process is *white noise*. It is a process that has all frequency components in equal proportion. In terms of Fig. 8.36, the generators g_i produce all possible frequencies and the distributions of the z_i are identical. This means, in particular, that the power spectrum $S(f)$ (we drop the subscript i from now on) is flat. White noise is the theoretical counterpart of perfect randomness and, as such, unattainable by any physical device. The term "white noise" comes from an analogy in optics in which the color white is the mixture of all colors (frequencies).

If we feed white noise with $S(f) = 1$ into a linear filter, the spectrum of the output will be simply $G^2(f)$. One can then view a stochastic process as white noise "shaped" by an appropriate filter.

Up to now, we have been considering univariate time series. When a multivariate time series is carried into the frequency domain, we can still consider each frequency separately. Thus, in the frequency domain, the strategy of Fig. 7.34a becomes legitimate due to the independence of each frequency. The use of complex variables introduces some complications, however. The covariance between two complex variables is now a complex number. The correlation between two time series is also a complex number, known as the *coherence*. Coherence values are computed frequency by frequency, giving coherence plots. What is actually plotted is the absolute value (the absolute value of $Z = (x,y)$ is $\sqrt{x^2 + y^2}$) *of the coherence, which is 0 for independent variables and 1 for perfectly dependent values as in ordinary, real-valued statistics.*

We may summarize, then, the strategy for multiple time series as follows:

1. Carry the situation into the frequency domain.
2. Analyze each frequency separately using complex multivariate statistics.
3. Carry the problem back into the time domain if necessary.

This method of analyzing time series is presented in Brillinger (1975). We illustrate this by considering linear regressions for time series. As may be remembered from section IV.B of this chapter, linear relationships may be measured using different types of correlation coefficients. In particular, if the effects of a group of variables were to be eliminated in order to study the interrelation of other variables among themselves independently of the first, then partial correlation methods were recommended (Fig. 7.26). Those ideas carry over to the frequency domain. The theory of *multiple and partial coherence* has been used by Gersch, Yonemoto, and Naitoh (1977) to study the localization of driving foci in epileptic patients.

Another advantage of working in the frequency domain is that phase shift phenomena, such as those in Fig. 7.35 can be dealt with effectively. The author of this chapter has developed a model, also based on multiple regression for time series, that is effective in estimating time shifting components of signals buried in noise.

Most neurometric results have used some sort of representation in the frequency domain.

3. Practical Problems in Estimating S(f)

The widespread use of frequency domain methods is the result of the availability of inexpensive computing power in the laboratory and the development of the Fast Fourier Transform (FFT). This algorithm, developed by Cooley and Tukey in 1965, has radically transformed time series analysis by cutting down Fourier analysis to a fraction of the time consumed by older programs.

The estimation of the spectrum is essentially a calculation of the FFT for a time series $Y(t)$. This is like finding out the particular values of z_i in a particular trail. What are needed are the variances of the z_i: $S(f)$.

In reality, one is faced with a finite record of a time series—that is, a single sample of a stochastic process. From this it is necessary to estimate $S(f)$ and, in the case of multivariate time series, the coherences. We only outline some of the more important problems; details are discussed in standard texts (Brillinger, 1975; Hannan, 1970).

The principal problems are as follows:

1. The time series is usually sampled at discrete time instants for digital processing. A well-known source of error is that of *aliasing*, in which high-frequency components appear as low-frequency components. An intuitive idea of how this can happen is shown in Fig. 7.38. This can be avoided by using a high enough sampling rate. It should be above the "Nyquist rate", two times the highest frequency component in the sampled signal. Another practical solution is to *prefilter* the signal, eliminating high frequency components.

2. Fourier methods are really devised for infinite time series. The analysis of short records introduces the phenomena of *leakage*. This consists in *smearing* of $S(f)$, the estimate for a certain frequency being contaminated by nearly frequencies.

This effect is more pronounced the shorter the record. Longer records and multiplying the time series by weighting functions called *tapers* can alleviate this problem.

3. Because only one replication is available, estimating $S(f)$ from the Fourier transform of a time series is like trying to estimate a variance with only two samples (the two components of x_i).

This leads to statistical instability of the estimates. Two alternatives are available. The first one is to count on stationarity and chop the record into overlapping or non-overlapping segments, calculate the FFT for each, and then average the estimated $S(f)$. The other procedure is based on the mathematical property (see Brillinger, 1975) that $S(f)$ is also estimated by the spectrum at close frequencies. This justifies smoothing the spectrum. In either case, more stable estimates are obtained.

Similar problems arise when estimating coherences, but these are not detailed here.

A last point is a comment on the data reduction that is obtained with a spectral analysis. The spectrum is indeed a summarization of data. It holds the same relation to the original time series as the variance does to the original univariate sample. More precisely, it is a sort of variance distributed across the frequency components. Two different signals might have exactly the same spectrum. And yet, the spectrum yields another graph that might aid, but

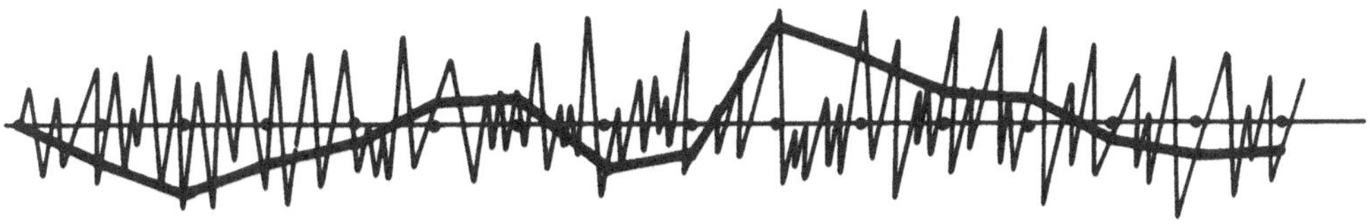

FIG. 7.38. *Aliasing effect.* A high-frequency content signal, sampled at a slow rate, shows the *aliasing effect*. This consists in the representation of high-frequency components as if they were low-frequency components. This must be taken into consideration in spectral analysis, either by prefiltering to eliminate high-frequency components or by choosing a high enough sampling rate.

does not substitute for visual inspection. The creation of a neurometric parameter does not end with a Fourier analysis.

4. *Linear Stationary Time-Series Models: Time Domain (Fig. 7.39)*

Another way of representing the structure of stochastic processes is in the time domain (Anderson, 1971; Box & Jenkins, 1970). The simplest models are the linear models, where the stochastic processes can be viewed as sums and multiplications of simplest events or past realizations of the stochastic process itself.

White noise in the time domain means a totally unpredictable random process. In other words, the correlation between any two time instants is zero. A realization of white noise may be considered a series of random shocks, totally uncorrelated with each other.

The first model we further discuss is the model known as Moving Average or MA (q) model, in which the stochastic process at time t is:

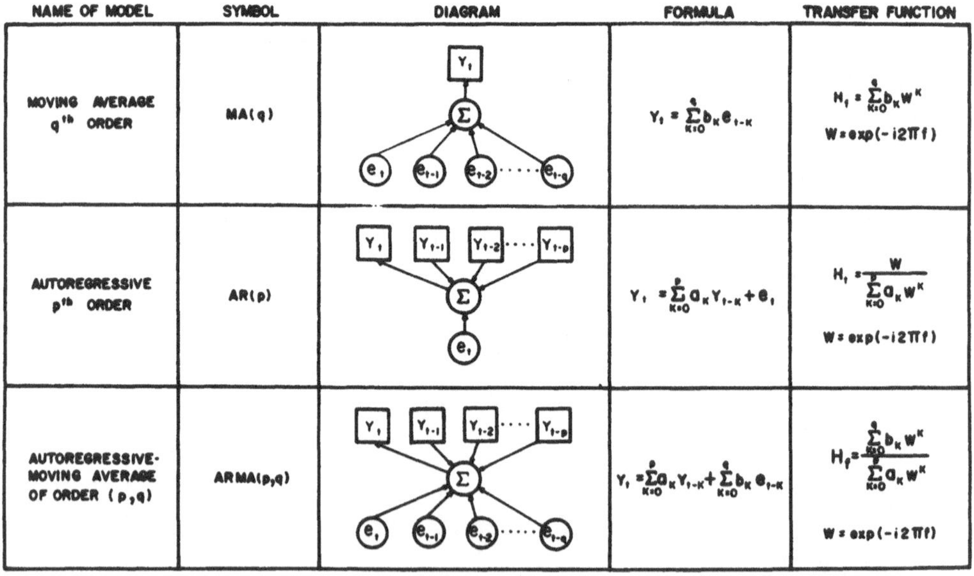

FIG. 7.39. ***Linear stationary time domain models.*** Squares represent observed variables, circles represent hypothetical variables. Arrows stand for linear combination, represented by circle with summation signs.

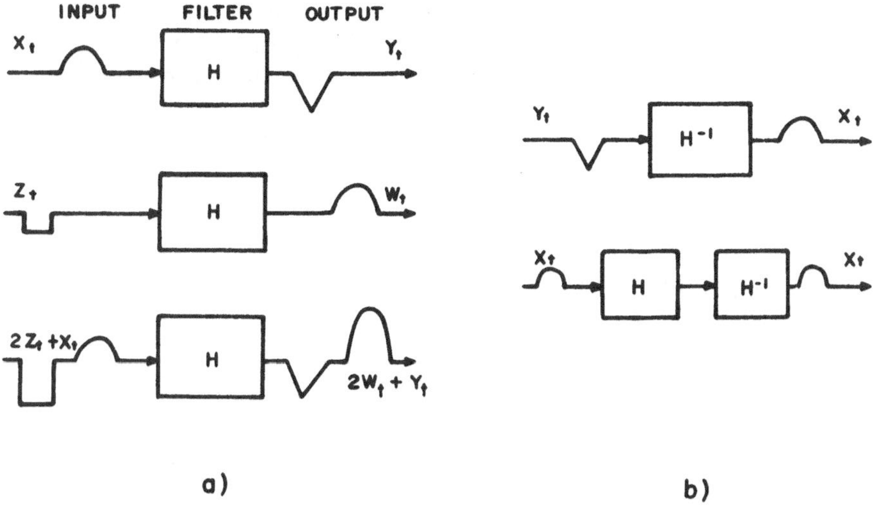

FIG. 7.40. *Linear filters.* A linear filter is a device that behaves as in (a). If input $x(t)$ produces $y(t)$ and $z(t)$ produces $w(t)$, any linear combination of $x(t)$ and $z(t)$ produces the same linear combination of $y(t)$ and $w(t)$. In (b) is illustrated the effect of the inverse filter of H. The inverse filter H^{-1} reverses the effect of H. H^{-1} coupled to H leaves the signal invariant.

$$Y(t) = \sum_{k=0}^{q} b(k)e(t - k) \tag{27}$$

In this formula $e(t)$ is a series of random shocks and $b(k)$ are ponderation coefficients of these random shocks that produce the stochastic process $Y(t)$. Note that for the realization of $Y(t)$, only the q past values of $e(t)$ are considered. Therefore, this model may be also viewed as the result of the influence of a series of random shocks in q-time instants, or in other words, this model reflects a system in a steady state, which means that afer q random shocks, the system returns to a base state.

Eq. 27 is representative of what is known as the effect of a linear filter $b(k)$ on a stochastic process $e(t)$. A linear filter (without memory) may be viewed as a device that, given an input, outputs a linear combination of the input, thus it only affects the input by sums and multiplications by factors (Fig. 7.40a). All linear filters have an inverse filter. The inverse filter is one that undoes the effect of a filter. H^{-1} is the inverse filter of H, if putting the output of H into H^{-1} produces as a result the original input to H (Fig. 7.40b).

A filter is completely specified by its *impulse response*, $h(t)$. This is defined as the output of the filter *H* at time t_0 if a unit pulse is fed into it. For example, consider a discrete time series $X(t)$ and suppose that we want to find another $Y(t)$, linear combination of the first one, in the following way:

$$Y(t) = 3X(t) + 2X(t - 1) + X(t - 2)$$

Then, the impulse response $h(t)$ is $h(0) = 3$, $h(1) = 2$ and $h(2) = 1$, since for each time instant t if we fed a unit pulse (1 in t_0, 0 in the remaining time instants), the output will be 3, 2 or 1 for $t = t_0, t_0 - 1, t_0 - 2$.

Eq. 28 in general becomes:

$$Y(t) = \sum_{k=0}^{\infty} h(k)X(t - k) \tag{28}$$

This is known as the convolution of $X(t)$ with the function $h(t)$.

In the frequency domain, $X(t)$ becomes $X(f)$ (the Fourier transform of $X(t)$), $Y(t)$ becomes $Y(f)$ (the Fourier transform of $Y(t)$). The Fourier transform of the impulse response function $h(t)$ is $H(f)$, the *transfer function* of the filter *H*. Eq. 28 then becomes:

$$Y(f) = H(f)X(f) \quad \text{or} \quad H(f) = \frac{Y(f)}{X(f)} \tag{29}$$

Compare now Eq. 27 with Eq. 28. It is clear that MA (q) model is the convolution of *qth* order of the impulse function $b(k)$ with the random shock series $e(t)$.

Let us consider now a system which depends in a linear form of its past values:

$$Y(t) = \sum_{k=0}^{p} a(k)Y(t - k) + e(t) \tag{30}$$

This formula represents a multiple regression on $Y(t)$ of its p past values. This model is known as autoregressive model of order *pth* or AR(p). Note that the effect of $e(t)$ (random shocks) is only at time t. The random shocks have no persistent effect.

A natural extension is to combine both $AR(p)$ models and $MA(q)$

models. This means we are considering systems that both depend on their past values in which the effects of random shocks have persistent effects.

The form of the model is:

$$Y(t) = \sum_{k=0}^{p} a(k)Y(t - k) + \sum_{k=0}^{q} b(k)e(t - k) \tag{31}$$

This is the autoregressive-moving average model of order (p, q) or ARMA (p, q). Its transfer function is a rational function with a q degree polynomial in the denominator and a p degree polynomial in the numerator.

We do not go into details on how to fit these models. It is enough to say that the objective is to fit the lowest order model compatible with the data. This is usually obtained fitting ARMA-type models.

We mentioned in the section on regression models that a very convenient way to check the validity of the models is to examine the "residuals" to see if they are compatible with the assumptions of the model. This is also true for AR, MA, and ARMA models. Because the basic heuristic idea is that of a filter that shapes white noise, one way of checking the model is to obtain the inverse filter. If the time series is fed in, and then if the model is adequate, the output of the inverse filter should be an approximation to white noise.

A point we would like to emphasize is that time domain and frequency domain descriptions are equivalent, as can be seen from Eq. 28 and 29. Some authors (Gersch et al., 1977) use time domain models to estimate spectra. The particular type of model, and whether to work in the time domain or the frequency domain, depends on the particular problem. Time domain models have also been extended to the multivariate case, and have been applied to the description of the EEG. Implications for neurometrics are discussed in Chapter 11.

5. *Linear Nonstationary Time-Series Models.*

Many times, "stationary" is a nonrealistic assumption. The nervous system exists to help the species cope with change. Transients rather than steady states appear to dominate the electrical activity of the brain. And yet, the theory of nonstationary processes is not as fully developed as would be desirable. Applications to the analysis of the EEG are scanty, those to neurometrics, nonexistent.

Nonetheless, the study of the nervous system at work will certainly impose in the future the use of techniques adapted to detect dynamic changes. For this reason, we now briefly review some methods for analyzing time-changing stochastic processes.

One obvious way of extending the types of models discussed previously is allowing their parameters to vary in time. Consider Fig. 7.36, the representation of a time series as the sum of outputs from sinusoidal wave generators. In the stationary case, the values c_i and s_i (the amplitudes of the cosine and sine generators of g_i) were fixed for any determined time series and only varied randomly from one realization to other. If, during the *same* time series, we allow these amplitudes to vary ($c_i(t)$ and $s_i(t)$), then instead of having sinusoidal waveshapes, we have *amplitude modulated sinusoidal waveshapes*. These would still be combined linearly to produce the realization $Y(t)$, but it would be a sample function from a *nonstationary* random process. The spectrum would theoretically be defined, now a function expressing power, or variance in terms of frequency and time, $S(f, t)$. This is the *time varying* or *evolutionary spectrum*. (For a critical discussion, see Loynes, 1968.) There are practical problems in estimating the evolutionary spectra. These and the statistical issues are discussed in Priestley (1965, 1966).

The time domain equivalent of this procedure is to allow the coeficients of the AR, MA, or ARMA model to vary with time (for example, they could also be time domain ARMA models). This approach has been discussed by Bohlin (1977); the comparison with the frequency domain representation is commented on by Rao and Tong (1972).

A particular type of time domain representation, which may represent a very wide class of stochastic processes, is *Kalman filtering* (Kalman, 1960). As with other types of time domain models, the Kalman filter shapes white noise into a particular type of stochastic process. Its peculiar feature, besides permitting the specification of time varying coefficients, is its *recursivity*. This means that values of the stochastic process may be recursively calculated form a limited number of previous values, thus facilitating the implementation of very efficient algorithms (Bohlin, 1977).

The ARIMA model (autoregressive, integrated moving average), described in Box and Jenkins (1970), complicates the ARMA model by introducing terms that are differences between successive values of the time series. This permits modeling the type of nonstationarity due to slow shifts of activity.

We mention one last approach, useful for time series defined in an interval of time. This is the *Karhunen-Loeve expansion*. This expansion expresses a particular stochastic process in terms of statistically independent time series, the first of which accounts for the major part of the total variance, the second for most of the variance left, and so on. In spite of the difference in terminology, this is essentially a *principal component analysis*.

It is interesting to see what happens to these models if the process studied is stationary. The evolutionary spectrum becomes constant for all time instants (in fact, this is the basis of Priestley's test for stationarity (Priestley & Rao,

1969). The coefficients of time domain models also do not vary and the Karhunen-Loeve expansion becomes the ordinary Fourier analysis. This last is an interesting result, that we will reword as follows: Principal components and Fourier analysis are equivalent for stationary processes if the number of variables (time instants) is large enough (Brillinger, 1975).

The converse situation is also noteworthy. If a nonstationary process is modeled with stationary models, then a sort of averaging is carried out and the estimates are not representative of the data. Applying the inverse filter to the actual time series will show highly nonstationary residuals. This has been used by Lopes da Silva, Dijk, and Smits (1975), Lopes da Silva, Ten Broeke, Van Hulten & Lommen (1976), Lopes da Silva, Van Hulten, Lommen, Storm Van Leeuwen, Van Vellen, & Viegenthart (1977) (see Chapter 12) as a means for detecting the type of nonstationarities of the EEG that are spikes.

6. Nonlinear Time-Series Models.

As with all types of nonlinear models, the subject for time series are less well developed for this subject than for the linear situation. There are many more possible types of models, and they are usually more difficult to fit. Neurometric applications are not yet evident. Nonetheless, for the sake of completeness, we refer to some types of analysis.

A well-known statistical relationship exists between the correlations of a stationary stochastic process and the power spectrum. In fact, the power spectrum is the Fourier transform of the autocorrelation function (the function that specifies the correlations between two different parts of the stochastic process; see section III of this chapter). It must be remembered that the first two statistical moments completely determine a Gaussian process. For non-gaussian processes, specifically those with nonlinear interactions, the spectral equivalents to higher order moments (like skewness and kurtosis) must be used. These are the *bispectrum, trispectrum*, and, in general *polyspectra* (Brillinger, 1975; Hannan, 1970). Examples of bispectra of EEG records are given in Dumermuth, Gasser, and Lange (1975) but due to their mathematical complexities and scant applications this topic will not be treated in greater depth here.

A somewhat more commonly used model is that of *complex demodulation* (D. O. Walter, 1968a). This model assumes that the observed signal is a sine wave that is both amplitude modulated and frequency modulated (Fig. 7.41). Its mathematical expression is:

$$Y(t) = A(t)\cos\,[f(t) + \phi(t)] \qquad (32)$$

In this equation, $A(t)$ is the amplitude modulating factor, $f(t)$ the frequency modulating factor, and ϕ is the phase variation factor. In terms of the

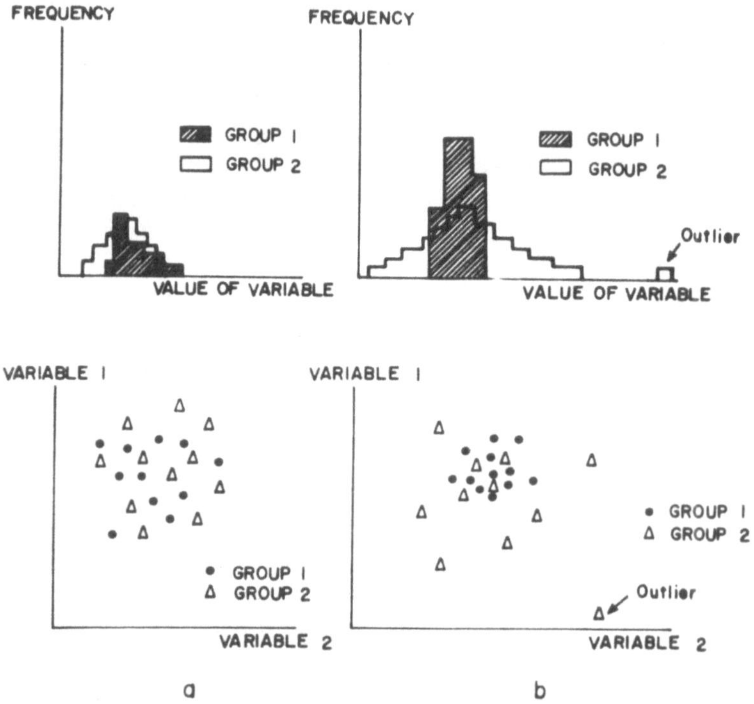

FIG. 7.41. *Use of histograms and scatter plots to analyze data structure.* (a) In top line on the left, two histograms, one for Group 1 and another for Group 2, are displayed. There are no noticeable differences for the two groups. The graph at the bottom left is a scatter plot for two variables. Once again, Group 1 does not differ appreciably from Group 2. In (b), similar graphs are displayed on the right, but now Group 1 is much more dispersed than Group 2. An outlier is detectable in both histogram and scatter plot.

model in Fig. 7.36, there is only *one* generator, a cosine generator, but frequency, amplitude, and phase change with time.

Other models are mentioned in Table 7.6.

7. Wiener Filtering.

Due to its occasional application in evoked-response analysis, we now outline Wiener filtering methods. This is a procedure for extracting a "signal" that is known from a time series, in which it is mixed additively with a different stochastic process to be considered "noise." The mathematical expression for this model is:

$$Y(t) = X(t) + n(t). \tag{33}$$

This equation expresses that the observed time series $Y(t)$ is the sum of the signal $X(t)$ and noise $n(t)$. The assumptions, overlooked all too frequently, are:

1 The spectra of the signal $S_x(f)$ and the noise $S_n(f)$ are both known or, at least, can be estimated.
2 The signal and the noise are both 0 mean *stationary* processes. If not, the spectrum does not have any meaning (see section IV E.5)

The *Wiener filter* is simply a linear filter based on the idea of suppressing those frequency components that have a high noise content. Consider the filter:

$$H(f) = \frac{S_x(f)}{S_x(f) + S_n(f)} \tag{34}$$

Remember that filtering $Y(t)$ can be expressed in the frequency domain as:

$$Z(f) = H(f)\, Y(f), \tag{35}$$

in which $Y(f)$ is the Fourier transform of the time series $Y(t)$ and $Z(f)$ that of the filtered series. The value of the filter $H(f)$, as seen from Eq. 34 will be near 0 when the noise component is high and the signal component is low, and near 1 when the signal component is predominant. This suppresses noise, because the filtered time series $Z(f)$ will have all high noise components attenuated. The signal may then be carried back to the time domain if necessary.

The questionable use of Wiener filtering for the study of evoked potentials is discussed in Chapter 10.

F. Methods for Studying Interrelationships Between Individuals

In our survey of methods to uncover the structure of the data, we have been focusing until now on interrelationships among the variables and on providing models to explain the interrelationships. We now turn to methods for studying the *relationships among individuals*. In terms of the data matrix (Fig. 7.24), this means that we are going to examine the data row-wise instead of by columns.

Consider the data once again as points in space. Though they appear to be scattered at random, experience shows that this randomness has some sort of pattern. Individuals tend to form clouds and clusters, to be distributed along curves, and so on. In other words, as discussed in section I of this Chapter,

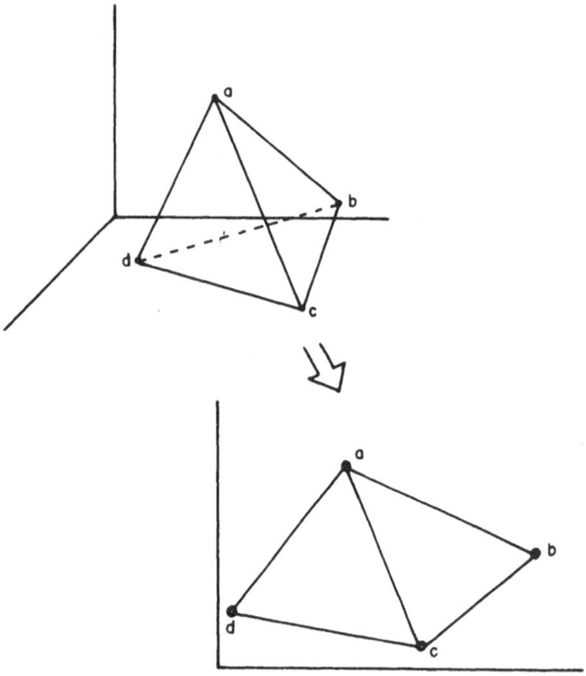

FIG. 7.42. *Mapping of individuals from original measure space to new low-dimensional representation.* The objective of the methods discussed in the text is to preserve the structure of the data, but to portray it in two or three dimensions to permit visual inspection. The structure of the data is characterized by the interpoint distances. An analogy is that of wires that join all points. The length of the wire is the distance. The transformation selected must compress the data into two or three dimensions without stretching, tearing, or shrinking the wires too much. The degree of deformation imposed upon a data set in representing it in a lower dimensional space is the *stress*.

there are very often consistent relationships, regularities present amidst the apparent randomness of the observed data. *The methods considered up to now presuppose some particular type of relationship. Those to be considered now try to reveal the existence of relationships.* To do this, the procedures to be discussed do either one of two things: They rely on the human capacity for pattern recognition and try to present the data in a way that this capacity may be exercized; or they try to formalize criteria for the existence of patterns and do the pattern recognition automatically. Let us give a typical example, so as not to be too abstract. Evoked responses to flashes differ from one individual to another. Is this variability totally stochastic? Or, are there certain "types," albeit variable, that constitute subgroups, but are not recognized because of the difficulty human beings have in comparing visually more than a few graphs? We see in the following discussion how this has been studied using the methods of this section.

Before reviewing the principal types of methods, it might be worthwhile to summarize the principal uses they may have in neurometrical applications. These are listed below.

1. *As a means for checking assumptions.* All too often, naive belief in statistical methods is followed by excessive skepticism (usually after an unsuccessful application). Frequently, this is not due to the statistical method employed, but to the fact that the data do not meet the requirements established to be able to employ the method legitimately.

Methods for analyzing the structure of individuals in the measurement space are especially helpful in checking assumptions and suggesting appropriate procedures. In particular, here are some typical situations:

One may check if the type of probability distribution assumed is correct. For example, the Gaussian distribution is a dome-shaped curve (Fig. 7.13); if the data distribute into two different groups, they certainly do not have a Gaussian distribution.

Before testing differences between two groups of sampled values or trying to construct a predictive procedure for assigning an individual to one of those groups, it might be worthwhile to see if the data points for the two groups tend to be separate.

Any one with experience in processing data knows about "outliers." These are aberrant individuals, so different from others as to constitute an exception. They may be due to faulty measurements, clerical error, or just inherent atypicality. In any case, their existence should be detected in order to eliminate them or to at least take them into consideration.

Before fitting some sort of functional relationship between variables, inspection of the data points might suggest the appropriate type of relationships to seek.

2. *As a means for elaborating hypotheses.* The subdivisions of a supposedly homogenous sample may lead to hypotheses about why these subgroups exist.

The methods discussed may be grouped according to their purpose, to the number of variables measured for each individual, and to the assumptions about probability distributions which are involved. Table 7.7 presents one possible classification.

1. Methods that Present the Data in a Form Amenable to Human Pattern Recognition: No Assumption About Distributions (Everitt, 1978).

When only one or two variables are measured per individual, traditional graphical methods are quite effective. The use of *histograms, cumulative*

TABLE 7.7
Methods For Studying Interrelationships Between Individuals

		Univariate	Multivariate
Methods which present the data in a form amenable to human pattern recognition	Non Parametric	Histograms Cumulative histograms Scatter plots	*Linear*: (Euclidean metric): Principal component analysis Factor analysis (Other metric): Correspondence factor analysis Principal coordinate analysis *Non linear:* Multidimensional scaling
	Parametric	Univariate probability plots	Multivariate probability plots Residual plots in regression and time series models Canonical coordinate analysis
Methods which substitute human pattern recognition	Non parametric		Cluster analysis
	Parametric	Sorting analysis Analysis of mixtures	

histograms, and *scatter plots* is well known from elementary statistics and can yield important information that should not be ignored because of the availability of complicated computer programs for analyzing the data in a multivariate fashion. A variable-by-variable inspection of the data is always recommendable. Fig. 7.41 illustrates the use of histograms for univariate data and of scatter plots for bivariate data. Two groups are plotted, in the top part a) for the univariate data and in the bottom b) for the bivariate data. In(a), there are practically no differences in how the data for the two groups are distributed. This can be formally tested, but the simple graphical procedure gives a pretty good idea of what the results will be. In (b), the distribution of the groups *is* different (or, rather, seems to be). This justifies testing for the difference. The graphs give more information, however. The differences between groups 1 and 2 (see Fig. 7.41) seem to be that group 2 is more variable. This suggests testing more for difference in dispersion measures than for differences in location measures (for example, the mean might be the same). The occurrence of an extreme value is also apparent, marked "outlier" in the Fig.

The construction of histograms is possible only for uni- and bivariate data, and that of scatter plots only up to three variables. Some rather complicated and ingenious methods have been devised in order to directly portray high-dimensional data in two dimensions, but we do not discuss them here in detail (see Everitt, 1978).

What is usually done is to abandon the original variables and look for a representation of the data points in a new, two or three dimensional space in such a way as to preserve the "structure of the data." Let us give a precise meaning to what the "structure of the data" is. In the space of original variables, the individuals form a "swarm" or constellation of points that can be characterized by the *distances* between all points.

We have already seen how the distance between two points measures the degree of "similarity" of two individuals: Zero distance means equality for all features measured and increasing distance means increasing difference on some or all features. The usual distance, known from everyday life and elementary mathematics, is *euclidean distance* (Eq. 7.6), but in what follows, other types of distances may be used. Changes of scale in the variables to give them unequal weightings may be performed before calculating the euclidean distance, or some other sort of measure with distance-like properties may be used, such as the number of different features for two individuals, and so on.

Whatever the type of distance introduced (or *metric*), one can imagine the data points united by wires; the length of each wire is the distance between two points. What is looked for is a way to compress the swarm of data to impose a minimum of distortions in the interpoint distances; that is, the "wires" joining the points should be stretched or compressed as little as possible (Fig. 7.12). The degree of deformation of the data swarm is quantified by a measure of "stress." If the stress is low, then one may look at the data in two or three dimensions without essential loss of information.

The methods discussed in section C of this chapter for forming hypothetical variables may be used for this purpose. *Principal component analysis* and *factor analysis* are widely used. They are suitable for data that are measured numerically and when the usual euclidean metric is used. Individuals are plotted using the first two or three components or factors. The use of numerical data and Euclidean metrics are relaxed in *correspondence factor analysis*, also discussed in section C. A method similar to these is *principal coordinate analysis*, a sort of principal component analysis applied to a pseudocovariance matrix ("pseudo" because a nonparametric measure of association is used, instead of the linear correlation coefficient that is conceptually related to the usual Euclidean metric).

All these methods (principal components, factor analysis, correspondence factor analysis, principal coordinate analysis) have in common the restriction that the transformations performed upon the original measure space are linear. In geometric terms, this means that the original axes are rotated, tilted, shrunk, or expanded, but they are still straight lines. These transformations are performed in such a way that the data represented on two or three axes give the minimum stress.

A major departure from these procedures is to permit nonlinear transformations. In this type of transformation, the axes may also be curved-sometimes giving a better chance to get a minimum stress in two or three dimensions. *Multidimensional scaling* performs nonlinear transformations of data measured in any type of scale to give low-dimensional representation of data configurations.

We will describe in some one such method, *nonlinear mapping*, so that the procedure may be understood. In nonlinear mapping, an initial, arbitrary configuration of points is assumed in 2 of 3 space, the number of points being the same as those to be mapped. This initial configuration may be random, but it is more usual to start off with the results of some linear method such as principal components. A measure of stress is defined as:

$$S = \sum_{i<j} \frac{(d_{ij} - d^*_{ij})^2}{d_{ij}} \Big/ \sum_{i<j} d_{ij} \qquad (36)$$

The parameter S measures the difference between the distances in the original space, d_{ij}, and those in the new two of three dimensional space, d^*_{ij}. At first, this measure might be quite large but the algorithm moves the points around in the new space until a minimal value of *S* is obtained. This is the nonlinear mapping.

Schwartz and John (1976) used multidimensional scaling procedures to study evoked-response waveforms. They report that a good representation is obtainable in two dimensions and that points representing evoked responses of normal subjects are separated from those representing evoked responses of patients with tumors.

2. Methods that Present the Data in a Form Amenable to Human Pattern Recognition: With Assumptions About Distributions

If a certain probability distribution is assumed, there are special methods for looking at the structure of the data. ***Univariate and multivariate probability plots*** are among the most useful. With univariate data, a rank ordering is performed and the empirical cumulative distribution function is computed. This is a plot of the percentage of members of the sample whose measure(s) are less than or equal to some value. It goes from 0% for very low values to 100% for very high values. The values of this graph, which are an estimate of the probability of the random variable having a value less than or equal to some fixed value are then interpreted as if they were probabilities. Using tables of computer-programmed functions the one looks for that value that would give the observed probability if a certain distribution is assumed. Two values are thus obtained for each measure, its actual value and the value it should have (according to the empirical distribution function) if the hypothesis of a certain distribution were true. These two values are plotted one against the other. If the sample is compatible with the hypothesis of a certain distribution, the points should fall more or less along a straight line. Breaks in the line or extreme values are easily detected (Fig. 7.43), being interpretable as inhomogenities in the sample or as the existence of outliers, respectively. In any case, flagrant deviations from a

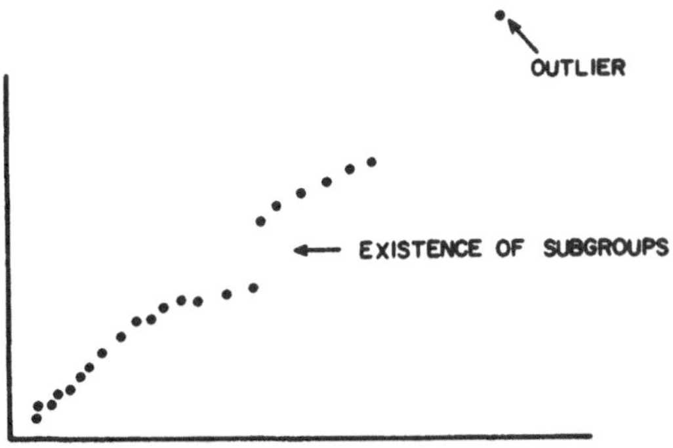

FIG. 7.43. *Probability plots.* The appropriateness of assumptions about distributions may be checked by using probability plots. The abscissa is the actual value of the individual, the ordinate the value it should have if the assumption that the sample comes from a population with a given distribution is true. The points should fall approximately along a straight line if the assumption is valid. If the sample is heterogenous, breaks in the graph may appear reflecting the existence of subgroups. Extreme values off the line, indicate the presence of outliers.

straight line can be considered evidence for rejecting the hypothesis of a certain distribution.

In the multivariate case, a single measure must be selected as representative of the multivariate vector. For example, in examining multivariate normality, Andrews et al. (1973) suggest using the Mahalanobis distance of the individuals from the sample mean. It is well known (Anderson, 1958) that these distances have a distribution known as Chi-squared if the parent population is multivariate normal. The same interpretations may be made as in the univariate case discussed previously.

The plotting of residuals, already mentioned in section C of this chapter may also be considered in this class of procedures.

Finally, canonical coordinate analysis (section D) is a way of plotting multivariate data in two or three dimensions when different groups are involved. The interesting point is that, in this type of representation, the ordinary distance of any point to another may be interpreted as a Mahalanobis distance. Thus, canonical coordinate analysis is useful in visualizing data sets when tests for differences of mean vectors or discriminant procedures are to be employed.

3. Cluster Analysis

Methods that rely on human pattern recognition abilities are very flexible and can cope with unusual situations. In some cases, however, it is not possible to apply these methods. This might happen because the intrinsic dimensionality of the data is so high that it is impossible to get a good representation in 2- or 3-space. In other words, the stress measure might be so high that substantial distortions in the representation of the data would be expected. Or, alternatively, the application might be such that subjective decisions should be excluded. In all these cases, automatic methods for determining the existence of subgroups in a given sample should be used. We term these methods *cluster analysis.*

The general objective of these procedures is, on the basis of measured features, to objectively decide if the sample should be considered as formed by subgroups, and to decide which members of the sample belong to which group. Cluster analysis is a vast subject (see, for example, Anderberg, 1973) precisely because there are so many possible definitions of what to call a "cluster" and many more procedures to divide a sample into clusters. Intuitively, a cluster is a group of objects that are similar to each other and different from the members of other clusters. This loose definition can be made a bit more precise by the use of the notion of distance that has already been encountered.

In this chapter, we have already considered a set of N individuals represented as points in p space (this might be the space of original variables or any transformation of it). Suppose that a distance has been defined between the points in the space (remember that this distance can be the usual Euclidean distance or any other type of distance). A cluster will be a set of points within which the interpoint distances are small compared to the distances to other points outside the cluster (Fig. 7.44).

To *cluster analyze* a sample is to divide it into sets that, on the basis of the idea previously given, are "clusters." Clustering methods can be *nonoverlapping*. In this case, each individual belongs or does not belong to a cluster, and the clusters partition the space of measurements into nonoverlapping sets. On the other hand, there are ways of defining *overlapping clusters*. In this case, instead of just "belonging" or "not belonging" a point may belong to a cluster with varying degree measured on some scale. For example, a point could belong with measure 1 (certainly does belong), or with measure 0 (certainly does not belong), or with measure .5 (might belong). In other words, the sets into which the space is divided are *fuzzy sets*. It is obvious that this notion is related to the theory of probability. The measure of membership might be interpreted as the probability of belonging to a given set.

Clustering methods also differ accordingly whether certain probability distributions are assumed (parametric methods) or not (nonparametric methods).

a. Nonparametric Methods. These are the most well-known clustering methods. Because they are not based on the assumption of any particular

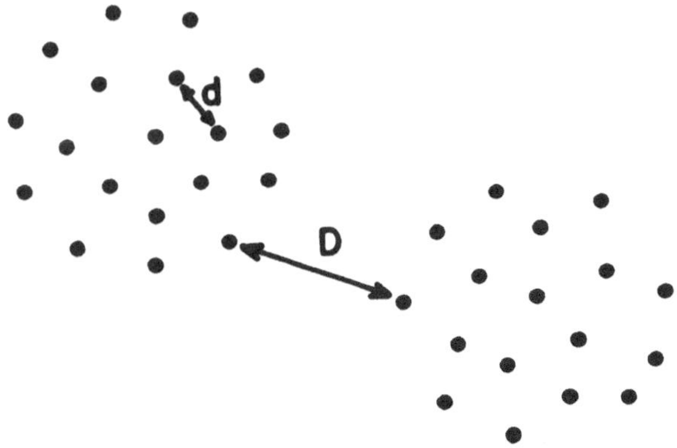

FIG. 7.44. *Definition of clusters.* In two dimensions, the idea of clusters can be grasped intuitively. Thus, here, the two separate clouds of points are different clusters. A more precise idea is that a cluster is a set in which the interpoint distances—(d) for example—are small in comparison with the distances between the members of the cluster to other clusters. This notion can be made still more precise and underlies a number of different clustering procedures.

probability distribution, some authors tend to consider the nonparametric methods as heuristic algorithmic procedures. Very little work has been done on tests for the significance of clusters and other aspects of statistical inference in nonparametric cluster analysis. The lack of theory has resulted in many equivalent methods being represented as different. For example, "single-link cluster analysis," "nearest-neighbor cluster analysis," and "minimal-spanning tree analysis" are all the same thing. Another problem is that, because different clustering procedures are based on different criteria (many times *not* stated explicity), the same data run with different programs usually give totally different results. This should not be a cause the data analyst to despair, because the different results may give insight into different aspects of the data. What is important is to have a clear idea of what types of clusters each method gives.

Nonparametric methods are usually subdivided into *hierarchical and nonhierarchical methods*. Hierarchical methods present, as a final result, a tree or *dendogram* of relationships between individuals (Fig. 7.45). The leaves of this "tree" are the individuals of the sample. Leaves are joined by small branches, small branches by large branches, and so on, following the

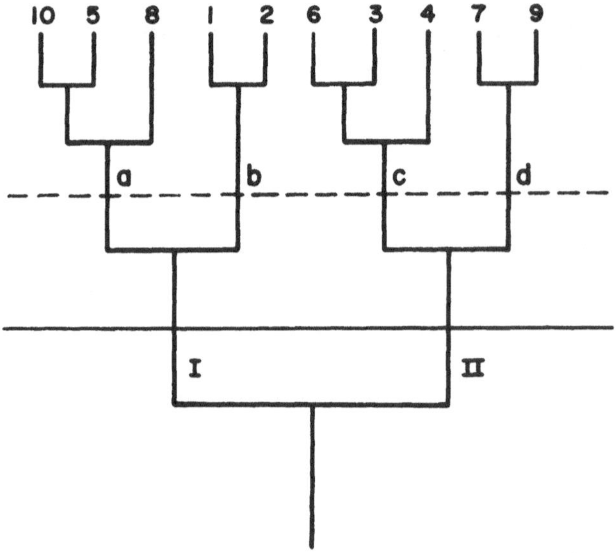

FIG. 7.45. *Output of a hierarchical clustering procedure:* a dendogram or tree of dissimilarities. Each "leaf" in the tree (numbered 10, 5, 8, . . .) is an individual. The branches join similar individuals and, then progressively, more and more dissimilar groups of individuals. The definition of the set of clusters to be selected is arbitrarily based on this tree diagram. For example, if the dotted line is used as a reference, then the branches marked *a*, *b*, *c*, and *d* are considered clusters. If the continuous line is used as a reference only, the two branches *I* and *II* are considered clusters.

rule that the length of the branches reflects the degree of dissimilarity of the individuals on the branch from individuals on other parts of the tree. The result is a sort of taxonomy of similarity. (As a matter of fact, one of the principal applications of hierarchical cluster analysis has been to provide a "numerical taxonomy" for biological work.) In this case, the division into clusters is made by considering different branches as different clusters. What results is a family of nested clusters. A certain degree of arbitrariness is present when a particular set of branches is selected as *the* division into clusters. For example, in Fig. 7.45, branches *a*, *b*, *c*, and *d* are considered as clusters, but, at another level, the division into clusters may be the two branches labeled *I* and *II*.

In spite of the difficulty in defining clusters, the hierarchical methods are very popular, because of their easy and efficient computer implementation (Enslein et al., 1977). We describe two examples of hierarchical methods here: single-link cluster analysis and Ward's method for clustering.

Single-link cluster analysis starts out by considering each individual as if it were a cluster. It then joins those two individuals that are nearest into a two-individual cluster. From then on, clusters may have more than one member. Step by step, clusters are "fused" using the following rule: Combine those two clusters for which the *cluster distance* is smallest.

Cluster distance is defined as the smallest of all distances between members of one set and those of another set. Single-link cluster analysis is very fast, but it presents the problem of "linking" (Fig. 7.46a). This happens when two well-defined, different clusters have individuals bridging the gaps between them. The method combines them into a single cluster, instead of keeping them separate.

Ward's method is similar, but uses a different definition of cluster distance, that results in clusters with the minimum total deviation from the cluster mean vector. This method tends to form compact spherical clusters, overcoming the problem of linkage. Yet, if the real clusters are ellipsoidal, the tendency to form spherical clusters may produce artifactual results (Fig. 7.46b). There are other methods, developed especially for detecting ellipsoidal and other queerly shaped clusters, such as those depicted in Fig. 7.46c.

Single-link cluster analysis and Ward's method have both been applied to the problem of identifying typical waveshapes in evoked responses. Work described in Chapter 10 tends to support the conclusion, also based on empirical computer simulations, that Ward's method clusters data in a fashion more acceptable to human intuition.

Both these methods are *agglomerative methods*, because they start with each individual as a cluster and then join them in a step-wise fashion. There are also *divisive methods*. These start with the whole sample as a cluster, then partition it into two subclusters, then partition these into further

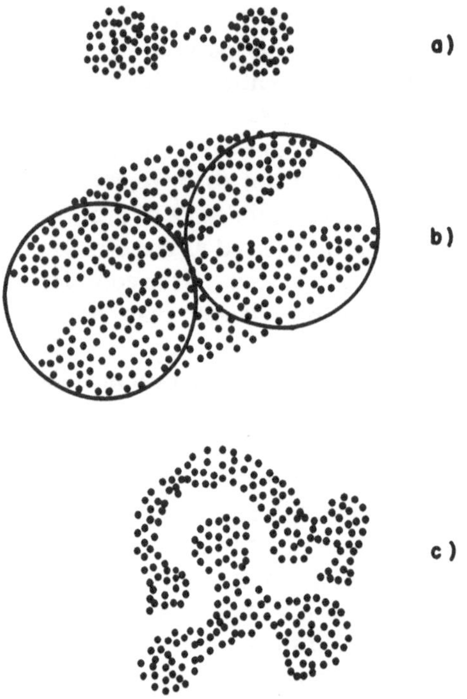

FIG. 7.46. *Difficulties inherent to some clustering procedures.* In (a), the phenomena of "linking" is illustrated. This is a pitfall of single-link cluster analysis. Two well-defined groups that have stray individuals bridging the gap between them are considered as a single cluster. In (b), the formation of artifactual clusters when applying Ward's method (which forms spherical clusters) to ellipsoidal clusters. (c) illustrates the possibility of queerly shaped clusters for which special methods should be used.

subclusters, and so on, also yielding a dendogram. Divisive and agglomerative methods do not give the same results.

Nonhierarchical methods do not yield a dendogram, just a partition of the sample into *k* clusters. The difficulty with nonhierachical methods is that one must input the approximate number of clusters one expects to find. Typical of nonhierachical methods is McQueen's *k*-means method. The process starts off with *k* points arbitrarily chosen by the data analyst as provisional cluster means. Each data point in the sample is assigned to the cluster with the nearest mean. After each point is assigned the mean is readjusted. This is done iteratively until stable cluster means are obtained. These are considered representative of the clusters.

We wish to stress the fact that many clusters programs are readily available. Suitable care in the selection and use of these procedures should be exercised. An important point is that *cluster analysis always clusters* the data. The emergence of clusters is automatic and might not have any meaning, because no statistical tests are available. Applying discriminant analysis or tests for differences of means *does not* provide a statistical basis for cluster validity, because the clusters are formed in a nonrandom way and tests of differences on this basis are so biased as to be useless.

b. Parametric Methods. These methods are based on the assumption that the observed sample has been obtained by taking at random items from different gaussian distributions. The result is *a mixture* of normal distributions. The problem is to estimate the means and variances (or covariance matrices in the multivariate case) of the original populations. Discriminant analysis methods (see section VI of this chapter) may then be used to assign each individual to the proper cluster. In spite of the existence of both univariate and multivariate procedures for the analysis of mixtures, with rigorous statistical tests, no neurometric applications have been made. The nearest approach to mixture analysis is the sorting procedure of Ruchkin (1971). This procedure scans the univariate marginal distributions of a multivariate vector (evoked responses in the original case) and tests for departures from univariate normality. Suppose the activity at a particular time instant, $x(t)$, has a larger variance than others, and the amplitude distribution at that point is non-gaussian as revealed by the existence of various peaks in the univariate histogram. Then the range of ER amplitude values is subdivided into regions corresponding to the peaks in the amplitude histogram at latency t, and the evoked responses are "sorted" into different groups on the basis of their amplitude at that latency. Each group of ERs is then examined to see if the variance is uniform across the analysis epoch and non-gaussianity has disappeared. This is a sort of informal, stepwise mixture analysis.

V. SAMPLE COMPARISON TECHNIQUES

When the following steps have been completed: 1) correct formulation of the neurometric problem; 2) selection of an adequate probability model; 3) study of the structure of the variables in order to select a correct descriptive model; 4) analysis of the structure of the individuals to identify outliers and ascertain the correctness of the definition of the groups; then it is possible to see if there are really any differences among the groups of interest and to assess the statistical significance of the observed differences. The ultimate objective of neurometric procedures is to provide predictions on the basis of quantitative parameters of brain activity. A necessary but not sufficient condition for predictive accuracy is that some neurometric parameter must vary when the brain condition of interest changes, be this change due to disease, effect of a drug or any type of physiological variation.

The statistical equivalent of this problem is the selection and application of statistical techniques to determine if a set of measures collected under one condition exhibits differences from one or more different collections of the same measures obtained under different conditions. Before treating the general problem, we will look at a specific example.

A. Differences in the Means of Neurometric Values

Because of the utility of predictive techniques based on the multivariate gaussian distribution (Eq. 17), we discuss an example based on the assumption of Gaussianity. In order to be specific, consider the following situation:

Two samples have been obtained, each of neurometric measures. The neurometric parameters are in the form of a two-dimensional vector. The first group consists of normal subjects, and N_1 such individuals have been subjected to the neurometric examination. N_2 sample vectors have been obtained from patients with, for example, brain tumors. In the geometric representation of these data vectors, the individuals from each group form a swarm or cloud. The question is: Do we have sufficient evidence to consider them different swarms?

Before answering this question, let us consider, the ideal situation in which we could infinitely sample many individuals from each group, so that the swarms would give a more complete idea of the probability distributions. We suppose that the distributions for the two groups are *multinormal* and that they have the *same covariance matrix*. It must be remembered (section III) that a multinormal distribution depends only on the mean vector, which specifies its position, and the covariance matrix Σ, which specifies the shape of the swarm of points. This means that we are assuming that the shape of the swarm of points from group 1 is the same as for group 2, but possibly displaced. In other words, the difference is exclusively in the mean vectors $\vec{\mu}_1$ and $\vec{\mu}_2$. Inspecting Fig. 7.47c, one can see intuitively that there are situations, in which multivariate differences might be much larger than any of the univariate differences. A measure of this difference could be the ordinary Euclidean distance between the mean vectors. If the distance is zero (Fig. 7.47a), the two swarms of points coincide—that is, there are no differences. The larger the distance between the mean vectors, the more different are the two groups (Fig. 7.47b and c). This is not a completely satisfactory measure, because a situation such as depicted in Fig. 7.47b shows that a certain degree of overlap between the two swarms might occur. In some sense, the distance between the means should be weighted so that the greater the intersection between the swarms, the smaller the measure of difference. This is accomplished by using the *Mahalanobis distance*:

$$D = |\vec{t}_1 - \vec{t}_2| \; ; \vec{t}_i = \vec{\mu}_i \Sigma^{-1/2} \tag{37}$$

This equation express that D, the Mahalanobis distance between group 1 and 2, is the distance between the standardized mean vectors t_i. The standarized mean vector t_i is obtained by multiplying the mean of group μ_i by the inverse square root of the variance and covariance matrix Σ. In terms of the geometric interpretation, this means that each swarm is turned into a

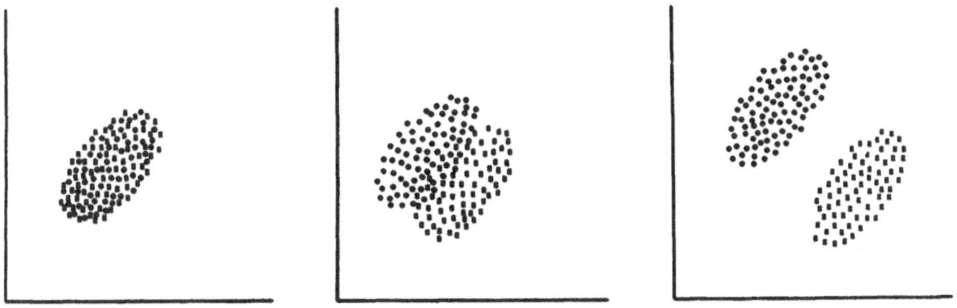

FIG. 7.47. *Differences between bivariate multinormal distributions with equal covariance matrices.* In the three graphs, individuals from two different groups are marked with points (.) or crosses (x). Samples from multinormal distributions assume approximately ellipsoidal shapes, which are determined by the covariance matrix, and the position by the mean vector. Because equal covariance matrices are assumed for both groups, ideally the shape of the cloud of points should be similar but placed differently in the plane. In (a), the mean vectors are the same and the two swarms of points are confounded. In (b), there is a certain degree of overlap, because the means differ, but not as much as in (c), where there is a large separation between the means. Two points should be noted. First, the difference between multivariate means may be much larger than that of the univariate means considered for each variable separately. Second, any measure of differences between samples must consider (b) in which, though there are differences between the means, there is also an overlap between the two distributions of individuals.

sphere-like cloud (Fig. 7.16) with unit variance in any direction and then the usual distance between the means is then measured.

Let us return to the Example, in which only N_1 and N_2 samples are available from group 1 and 2 respectively. We may compute the *sample Mahalanobis distance* D by substituting, in Eq. 37, the population covariance matrix Σ by the sample covariance matrix S, and the population means μ_1 and μ_2 by the sample means $\bar{\mathbf{x}}_1$ and $\bar{\mathbf{x}}_2$, we can then try to assess the difference between the two groups. We must take into account that the sample means and covariance matrix are imperfect estimates of the population quantities, based on limited samples, and the value of D will fluctuate from sample to sample. This compels us to use probabilistic decision-making procedures.

We postulate the *null hypothesis* of no difference between the means ($D = 0$), and then calculate the probability of D being equal to or larger than its observed value. If this is too improbable, then we may safely reject the null hypothesis and assume that there exist real differences between the two groups. The procedure just outlined very roughly is Hotteling's T^2 test for differences between vectors.

If only one variable is studied, this reduces essentially to Student's t test, familiar from elementary statistic courses.

Before we turn to a more general description of sample comparison techniques, it might be of interest to examine the methods already explained in connection with one other neurometrical examples. It is shown elsewhere in this book that asymmetry of evoked response from homologous right–left derivations is an important indicator of brain lesions. It is then important to devise reliable measures of evoked-response symmetry. Due to the prevalence of average response computers, in many applications, only the average evoked response is available. Measures such as correlation, signal energy ratio, mean square differences are then computed. Although these provide valuable information, they ignore the degree of single-trial evoked response variability. The Mahalanobis distance would be an ideal measure of symmetry, but it requires substantial further computer processing. This illustrates that there are current problems in which a balance must be struck between the ideal theoretical statistical approach and practical constraints. Neurometrics has not yet extracted the utmost from the information available in the EEG or in the ER.

B. General Formulation of the Problem

In a more general formulation, the question is: Given two or more samples of univariate, multivariate, or time-series measurements, do they come from the same population or from different populations? More formally, if the items of sample i are samples from a population with probability distribution F_i; should we consider the F_i identical or different?

If we specify the general form of the F_i and suppose that the only difference may be in a parameter or group of parameters, then the question is *parametric*. The most important case is the gaussian distribution. The only parameters that can vary here are the means, the covariances, or both.

If we do not specify the general form of the F_i, then the differences sought for are both of type of distribution and possibly of parameters (because we do not know the form of the distribution, they could be of the same type). The question and the techniques developed for answering it are termed *nonparametric*.

In either case, testing for differences in parameters of distributions, the procedure is to set up the *null hypothesis* (H_0) of no differences. This contrasts with the *alternative hypothesis* (H_1) of some sort of difference. *Test statistics* are measures that are computed from the collected samples and that reflect, in some way, the differences between the distributions. These test statistics, being computed from samples, vary depending on the particular items that happened to be selected at random from the total population. One must know the probability of the occurrence of different values of any statistics when H_0 is true and when H_1 is true. Using this information, a criterion is established as to which test statistic to use and at which value of this test statistic compels a rejection of H_0—that is, when is one to accept that there are differences. The random nature of the observations under study ensures us that no decision will always be totally sure. The problem is to select a test and a *critical value* of this statistic that will minimize our probabilities of error.

In testing the null hypothesis, there are two types of error: accepting the existence of differences when no differences are present (Type I error) and accepting the null hypothesis when, in fact, there are differences (Type II error). Let us call the probability of Type I errors α and that of Type II errors β. The preceding criteria must, then, minimize both types of errors. It is demonstrable, however, that decreasing the probability of one type of error increases that of the other. What is usually done is to fix the probability α at some small conventional level. (.05 as significant, .01 as highly significant) and then to select the test statistic and the critical value to make β as small as possible.

One way of doing this is to choose an adequate test statistic. Another is to increase the sample size. The planning of what samples to select, what tests to apply, which sample sizes to use, and how to interpret the results are a subspeciality of statistics known as *experimental design*. (A better name would be "statistical design of experiments with standard techniques." because what is covered in texts on the subject is only a fraction of possible designs for experiments with stochastic events.)

The particular test statistic to use depends on many factors. These are:

1. The type of measurement (single value, vector, or time series).
2. The number of different samples. There are special techniques for only two samples and others for the general multisample case.
3. Is the difference to be assessed only a difference in one paramater? If so, which one? Or, alternatively, are difference in the whole distribution to be tested?
4. Are the samples obtained related or not related? Unrelated samples are obtained from statistically independent situations, for example, measurements in two totally different groups of people. Related samples are correlated in some way. The measurements performed on two different occasions for the same patients is a typical situation of this type. Special methods are available to consider the relatedness of the samples.

Based on these distinctions, Table 7.8 has been constructed to illustrate the great diversity of procedures that have been developed to test for such

TABLE 7.8
Sample Comparison Techniques[a]

Type of Model		*Two Groups* — *Independent*	*Two Groups* — *Related*	*K Groups* — *Independent*	*K Groups* — *Related*
		Number of Groups			
One Variable (Univariate)	Nonparametric	Fisher "exact prob" Chi-squared test Two sample Kolmogorov-Smirnov test Mann-Whitney *U* test	Sign test Wilcoxon's test	Kruskal Wallis test Chi-squared	Frieman's χ^2_R test
	Parametric	*t* test *F* test	Paired *t* test	Analysis of variance (ANOVA) and of covariance Bartlett's test for homogeneity of variance	Repeated measurement analysis

More than One Variable (Multivariate)	Non-parametric			Contingency table analysis	Multivariate generalization of Frieman's χ^2_R test
	Parametric	Hotelling's T^2 test Equality of regression lines lines	Paired T^2 test	Multivariate Analysis of Variance and Covariance (MANOVA, MACOVA) Likelihood test for equality of covariance matrices Graphic methods for MANOVA	
Time Series	Until now, only parametric models well developed	Comparison of power spectrums Comparisons of parameters of time domain time-series models		ANOVA for univariate time series	MANOVA for multiple time series

[a]This table presents examples of different, commonly used techniques for the comparison of samples. These techniques test for the equality of some parameter. The examples are classified according to the type of model and to the numbers of groups compared.

differences. This table is by no means exhaustive; it is only intended to provide a guide in the selection of techniques. Once again, we repeat that the mechanical use of standard technique may not be adequate for the particular problem considered, so tables like those presented here should only serve to indicate possible solutions.

C. Methods for Testing Differences Between Samples Obtained from Gaussian Distributions

What follows is not intended as a detailed explanation of the basis and practical details of different tests, but rather as an overview of what can be asked using standard techniques.

Because multinormal distributions differ only in the mean vector and covariance matrix, one can ask the following types of questions:

1. Are the distributions from which the samples are obtained different in any way? This question requires evaluation of *both* differences in mean vectors and in covariance matrices.
2. *Assuming* equal covariance matrices, are the mean vectors different?
3. Are the covariance matrices different?

As can be seen, questions about mean vectors are not independent from assumptions about the equality of covariance matrices; in fact, this assumption is essential. The general problem of testing differences between mean vectors when the second-order moments are different is called the Behrens-Fisher problem and has a long, controversial, and unresolved history. Therefore, answering question 3 with the appropriate test is the logical first step. An example of what may happen is given by Valdés (1978; see Chapter 10). Covariance matrices for different sets of single-trial evoked responses were found to be different. This should help to eliminate the unconcern with which tests of type 2 are applied in this field, since in such instances the results can be severely misleading.

Question 1 is rarely asked, but is important for prediction, a situation in which any sort of difference is information useful for decisions.

Question 2 is the most frequent asked. For one variable and two groups, the standard *t test* is used. When one variable is measured for many groups, the method of *analysis of variance* or ANOVA (which examines mean difference in spite of the name) is available. This is a well-developed area useful in statistical experimental design.

The extension of these methods for multivariate observation is the *T^2 test* (due to Hotteling) and *Multivariate Analysis of Variance* (MANOVA), for two and more than two samples, respectively. Using the strategy outlined in section IV of this chapter for the analysis of time series—that is, applying complex number adaptions of standard statistical techniques to the complex coefficients of the Fourier transform—*complex ANOVA* may be used in the analysis of experimental designs with univariate time series. Similarly, *complex MANOVA* may be used for the analysis of multiple time-series experimental designs.

Two special situations merit attention when comparing means. There may be a set of variables that are identified as influencing the parameters under study, but that are not of particular interest. The effects of these *concomitant* variables may be partialled out, using regression techniques and then the methods for testing differences in means applied. This combination of regression methods with tests for differences in means is known as *Multivariate Analysis of Variance and Covariance* (MANCOVA). We mention this particularly because of its potential neurometric use. For example, the effect of age-related changes may be eliminated from a set of neurometric parameters and then tests for differences in means carried out, in order to assess the possible usefulness of these measures for diagnosis.

The other special situation occurs when related samples are collected. This happens frequently in clinical studies when patients are followed up, possibly to evaluate the efficacy of some therapy. For example, evaluation of interhemispheric symmetry in epileptics, before and after drug therapy, should not be compared using the t or T^2 test. There is a bias because the measurements are made on the same person for both samples. Thus, if before therapy, the values of symmetry were high, they might tend to continue high after therapy; the same situation might hold for low values. One example of something that can be done in this type of situation is to use the *paired or* T^2 *test*. This consists of working with the *differences* of the measures before and after treatment for each individual. This is now a one-sample problem, to test that the differences randomly vary around the value zero.

Finally, we wish to mention the use, made by some authors in the EEG and evoked-response literature, of *step-wise discriminant analysis methods* for assessing differences in means. Though we treat this topic in its proper context, that of prediction, it is important to point out that the objective of this method is to *predict*, not to give an ordering of the values according to their difference. In any case, many authors have pointed out that step-wise methods are biased and that the nominal significance levels supposedly used are really unknown. Thus, though there might be a justification for using this sort of procedure for prediction, depending on the empirical efficacy obtainable, inferences based on the output of these methods should be considered with extreme caution.

VI. STATISTICAL PREDICTION

The objective of neurometrics is to provide predictions about states of the central nervous system. These predictions must be based on the available knowledge about the distribution of quantitative parameters of brain electrical activity. The types of predictions may vary. Presence or absence of brain damage, probable disease or localization, prognosis, suggestion as to possibly optimal therapy, forecast of academic achievement, these and many more are the potential types of predictions that might be attempted. What all the types of prediction have in common are the following features:

1. Individuals are grouped according to some practical or theoretical criteria.
2. Neurometric parameters are defined and measured for samples of each of the defined groups.
3. After assessing whether or not there are differences between the groups (section V of this chapter), the information available is used to set up some type of automatic decision-making procedure. This procedure specifies into which group an individual should be placed, depending on how the neurometric parameters measured for that individual relate to the available data base.

The prediction need not be about a finite and discrete number of groups. In fact, regression methods (section IV of this chapter) may be used to predict continuous quantities (such as age; for prediction of "EEG age," see Chapter 11). The issue studied here, however, is that of predicting the membership of an individual in one of a finite number of groups. This is known in statistical theory as *discriminant analysis.*

There are many procedures for statistical prediction and for discriminant analysis in particular. As with all statistical methods, the assumption of a specific probability distribution is the basis of parametric techniques as contrasted to nonparametric techniques. A further distinction is possible depending on way predictive procedures behave with respect to extremely atypical individuals. If they are assigned to a group of "unclassifiables," then the procedure is called *partial. Forced predictive procedures* allot the outlier to one of the preestablished groups, even if they have a very low probability of belonging there.

A classification of some predictive methods, following the preceding criteria, is given in Table 7.9.

We deal here only with the parametric, gaussian type of discriminant analysis. This should not bias the reader against considering other types of discriminant procedures, even totally empirical ones. Our own emphasis on parametric methods stems from the belief that well-known procedures, studied from both the theoretical and empirical points of view, will, in the

TABLE 7.9
Methods For Statistical Prediction

	Continuous Prediction: Regression	Discrete Prediction: Discrimination
Empirical Methods	Graphical Regression	Convex Hull Method
Statistical Methods *Non Parametric*	Least Squares Regression Least sum of absolute values	Discrimination based on multinomial
Parametric	Maximum likelihood regression	Fishers linear discriminant function Non linear discrimination

long run, give better results, because they permit rational choices of strategy. Their totally explicit nature discourages haphazard decisions that may camouflage unnoticed assumptions. Nonetheless, there is a vast literature on the subject, sometimes published under the heading of "pattern recognition." In pattern recognition terminology, a "feature" is a variable as originally defined or in some new space obtained by the methods described in section IV of this chapter. The establishment of patterns, "learning without a teacher," and so on, are what we call analysis of the structure of individuals. Pattern recognition proper, learning with a teacher, and classification, are synonymous with discriminant analysis.

A. Basic Ideas Underlying Discriminant Analysis

Let us recall once more the geometrical representation of sampled individuals in the space of measured variables. We are now working with various groups (demonstrated to be different) that constitute separate clouds or swarms. What is needed is a procedure for assigning a new individual to the correct cloud. There may be a certain overlap between clouds. This means that we will not get a 100% perfect classification of all new individuals, but we will try to do the best possible. In fact, "the best possible" must be evaluated in order to know if using the procedure is worthwhile. The decision procedure consists of establishing surfaces or boundaries that separate the clouds in such a way as to minimize the errors of misclassification. Fig. 7.48 represents a situation in which two variables are being used, and the probability density for two different populations is completely known. Though the mountain range-like densities overlap to some extent, it is undoubtable that population I and population II are concentrated differently on the measurement plane. A boundary may be drawn defining a region (I) that encompasses most of population I with a minimum of encroachment by population II. The same way be done for

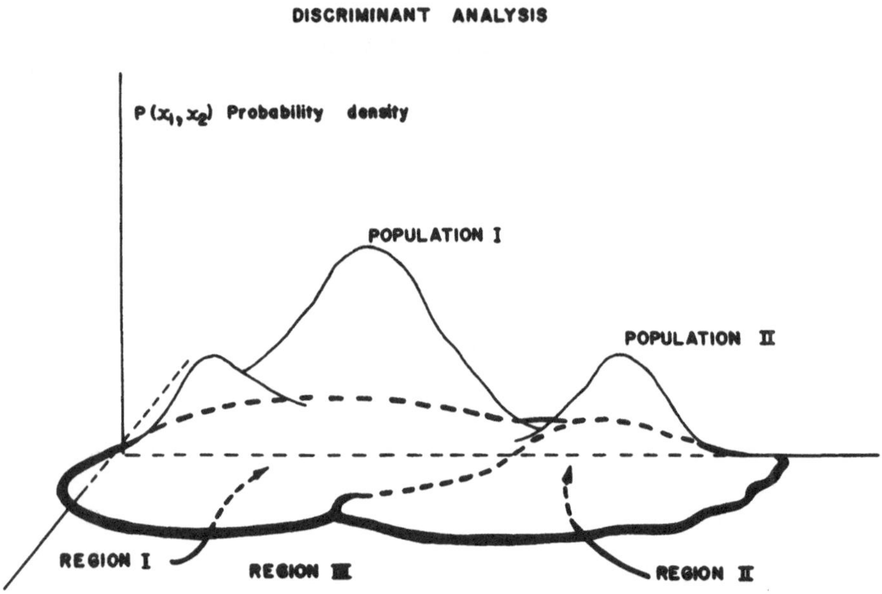

FIG. 7.48. *Graphical representation of discriminant analysis.* If the probability densities for two populations are known, then boundaries may be drawn that separate regions of the measurement space (two-dimensional in the Fig.) on which the different populations are constructed. The discriminant procedure consists of classifying a new individual according to the region in which he or she falls. In this case, Region I defines the individuals who are to be classified as belonging to Population I and Region II, the individuals to be put in Population II. While Region III is the region of "unclassifiables." The boundaries are chosen in such a way as to minimize the probability of misclassification.

population II, by defining region II. A third region (III) is that portion of the measurement plane for which neither population has a high probability density. The decision procedure for prediction may be stated as follows: If the point representing an individual falls in region I, assign it to population I; if the point falls in region II, classify it as belonging to population II; and if the point falls in region III, label the individual as "unclassifiable."

There are three types of errors:

1. Individuals belonging to population I are put into population II.
2. Individuals belonging to population II are put into population I.
3. Individuals belonging either to populations I or II, but are "queer" and are put into the "unclassifiable" group.

Some methods of discriminant analysis try to minimize all three probabilities. Others take into consideration the relative "costs" of misclassification. It is certainly more serious to assure a patient with a brain tumor that he or she is normal than to make a healthy individual undergo a thorough examination. These costs might not only be ethical, sometimes they may actually be measured in monetary units. In many cases, it proves difficult in practice to assign costs, so cost weighted discriminant analysis has not been used very much in neurometrics.

Another consideration is that of the relative prevalence of the conditions pertaining to the two populations. There are certainly more normals than any particular disease. This is reflected by a priori probabilities of belonging to different populations that may also be considered when drawing the boundaries. As with cost, the estimation of a priori probabilities is difficult and has not been used much to date.

In practice, there are many more than two variables, and there may be more than two groups. Instead of a graphical procedure, the boundaries are embodied in mathematical formulae, so that evaluation of an individual by an equation or a set of equations serves the purpose of defining the region of hyperspace into which the individual falls.

The principal complication in discriminant analysis is that, contrary to the ideal picture given in Fig. 7.48, we do *not* know the probability densities for the populations, but rather have to estimate them from sometimes relatively small samples.

B. Discrimination When the Populations are Gaussian: Ideal Case of Knowledge of Population Parameters

We first consider the ideal Gaussian case with perfect knowledge of means and covariance matrices and then turn to practical problems in dealing with actual data.

Consider the case of one variable. Suppose we only know the values of the mean μ and variance σ^2 of the normal subjects. A possible discriminant procedure is to use Eq. 16 for the univariate Gaussian density to evaluate the probability that the individual does or does not belong to the normal population. This is facilitated by the *z score*:

$$z = (x - \mu)/\sigma \tag{38}$$

Which transforms the individual value into distance from the mean in σ units, by subtracting the mean and dividing by the standard deviation. This permits working with the *standard Gaussian density*. For this density, the probabilities for any particular value are easily found in any statistical table. For example, $z = 1.96$ corresponds to a probability of .05 of belonging to the normal population.

This procedure does not use the information available about the other populations (in real situations, the information about other populations is sometimes so scanty that this is an advantage). Let us see what happens when two populations are being studied, because the arguments involved generalize readily to more than two populations.

There are three possible cases: The two populations differ in mean only, they differ in variance only, or they differ in both variance and means (Fig. 7.49a, b, and c). In all three cases, a criterion that gives good results is: Evaluate the density corresponding to the individual value for each of the populations and assign the individual to the population for which the density at that value is highest. This is equivalent to locating the individual value on the x axis in Fig. 7.49 and drawing a vertical line upwards. The line crosses successively the two densities. The last density encountered determines the population to which the individual is assigned. For the equal variance and unequal mean situation, this criterion determines that all points to the right of the point labeled z in Fig. 7.49a will be assigned to population II and those to the left of z will be assigned to population I. Note that z is simply the average of the two means. In the other two cases, when variances are unequal, *two points*, z_1 and z_2, define an interval in which the individual is assigned to population I or otherwise, if the measured value falls out of the interval (Fig. 7.49b and c). An important point is that the individual, on the basis of this rule might be assigned to population II—and yet be an outlier—for example, Fig. 7.49c. The examination of the z-core for each population can help to detect this situation.

When considering more than one variable, the *z vector* might be used when only information about the normal population is available. The *z vector* is defined (John et al., 1977) as the vector of z scores for different neurometric parameters. It has been demonstrated to be useful as a rough measure of the presence of disease. In addition to the disadvantage of not using the available information for abnormal populations, that the intercorrelations of variables are ignored is a statistical drawback. If the decision is to consider a person abnormal if any of the individual z scores are abnormal, then the decision regions for normality looks like the one in Fig. 7.50, in the form of a square. An overall measure of normality is best given by the Mahalanobis distance. Given the value of the Mahalanobis distance for a certain individual, the probability of that person being normal may then be calculated. This gives a decision region that is an ellipse for two dimensions and is the statistically correct solution.

In multivariate discrimination, when considering, the information available for groups other than the normal, a situation occurs similar to that in the univariate discrimination problem occurs. The populations to be discriminated may differ only in the mean (Fig. 7.51a), or both in the mean and the covariances (Fig. 7.51b). The same rule is used: Assign the individual to that population for which the probability density is highest. This gives a *linear* boundary in two dimensions and a *hyperplane* in p dimensions. When the covariance matrices are different, then the boundaries are nonlinear in shape. Thus, a distinction between *linear* and *nonlinear* discriminant analysis may be made according to the equality or inequality of the covariance matrices. The use of linear boundaries in the unequal covariance case can lead to substantial errors in classification (Fig. 7.51c). Remember that we are discussing the case of perfect knowledge about the population densities. The situation changes when real data is used, the advantages of nonlinear methods being offset by other factors.

Individuals far off the graph (outliers) may be detected by using the Mahalanobis distance to the population means and, if present, are not included in any group.

C. Practical Discriminant Analysis

In practice, when population parameters are *not* known, two solutions are presently available. The standard solution (Anderson, 1958) is to estimate the population parameters by the sample means and sample covariance matrices. Aitchinson, Habbema, & Kay (1977) call this procedure *estimative* discriminant analysis. They further divide estimative methods according to the assumption that covariance matrices are equal (Ee, in Aitchinson's notation) or unequal (Eu). The authors discuss another type of procedure in which the sample estimates are not substituted into the multinormal density equation, but rather into the *multivariate t* distribution. The bivariate graph of this distribution is also bell-shaped, but is more widely spread. This wider spread takes into account our degree of ignorance about the actual distributions (in fact, the sample size, which is not used in the Gaussian formulae, is an explicit parameter of the multivariate t density). Procedures based on the multivariate t distribution are called *predictive*. As with estimative procedures, we may distinguish the equal covariance (Pe) and unequal covariance (Pu) case.

Aitchinson et al. (1977) report an interesting series of empirical computer simulations that not only support theoretical arguments in favor of predictive methods, but also agree with other results on comparisons of discriminant methods. These authors report that the worst method is Eu (contrary to conclusions in the ideal case (Fig. 7.51c). When the covariance matrices are really equal, the Pe is the best method. When the covariance matrices are unequal, then Pu is best, but for small sample sizes, the advantage over Pe is not great. This bears out the conclusion, reached by other authors, that for small sample sizes, linear discrimination is preferable to nonlinear discrimination. The advantage of linear methods probably consists of the increased number of samples used to estimate the common covariance

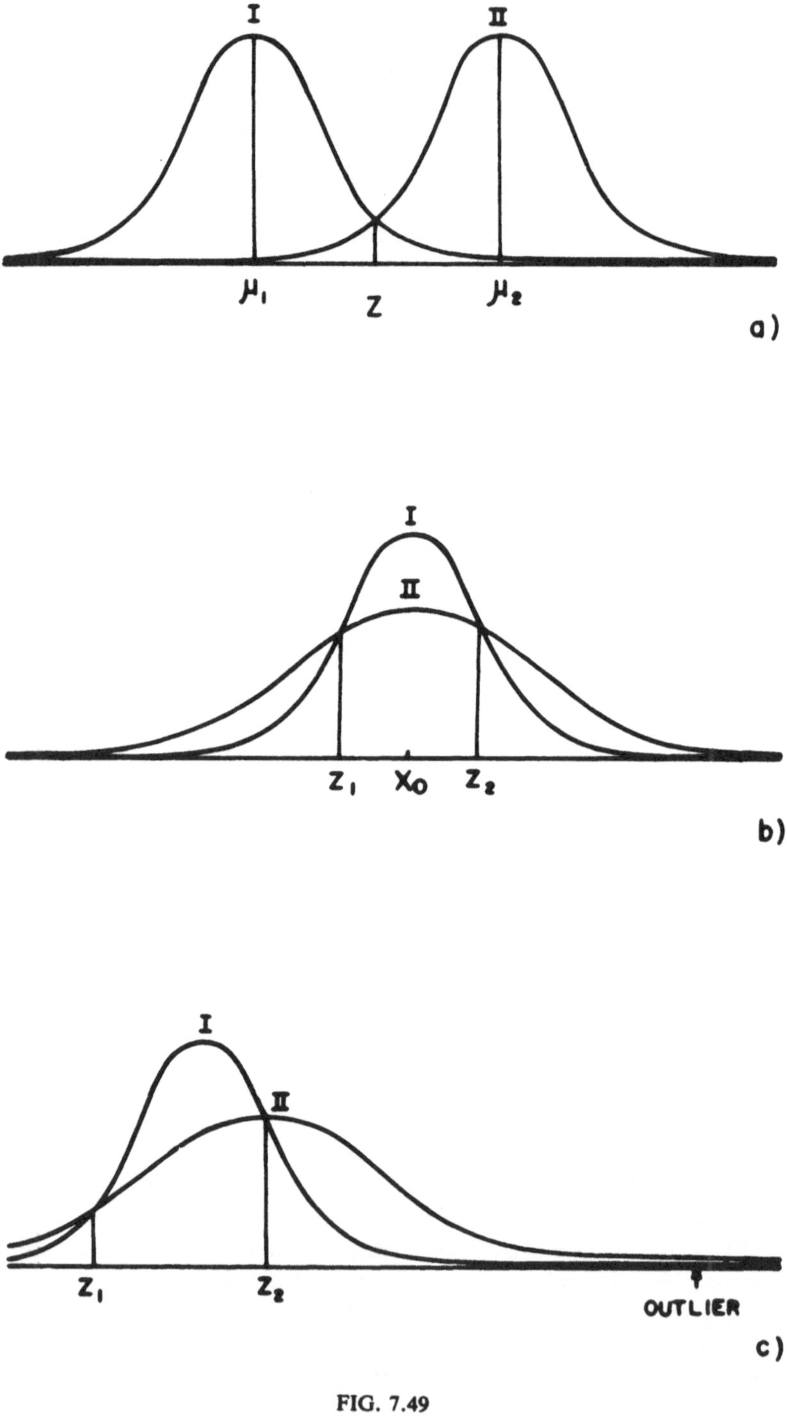

FIG. 7.49

matrix. In discriminant analysis, the concept of "small" sample size is relative to the number of variables used for discrimination. Roughly, a rule of thumb is that there should be 5 times as many subjects as the number of variables used for discrimination. The sample size rapidly becomes "small" (for the purpose of discrimination) as new variables are included. This should caution to those who use a "try-them-all" philosophy in selecting variables for discrimination.

When preparing for a discriminant analysis, several points should be kept in mind:

1. Use well-defined groups. A lot of effort may go into getting "almost good" discriminant equations because of faulty group definition. This is especially dangerous because the classification of the initial sample from which the equation is constructed is almost always very impressive (see next section). The methods described for studying the structure of the individuals may be of help in solving this problem.
2. Try to select variables on a rational basis. Too many variables add noise, not information. They favor the odds that variable selection methods will do well by capitalizing on chance features of the particular data set. They also introduce the problem of zero covariance matrix determinants, which arises with highly redundant data sets (Visual variable sets discriminant programs do not work with zero covariance matrix determinants.)
3. Test for the equality of the covariance matrices. Use nonlinear discriminant methods if the sample sizes or the nature of the data make it advisable.
4. Test for multinormality and the presence of outliers, because discriminant methods are sensitive to the violation of assumptions if using nonlinear discriminant analysis.

D. Evaluating Discriminant Functions

An important practical problem, that cannot be underrated is the evaluation of the future accuracy of the discriminant equations obtained. It is well known that all discriminant analysis programs do rather well when classify-

---

FIG. 7.49. *(Opposite page) Gaussian discrimination for one variable.* (a) Two Gaussian populations differing only in the mean. (b) Two Gaussian populations differing only in the variance. (c) Two Gaussian populations differing both in the mean and the variance. The discriminant analysis rule is to classify the individual to the populations for which it has the highest density [individual x_0 in (b) will be classified as belonging to Population II]. This defines a point z in (a). Individuals falling to the right will be classified as Population II and to the left as I. The same rule (highest density value) defined an interval (z_1, z_2) in (b) and (c). Individuals falling in the interval belong to I, out of the interval to II. In (c), an outlier is shown.

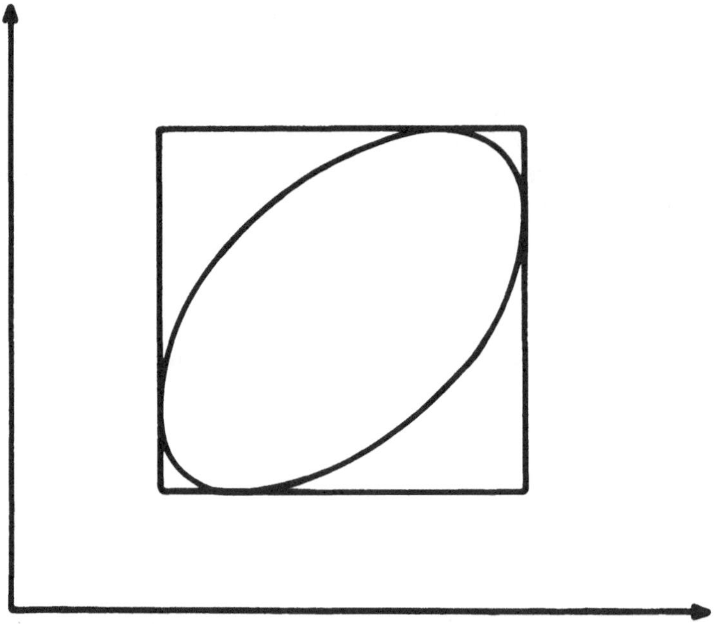

FIG. 7.50. *Z-vector and Mahalanobis distance in two dimensions.* The regions for acceptance of normality using the Z-vector criterion (see text) and the Mahalanobis distance are shown. The square region is the Z-vector region and the ellipse, the Mahalanobis distance. The latter corresponds better to the multinormal distribution.

ing the individuals with which the equations were constructed. This is especially the case when using step-wise methods. In our experience, equations that had 97% accuracy when classifying the original sample often fell to worse than chance discrimination when tested with a second, independent set.

Methods for evaluating discriminant functions are principally of the following types:

1. Theoretical methods that calculate the probability of misclassification. These are currently still being developed and are quite difficult to apply.
2. Split-sample methods. The sample is divided into two roughly equal subsamples. The first subsample, "the training set," is used to compute the discriminant equations. The second subsample, "the test set," is used to evaluate the equations obtained. This method is good but wasteful of data and impractical when small sample sizes are available.
3. The "hold one out" or "jacknife" procedure. This method successively extracts each individual from the sample. Using the rest of the

sample, an equation is obtained and used to classify the extracted individual. Thus, each individual is classified by an equation based on samples to which he or she does not belong. This method can be easily implemented to run at the same computer time needed to classify the whole sample in the usual way. It has much to recommend it, because it gives a conservative estimate of misclassifications without wasting information.

E. Selection of Variables

There is not at the moment a completely satisfactory solution to this problem. It is very common that the exact variables that will have discriminatory value are not known in advance, especially when the

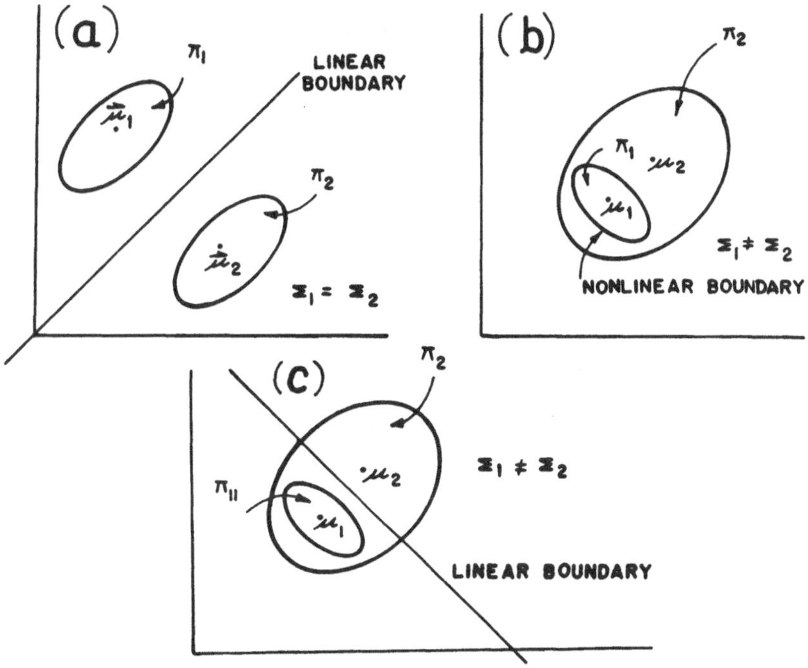

FIG. 7.51. *Effects of covariance matrix on discriminability.* (a) When multinormal populations have the same covariance matrices ($\Sigma_1 = \Sigma_2$) and differ only in their means ($\mu_1 \neq \mu_2$), then the boundary for discrimination is *linear.* The rule is: Individuals above the line beong to population π_1 and those below the line to π_2. (b) When the covariance matrices are different ($\Sigma_1 \neq \Sigma_2$), then the boundary for discrimination is nonlinear. Here, it is ellipsoidal in form. Individuals falling within the ellipse are classified as π_1. (c) Effects of using linear discriminant criteria when the covariance matrices are unequal. The linear discriminant boundary would be the straight line giving a much worse discrimination than the elliptical boundary.

parameters defined are still based on empirical models. The only thing to do is to gather enough information and find out which variables are useful. Some of the solutions used are the following:

1. Reduce the dimensionality of the variable space by using some of the methods described for analyzing the structure of the variables. In particular, a principal component analysis is sometimes carried out and the principal component scores used to discriminate. This is a possible solution, but there is no guarantee that the particular linear transformations that form principal component scores will give good discriminators. If variable reduction is to be carried out by transformations factorial discriminant analysis, or canonical, coordinates should be utilized (section IV of this chapter). The problem with this type of analysis is that the same number of original measurements must be made; many times, this is what must be reduced.

2. Test all possible combinations of variables. This means finding 2^p discriminant functions (p is the number of variables). This solution is feasible only for small sets of variables, even in spite of recent, very efficient computer methods (Enslein et al., 1977).

3. Step-wise methods. These are the most popular, methods, so they are described in detail next.

Linear step-wise discriminant analysis, as embodied in many computer program packages (Enslein et al., 1977), proceeds in a step-wise fashion to examine the entry, or extraction of variables into the discriminant equation one variable at a time.

Roughly, the method proceeds as follows:

1. The single variable for which the greatest difference in means exists (measured by some test statistic) is entered into the discriminant equation.
2. The portion of the variation correlated with this variable is partialled out of the rest of the variables.
3. The next step is to look for the variable, not yet in the discriminant equation, for which the differences in means is highest and to enter it into the equation.

From this point on, variables are: (1) either entered, if they are not in the equation and have the highest value of the statistic used to assess mean differences (after partialling out the effects due to the variables already in the equation); or (2) taken out of the equation, if the value of the test statistic is too low after partialling out the effect of the rest of the variables in the equation.

If, at any step, a variable has too high a multiple correlation coefficient with those in the discriminant equation, then it is not put into the equation, and is considered as redundant. This eliminates the possibility of 0 covariance matrix determinants.

A nonlinear step-wise discriminant analysis was developed by Valdés & Baez (1977), along similar lines as the linear step-wise procedure just described, using a test statistic for testing both means and variances.

Step-wise methods have been criticized severely in the last few years for many reasons. In the first place, a variable-by-variable examination is *not* equivalent to comparing all 2^p equations, so possibly a suboptimal discriminant equation is obtained, instead of the optimal one. Also, the sampling properties of these procedures are unknown making precise statistical tests impossible.

In the third place, step-wise methods tend to be highly biased: They tend to capitalize on chance features of the particular training sample. In spite of these criticisms, sometimes there is no other solution. It has been our experience, after many years of using different methods for variable selection, that the sets of variables selected by step-wise methods perform better, or at least as well, as those selected by any other procedure.

In general, there is no substitute for clear definitions of groups, rational, neurophysiological (not automatic) variable selection, and the use of large sample sizes. The blunderbuss–shotgun approach, regardless of which sophisticated computer algorithm supports it, is apt to end up bogged down in reams of undigestable computer output which cannot be evaluated statistically.

8 Fundamental Considerations In Automatic Quantitative Analysis

In the quantitative analysis of either the EEG or the evoked responses, similar technical problems arise that must be considered in detail. One extremely important aspect that should be taken into account during data acquisition is the change of the internal state of the subject, because such changes produce marked variations in brain electrical activity. The presence of artifactual signals mixed with true data is probably the single most difficult problem, and may be solved by different methods of artifact rejection. Quantitative analysis of brain electrical activity may be done on analog or digital computers. The use of digital computers in neurophysiological laboratories requires analog to digital conversion. Therefore, problems arising from sampling, multiplexing, and digitizing continuous multichannel bioelectrical data should also be considered. The procedures used to cope with all these different aspects may vary from very simple to highly sophisticated automatic systems, but in all instances, these problems must be taken into consideration in order to obtain accurate data. Such procedures should always be evaluated in the context of the type of analysis that is intended, with an adequate knowledge of the assumptions and limitations involved (see Chapters 9 and 10).

I. ANALOG TO DIGITAL (AD) CONVERSION

After amplification of the EEG signal, AD conversion is the first step in automatic digital analysis. The EEG signal may be stored on an analog tape, in which case the analysis will be "off-line" or it can be directly analyzed "on-line." The bioelectrical signal may be considered as composed of relevant and irrelevant components; the later should be eliminated as much as possible before digital processing. The frequency range of the relevant activity should be estimated in order to fix the highest frequency component of interest, which determines the necessary sampling rate and, thus, the amount of digital data to be processed. Digitizing a continuous signal means sampling its amplitudes at certain predefined and generally equidistant time intervals (Δt) and transforming it into a series of consecutive numerical values. In this way, a new representation of the signal is obtained, consisting of a series of numbers whose sign and magnitude correspond to the sampled amplitudes (Fig. 8.1). This series of numerical values has the same information as the continuous analog activity *only if the sampling frequency is equal to or greater than twice the highest frequency of interest.* This means that if the equidistant time-sampling intervals are represented by Δt and the highest frequency of the signal is f, only if $f \leq f_N = ½ \Delta t$ may the analog signal be completely recovered from the series of numerical values. f_N *is called the Nyquist frequency. If the signal contains frequency components higher than the Nyquist frequency, then those frequency components will be aliased* into frequencies less than the Nyquist frequency (see Fig. 7.38). As a result, not only will recovery of the higher frequency components become impossible, but they will appear as subharmonics at lower frequencies, where they may cause drastic distortions of actual low frequency components of the signal. The practical implication is that if frequency components above the Nyquist frequency are considered irrelevant, they must be eliminated before sampling by appropriate low-pass filtering. *After sampling, there is no procedure to compensate for aliasing errors.*

The accuracy of the numerical representation of analog values is obviously limited by the number of quantizing levels—that is, the number of divisions into which the voltage range of the analog signal can be divided. It is necessary to achieve adequate precision in A/D conversion to take advantage of quantitative analytical procedures. This requires A/D converters with 8 to 11 bit resolution, which is equivalent to ± 127 to ± 1023 binary levels. EEG data is generally recorded in parallel channels that must be digitized concurrently. Fortunately, this need not require a separate A/D convertor for each EEG channel. The problem may be solved by multiplexing the analog data channels before digitizing. The multiplexer consists of an array of electronic switches that sequentially connect the analog imputs to the digitizing device. This sequential sampling introduces a systematic phase error, which can be reduced to a minimum by rapid sampling of each analog EEG channel. For a more complete review of this topic, the reader may consult Dumermuth (1976).

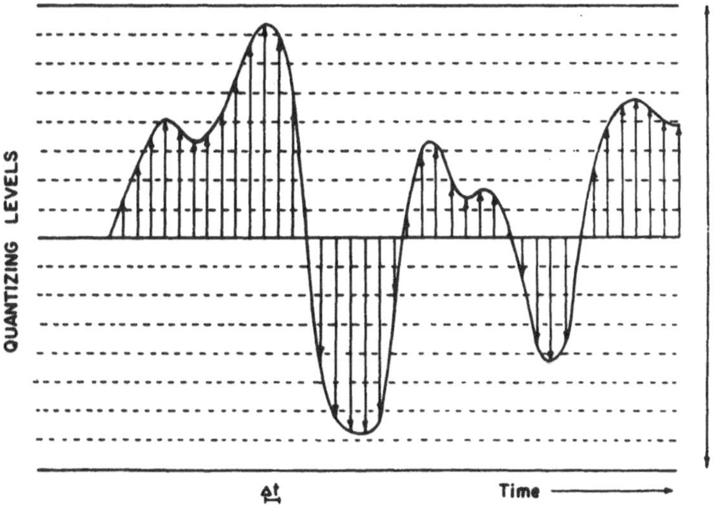

FIG. 8.1. Analog to digital conversion. The amplitude of the EEG is sampled at regular intervals Δt. This transforms the continuous electrical signal $V(t)$ into a series of analog values $V(t_1)$, $V(t_2)$, $V(t_3)$, etc., in which the time interval between any successive values $V(t_i)$ and $V(t_{i+1})$ is Δt. Many types of analog to digital (AD) convertors exist; they share the general property that each sample $V(t_i)$ is retained in a "sample-and-hold" circuit until a digital representation of that voltage, which we will call $V(t_i)$, is constructed. The number $n(t_i)$ is then output for storage in an identifiable location, and the process repeated with the next sample, $V(t_{i+1})$. The product of this AD conversion is the series of numbers $n(t_1)$, $n(t_2)$, $n(t_3)$, etc., stored sequentially on some mediums.

II. ARTIFACT REJECTION

Artifact rejection can be done by previous visual inspection and editing of the EEG data that is going to be analyzed. This procedure has serious disadvantages. It is very tedious and time consuming and undesiderably dependent for accuracy on the skill and sustained attention of the visual editor. Sometimes, such as during the on-line averaging of evoked responses by a computer of average transients, it is practical to interrupt data acquisition manually when artifacts are detected on a visual monitor, before serious contamination of the data. This procedure is practical in many circumstances, for example, when recording from uncooperative subjects who yield only brief intervals of usable data, or when small segments of EEG activity are being analyzed on-line.

Automatic rejection of artifacts is a very complex problem. It has been tackled in two different ways. The simplest technique consists of determining if the incoming signals exceed some fixed voltage (Low, 1977). This can be done by using special-purpose devices or computer programs. In the first case, interruption of data acquisition is made by signals coming from special transducers to detect eye or head movements (Papakostopoulos, Winter, & Newton, 1973). When using the computer for discrimination of high-voltage levels on EEG data, it is also very useful in special channels to record eye movements, eye blinks and head movements as an aid for artifact rejection. Fig. 8.2 shows an example of a recording obtained from a child by two different options, according to the system developed by John (1977). The first option accepts the data, but enters a protocol note commenting that the data in a particular channel is contaminated by an artifact, and thus the data is plotted and the artifactual signal will be underlined in any channel in which it occurred. Option 2 refuses to accept data while any EEG channel displays artifact, or if eye movement, eye blink or head movement has occurred within the last 2 seconds. This procedure has successfully yielded good data from infants, hyperkinetic children, and patients incapable of cooperating, in whom it is simply impossible to obtain reliable EEG or ER data without the capability for automatic exclusion of artifact periods while brief, interspersed intervals of usable data are accumulated. According to Gevins, Yeager, Zeitlin, Ancoli, & Dedon (1977a), artifact rejection by high-voltage levels adequately detects large electroculogram and movement artifacts in normal waking EEGs, but is less effective when it is used on abnormal or sleep EEG recordings, because high-voltage paroxysmal electrical events occur in the brain.

The other strategy that has been used for artifact detection is a type of pattern recognition. The algorithm most widely applied is based on the frequency characteristics of the artifacts: eye movements or head movements usually produce artifacts between .1–1.0 Hz, whereas EMG is characterized by high-frequency components. Thus, such artifacts can be eliminated by setting fixed thresholds of the amount of activity below and above some critical values (.5 and 35 Hz have been used by Viglione 1975; 2 and 30 Hz by Hartwell & Erwin, 1976), or assigning lower weights to features computed in those frequencies (Gotman et al., 1973, 1975). Whitton, Lue & Moldofsky (1978) have subtracted the electroculogram spectra from the EEG spectra. Matousek and Petersén (1973b) and John (1977) compute low delta (.5–1.5 Hz) and high delta (1.5–3.5 Hz) separately in spectral analysis. Markedly greater values of low than high delta are automatically interpreted to indicate the presence of artifact. The programs issue a cautionary statement and analysis bandwidths are reduced.

Gevins et al. (1977a), in artifact-free 1-second EEG segments, estimated the mean and standard deviation of spectral intensity for each channel in the frequency bands associated with three major types of artifacts: (1) head and body movements, perspiration, and low frequency instrumental artifact (under 1 Hz); (2) high frequency artifact including gross EMG (34–44 Hz);

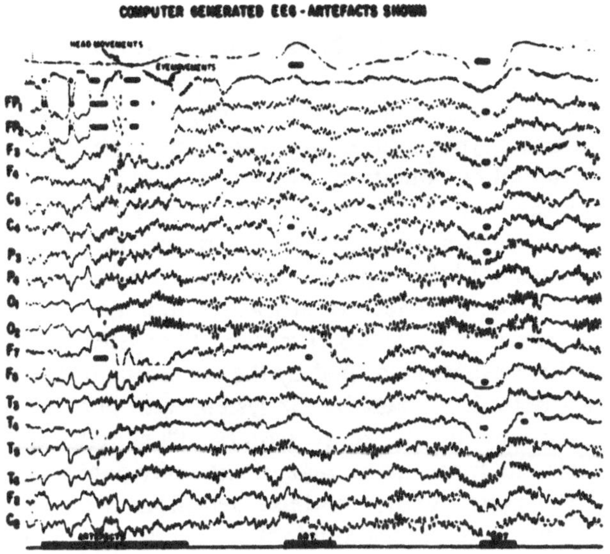

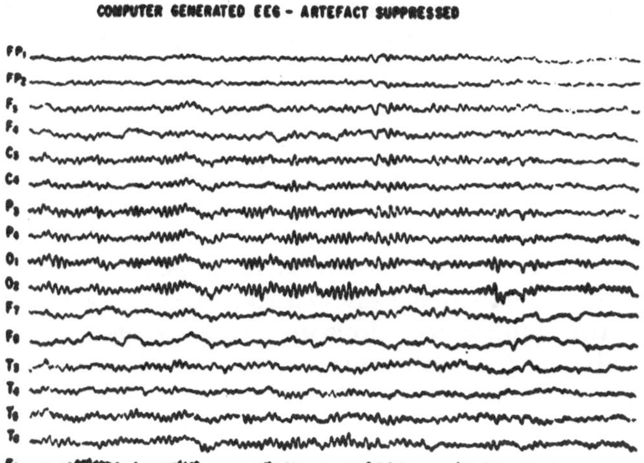

FIG. 8.2. Examples of EEG that were digitized by DEDAAS and then reconstructed by the matrix printer. *Top*: example of recording obtained from a child, without using the program option to suppress artifacts. Under this option, artifact-contaminated data is accepted for recording, but is underlined on the reconstructed record. The first channel shows artifacts from head movements, detected by a small accelerometer; the second channel shows artifacts produced by blinking and eye movements. *Bottom*: example of data recorded from same child using option to suppress artifacts. Under this option, only segments of artifact-free data at least 2.5 seconds in duration are accepted for recording and are joined to construct a "continuous" record. (From John, 1977.)

and (3) electroculograms (under 4 Hz in frontal channels only). For each channel and artifact type, a threshold was set at 2.5 SD above the mean. Following this initial computation, the power spectrum of the subsequent EEG segments are compared with their respective thresholds. If any threshold was exceeded during EEG data acquisition, data from all channels were discarded until the appropriate value fell below its threshold. The system's performance in detecting artifact-contaminated EEG was compared with the criteria of three expert scorers. The system correctly detected 65% of the artifact events identified by the consensus of the three scorers, and 27% of the detections made by the system were of events that had not been marked by any of the three scorers. This performance was not statistically different from the average of the individual scorers versus the consensus. The largest number of false detections were of intermittent, high-amplitude events of cortical origin that did not occur during the supervised calibration period, during which the criterion values were obtained. Hartwell and Erwin (1976) used combined criteria: rejection of eye-movement artifacts was made when the electroculogram channel contained excursions greater than a preset amplitude; significant contamination of muscle potentials was inferred when the power spectrum computed for any channel was found to contain more power above 30 Hz than in the band from 2–30 Hz.

Arvidsson, Friberg, Matousek, and Petersén (1977) used, for the automatic selection of EEG data, a classification procedure for five different classes of activity: background activity, paroxysmal activity, sleep activity, slow artifacts, and muscle artifacts. EEG epochs of 2.5 seconds of 20 different subjects were visually assessed and classified, according to these classes, by two experienced electroencephalographers. In those EEG epochs, 10 different features were computed. The features used were computed in the time domain and included, for instance, the average amplitude of the epochs and the total number of waves. After these calculations, a discriminant equation, using the 10 features, was computed. Later on, this equation was applied to new EEG epochs, in order to assign them to one of the five different classes. The automatic classification of these new epochs was compared with the visual assessment of the electroencephalographers. Slow artifacts and muscle artifacts were correctly rejected in 80% of these epochs.

Quilter, Wadbrook, & MacGillivray (1977) used a correlation factor to provide a weighted linear superposition of ocular and contaminated EEG signals to eliminate eye-movement artifact. They used the measurement of two components of the eye-movement signal, ideally orthogonal to one another. The voltage measured at some position of the scalp is considered to be composed of the EEG signal plus the two eye-movement signals. Correlations between the voltage measure at the scalp and the two eye-movement signals are used to calculate the coefficients for the eye-movement signals. The process is self-calibrating and automatic, eliminating the need for editing, and has been used for the assessment of EEG background activity as well as for spike detection (MacGillivray & Wadbrook, 1977).

The procedures just described are an invaluable adjunct to automatic data acquisition, reducing the need for time-consuming editing by skilled personnel and permitting the recording of many cases in which it is impossible to obtain reliable data with routine techniques. However, as there are a great variety of normal and abnormal EEGs, these procedures may fail in some circumstances. Thus, it is desirable to assess by visual inspection all the EEG epochs that have been accepted by the artifact rejection program until enough experience is obtained. Of course, this does not offer protection against the danger that important biological phenomena will sometimes not be erroneously excluded from the record. One safeguard against this danger is to subject EEG segments rejected by amplitude criteria to scrutiny by a spike detector algorithm before classifying them as unacceptable (John, 1979).

III. VARIATIONS OF THE INTERNAL STATE OF THE SUBJECT

It is important to record the brain electrical activity of a subject in standard conditions in order to reduce variability and enhance reliability. Ideally, data should be gathered promptly after the patient is prepared, and recording sessions should be no longer than the few minutes needed to obtain reliable spectral estimates. In certain situations, unfortunately, this may not be practical. The variations of the internal state that are most frequently observed are those related to alertness, drowsiness, and sleep. In order to analyze the EEG activity in similar conditions, one can try to control the state of the subject by the performance of some tasks, as is done in psychophysiological studies, or one can record all artifact-free epochs and discriminate those characteristic of drowsiness by some features. According to Kellaway and Maulsby (1967), drowsiness is characterized by a decrease in alpha amplitude, increased amplitude and abundance of theta activity and slow left–right eye movements. Matousek (1967) considered as sensitive indicators of drowsiness the increased ratios of theta to alpha activity, increased activity in the 17.5–25 Hz range, and increased alpha variability. Volavka, Last, and Maynard (1969) found that activity between 10–20 Hz greatly decreased with increasing depth of drowsiness. The most difficult task has been the adequate discrimination between waking and stage 1 sleep in low alpha subjects (Johnson, Lubin, Naitoh, Nute, & Austin, 1969; Martin, Johnson, Viglione, Naitoh, Joseph, & Moses, 1972). Larsen and Walter

(1970) achieved 91% correct recognition of the waking state and 79% correct sleep-stage classification using a two-layered multiple step-wise quadratic discriminant analysis, based on frequency characteristics of the EEG. For detection of REM sleep, several systems based on the computation of polygraphic signals, such as EOG and EKG, have been developed (Meienberg & Gerster, 1977).

Friberg, Magnusson, Matousek, & Petersén (1976) defined drowsiness (or, to be precise, desynchronization of background activity) as a decrease to 20% or less of the maximum amplitude within the corresponding alpha frequency; with this criterion, the computer made correct decisions in nearly all cases. The only exception was one set of EEGs with low-voltage background activity without any other changes in the frequency distribution.

Gevins, Zeitlin, Ancoli, & Yeager (1977b) selected the ratios of the delta band (1-3 Hz) to alpha band (8-13 Hz), and theta band (4-7 Hz) to alpha band for spectral intensity in four posterior electrode placements (C_3P_3, P_3O_1, C_4P_4, P_4O_2), and the occurrence of slow eye movements (SEM) as features sensitive to drowsiness. In this study using a small subsample, they found that SEM activity was not useful in discriminating drowsiness, and, thus, they only used the previously mentioned ratios. These ratios were computed for each derivation during the occurrence of drowsiness and waking and were tabulated separately, as normalized functions, for the drowsy and waking states. After this, overall average distributions were formed to characterize each state in the training data set. The distribution functions were composed of the percent of epochs in which the ratios exceeded values from 1 to 10. With these distribution functions of each ratio for each derivation, the conditional probabilities of missing drowsiness and of falsely identifying the waking state as drowsy were computed. Then, the drowsiness threshold was set to minimize: [(cost of miss) x P (miss/drowsy) + (cost of false drowsy) x P (false/awake)]. The cost of miss was arbitrarily set to 1.5 and the cost of false identification was set to 1.0. In this manner, a drowsiness threshold for each ratio for each derivation was obtained. If the threshold was exceeded in both channels of a homologous pair, a mark was set. The final decision of drowsiness onset and offset was then made by the total mark count: If the current state was awake, it was changed to drowsy if the sum of the marks was equal to or greater than 7. The onset of the drowsy state was defined as the first nonzero mark count. If the current decision state was drowsy, it was changed to awake if the sum of the marks was less than 6, and the onset of the awake state was defined as a first epoch having a zero count. With this procedure, Gevins et al. (1977b) were able to detect 84% of 85 episodes found by three or more of five experts, and 89% of the 62 episodes found by all five scorers. Only one event was found by the system that was not reported by any scorer.

Broughton, Healey, Maru, Green, & Pagurek (1978) defined sleep spindles as 11.5 – 15 Hz rhythmic bursts of central activity, over 25 μV in amplitude, and .5 seconds duration. They compared the reports of three experienced scorers with an automatic spindle detector, and found that from EEG events designated as spindles by all three, two, and only one human scorer, 86%, 68%, and 50% were detected respectively by the system. An overall false positive rate of 47% was present, usually representing detection of spindle frequency activity superimposed upon delta waves. Concerning sleep staging, when the spindle amplitude criterion increased to 100 μV, concordance was 96% for epochs designated as stage 2 by all three scorers and 92% for all epochs so designated by one or more scorers, with only 3% false positives.

Those results show that it is possible by automatic analysis to provide reliable data acquisition of the EEG activity during specific conditions of alertness in the subject.

IV. DATA PROCESSING: OFF-LINE VERSUS ON-LINE ANALYSIS

The major methods of quantitative analysis of the EEG and of the ERs, emphasizing their mathematical assumptions and applications, are described in the next chapters. Here, we only comment on the convenience of on-line analysis. Off-line procedures are widely used. The data are storaged in analog magnetic tapes and the analysis is performed later. This procedure is too time consuming, because artifact-free intervals must be identified, although some procedures have been described to edit magnetic tapes free of artifacts before the analysis (Debecker & Carmeliet, 1974). But, the most important inconvenience of analog storage is further processing of the data of large populations. Then, the intervention of an operator and consultation of a protocol written during the recording session is necessary, which takes approximately as much as 10 times as long as that required for the original recording.

A further advantage of direct on-line analysis is the immediate production of results, which are necessary in some cases, such as in intensive-care patients. On-line analysis permits an active interaction between the researcher and the computer system in order to provide conclusive results. The ideal combination is on-line data acquisition and real-time analysis with simultaneous storage of the information in a digital encoded form on a digital tape; this is feasible in the system that is described in the last part of this chapter. By this procedure, it is possible to have, in real time, some results that are going to be used immediately and to maintain a data bank that can be processed again with as many complementary programs as is desirable. This also permits automatic analysis of population features without consultation of the protocols of the recording sessions.

The advantages of storage on digital tape have been discussed by Vos (1977): (1) the data on the tape are already in a form suitable for entry into a computer; (2) the signal-to-noise ratio of the recording reproducing system can be made arbitrarily high by choosing a sufficiently large word length in bits; (3) noise inside the tape material is relatively unimportant because only 1's and 0's have to be recorded or reproduced; (4) the recording–reproducing system is insensitive to tape speed variations within a relatively wide range; (5) a separate time code is not necessary because the position of a number on the list completely defines the instant of time to which it belongs, because the sample interval is known; (6) mass-produced computer tape drives and tapes can be used, with a consequent reduction in cost.

V. DISPLAYS

Bostem (1977) analyzed the reasons why the quantitative analysis of EEG activity has not yet replaced conventional EEG visual interpretation in routine clinical work. According to him, one of the most important reasons is that, frequently, the quantitative analysis does not really provide a data reduction, but only a different representation of the original data. He argues that initial data processing should not be considered as a final, but rather an intermediary step, and that the real advantages of the computerized methodology only appear after production of reduced data and display of the computed results in a simple, understandable manner that allows the clinician to reach a conclusion. Examples of this type of display are those provided by the group headed by Ingemar Petersén in Goteborg, in which a verbal description and interpretation or the EEG record is given. From the same group, Friberg (1977) described a procedure that gives an oral report, generated by the computer, as a fast and inexpensive way for immediate answers to laboratories that use telephone EEG transmission to the computer center. Those displays, which give the result of the analysis with conclusions about the type of alteration and the evaluation of every subject according to individual electrophysiological characteristics, demonstrate the most desirable features of neurometric displays. There are other types of displays that provide a visual impression of some features of the brain electrical activity, such as EEG topography (Harner, 1977), which are also useful for a quick interpretation of the analysis.

VI. SELECTION OF THE COMPUTER SYSTEM

Digital computers may be classified as special-purpose computers and general-purpose computers. The general-purpose computers may be divided into large computers, microcomputers, and microprocessor-based microcomputers. Selection of the system to be used depends on the goals of the laboratory, because each type has its own merits and demerits. Special-purpose computers are fixed-program machines, such as average response computers, and their merits and disadvantages are obvious: They are very simple to operate, no programming is necessary, but they are only useful for the special task for which they have been built. Their use is recommended in routine clinical work, in which a well-documented literature allows a conclusion to be reached immediately. Mass screening of neurological diseases in the absence of skilled personnel will only be possible with the development of special-purpose computers.

Microprocessors are now invading our laboratories. They are very inexpensive and the technical improvement is so accelerated that, in the near future, it is likely that they will replace minicomputers. Microprocessors are also being used for the construction of special-purpose machines in different scientific branches. Today, minicomputer systems are the conventional laboratory general computer. They have the great advantage of being readily accessible, and, therefore, on-line data collection and analysis is possible, as well as rapid program modification. They usually have a relatively small capacity. Complex analyses of a huge amount of information are not possible with them. This type of analysis can only be performed in large installations, which have the disadvantage of limited access and, thus, only off-line analysis is economically practical with them.

Several systems have been developed for the automatic assessment of EEG activity. Among these are: the system developed by the group headed by I. Petersén, which is described in Chapter 11; the ADIEEG system, an interactive, real-time system (Gevins, Yeager, Diamond, Spire, Zeitlin, & Gevins, 1975; Gevins et al., 1977a & 1977b); the system developed by Gotman et al. (1973, 1978), which is also described in next chapters. All these systems provide automatic artifact rejection, selection of the waking EEG activity, automatic analysis of the EEG directly on-line and in real time, and displays in a compact and understandable form.

John and his co-workers developed one of the most advanced systems for automatic digital electrophysiological data acquisition and analysis (DEDAAS), which was fully described in the second volume of this series (John, 1977). With it, it is possible to analyze the EEG and evoked responses to different types of stimuli in standardized conditions, using a detailed test battery also developed by this group. The major features of the DEDAAS system are:

1. 24 amplifiers of precise, fixed gain, with a very high CMRR and a sharp 60 Hz notch filter to eliminate any need for a shielded room. The full 10–20 system is recorded monopolarly, using linked ear lobes as a reference,

occupying 19 channels. The remaining channels are used for detection of eye movements, head movements, and EKG or other measures desired.

2. To every electrode position corresponds a light-emitting diode (LED), arranged in the form of a head in a display system. If the output voltage of the amplifier swings positive, the LED turns red; if the output is negative, the LED turns green. A circuit included in the amplifier itself permits the computer to interrogate each electrode for impedance testing, performed periodically. If this reveals unacceptably high impedance at any electrode, the LED at this location on the display turns and remains red until the undesirable condition is corrected by the technician.

3. The output of the amplifier system leads into an A/D conversion system. Each of the 24 channels is digitized in sequence, at a rate of 200 samples/channel/second, and the resulting 10 bit words are multiplexed as input to the computer.

4. Automatic artifact rejection is accomplished by amplitude threshold values, as has been described previously in this chapter.

5. Station multiplexing. The four previously mentioned components constitute a "station." The computer may gather data simultaneously from two or three stations. Any station can begin, interrupt, or end data acquisition independently.

6. Digital recording, encoded protocols, and automatic analysis. We have mentioned that processing EEG data initially recorded on analog tapes requires several times more than the time required for the original recording. Therefore, it is a unique advantage to achieve on-line transformation of all data into digital representation, using a format that permits subsequent automatic analysis without the need for operator intervention or consultation of a written protocol made during the recording session. DEDAAS accomplishes this by incorporating a gain protocol and an artifact protocol directly on the digital recording constructed for each EEG channel during the data-acquisition session. Further, a stimulation protocol is also stored on the tape whenever any instruction is sent to the stimulator by the computer. As a consequence of the presence of all these protocols encoded directly upon the data tape itself, the computer can be self-instructed how to process the data on any segment of tape by decoding these protocols. In this way, DEDAAS eliminates the need for operator intervention to locate any desired type of data, to monitor or edit during A/D conversion, or to make scaling corrections in order to compensate for changes in amplifier gain. Analytic programs automatically select appropriate portions of data for analysis, using tape-recorded protocols.

7. Computation of all bipolar montages. During data acquisition, the full 10–20 system is recorded monopolarly. In addition, for data analysis, the conventional sagittal and coronal derivations or any multielectrode derivations are constructed in the computer by simple arithmetic operations

performed on data from pairs or appropriate groupings of monopolar channels. Routinely, the system computes 19 monopolar, 19 coronal bipolar, and 19 sagittal bipolar leads.

8. Computer-controlled stimulation. The computer controls different types of stimulators, to ensure that stimulation is delivered in a reproducible fashion. The stimulation protocol is encoded onto the digital data tape in order to be able to process separately the evoked responses to different stimuli and different conditions.

9. The computer system is comprised of a general-purpose minicomputer with 16K of memory core, a 1.2 million word disk, a digital display oscilloscope, a teletype, and an industry-compatible digital tape drive operable at either 800 or 1600 bits per inch.

10. Plotter. All hard-copy data output is provided from an electrostatic matrix printer. This device outputs alphanumeric or graphic data at a rate of as much as 7 linear inches of full-width (8 inches) data per second. Data are represented by spots with a density of up to 200/inch. The EEG example shown in Fig. 8.2 was produced by this plotter.

With the evolution of microprocessor technology, it became practical to separate the acquisition and analysis functions of DEDAAS (John, 1979). Data acquisition, A/D conversion artifact rejection, impedance testing, calibration, stimulation, protocol construction, limited data reduction and on-line analysis, digital recording of raw data and intermediate results, and display of raw data and intermediate results are all accomplished by a small, economical microprocessor-based terminals.

Reconstruction of EEG hard copy with automatic spike detection, displays of average evoked response waveshapes, extraction of neurometric features, multivariate statistical evaluations, population analysis, and automatic generation of visual displays and written reports are subsequently performed in a minicomputer.

This division of functions between micro- and minicomputers permits one minicomputer system to process data gathered by several terminals, each independently capable of sufficient on-line data analysis to provide enough immediate results to satisfy most clinical requirements. Great increase in economy and efficiency can thereby be achieved. With further advances in microprocessors, it seems probable that more and more of these functions will be transferred from the minicomputer to the microprocessor.

9 Review of Major Methods of EEG Analysis

I. INTRODUCTION

Several attempts have been made to describe EEG signals mathematically to supplement the diagnostician's visual inspection of EEG recordings with quantitative features extracted from the EEG, in order to improve consistency and accuracy, to achieve greater reliability, and to increase the precision and sensitivity of electrophysiological evaluation of brain functions. According to Bohlin (1977), two kinds of descriptions have been tried:

1. The EEG is considered as a stationary, stochastic process. The information obtained comprises time invariant statistical characteristics of the EEG signal, such as the power spectrum or amplitude distribution, or other characteristics derived from these. To this category belong methods that analyze one single channel such as autocorrelation analysis, frequency analysis, and the fitting of time-series models, and procedures that look for interrelationships of EEG activity in different channels, such as, for example, cross correlation analysis, the cross spectrum, the analysis of coherence, and coupling analysis. In recent years, procedures have been developed that allow the study of the statistical characteristics of the EEG, even if it changes in time. Examples are adaptive segmentation and those based on Kalman filtering.
2. Wave patterns are analyzed to obtain the frequency of occurrence and the form of a particular, characteristic pattern. In principle, any waveshape is allowed. However, to render the analysis practical, the waveforms belong

to one of a few restricted classes. In this category are sequential analysis, mimetic analysis, and procedures for transient detection (i.e., spike detection). Topographic methods, which study the spatial distribution of the electrical potentials, also look for interactions between different brain areas. They provide a compressed pictorial description, which must be interpreted by visual inspection, but in which it is possible to observe the organization of the EEG activity throughout the montage, giving information about the location of current sources and sinks (spatio-temporal maps).

In this chapter, we review the major methods of quantitative analysis of EEG background activity and their applications. Mathematical terms for the procedures that are discussed, as well as the mathematical bases of such procedures, were provided in Chapter 7. The term EEG background activity refers to a more or less general and continuous activity, in contrast with paroxysmal and focal activities (Terminology Committee of the International Federation of Electroencephalography and Clinical Neurophysiology, 1966). These procedures constitute the basis for the development of neurometric methods. Neurometric assessment is more than the pure mathematical description of the EEG characteristics. The neurometric procedures must extract those features of interest and provide criteria for adequate decisions in individual cases. Thus, all neurometric procedures are quantitative, but the inverse does not hold true. A huge literature exists on quantitative analysis of EEG background activity. The reader may consult books by Livanov and Rusinov (1968), Kellaway and Petersén (1973, 1976), Matousek (1973), Dolce and Künkel (1975), Rémond (1977), and John (1977).

II. STOCHASTIC PROPERTIES OF THE EEG

The probabilistic approach, which seeks to estimate statistical properties, makes two important assumptions about the EEG activity: stationarity and Gaussianity. It is important to discuss these properties before initiating the description of the different procedures of analysis.

The assumption of stationarity, demanding that the average statistical properties of a random process do not change with time, is a very important aspect in the application of different analytical procedures. In general, inferences are drawn from the study of a particular segment of the EEG. It is well known that the EEG changes in time spontaneously—that is, due to variations in the state of alertness or to the presence of some pathological conditions. Thus, it is necessary that all studies of the EEG that assume stationarity must be done in standardized experimental conditions and with careful artifact rejection.

Evaluation of stationarity of the EEG has been carried out by the comparison of some statistical parameters in successive segments of the EEG. As was seen in Chapter 7, nonstationarities may be due to a time-varying mean or a time-varying covariance matrix. Cohen (1977) studied the stationarity of the mean amplitude values and of the frequency values, obtained by period analysis, according to the epoch length. He concluded that the EEG in general may be considered as stationary for epochs up to about 12 seconds. Gasser (1977) suggests a test for homogeneity over time by a two-way analysis of variance of the ordinary spectrum of EEG segments. If stationarity is rejected, the test should be repeated in overlapping sections of the total records, and so on. Other procedures have also been used (see Dumermuth et al., 1975; Gasser, 1977) and there is a general consensus that it is possible to select segments of the EEG with stationary characteristics.

The study of invariate Gaussianity of the EEG amplitude distribution has provided very dissimilar results. Lion and Winter (1953), Koshevnikov (1958), Saunders (1963), and Sato, Keiich, Sata, Ochi, & Ishino (1970) found Gaussianity of EEG records, whereas Campbell, Bower, Dwyer, & Lodo (1967), Dumermuth (1971), Voitinsky, Livshitz, & Romm (1972), and Weiss (1973) have reported pronounced deviations from a Gaussian amplitude distribution in the spontaneous EEG of adults. Elul (1969) observed that changes in cerebral activity were accompanied by modifications of the statistical organization of EEG amplitudes, because Gaussian distribution of the EEG was found during mental rest, but was absent during mental tasks. Grosveld and De Rijke (1977) described that in subjects in whom a modulation of the alpha exists, the amplitude histogram of the parieto-occipital EEG amplitudes is unimodal and bell shaped, whereas in subjects in whom the alpha rhythm is continuous and regularly shaped, the amplitude histogram is broad, bimodal, and has a negative kurtosis.

Persson (1974) remarked that these univariate statistical studies are based on the assumption that the EEG is stationary and that in these procedures the correlation between the different time samples is ignored. From the statistical point of view, a test is more powerful with a larger sample. In EEG analysis, this can be obtained in two ways: increasing the sample frequency, which produces an increment in the correlation between samples, or increasing the time epoch, with the risk of appearance of nonstationarities. Gasser (1977) suggests a more complete test based on the computation of the skewness and kurtosis in the distribution of frequency-domain measures. This solves the problem of the correlation within the sample, but it has a high computational cost. As was discussed in Chapter 7, the assumption of Gaussianity is important in frequency analysis: Spectra and cross spectra provide us with completed probabilistic information in the Gaussian case. In other cases, they provide relevant, but not complete, information; exact tests for autoregressive models of the EEG are also based on a Gaussian distribution.

III. TIME-DOMAIN ANALYSIS

A. Amplitude Analysis

Amplitude is one of the features considered in the EEG signal. In routine electroencephalography, the term amplitude refers to the maximal peak-to-peak voltage in the recordings. In automatic EEG analysis, in general, all instantaneous values of amplitude are considered, although a variety of indices of amplitude may be also chosen: peak-to-peak voltage, root–mean-square voltage, or squared voltage. Amplitude analysis considers only the size of all waves and ignores their frequency. There are two different basic types of amplitude analysis: amplitude integration and amplitude histograms.

The integrative estimates of the amplitude of the EEG activity can be obtained by special purpose devices, such as, for example, Drohocki's integrator (1948), which sums the instantaneous values of amplitude across successive time periods. The output of such devices may be expressed as pulses per time unit (Fig. 9.1). According to Etévenon & Pidoux (1977), this is a highly valuable method because it takes into account the variance or mean power value of the EEG over the entire period T of analysis. This procedure has been applied to the study of drug effects (Goldstein, Murphree, Sugerman, Pfeiffer, & Jenney, 1963), for the automatic control of the depth of narcosis (Bickford, 1950), for the study of sleep stages (Agnew, Parker, Webb, & Williams 1967), and in long-term monitoring of EEG in patients suffering from brain anoxia (Prior, Maynard, & Scott, 1970).

For the construction of amplitude histograms, the range of amplitude is divided into different intervals. The histogram is a plot of the number of amplitude values in each interval that occur in a selected period of analysis. These instantaneous amplitude histograms are dependent on the sample frequency and the length of analysis. They can be computed by automatic amplitude distribution analyzers (Drohocki, 1969) or general-purpose computers. Amplitude distributions of the EEG have shown to be different in normal and schizophrenic patients: Although no differences in mean amplitude of occipital EEG recordings were found, highly significant differences in the variances of the distribution of values were observed, with lower coefficients of variation (CV = SD/mean) in psychiatric patients (Goldstein, Sugerman, Stolberg, Murphree, & Pfeiffer, 1965). Behavioral improvement of this type of patient, by administration of phenothiazines, was highly correlated with an increase of variability in the amplitude distribution of the EEG (Sugerman, Goldstein, Murphee, Pfeiffer, & Jenney, 1964).

The forementioned results indicate that although amplitude analysis is a

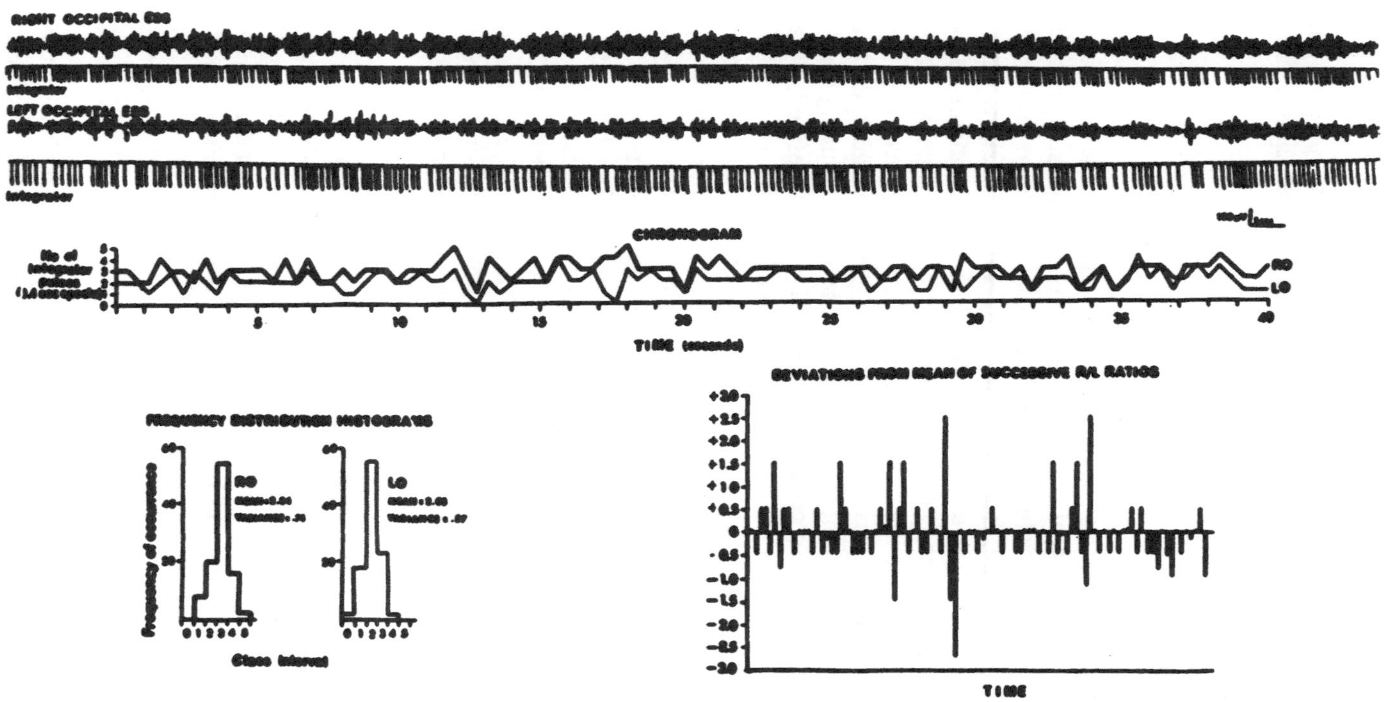

FIG. 9.1. Review of some methods used in amplitude analysis of the EEG. *Top*: direct tracings from right and left occipital areas and the output pulses from the integrators. *Directly underneath the tracings*: chronogram of the variations of right and left occipital amplitudes. *Bottom right*: successive deviations of the individual R/L amplitude ratios (i.e., number of pulses for the right/number of pulses for the left). *Bottom left*: histograms of the frequency distribution of the integration pulses into six classes: going from 0 to 5 pulses per epoch. (From Goldstein, 1975.)

simple procedure, it is very sensitive to changes in cerebral activity due to different causes. It also provides well-defined parameters suitable for further statistical treatment.

B. Period Analysis

Another important characteristics of the EEG signal is the wave length. Wave length is the inverse of the frequency; thus, period-analysis techniques are referred to as procedures in the time domain, whereas those analyzing frequency are in the frequency domain. Period analysis (interval analysis, base line-crossing analysis) is based on measurements of wave lengths (Saltzberg & Burch, 1957). It measures the time intervals between critical data points. The critical data points of the EEG waves are its zero crossings. Primary zero crossing points are the times at which the signal passes through its average amplitude value or base line, producing the "major" periods. Levels of zero crossings must be rigorously defined, because slight shifts in the base line produce a large change in the intervals detected. Also, data must be digitized at about 250 per sec or faster, in order to resolve differences in wave length that correspond to .5 Hz in the alpha range. The use of zero crossings produces a weighting of the frequency components of the EEG toward those of higher amplitude, because large waves are more likely to cross the base line than small waves (Saltzberg, 1973).

Because the method just described detected superimposed higher frequencies with lower amplitude inadequately or not at all, Saltzberg (1973) also obtained the zero crossings of the first two derivatives of the EEG signal, forming the secondary periods (intermediate and minor periods). The first derivative measures the rate of voltage change, whereas the second derivative measures the rate of the rate of voltage change. Several objections have been raised to this procedure: the noise component of the EEG signal can lead to difficulties because the signal-to-noise ratio decreases progressively through successive differentiation (Künkel, 1977); the intermediate period or its inverse, the mean frequency of the first derivative of the EEG signal, is difficult to compute with accuracy, and depends on the A/D converter precision (15 bits are needed for good precision); and the minor period, or its inverse, the mean frequency of the second derivative of the EEG signal, is obviously more affected by the lack of precision of the incoming digitized EEG amplitudes, and also by the high frequency noise of the EEG amplifiers (Etévenon & Pidoux, 1977).

According to Zetterberg (1974), period analysis is a highly nonlinear operation and it is very diffcult to analyze it theoretically. It does not depend on amplitude distribution. The procedure is very simple and various types of automatic devices that registered the periods of the waves have been described (Demetrescu, 1957; Koshevnikov, 1955; Saltzberg & Burch, 1957; Spunda & Radil-Weiss, 1972). The method is very effective and efficient when using digital computers (Burch, 1964). Saltzberg (1973) also found a remarkable degree of correspondence between the autocorrelation functions computed from the square-wave train derived from the zero crossing points alone and the autocorrelation functions computed by normal procedures for stationary background activity. Also, power spectra derived from each of these correlation functions showed only minor differences in the spectra obtained using the two approaches. Similar results have been described by Tchavdarov & Matveev (1977) and Takahashi (1977). Just as with amplitude analysis, period analysis measures are suitable for further statistical treatment (Fink, 1975).

Cohen, Bravo-Fernández, & Sances (1976) found a substantial increase in low-frequency activity with a concomitant decrease in high-frequency activity in cerebrovascular disease patients, when compared with a control group. The patients were followed up to 1 year postictus. Computerized evaluations of serial records in these patients showed trends that were similar to the percent disability of the patients, who were also assessed neurologically. These results show the efficacy of the procedure for the evaluation of serial EEGs.

The interval histogram from measurements of 780 half waves recorded on left parieto–occipital derivation in 15 hyperactive children during performance of a simple reaction task, while on medication with stimulant drugs and after being free from medication, were studied by Surwillo (1977b). The first four moments (mean, variance, skewness, and kurtosis) were computed during and without stimulant medication and compared by a Wilcoxon matched-pairs signed-rank test. The four moments have lower mean values during medication. In an earlier study, a multiple regression equation was developed for predicting the age of normal boys 5–17 years old from the second, third, and fourth moments of their EEG interval histograms. The equation was:

$$\log \text{age} = -.0206 \quad \sqrt{M_2} + .0631 \quad \sqrt[3]{M_3} - .0463 \quad \sqrt[4]{M_4} + 2.6351$$

The age of the group of hyperactive children predicted by this equation was 91 months when the children were free from medication, 9 months less than the groups' actual mean age. Age predicted in the same way when the children were on medication was 97 months. These results led the author to infer the presence of a maturational lag in hyperactive children, and to suggest that this lag is overcome, in part, by the use of stimulant drugs.

Determination of the percentage of time spent in several frequency bands in both the primary wave and first derivative measurements, the average frequency for primary wave and first derivative, the frequency deviation for the primary wave, and the average absolute amplitude and amplitude variability in a group of schizophrenic patients showed that patients who have more fast activity and a lesser degree of alpha and slow waves before treatment have a better therapeutic outcome to treatment with major neuroleptic drugs. Itil, Marasa, Saletu, Davis, & Mucciardi (1975) also made a cluster analysis based on clinical data obtained by 18 items of the Brief Psychopathological Rating Scale (BPRS) and found that a great percentage of subjects with similar BPRS profiles also had similar EEG profiles.

Period analysis has also been used in the study of drug effects (Fink, 1975; Fink, Itil, & Shapiro, 1967; Saltzberg, Lustick, & Heath, 1970), electroconvulsive treatment effects (Volavka, Feldstein, Abrams, Dombush, & Fink, 1972), sleep (Burch, Greiner, & Correl, 1955; Klein, 1976; Saltzberg, 1973), during mental tasks (Cohen, Silverman, & Shmavonian, 1963), in monitoring the EEG of patients during open heart surgery (Pronk, Simons, & de Boer, 1977), and in the study of the EEG of patients with cirrhosis (Kardel & Stigby, 1975).

C. Interval-Amplitude Analysis

Interval-amplitude analysis combines the information of amplitude and wave length. Marko and Petsche (1957) used an oscilloscopic display for representation of each EEG wave as a point located on a graph of amplitude versus the zero crossing interval. Since then, many procedures have been described based mainly on the measurements of amplitudes and wave lengths of waves and half waves (Kaiser & Sem-Jacobsen, 1962; Legewie & Probst, 1969). According to Harner (1977), the first step in interval–amplitude analysis is the definition of occurrence of a wave or a half wave. Some methods, based on zero crossing, define a peak as the highest value between an up zero crossing and a down zero crossing. Other methods avoid the use of zero crossings as a primary detector and, instead, perform a smoothing function on the wave to reduce the effect of small wave "ripples" when attempting to describe the wave length and the amplitude of a larger wave upon which such ripples are superimposed. In all these methods, classification of each portion of the EEG signal into a particular interval-amplitude class is done in real time.

Interval-amplitude analysis, in general, represents a method of data reduction that retains a large amount of information about the original EEG. If the sequence of waves is also retained, the description of the EEG is more accurate. Goldberg & Samson-Dollfus (1975) proposed a method that also uses the sequence of the waves to recognize the rhythm present in the EEG. Results obtained by the computer were highly correlated with traditional visual evaluation of EEG recordings.

1. Sequential Analysis

Harner (1975, 1977) and Harner & Ostergren (1976, 1977) developed a method called sequential analysis. They compute peak-to-peak intervals and peak-to-zero crossing amplitudes for eight channels of EEG data and store those parameters sequentially in computer memory, monitoring their temporal order. Such data are displayed in real time according to location, amplitude, and wave length (frequency equivalents are preferred). An estimate of "average peak amplitude" is obtained in real time by using a measure that will increase by one count when it is exceeded by wave amplitude (within a specified frequency band and channel), but requires 20 smaller waves in order to decrease by the same amount. The average peak amplitude is used as a criterion for detecting nonstationarities or paroxysmal events (see Chapter 12). Further statistical treatment provides a display with mean frequency for each area, percent time of occurrence, amplitude, frequency, and number of paroxysmal events for the delta, theta, alpha, and beta bands, as well as for a high-frequency band that contains mostly muscle artifact and other high-frequency noise (Fig. 9.2).

The same authors have developed the Computed EEG Topography Display (CET). The display looks like a head from above and its final form has some resemblance to computerized axial tomography (see Fig. 9.3). The display of each wave is made by the comparison of successive wave length data from eight channels. If the preceding wave in another channel is of nearly identical wave length to the wave on study, then the display of the latter wave will be located halfway between the location of the preceding wave and the location of the wave on study. Thus, a 100 msec wave recorded from the right occipital area would be displayed midway between the right occipital and the right parietal leads, if the preceding wave in the right parietal area was also 100 msec in duration. Paroxysmal events are represented as vertical lines, to distinguish them from background activity, with the height of the line proportional to the amplitude of the paroxysmal event.

Harner's procedure and display is one of the most advanced methods described in EEG analysis for the study of brain lesions. It provides a quantitative description of various features in different channels in a form suitable for further statistical treatment in the study of diverse populations, a spike detection procedure based on the average peak amplitude, the interrelationships of the EEG activity in many areas by the comparison of successive wave length data from eight channels, and a clear and beautiful display easily understood by any clinician. Thus, the procedure also gives important information about the localization of the lesion. Although the goals of this procedure have not been the statistical discrimination between "normality" and "abnormality" of the EEG activity or the classification of the subject according to the measured EEG parameters, we consider it a procedure with potential neurometric utility, because those parameters

G7X16806   L.N. 21M MAIN29   5/12/77
58.0 SECS

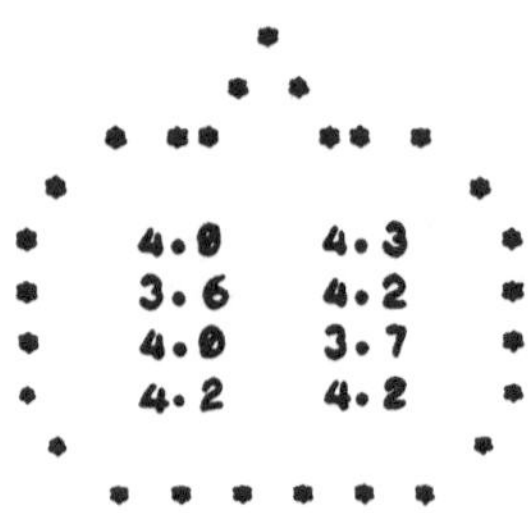

F7-F3	F8-F4
T3-C3	T4-C4
T5-P3	T6-P4
O1-PZ	O2-PZ

% TIME		MEAN UV		FREQ		PAROX #	
			NOISE				
00	00	06	03	0.0	46.7	00	00
00	00	00	00	0.0	0.0	00	00
00	00	00	00	0.0	0.0	00	00
00	00	00	00	0.0	0.0	00	00
			BETA				
00	00	03	05	21.7	17.6	00	01
00	00	02	05	17.8	20.8	00	00
00	00	00	00	0.0	0.0	00	00
00	00	00	00	0.0	0.0	00	00
			ALPHA				
02	06	06	06	10.5	10.7	01	02
00	03	04	07	10.3	10.8	05	01
01	02	07	06	9.6	9.5	01	00
02	02	08	07	9.3	9.5	01	01
			THETA				
40	40	12	13	5.1	5.0	03	04
35	44	08	13	5.0	5.1	03	02
43	37	12	12	5.3	5.1	03	04
47	48	16	17	5.3	5.2	04	05
			DELTA				
49	41	14	16	2.8	2.6	07	09
53	50	10	18	2.5	2.8	10	01
50	55	16	17	2.6	2.5	04	04
46	43	19	20	2.7	2.7	02	04

FIG. 9.2. Numerical data calculated from interval-amplitude data. Mean frequency for each area is displayed in a head diagram. Percent-time occurrence, amplitude, frequency, and number of paroxysmal events are recorded for each of the four commonly recognized EEG frequency bands, as well as for a high-frequency band that contains mostly muscle activity and other high-frequency noise. (From Harner, 1977.)

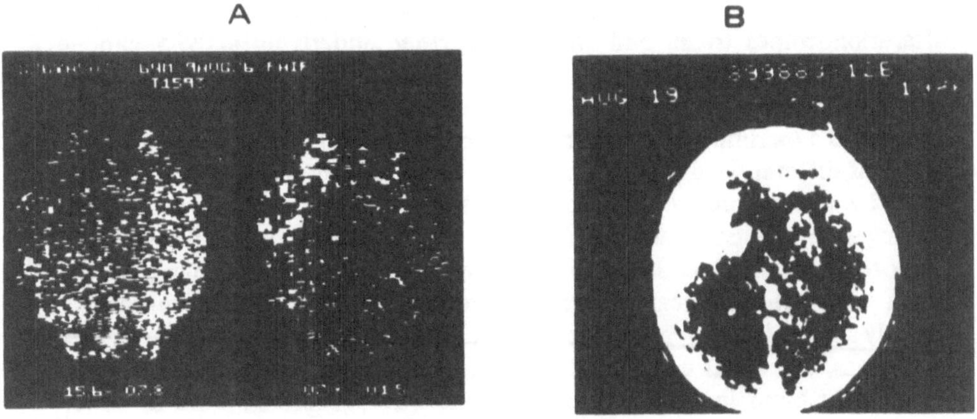

FIG. 9.3. (A) CET in cerebral infarction. On the left side, frequencies from 7.8–15.6 Hz are displayed. On the right side, waves with frequencies from 1.5 to 7.8 Hz are displayed. It is possible to observe marked left fronto-temporal slowing with depression of alpha activity throughout the left hemisphere. (B) EMI scan shows a circumscribed area of contrast enhancement. (From Harner, 1977.)

might be used in the elaboration of statistical criteria for the assignment of individuals to different groups.

2. *Iterative Time-Domain Analysis*

Iterative time-domain technique (ITDT; Matecjek & Schenk, 1973; Schenk, 1972, 1976) and mimetic analysis (Findji, Renault, Baillon, & Rémond, 1973; Rémond, 1975; Rémond & Renault, 1972; Rémond, Renault, Baillou, & Bienenfeld, 1975) are automatic time-domain analyses of EEG waves that share a common assumption: The human EEG is composed of many types of patterns, characterized by a temporal sequence and superposition of various waves with a variety of amplitudes, which are identified in the visual EEG analysis. Using this viewpoint, both procedures quantify the EEG in a multipurpose and pattern-oriented EEG description, closely related to visual EEG interpretation.

In ITDT, the following steps are followed: First, extremes (points of maxima and minima) are obtained and elementary vectors between the extremes are formed. Next, the slower underlying component is estimated as the average of the maxima and minima of the envelope of the elementary vectors. Thus, vectors of the underlying base component are generated. Afterwards, an iterative procedure continues that performs, in similar way, estimates of the next slower underlying component, using the result of the preceding analysis for the generation of the superposition components. Iteration comes to an end when no further underlying activity can be detected or when a defined number of iterations is reached. The basic parameters used are interval and amplitude of quarter or half waves of the basic and superimposed components. Applying ITDT to the study of the effects of different drugs and comparing the results obtained by this analysis and by power spectra showed that ITDT was more sensitive to small changes in the EEG activity (Schenk, 1976). Matejcek & Devos (1976) reported that spectral analysis failed to detect any essential change in the beta band after medication, whereas iterative interval analysis revealed a highly significant increase in the number of waves. Despite the large number of waves, there was not a significant increase in the energy content of the frequency band in question, because the wave generated were of lower amplitude than those present before treatment. Conversely, interval analysis showed a relatively small number of slow waves, which, with their high energy content and greater variability, were more accurately represented by spectral analysis.

3. *Mimetic Analysis*

Mimetic analysis is based on the theory of "electrographic objects." It considers the EEG as entirely composed of graphic objects that are arranged in a more and more complex series of classes, each one defined as a particular grouping of the preceding classes. Six increasingly complex classes of objects have thus far been identified: (1) points of measurement (extreme of the signal); (2) pairs of points or elements (which define half waves); (3) couples of elements (defining the waves); (4) series of couples of elements (for example, bursts and complexes); (5) groups of series; and (6) sets of groups. Application of the procedure has shown that it is possible to find significant differences between different groups of subjects (Renault, Joseph, Lagarce, Baillon, & Rémond, 1975). More experience with this method is needed for its final evaluation.

D. Correlation Analysis

In the study of one EEG signal, correlation analysis is used to demonstrate periodic activity (autocorrelation functions; see Barlow, 1973) and temporal patterns of different rhythms (reverse or echo correlation; see Kaiser, Magnusson, & Petersén, 1973). For the comparison of two EEG signals, cross correlation analysis emphasizes those components that occur in both signals simultaneously or with a constant phase shift, giving very accurate information of the waveform similarity between two curves. From the historical point of view, auto- and cross-correlation methods were the first procedures that considered the EEG as a stochastic signal and gave a statistical treatment of the results of quantitative EEG analysis. The mathematical bases of these procedures were discussed in Chapter 7.

1. Autocorrelation

In the autocorrelation procedure, the EEG is compared with a shift version of itself. Thus, the voltage of the EEG signal is sampled at successive points, separated by equal time intervals, Δt. The voltage values of the EEG signal at each interval Δt are multiplied by the corresponding voltage values of the shifted signal, and summed. The sum of these products yields the covariance function. This covariance function is computed for each of a range of values of the lag introduced between the original signal and its shifted version, yielding the autocorrelogram (Fig. 9.4). If the signal contains some periodic components, the autocorrelogram will oscillate at the frequency of that component.

This procedure was first applied in electroencephalography by Imahori & Suhara (1949) and by Brazier & Casby (1951). The method has been useful for demonstrating the periodic activity of the normal EEG (Barlow & Freeman, 1959); pathological activity showed an irregular aperiodic pattern (Abrakov, Vedenskaya, & Dilman, 1962; Bergamini, Bergamasco, Mombelli, & Mutani, 1966b; Brazier & Barlow, 1956). Matousek (1973), in

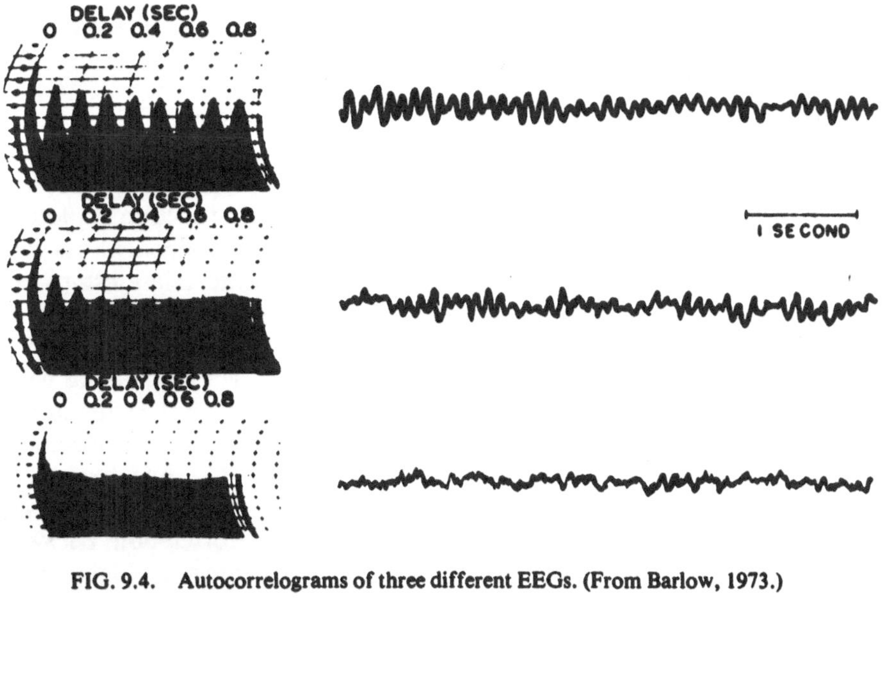

FIG. 9.4. Autocorrelograms of three different EEGs. (From Barlow, 1973.)

his evaluation of the method, mentioned several disadvantages: The technique is relatively complicated, and the evaluation of the results and further statistical treatment of resulting data is difficult, with the final evaluation often being dependent on visual inspection of the correlograms. Maybe these reasons explain why, at present, this technique is not widely used. The autocorrelation function remains in the time domain, but it is closely related to the power spectra, because its Fourier transform gives the power density spectrum and vice versa. This property was used for computation of the power spectra for many years, until the development of the fast algorithms that are presently in use.

2. Reverse Correlation

In order to investigate the periodicity and the temporal pattern of different rhythms, a special method was introduced by Kaiser and Petersén (1968) named reverse (or echo) correlation. All phase interrelations are preserved in this method, which looks for changes in the temporal pattern (nonstationarities). The reverse correlation method has been applied to the detection and analysis of the pattern "14 and 6 per second positive spikes" (Kaiser & Petersén, 1968) and in the study of slow posterior rhythms in adults. A strong interharmonic relationship was revealed between the alpha activity and the slow posterior rhythmic activity, indicating subharmonic waves at one-half or one-third of the alpha frequency (Kaiser et al., 1973).

3. Cross Correlation

Cross correlation analysis is used to compare two different EEG signals. In autocorrelation analysis, the EEG signal is correlated with a shifted version of itself. In cross correlation analysis, the same procedure is used, but comparing two different signals. When this covariance function is plotted as a function of the shift time, the cross correlogram is obtained. Cross correlograms have been used for the study of mutual linear relationships between different brain areas. In tis case, it is assumed that the presence of common components that occur in both signals simultaneously, or with a constant phase shift, is a sign of mutual relationships. The method has been applied to the study of propagation of waves induced by photic stimulation (Barlow, 1960), to study the interrelationships between different structures during spontaneous sleep (Krekule & Radil-Weiss, 1966), and to predict correctness of the responses during learning (Adey, Dunlop, & Hendrix, 1960). Some publications have described the low correlation between pathological EEG activity and activity derived at the same homologous area of the opposite hemisphere (Brazier & Barlow, 1956; Grindel, Boldyreva, Burashnikov, & Andrevski, 1964; Zhirmynskaya, Voitenko, & Konyukhova, 1970). Cross correlation has been also applied to the detection of some special patterns; it is possible to construct an analog template of a spike and then compare this template with the EEG by successive cross correlations. When a higher correlation develops, then a spike of the same shape may be detected (Barlow, 1975; see Chapter 12). Although this method is computationally efficient, its efficacy depends on the prior knowledge of waveshape of the potential we desire to detect.

4. *Polarity Coincidence Correlation Coefficient (PCC)*

For the analysis of interhemispheric waveshape symmetry of the EEG, John & Laupheimer (1972) devised a symmetry analyzer in which the computation of the waveform symmetry was based on utilization of polarity coincidence correlation methods. PCC consists of making a large number of comparisons of the polarity (positive or negative) of two simultaneous electrical signals. If A stands for the number of instances when the signals were of the same sign, B stands for the number of instances when the signals were of the opposite sign, and M for the total number of measurements, then the PCC = $(A - B)/M$. If the two signals are identical and inphase, then $A = M$, $B = O$ and PCC = $(M - O)/M = 1$. If the two signals are identical, but 180° out of phase, then $A = O$, $B = M$, and PCC = $(O - M)/M = -1$. If the relation between the signals is random, then, on the average, $A = B = M/2$, and PCC = $(M/2 - M/2)/M = O$. Ruchkin (1965a) has shown that the PCC is equal to the arc sin of the Pearson product moment correlation coefficient, so it can be considered as an approximate estimator of the cross correlation. Results obtained using the PCC index in different groups of neurological patients are described in Chapter 11.

E. Coefficient of Information Transmission of Uncertainty Reduction (CITUR)

On the assumption that when two areas of the brain are in active, functional communication with each other, then some meaningful relationship should exist between the EEGs from these two areas, Callaway & Harris (1974) measured coupling between two areas by the CITUR. Each of the EEG channels were sampled every 4 msec, and every sample was classified as to whether its polarity was positive (+) or negative (-) and whether the first derivative was positive ($d+$) or negative ($d-$). Thus, there were four possible categories: +, $d+$; +, $d-$; -, $d+$; -, $d-$. Two random variables, X and Y, are said to be jointly distributed if they are defined as functions of the same probability space. It is then possible to make joint probability statements about X and Y—that is, probability statements about the simultaneous behavior of the two random variables. In this procedure, four possibilities exist for any sample of each channel. Therefore, a 4 x 4 contingency table was constructed, in which the four rows corresponded with the four possible categories of channel X and the columns with the correspondent categories of channel Y. Every time the sample fell in channel X—that is, in the (+, d+) category, and the simultaneous sample in channel Y was classified in the (-, d-) category, an event in cell (+, d+ and -, d-) was marked.

Information transmission is considered to be equivalent to uncertainty reduction. Uncertainty (H) is (Shannon & Weaver, 1949):

$$H = - \sum_{i=1}^{N} p_i \log_2 p_i$$

where p_i is the probability of an event in each of the four categories and it is estimated from the relative frequency of EEG samples classified into each of the four (N = 4) categories. From the contingency table, it is possible to compute the probability distribution of events in channel X, $p(X_i)$, and in channel Y, $p(Y_j)$ (the marginal distributions), and uncertainty for channel X, $H(X)$, and for channel Y, $H(Y)$. The joint probability distribution of events x_i and y_j, is defined by:

$$p(x_i, y_j) = Pr(X = x_i \text{ and } Y = y_j) \quad i, j = 0, 1, \ldots$$

and uncertainty for the joint events:

$$H(X, Y) = - \sum_{i=1}^{N} \sum_{j=1}^{N} p(x_i, y_j) \log_2 p(x_i, y_j)$$

The average mutual information is equal to:

$$H(X) + H(Y) - H(X, Y), \text{ where } H(X, Y) \leq H(X) + H(Y)$$

The coefficient of information transmission is:

$$100[H(X) + H(Y) - H(X, Y)] \,/\, (\text{minimum } H(X), H(Y))$$

where minimum of $H(X)$, $H(Y)$ is the minimum certainty value obtained from channels X and Y.

In this approach, the goal is to know whether the two EEG signals are at all related. It resembles the use of the Chi-square statistic: If events in channels X and Y are randomly distributed, no significance will be observed.

However, if some type of relation exists between channels, a significant Chi-square value will show it.

CITUR has been used for the study of hemispheric lateralization during complex behavior (Yingling, 1977). It has been shown that it changes as a subject's cognitive operation changes (Yagi, Ball, & Callaway, 1976).

F. Normalized Slope Descriptors

Hjorth (1970, 1973) described a method for continuous time domain EEG analysis that selects parameters that have interpretations in the frequency domain as well. The normalized slope descriptors (NSD) are derived from three basic aspects of any curve: the amplitude or deviation from the baseline, the slope measured by the first derivative, and rate of slope change, measured by the second derivative (see Fig. 9.5). As descriptive parameters, the derivatives have the disadvantage that they change with amplification. In the NSD method, normalization of the derivatives is implemented by using the amplitude as scale factor. For each epoch, the squared average values for amplitude, σ_a^2, slope σ_s^2, and rate of slope σ_{sc}^2 are calculated.

From these averages, the NSD are derived:

1. *Activity* (σ_a^2): quantified by means of amplitude variance. The transformation of the parameters between the frequency and the time domain is based on the energy quality within the actual epoch—that is, the total power in the frequency domain is identical to the amplitude variance or mean power in the time domain (the mean power of the time function is recognized as its variance σ^2).

2. *Mobility* (σ_s/σ_a): giving a measure of the standard deviation of the slope with reference to the standard deviation of the amplitude. It is expressed as a ratio per time unit and it measures the relative average slope. In the frequency domain, mobility corresponds to an average frequency in Hz (Saltzberg & Burch, 1971).

3. *Complexity* $[\sqrt{(\sigma_{sc}^2/\sigma_s)^2 - (\sigma_s/\sigma_a)^2}]$ measures the slope variability. It may be said that complexity describes the frequency spread during the measured epoch.

When applied to sine waves, the NSD yield a mobility equal to the wave frequency, and a complexity equal to zero. This procedure provides an extreme reduction of information, because the EEG signal is described by only three parameters. However, the same objections as those discussed in period analysis may be made in relation to successive differentiations and the reduction in signal to noise ratio. Denoth (1975) has shown that NSD

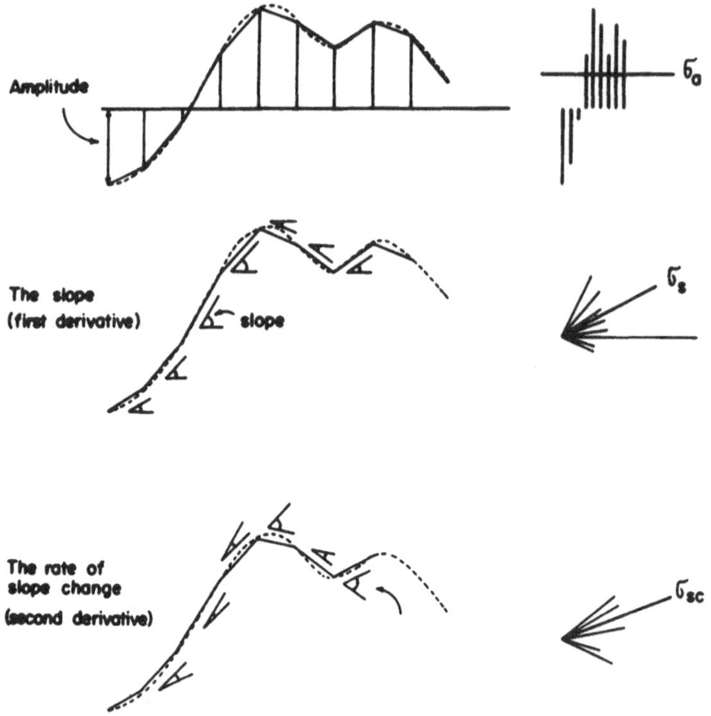

FIG. 9.5. The normalized slope descriptors are derived from three parameters of the EEG: amplitude, the slope (first derivative with respect to time), and the rate of slope change (second derivative with respect to time). The EEG is digitized at equally spaced intervals. At each sample, the three parameters are computed, as indicated in the left side of the Fig. The right side shows the amplitude distribution, the slope distribution, and the distribution of slope changes for an EEG epoch and their standard deviation (σ). The normalized slope descriptors are calculated from these standard deviations.

are excellent for describing EEG recordings with a great alpha content, but that they are not sufficient and are biased when corresponding spectra have more than one well-defined peak outside the low-frequency range.

The clinical applications of these descriptors have shown that it is possible to differentiate normal and pathological background activity or localized abnormalities with continuous differences in frequency or amplitude. Nevertheless, short latency episode or paroxysmal abnormalities could not be reliably detected (Elmquist, 1974; Lütcke, Meitins, & Masach, 1974). An increase in mobility and a decrease in complexity (the EEG became faster and less variable) has been observed after hemodialysis. These parameters were also correlated with performance in a visual discrimination task (Spehr, Sartorius, Beiglund, Hjorth, Kablitz, Plog, Wiedemann, &

Zapf, 1977). Hjorth's parameters, calculated for the delta and theta bands, have been useful in the discrimination between different sleep stages in the newborn (Marciano, Monod, & Nalfe, 1977). NSD have been also used for monitoring vigilance, tracing the time course of drug action, and detecting effects of drugs on sleep (Matejcek & Devos, 1976). A comparison between these parameters and those provided by frequency analysis for the discrimination of abnormal EEG records is presented in Chapter 11.

IV. FREQUENCY ANALYSIS

According to Matousek (1973), there are two practical differences between frequency and period analysis. In the first place, both dominant and superimposed activity are evaluated independently in frequency analysis. Secondly, information on amplitudes is included in the results of frequency analysis. Most of the early work on frequency analysis of the EEG used active or passive filters to separate the frequency components, which were then integrated and stored in capacitors. Most analog instruments perform the analysis on line, either writing the outputs of the filters without integration, or writing the integrated activity over different time epochs (5, 10, 20 secs) immediately after the collection of the data (W. G. Walter, 1943). Dietsch (1932) and Grass and Gibbs (1938) applied the Fourier transform to the EEG, demonstrating the technique to be a useful way to characterize background activity. With the introduction of minicomputers to the EEG laboratories, frequency analysis became a widely used procedure. Frequency analysis may be made in narrow or broad bands. A narrow-band frequency analysis uses 20 or more filters, each unit with a bandwidth not exceeding 1-2 Hz. In broad-band filter analysis, the EEG activity is divided into several frequency bands (alpha, beta, theta, delta). It is important to note that the empirical divisions between frequency bands of the EEG, made at the beginning of the study of the EEG, have found powerful support in the results of Elmgren & Löwenhard (1973) and Defayolle & Dinand (1974). These authors have demonstrated, by principal-component analysis of basic EEG frequency spectra, that the factors that are obtained have a very good correspondence with those bands currently used in clinical EEG.

A. Power Spectrum

In Fourier analysis, approximation of a given function is possible by its decomposition in series of sine and cosine waves, as has been described in Chapter 7. These sine and cosine waves are harmonically related, beginning with the fundamental frequency that has a period equal to the sample length (i.e., if we analyze an EEG epoch of 1 second, the fundamental frequency will be 1 Hz and its harmonics 2, 3, 4, 5, etc. Hz; if the epoch is of 2 seconds, the fundamental frequency will be .5 Hz, with harmonics at 1, 1.5, 2, 2.5, 3, etc. Hz). The component at each frequency can be represented as the sum of a sine and a cosine wave of that particular frequency. If the sine and cosine components of a particular frequency are squared and added, the amount of power at that frequency is obtained. Thus, the phase relationships are lost and only the frequency components are obtained. Power spectra, also known as autospectra or variance spectra, give an estimate of the mean square value or average intensity of the EEG as a function of frequency. It can be computed by the Fourier transform of the autocorrelation function (Blackman & Tukey, 1958; Walter & Adey, 1963) or by the fast Fourier algorithm described by Cooley & Tukey in 1965. This is a very rapid procedure that can be performed in real time, using general or special-purpose computers.

Spectral analysis is now widely applied and many computerized systems for the analysis of the EEG have included it (Bickford, Brimm, Berger, & Aung, 1973; Dumermuth, 1971; Gevins et al., 1975; Gotman et al., 1973; John et al., 1977; Massone, Gasparetto, & Rodriguez, 1977; Matousek & Petersén, 1973b; Maynard, 1977; Spoelstra, Wieneke, & Storm Van Leeuwen, 1977).

An extremely important feature of power spectrum, which has been emphasized by Dumermuth et al. (1975), is that the primary output of spectral analysis, in general, gives no effective data reduction. On the contrary, it provides a large mass of new data to be evaluated and interpreted. It is necessary to condense the output and extract the relevant information for further statistical treatment. This problem has been solved by different neurometric procedures that are discussed in Chapter 11. A more detailed discussion about the advantages and limitations of power spectrum has been presented in Chapter 7. Many authors have described synoptic displays: contour maps (Walter, Rhodes, Brown, & Adey, 1966); scalp maps (Adey, Kado, & Walter, 1967); spectrograms (Dumermuth, 1971), and compressed spectral arrays (CSA, Bickford et al., 1973). In the spectrograms, the X axis corresponds to the different frequencies and in the Y axis, the power spectra of different EEG segments are displayed continuously. Bickford et al. (1973) modified this type of display, following a procedure that consists of computing the power spectral analysis by the FFT in successive 4-second segments of the EEG. The successive spectra are then displayed sequentially, one above the other, using the technique of "hidden line suppression." This technique ensures that no subsequent line spectrum crosses a previously plotted spectrum, and provides a three-dimensional display. This procedure is shown in Fig. 9.6. In CSA, the displays from single EEG channels are arranged in an array corresponding to the relative

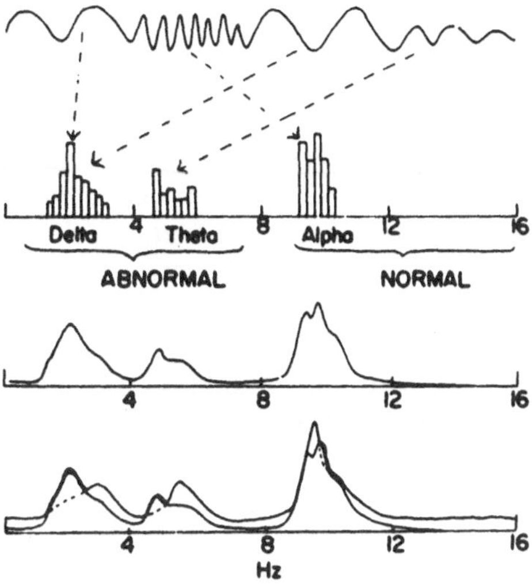

FIG. 9.6. Row one shows the original EEG tracing with mixed pathologic and normal frequencies. In the second row are the results of power spectral analysis, which tends to separate abnormal from normal frequencies, because the former tend to be at the lower end of the spectrum in the waking state. The power spectrum is now smoothed (row 3) in preparation for the plotting shown in row 4. Here, spectra from successive 4-second periods of primary data are compressed sequentially down upon each other using the technique of "hidden-line suppression." This technique ensures that no subsequent line spectrum crosses a previously plotted spectrum and thereby provides the display with three dimensions for easy comprehensibility. In the CSA type of disply, time rises vertically in 4-second spectral increments. (From Bickford et al., 1973.)

positions from which they were sampled in the head, yielding a display of the distribution of EEG frequencies related in space and time. An example from a normal subject is illustrated in Fig. 9.7. The symmetry of the array and a clear alpha peak can be observed. CSA has been shown to be useful in many different types of lesions (Chiappa et al., 1976). Tumors, characterized by slow-wave foci, are easily detected. Fig. 9.8 shows a CSA from an infant with a cyst formation in the left temporal area. A localized increase in delta activity in the left temporal area appears, with the absence of any alpha peak because the patient was an infant. According to Bricolo, Turazzi, Faccioli, Odorizzi, Sciarretta, & Erculiani (1978), CSA provides useful elements for assessing the comatose state in individual cases and for adjusting treatment.

Spectrograms and CSA permit a clear visualization of the results of spectral analysis, but qualitative judgments and impressions are nevertheless necessary to interpret them. The same happens with all displays of spectral analysis, in which visual inspection of the original EEG tracing is replaced by visual evaluation of the new graphs. Storm van Leeuwen, Arntz, van Hulten, Spoelstra, & Wieneke (1977) summarized their experience in the comparison of traditional EEG evaluation and interpretation by visual inspection of the corresponding spectral analysis: In 30% of the cases, the analysis did not contribute to a better final evaluation of the EEG, in another 30% of the cases, both procedures were equally useful, and in 40% the spectral analysis improved the evaluation, giving new information not available by visual inspection of the EEG raw data in 15%. Magnus, van der Wulp, Holst, Huffelen, & Heimans (1977) reached similar conclusions when comparing the traditional interpretation of the EEG recording with the evaluation of power spectra from homologous left and right areas presented in a mirror fashion with regard to the axis, with the difference between both channels inbetween. Yeager, Gevins, & Henderson (1977) compared the classification in six different descriptive categories of three different procedures of visual EEG interpretation and the CSA interpretation. Significant differences were obtained for all descriptive categories with the exception of the localization criteria. When only the visual interpretation procedures were compared, no significant differences were found. The authors concluded that CSA takes into account the low-amplitude slow activity that is not observed by the electroencephalographer when estimating high values in the delta band.

Dumermuth et al. (1976) defined, by spectral analysis, different types of beta activity: broad and narrow band and peakless beta. In the broad-band type, a major part of the beta band is covered with a clearly defined peak. This is almost always observed in cases treated with diazepines or barbiturates. It is also characterized by insignificant coherence (see IV-B) be-

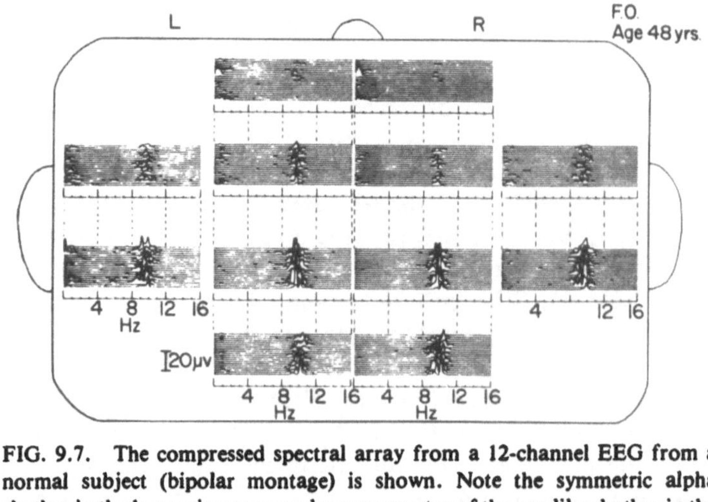

FIG. 9.7. The compressed spectral array from a 12-channel EEG from a normal subject (bipolar montage) is shown. Note the symmetric alpha rhythm in the lower six arrays and an asymmetry of the mu-like rhythm in the motor regions. There is no appreciable slow activity present. (From Bickford et al., 1973.)

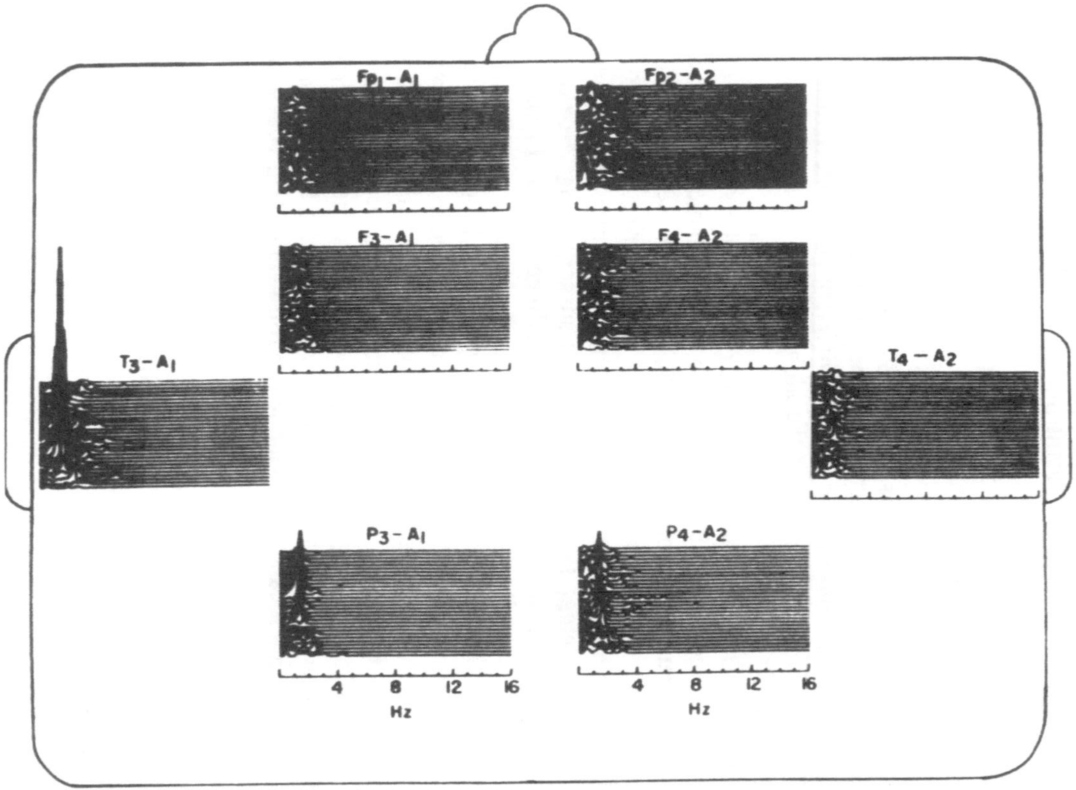

FIG. 9.8. Compressed spectral array on an infant with a congenital malformation (cyst formation) in the left temporal area. Note the clearly defined slow-wave delta discharge appearing from the left temporal region. No adult type of alpha peak is seen because the patient was an infant. (From Bickford et al., 1973.)

tween anterior and posterior channels of the same hemisphere and between homologous regions. In narrow-band beta, a sharp peak appears in a narrow part of the band. Its intensity is very low, it presents a high anteroposterior coherence and an insignificant one between homologous regions. It has been observed in minimal brain dysfunction. Some subjects show a mixed beta type characterized by a complex spectral shape in the beta band.

Broad-band frequency analyses have shown that interindividual variability is greater than the intraindividual one. Reproducibility of each subject profile could be improved by using percentage amplitude scores instead of the absolute values (Van Dis, Corner, Dapper, & Hanewald, 1977). In a study of two subjects, it has been found that different circadian rhythmicity in dominant frequency and power of the alpha band is present in normal subjects (Pruell, 1977a).

Spectral analysis has been shown to vary in frontal regions during mental tasks (Kamp & Vliegenthart, 1977). It is also a valuable indicator for modifying the therapy during hemodialysis (Knoll, 1977); for the control of intravenous infusion in anesthesia (Bickford, 1977; Prior, Maynard, & Brierley, 1977); for monitoring the EEG activity during carotid endarterectomy (Chiappa & Young, 1977) and high risk surgery (Sulg, Hokkanen, Saarela, Arranto, Sotaniemi, Reunanen, & Hollmen, 1977). In ischemic cerebrovascular disease, Van Huffelen, Van der Wulp, Poortvliet, Van der Holst, & Magnus (1977) were able to detect asymmetries in spectral analysis in patients with unilateral ischemic cerebral changes, even in those in which no changes were observed in visual EEG interpretation. Stenberg, Sainio, & Kaste (1977), in a follow-up of patients with ischemic brain infarction, observed a generalized slowing of the EEG, measured by the alpha percentage and the median frequency of the spectrum during the first two weeks after the stroke, with a localized slowing in the following weeks that agreed with clinical findings. They did not find the amplitude values useful. Pruell (1977b) reported great correlation between the spectral analysis and the clinical course of the illness, suggesting its prognostic value in the follow-up studies of acute brain infarction. Similar findings have been observed by Sainio, Kaste, & Stenberg (1977).

In psychiatric patients, Giannitrapani & Kayton (1974) found significantly higher values at 19 and 29 Hz in schizophrenic than in healthy subjects. Fenton, Fenwick, Dollimore, Hirsch, & Dunn (1977) reported no significant differences in the power spectrum of the EEG between neurotics and healthy subjects, whereas significant differences between various groups of schizophrenic patients and the control group were apparent in terms of the relative amounts in delta, alpha, and beta frequency ranges. Colon, van der Veer, & de Weerd (1977), in a study of 100 EEGs of neurological and psychiatric patients, concluded that new information always has been provided by power spectra, and is especially useful in asymmetries and slight abnormalities missed by visual assessment. O'Connor, Shaw, & Ongley (1977), in the study of three different groups of old patients (arteriosclerotic, senile dementia, and depression), in which no differences were observed by the routine EEG assessment, showed significant differences in the frequencies between 4 and 16 Hz between the three groups, concluding that power spectrum is a highly sensitive procedure for the analysis of the EEG of geriatric patients.

Power spectrum has also been shown to be useful in the study of different sleep stages (Dumermuth, Walz, Scollo-Lavizzari, & Kleiner, 1972; Havlicek, Childiaeva, & Chernik, 1975; Sterman, Harper, Havens, Hoppenbrouwers, McGinty, & Hodgman, 1977) and in the maturational changes of the waking EEG (Hagne et al., 1973; Matousek & Petersén, 1973a). On the basis that any drug that reversed age-related EEG changes should also produce improvement in the clinical state of geriatric patients, Matejcek & Devos (1976) used spectral analysis to quantify age-related EEG changes and to test different drugs.

The forementioned results demonstrate that spectral analysis is a very powerful method for the evaluation of small changes in brain electrical activity. Nevertheless, in order to increase objectiveness and accuracy, it is extremely important to extract well-defined parameters that are susceptible to further statistical treatment; examples are values for intensity, frequency, bandwidth of significant features, and so on. Quotients between different parameters have been also used (Gotman et al., 1973; Matousek, 1968). The Age Dependent Quotient (Matousek & Petersén, 1973b) is a combined quotient resulting from the combination of 20 spectral parameters. These procedures, which have yielded powerful neurometric procedures for the evaluation of the EEG background activity in the presence of brain lesions, are presented in detail in Chapter 11. Parameter extraction and their further multivariate statistical analysis have made discrimination between different states of consciousness (Walter, Rhodes, & Adey, 1967) and sleep stages (Larsen & Walter, 1969) possible. Hanley, Rickless, Crandall, & Walter (1972) carried out a discriminant analysis with the spectral values of the EEG recorded in a schizophrenic patient with subcortical implanted electrodes during 10 different behaviors (two were normal appearing and eight bizarre). A success rate of 93% was achieved in separating different behavioral groups, and no instances of bizarre behavior were misclassified as normal or vice versa. The most successful of the discriminating parameters was the bandwidth in the 25–28 Hz range from right septal–right amygdala. These results demonstrate how, by the use of proper neurometric procedures, it is possible to demonstrate strong relationships between brain electrical activity and behavior.

B. Cross Spectrum and Coherence

Another technique for measuring the statistical interrelationships between two simultaneous EEG signals is provided by cross spectrum. Whereas spectrum analysis computes the amplitude or power in one signal as a function of frequency, cross spectrum computes the amplitude or power common to two signals (phase-locked) as a function of frequency.

If two signals contain a component at a particular frequency with a constant phase difference, this component will make a contribution to the cross spectrum; if only one signal has components at this frequency (or if the phase difference varies), it will not. Computation of the cross spectrum thus gives information about the phase relationships of the common frequency components of the two signals (D.O. Walter, 1963), as discussed in Chapter 7.

Another related function is the coherence function. The coherence is derived from the cross-spectral amplitude and the two corresponding spectra and gives a measure of the square of the correlation between two EEG channels for each frequency. Computation of cross spectrum and coherence yields a large amount of data that should be compressed, extracting the relevant information. D. O. Walter et al. (1966) developed contour maps as synoptic displays in which the axes are frequency and time, and the contour levels represent different intensities of coherence.

The application of cross-spectral analysis has been directed towards experimental work in animals and humans. Giannitrapani (1970) used cross-spectral analysis to compute phase differences between recording sites and their response to various kinds of auditory stimulation (voice and music), in order to study the association between EEG and cortical functions. Suzuki (1974) has used this analysis for the study of phase relations of the alpha rhythm recorded from midsagittal anterior–posterior leads.

In all stages of slow sleep, as well as in paradoxical sleep in normal adults, high coherence between bilateral homologous derivations for all frequencies between .25 and 40 Hz was found, whereas between anterior and posterior derivations, significant coherences were restricted to the theta band (Dumermuth et al., 1971). O'Connor et al. (1977) reported that coherence values differed significantly between different groups of geriatric patients. Dobronravova, Grindel, & Bragina (1977) observed a continuous decrement of coherence of the EEG activity during development of coma. Sklar, Hanley, & Simmons (1973) recorded the EEG in 10 channels of 12 dyslexic and 13 normal children, sex matched and ranging in age from 6 to 18 years, during five different situations: rest, eyes closed, attentive with eyes opened, performing mental arithmetic, reading word lists, and reading a text. Autospectra and cross spectra with coherence calculations were made over the spectrum 1–32 Hz with a resolution of 1 Hz. The spectral data from 1–22 Hz were tabulated as 152 variables, which were then subjected to discriminant analysis. The most prominent differences appear in the parieto-occipital region at rest with eyes closed. Dyslexics have a higher energy at 3–7 Hz and 16–32 Hz, whereas normal children showed highest average energy at 9–14 Hz. During reading tasks, autospectral disparity between the two groups was reversed at 16–32 Hz, with normal children tending to higher energy levels. The coherences of all activity between various scalp leads displayed distinctive patterns during reading and provided the most prominent discriminating features. In the dyslexics, coherence between leads were typically higher within the same hemisphere than in normal children, whereas coherences between the two hemispheres were higher in normal children.

C. Bispectral Analysis

Power spectrum provides complete information about the statistical properties of time series only with the assumption that the underlying process is stationary and Gaussian. However, deviations of the amplitude from a normal distribution are a common EEG feature, as has been previously discussed. Whereas the variance—that is, the second central moment—is analyzed by power spectrum, the bispectrum allows a detailed analysis of the third moment of a random signal, which is influenced either by interrelations between different frequency components or by nonstationarities. The power spectrum is the Fourier transform of the autocovariance function. We have defined the autocovariance function as the sum of the products between the signal and the same signal with a specific delay. Analogously, the bispectrum represents the spectral counterpart of the second order autocovariance function, which is a function of two different mutual time delays (the sum of the products between the signal, the signal with a delay Δt_1, and the signal with a delay Δt_2). The bicoherence gives an estimate of the mutual relationships between different frequency bands within the same time series. This procedure, described by Dumermuth, Huber, Kleiner, & Gasser (1971), has been shown to provide interesting additional information about the properties of the EEG, especially about certain special patterns in which phase locking between harmonic frequency components is obvious.

D. Complex Demodulation (CD)

This method was first introduced to quantify EEG signals by D. O. Walter (1968a). According to Papp & Ktonas (1976), CD may replace crossing and peak-amplitude measurements of visual analysis. It is recommended for use in all the cases in which a narrow-band component of a signal is to be analyzed for its amplitude and instantaneous frequency time variations. For a stationary process, the amplitude spectrum may show the presence of bands of well-defined activity. In this case, CD can be used to modulate this particular band and quantify the respective time-domain activity. For nonstationary processes, CD is particularly useful for the detection of transient wavelets and for the quantification of time nonstationarities in a particular band in terms of envelope and instantaneous frequency variations. The envelope function is, in a more detailed form, the same envelope of the signal that the human eye extrapolates by following the path of the positive peaks of the signal. CD is based in the fact that any signal can be expressed as originating from a modulation of the amplitude (envelope) and the phase of a cosine wave. If the signal is known, the problem consists in the calculation of the envelope and of phase functions. This is obtained by multiplying the signal (EEG) by a "demodulating" function that can be considered as a "local oscillator" set at some frequency of interest in the EEG spectrum. The resulting products of both sine and cosine phase of the local oscillator with the EEG signal is a complex function and its argument is the phase function. The envelope function has the interesting property that its total energy is twice the total energy of the signal for the particular band that has been modulated. Computation of the envelope function by CD is more precise than by a computer program that searches for consecutive peaks of the signal (Papp & Ktonas, 1976). The time derivative of the phase function is defined as "instantaneous frequency" and is commonly used. CD provides a more accurate estimate of the instantaneous frequency than zero-crossing computation.

CD has been used for evaluating the changes in alpha activity during photic stimulation (Nogawa, Katayama, Tabata, Ohshio, & Kawahara, 1976) and for the quantification of dynamic changes in sleep spindles of drug abusers (Papp & Ktonas, 1976).

E. Autoregressive Models of the EEG

1. Introduction

Regression analysis deals with the problem of estimating the value of some dependent variable, Y, on the basis of information about one or more fixed or independent variables, $X_1, X_2, \ldots, X_p$. Usually, the measured values of Y deviate from the regression curve of Y on X. Such deviations represent a residual or error. Thus, in linear regression, Y may be expressed as a linear function of p fixed variables and a residual term. It is assumed that the regression curve is selected so that residuals are of a random nature, normally distributed with zero mean and variance σ^2. The error should be as small as possible, and procedures such as the method of least squares, which minimizes the sum of the squares of the residuals, are frequently used.

In a time series, such as the EEG, autoregressive analysis is used. Autoregression is based on treating each sampled value of an EEG signal as the dependent variable and the independent variables are any or all of the preceding sampled values in that same EEG signal. More precisely, the EEG signal can be described as a function of its own past and a noise term.

Autoregressive models (also called parametric models) of the EEG constitute a physically motivated approach based on the fact that any random process with a rational power spectral density can be modeled as a white noise sequence passed through a time-invariant system. Thus, the EEG is represented as the output of a linear time-invariant network (filter) driven by some noise source. The generator (considered to be uncorrelated noise with zero mean) will have a flat spectrum; thus, the characteristics of the filter will define the output. If the filter is so constructed that its output signal has the same statistical characteristics as the EEG analyzed, which means that the autocovariance functions and spectral densities must be as similar as possible, the filter can be viewed as providing the best fit fo the ongoing EEG activity.

In the simplest case, the filter will be of the autoregressive (AR) type. The coefficients of the independent variables will be the parameters of the filter. The number of parameters used will yield the order of the model or filter. The choice of the order of the model is comparable to the choice of the bandwidth constant in spectrum estimation. According to Lopes da Silva, Dijk, & Smits (1975), there is not much profit in having a model of order higher than 12. Therefore, this approach tries to describe the EEG signal by a small set of parameters representative of the structure of the process. There is no more information in AR parameters than in spectrum, but there may be less redundancy.

In the ordinary AR model, the effect of the random term is to produce an error between the actual observed time series and what would have been predicted from postvalues to influence the actual time series; then, a more complex model, an autoregressive moving average (ARMA) model is used. Thus, the error or residual term of the AR model is substituted by a polynomial with coefficients that express the weight attributed to errors at different sampled times (MA parameters). The order of the ARMA filter is defined by the number of AR parameters and the number of MA parameters used.

The interest in the AR and ARMA models of the EEG is that if exactly the right model is postulated, we have parameters with possible biophysical significance, which may yield great insight in our knowledge of the EEG. According to Gasser (1977), several disadvantages must be taken into account: linearity of the process and/or normality of the source are often not fulfilled, difficulties with numerical convergence to fit the model are expected, and computing costs are high.

AR models (Fenwick, 1975; Fenwick, Mitchie, Dollimore, & Fenton, 1971) have been used to describe the spectral parameters of the EEG background activity.

In Chapter 11, a procedure developed by Sato is discussed. It shows that, on the basis of AR analysis, it is possible to obtain statistical criteria suitable for clinical diagnosis. For large sample sizes, the estimated coefficients of the independent variables have an asymptotially Gaussian distribution and can be used in any standard multivariate test. Lopes da Silva et al. (1975) and Lopes da Silva, Ten Broeke, Van Hulten, & Lommen (1976) have introduced another interesting approach, based on the description of the EEG in terms of AR models, for spike detection. Results obtained with this procedure are presented in Chapter 12.

2. *Spectral Parameter Analysis (SPA)*

This method, introduced by Zetterberg in 1969, is based on the ARMA model. Wennberg (1975) made a complete review of this procedure. The power spectrum is divided into delta, alpha, and beta components. Each component is described by two or three parameters: peak or center frequency (f), bandwidth (σ), and power (G). To produce the delta component, a first order model suffices, defined by the bandwidth (σ_δ) and the power (G_δ). The peak frequency is equal to zero. A filter of the second order is needed to describe a signal with only one type of rhythmic activity; the parameters used are the bandwidth and the peak frequency. For EEGs from infants, a model of the first order is usually the most suitable. For normal EEGs from adults, the best results are obtained with a model of the third or fifth order (Isaksson & Wennberg, 1975a, 1975b; Wennberg & Zetterberg, 1971). In such cases, the power spectrum contains a low-frequency component (delta) and one or two peaks (alpha and beta). A description of a spectrum of the fifth order requires eight parameters (see Fig. 9.9).

Gersch et al. (1977) applied several features derived from the ARMA modeling of multichannel EEG to the discrimination among different sleep stages.

From the forementioned results, it may be concluded that SPA makes an adequate description of normal EEGs in different conditions. More ex-

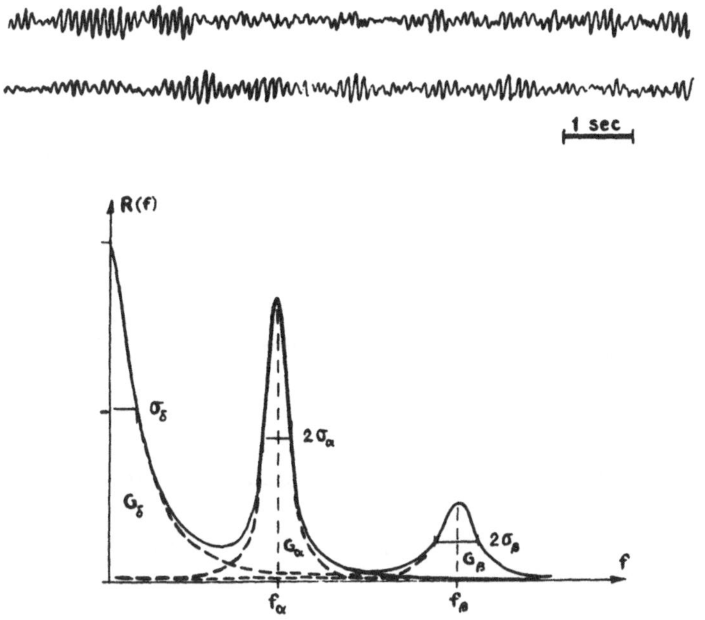

FIG. 9.9 Spectral power of an EEG signal analyzed with a model of the fifth order. It consists of a low-frequency component (delta) and two resonance peaks (alpha and beta), and it is described by the parameters G (power), σ (bandwidth) and f (peak frequency) for the corresponding components. Broken lines denote the individual spectral components; the solid line, the total spectrum. (From Isaksson & Wennberg, 1975a.)

perience is needed with the application of SPA to EEGs from neurological patients to make a final evaluation of the clinical utility of the procedure possible.

3. *Kalman Filtering*

In routine visual EEG interpretation, great importance is given to episodic and paroxysmal changes in the EEG record. Thus, description of the variation in spectral properties of the EEG signal may be useful for the clinical diagnosis. To describe a nonstationary signal requires a model that permits the spectral properties of the signal to vary with time. Recently, methods for description of the nonstationary EEG have become into use, and Kalman filtering (Kalman, 1960) is one of them.

Kalman filtering not only constitutes a more efficient, recursive, algorithm that allows that each up-to-date estimate of the function can be computed from the last previous estimate and the newly received data sample, but it also allows the AR parameters to vary in time:

$$a_i(y) = a_i(y - 1) + d\epsilon_i(y)$$

in which a_i are the AR parameters; y is the sampled EEG signal $Y(t)$; $\epsilon_i(y)$ forms an independent sequence of uncorrelated normal variables with zero mean and unit variance. The parameter d determines the average rate of change for the variables $a_i(y)$. By minimizing $\epsilon_i(y)$ with respect to d numerically, it is possible to get the optimum Kalman filter—that is, a filter that models the signals in the best achievable way. According to Isaksson & Wennberg (1976), a time-invariant process corresponds to $d = 2^{-15}$; a slightly time-variable model to $d = 2^{-11}$; a moderately time-variable model to $d = 2^{-9}$, and a strong time-variable model to $d = 2^{-7}$. Thus, it is possible to classify EEG signals with respect to the time variability of their spectral properties. Isaksson (1975) observed that normal EEGs from healthy people are generally stationary, so fixed models such as SPA are favorable to use. The abnormals EEGs from patients with brain lesions frequently presented time-variable spectral properties. Bohlin (1977) also defined an "index of nonstationarity" and developed a procedure, based on Kalman filtering, for the analysis of nonstationarities of the EEG.

4. *Adaptive Segmentation*

Praetorius, Bodenstein, & Creutzfeldt (1977) and Bodenstein & Praetorius (1977) developed a procedure called adaptive segmentation that is able to perform three tasks simultaneously: segmentation, transient detection, and spectral estimation. It is based on the AR model of the EEG signal. The EEG is considered to be composed by quasistationary segments of variable length, on which transients may be superposed. Quasistationarity means here that a short-term spectral estimate does not change appreciably with time, and transients are short-term nonstationarities consisting of a single wave or two. Nonstationarities are represented by either transients or segment boundaries. This procedure looks for spectral changes for the definition of a segment: When a new spectral component appears in the signal, the AR filter is no longer adapted to the signal. If the error passes a certain preset threshold, it is assumed that a new pattern has appeared and so a pattern boundary is marked. Transient detection is made in a similar way to that described by Lopes da Silva et al. (1975). The goal of this procedure is to obtain an automatic assessment of the EEG for clinical purposes, in which the information of the EEG background activity will be represented by the spectra of each segment and the description of the characteristics of the EEG transients. In this way, time structure, as well as the frequency content of the signal, is preserved. Investigation related to the application of this procedure to diagnostic classification of EEG segments is now in progress.

V. TOPOGRAPHIC METHODS

According to Petsche (1972), the aim of topographic methods is the full description of the EEG, which requires at least a five-dimensional system:

1. Two dimensions (*X* and *Y*) are required to identify each point of the skull. Conventional EEG methods only sample the electrical activity at the skull at discrete points because there is a limitation on the number of electrodes that can be placed. One aim of topographical methods is to interpolate this sampled activity, so that a picture of the continuous electrical surface over the skull can be built up.
2. The *Z* dimension indicates the depth of the grey matter. It is only possible to study this parameter with implanted electrodes.
3. The electrical parameter. The electrical processes are due to movement and exchange of ions. Ideally, what should be measured is the current density, but it is very small; therefore, it can only be measured indirectly by the potential differences that are produced in the tissue impedances. Another aim of topographical methods is to make some inferences about the current fields by suitably transforming the measured potential differences.
4. The last parameter is time. This is the only one that might be represented continuously. However, many methods of topographic analysis also sample activity in the time domain.

In summary, the discontinuous information about the three spatial dimensions limits our knowledge of the continuum of bioelectrical activity. Therefore, topographic methods aim to derive information about these parameters by using interpolation methods. Two main procedures are discussed, the toposcope and contour-mapping techniques.

A. Toposcopy

The toposcope, described by W. G. Walter & Shipton (1951), registers the EEG activity as a function of time, and also plots it on a spatial coordinate system in such a way that a "map" of the brain function is formed. At the same time, the information content of the EEG, which is redundant for interpretation, should be compressed as far as possible. The toposcope compressed 22 channels, each with a two-phase preamplifier and an oscilloscope on which the signals were photographed. In the early models, the display on each tube was a rotating vector going round like the hand of a clock. The brilliance of this vector was modulated by the amplitude of the signal, so that if the speed of rotation was equal to the frequency of the signal, one segment of the tube was consistently bright. When the speed of vector rotation was a quarter of the signal frequency, there were four bright segments.

Therefore, the frequency of the EEG rhythms and their topographical phase relationships could be interpreted using this instrument, although only visually and only for short intervals of a few seconds per image. This system was extraordinarily complex, difficult to operate, and not amenable to quantification. As Shipton (1963) observed, the system did not find wide applications, although it doubtless provided a highly compressed representation of the EEG. Other toposcopic systems were developed by Petsche (1952), Livanov & Ananiev (1955), and Bechtereva (1960). Although these procedures are of value in the hands of experienced observers, quantitative evaluation of the filmed material obtained is difficult and time consuming.

Livanov, Gavrilova, & Aslanov (1964) developed a procedure for quantifying the data from the electroencephaloscope. They studied the intercorrelations between different brain areas during rest and during mental arithmetic in a group of healthy subjects and in a group of psychiatric patients. Normal subjects have lower correlations at rest than during mental activity, with a most important increment in the frontal areas during the arithmetic task. In schizophrenic patients, frontal correlations were very high at rest and decreased after the administration of chlorpromazine.

B. Contour-Mapping Techniques

Toposcope methods are currently being replaced by contour-mapping techniques. Because space is only sampled discontinuously by finite numbers of electrodes, interpolation methods must be used to estimate the way in which the potential changes between the sampled positions. Because time is still a relevant parameter, this variable must also be retained. Two methods are used to solve this problem (Petsche, 1972): One is to record from a linear array of electrodes, measure the amplitude of the signals at successive identical time instants, and construct potential distribution graphs by interpolation. Time is then included by showing a sequence of distribution in such a way that temporal changes are visible, converting the information into contour maps where the Y axis represents distance along the line of electrodes and the X axis represents time, and the contour lines represent potential. The other method consists of recording the signals from a two-dimensional array of electrodes, measuring the amplitudes of the signals at successive time instants, and constructing separate contour maps for each time instant at which the signal is sampled.

Fig. 9.10 shows construction of linear potential distributions by the first method. The measured amplitudes are joined by straight lines in this sample (first-degree interpolation), but other methods of interpolation are also used, for which computation is needed (Bostem, 1977). The maps resulting from such procedures are only represented by a family of curves. Addi-

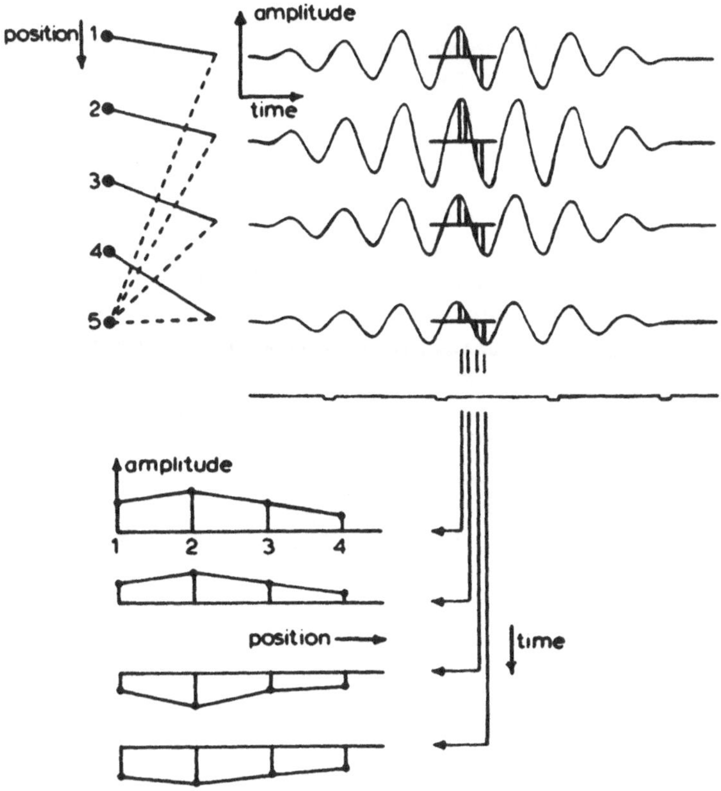

FIG. 9.10. The derivation of linear potential distributions. The four signals are derived from the common reference electrode array to their left. Wave amplitudes from the zero line are measured at different time instants and are converted to corresponding plots of amplitude versus position along the line of electrodes. (From Petsche, 1972.)

tional processing is still necessary to reach a meaningful representation: Zero levels must be distinguished, and the positive and negative surfaces must be identified. The regions between levels can then be represented by gradations on a grey scale or in various colors, such as the new display used in computerized axial tomography.

According to Petsche (1972), there are two important things to take into account when constructing linear potential distributions. The first is that if temporal changes are to be accurately followed, then the sampling interval in the time dimension should be determined by the Nyquist criteria of sampling frequency. The second is that this criterion may also apply in the spatial domain: Electrodes must be close enough together for the curvature in the potential distribution to be adequately sampled.

Contour-mapping methods have been used in the time domain and in frequency domain. Rémond (1961) was the first to work on a synoptic representation in the time domain of averaged evoked responses and of the EEG spontaneous activity. If bipolar records are obtained from a line of electrodes along an axis of the sagittal plane for each given value of time, there exists a set of electrical values (coming from each of the respective derivations) for each poststimulus time in the case of the evoked responses, or for the time after a characteristic value of the alpha wave from one derivation, which will be considered as the time reference for the study of the spontaneous EEG activity ("alpha average"). At each instant, the instantaneous electrical potential differences between derivations are transformed to gradients (μV/cm). By interpolating those discrete values and drawing a line to connect regions in space time that are at the same potential, it is possible to construct isogradient curves. These curves are plotted, with the time in the X axis and distance in the Y axis (chronotopograms). Contour maps are positive in the white areas, negative in the black areas (Fig. 9.11). In such a picture, it is possible to observe the organization of the EEG activity throughout the montage, and to see that at a certain time, a negative gradient is spread over several electrodes while at the same time, a positive gradient is spread over several other electrodes, giving information about the location of current sources and sinks. This method has been used for the study of the spatio-temporal organization of the EEG in adults and infants (Joseph, Lesèvre, & Dreyfus-Brisac, 1976; Rémond, 1968).

Lehmann (1971) developed a technique for deriving contour maps using a system having 48 independent amplifiers and recording channels, with a common-average reference derivation. The results are displayed as sequences of isopotential plots. A study of the alpha activity with this system showed that the EEG field maxima were located in three preferred scalp areas: left occipital, right occipital, and precentral–central. These maxima are seen to rotate in a clockwise or counterclockwise direction from area to area (Fig. 9.12).

In conclusion, topographic methods are very useful in two aspects: as an important contribution to the study of the distribution of the electrical brain potentials, and as display procedures that, in a synoptic representation, compress a huge amount of information.

VI. CONCLUSIONS

The EEG is a very complex signal. A point that emerges from the review made in this chapter is that each different procedure highlights a peculiar characteristic of the EEG. Those workers who have compared different techniques for the analysis of the same signal usually concluded that dif-

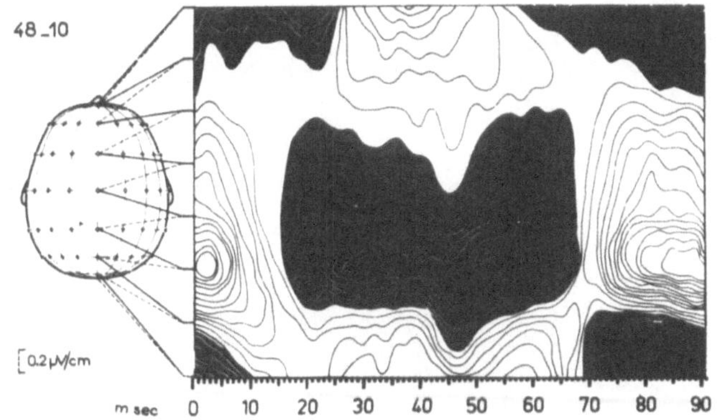

FIG. 9.11. Chronotopogram. Time, horizontally; distance, vertically. At each instant, the instantaneous electrical potential differences between derivations are transformed to gradients (μV/cm.) In locations between two electrodes, the recorded potential differences can be interpolated as an estimate of their values everywhere along the line of electrodes. Isopotential contours in space and time are joined by lines, indicating the change in voltage as a function of time. Positive potential differences are shown in white, negative in the black areas. Here, it is possible to observe the spatio-temporal organization of the EEG activity: At a certain time, a negative gradient is spread over several electrodes, while, at the same time, a positive gradient is spread over several other electrodes, the distribution changing with time. (From Rémond, 1964.)

ferent methods supply information that is not available using only one procedure. The ideal system for complete automatic evaluation of the EEG may have to combine mutually supplementary procedures, which take into account frequency, time, and pattern-recognition domains. Such a system will be very complex and expensive. Three different lines of investigation may be considered to solve this problem: to continue the search for new and better mathematical models that may provide more complete information about the EEG signal, to perform more comparative studies between different procedures in order to obtain an empirical answer for the optimal selection of those features to be used in different applications, and to identify those features that have reliable functional implications or clinical correlates. All of these should be encouraged for the purpose of improving the applications of EEG analysis. A great advance in the investigation of methods that may deal with nonstationary signals has been made in the last few years. Applications of time and frequency-domain techniques have been mainly directed to the study of sleep and maturational and aging changes in healthy subjects, the effects produced by different types of diseases and for characterizing the central effects of psychoactive compounds. The results obtained are clear evidence that quantitative analysis of

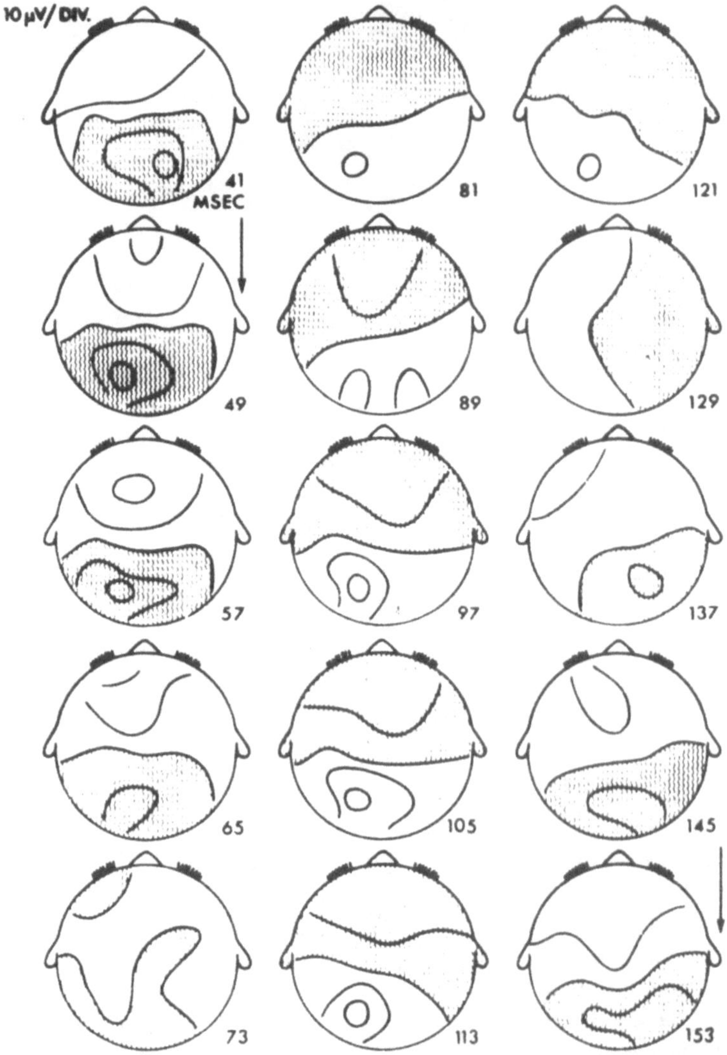

FIG. 9.12. Semischematic equipotential maps of alpha EEG sampled in 8-msec intervals. Head seen from above. Sequence from top to bottom, left to right. Negative areas are gray, positive areas are white. Reference is the average potential. Equipotential lines at 10- μV intervals. The field distribution is simple and shows one to two positive and negative maximal values in each map. The maximal values stepped clockwise from preference area to preference area. (From Lehman, 1971.)

the EEG is an important tool for the detection of subtle changes in brain state. Attention has also been put in synoptic displays and beautiful and easily understandable displays are available. The results obtained with many of the procedures, which provide parameters able to be submitted to further statistical analysis for the extraction of relevant information, can be the basis of powerful neurometric procedures. Some examples have been presented in this chapter. In Chapter 11, we present those neurometric procedures that have been used for the assessment of neurological patients.

10 A Review of Major Methods of Evoked Response Analysis

I. INTRODUCTION

Four different types of statistical problems are encountered in the quantitative analysis of the Evoked Responses (ERs). The first one, or *estimation* of the ERs, deals with the extraction of the stimulus-dependent activity. Averaging has been the most common procedure for estimation of the ERs, but there are many other methods, as we shall see later in this chapter. The second problem, or *hypothesis testing*, evaluates the validity of hypotheses, for example, seeking differences between different groups of ERs. The third problem involves the *structure* of the data; in other words, it focuses on the search for underlying features that are not easily observable in the time-voltage curve of the ERs. The final problem relates to the possibility of making adequate *predictions* as to the group to which an individual ER belongs. In order to solve all these problems, the ERs are modeled as realizations of a stochastic process dependent on time and represented by a series of numerical values of voltage at sequential time points. *All the procedures for the quantitative analysis of ERs are based, explicitly or implicitly, on a definite mathematical model with precise assumptions.* Violations of those assumptions produce inaccuracies and difficulties in interpretation.

Until now, we have mainly discussed the differences observed between the average evoked responses of healthy subjects and of neurological patients. We have used averaging as an estimation procedure of the ERs and we have described the effect of different alterations of the nervous system on the ERs, in terms of peak amplitudes and/or peak latencies. We see in Chapter 13 that, on the basis of such measurements (amplitudes and latencies), it is possible to develop neurometric procedures that accurately predict if a given average ER is normal or abnormal. These measurements have been useful for the assessment of brain dysfunction, especially when the components are very stable, such as, for example, when they reflect the activation of sensory specific pathways. However, the majority of the components of the ERs are of unknown origin and the particular meaning of each of them is not known. Therefore, methods intended to extract all of the useful information contained in the ER and not just specific characteristics of each component must examine these potentials over the whole latency domain. Many of the procedures that are discussed in this chapter were developed and applied in psychophysiological studies and have not yet been used for the assessment of neurological patients. Nevertheless, they may be suitable for this purpose and for this reason are included in this chapter. We have emphasized that application of a given procedure implicates precise assumptions, and, therefore, we first give an overview of the stochastic properties of the ERs.

II. STOCHASTIC PROPERTIES OF THE EVOKED RESPONSES

Valdés (1978) reviewed the basic assumptions underlying the different methods for analysis of the ERs. On the basis of a general additive model, which defines the ER to be a combination of (1) the stimulus dependent evoked activity (SDA) of the brain or signal; and (2) brain activity not related to the stimulus, considered as "noise" or stimulus-independent activity (SIA), he analyzed the different mathematical models that have been proposed for the SDA and the SIA. In this model, nonlinear interactions between both activities are not taken into account. With respect to the SDA, various models consider it to be constant or invariant (Dawson, 1947a) or to vary depending on known or unknown factors. These variations may be of different types: The whole SDA may shift in latency, the SDA may undergo amplitude variations, the SDA may vary both in amplitude and latency, the different components of the SDA may vary in a nonlinear way, or the different components of the SDA may have independent variations in amplitude and/or latency. With respect to the SIA, several models have also been considered; some of them require precise statistical assumptions, such as a Gaussian distribution with 0 mean, whereas for others the SIA characteristics are not important, or they have the same properties as the background activity.

Valdés (1978) developed procedures for the analysis of Gaussianity, stationarity, and homogeneity of the covariance matrices of an ensemble of single-trial evoked responses and he applied them to the study of the visual evoked responses in man. As has been discussed in Chapter 7, a normal distribution for each variable (the amplitude at any defined latency) does not imply that the set of variables has a multinormal distribution, because for a multinormal or Gaussian distribution, it is also necessary that all joint distributions must be normal. Valdés modified the test of multinormality proposed by Mardia (1970), based on the measurement of skewness and kurtosis, in order to apply it to a greater number of variables. He concluded that visual evoked responses to flashes and to pattern stimuli, presented to subjects in different states and presumably processed in different manners, have a multinormal distribution. Thus, it is possible to apply to them all procedures that are based on the assumption of multinormality.

Many procedures for estimation and analysis of the structure of the ERs assumed the stationarity of the signal; therefore, it is extremely important to analyze if this assumption holds. As was stated in Chapter 7, nonstationarities may be due to a time-varying mean or to a time-varying covariance matrix. In relation to stationarity of the ERs, it is obvious, from the very existence of the averaged evoked response, which clearly indicates a time-varying mean, that a nonstationarity of the mean exists. This problem can be avoided by subtraction of the mean value, yielding a zero mean vector that does not change with time. A very low-frequency component may be also eliminated by regression analysis (McGillem & Aunon, 1977). However, nonstationarities of the covariance matrix cannot be easily solved. We have seen (Chapter 7) that a stationary process of the second order has a covariance matrix of the Toeplitz form. Valdés developed a test for the hypothesis of stationarity for multiple observations, based on the analysis of the covariance matrix of the ensemble of single ERs. In every case, nonstationarity of the second order of the visual evoked responses to different types of stimuli and in different conditions of the subject was observed. The implication of this finding is that all procedures of analysis that assume the stationarity of the ERs, like Wiener filtering, adaptive filtering, amplitude sorting, Fourier transform, and so on, are severely handicapped if this assumption does not hold.

In a group of subjects, the equality of the covariance matrices of single VERs to the same stimuli processed in different manners was tested. It was observed that such equality does not hold for the majority of comparisons. Fig. 10.1 shows the correlation matrices of the VERs recorded in three different leads while the subject performed tasks requiring a spatial or a verbal strategy. It is possible to observe differences in the distribution of the significant correlation values depending on the strategy used by the subject. This result indicates the necessity of the analysis of the covariance matrices between ensembles of ERs before the computation of linear discriminant functions for the assignment of single-trial ERs to a particular group. Similarly, for application of linear discriminant analysis to different groups of averaged evoked responses, it is necessary to test the equality of the

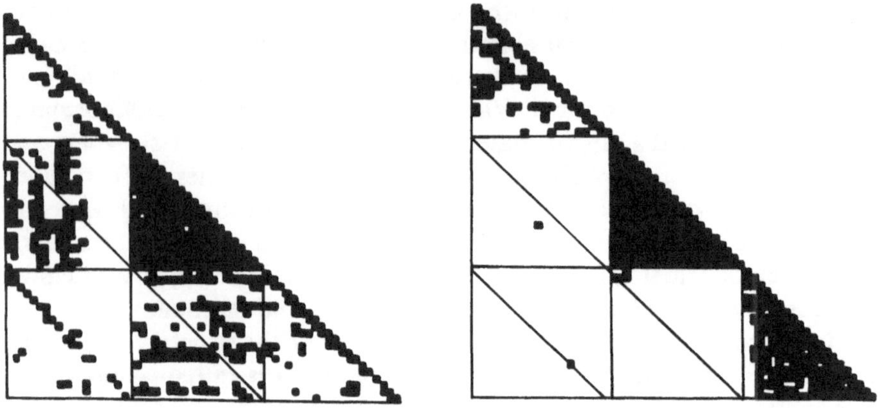

FIG. 10.1. Correlation matrices of an ensemble of single-trial VERs recorded in three different leads (O_1, P_3, and P_4) to the same type of stimuli processed according to a spatial (left) or verbal (right) strategies. Only half the matrix is plotted because correlation matrices are symmetrical. The triangular matrices present the results for the two different processing strategies. Each sector represents a different lead, from left to right and top to bottom in the order O_1, P_3, P_4. Each cell represents the correlation between values of VERs at two different time points and/or leads. The rows of the matrices correspond to the correlation of the successive time points of O_1, then P_3, then P_4 with all other time points of other leads. Block cells denote significant ($P < .01$) spatio-temporal correlations. Note the great difference in the distributions of the significance correlation values according to the strategy used by the subject. (From Valdés, 1978.)

covariance matrices of the different groups. If this assumption does not hold, nonlinear discriminant analysis should be used, as was discussed in Chapter 7.

III. ESTIMATION OF THE EVOKED RESPONSES

Two major groups of estimation procedures may be defined: (1) those that have as a basic assumption that the SDA is constant (homogeneous) or, in other words, that the single evoked responses recorded in different trials come from the same statistical distribution; and (2) those that consider the SDA variable, because it arises from a continuous, very complicated multimodal distribution or from different distributions (nonhomogeneous) that are mixed upon sampling. The estimation procedure should be selected according to the purpose of the experiment and the basic assumptions that are made in relation to the signal and the background activity. The existence of well-known relations between the ER morphology and the characteristics of the stimulus (frequency, intensity, temporal sequence, etc.), as well as between the ER morphology and the internal state of the subject (arousal level, motivation, attention, etc.), produce an undesirable increase in the variability of the ERs if there is not adequate control of the experiment. This cannot be solved by statistical analysis. Therefore, well-controlled experiments that consider standardization of the stimuli and relevant environmental conditions, as well as the state of the subject and artifact rejection, are necessary in order to obtain more homogeneous samples of ERs. It is known that there are also variations of the ERs due to events that cannot be controlled or that have not been identified, such as those related to purposeful activity (John et al., 1978). If it is of interest to study such variations, then the estimation of ERs may be done by classification procedures such as cluster analysis. The purpose of cluster analysis is to find sets or "clusters" such that the members of each cluster are similar to each other and different from those belonging to other clusters (see Chapter 7). Although not yet applied to the study of the ERs, estimation procedures for mixed distributions may also be used for the identification of the distributions from which the different ERs come.

A. Procedures That Assume That the Stimulus-Dependent Activity is Invariant

1. Averaging

The basic assumptions underlying averaging are that the ER consists of the sum of an invariant SDA and an SIA that has at least a symmetrical statistical distribution. Thus, averaging is most valid for short-latency contributions to ERs that reflect sensory processes and therefore are more constant, and least valid for the longer latency components related to cognitive activity. The averaging procedure, as well as the clinical applications of the averaged ERs, were described in Chapters 3 to 6. Fig. 10.2 shows the effect of averaging waveshapes with different latencies, in order to illustrate the risk of using inadequate procedures for the estimation of ERs.

An important fact to consider in averaging is the interval between stimuli (Ruchkin, 1965b). If it is large, the SIA activity associated with each epoch following a stimulus will be uncorrelated with SIA from other epochs, and it is reasonable to expect its cancellation. However, with short-stimuli intervals, problems may arise, particularly if periodic stimuli are used. When using frequencies of stimulation close to the fundamental or to the harmonic of the

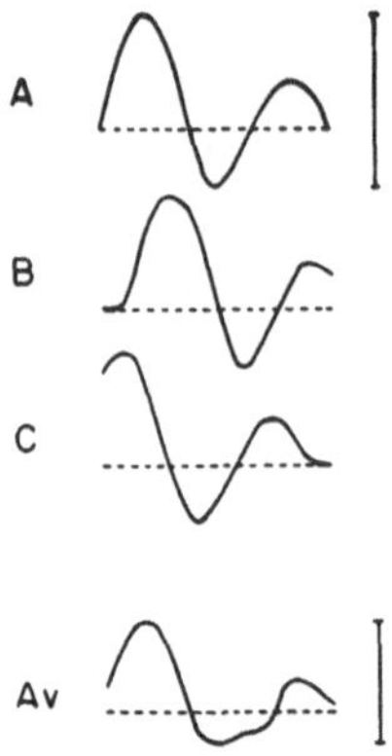

FIG. 10.2 (A), (B), and (C): signals with similar amplitude and waveshape, but shifted in latency. (Av): the average of the three signals is of smaller amplitude and distorted waveshape.

EEG background activity while averaging, rhythmic EEG activity such as alpha will be less attenuated (less SIA cancellation) than for statistically independent SIA. Problems will also arise if the ER persists beyond the time of occurrence of subsequent stimuli. With periodic stimuli, the overlapping late components will be time-locked to the subsequent stimuli. Such overlapped late components will not be canceled by averaging and so will appear as spurious short-latency components of the extracted signal. Interference due to rhythmic SIA and overlapped components may be attenuated if the stimuli are suitably aperiodic. The overlapping components and rhythmic SIA will then be asynchronous with respect to the stimuli, and effective cancellation can occur. As a rule, the effective time span of the range of variation of the interstimulus intervals should be greater than the period of the lowest frequency components of the rhythmic or overlapping activity to be attenuated (John et al., 1978).

One of the most extensive uses of ERs has been in the evaluation of sensory acuity, in particular Evoked Response Audiometry. The difficulties that appear in the definition of presence or absence of ERs in such cases were discussed in Chapter 4. An objective method of SDA detection in averaged EEG epochs has been described by Wicke, Goff, Wallace, & Allison (1978). The statistical properties of the subject's averaged background activity are summarized by making a set of comparisons between two consecutive EEG epochs immediately preceding each stimulus presentation. After stimulus presentation, a second set of comparisons is made between the poststimulus EEG epoch and the immediately preceding prestimulus epoch. The comparisons are performed by Sandler's *A parametric statistic*, mathematically equivalent to Student's *t test*. These two sets of comparisons are then examined to determine whether the latter differ significantly from the former. The technique has been used for Evoked Response Audiometry threshold determination in young children, with greater efficiency than subjective evaluation of the averaged evoked responses.

2. Median Evoked Response

Borda & Frost (1968) demonstrated that the median ER is appreciably less sensitive than the averaged ER to large artifactual disturbances. For the estimation of the median, the signal is considered to be constant and no assumption is made with respect to the distribution of SIA. If the SIA distribution is symmetrical, the mean and the median will coincide. It has been reported that for small sample sizes, when the SIA consists predominantly of quasisinusoidal waves, the resulting median ER will be contaminated by additional noise and harmonic distortion (Cooper, 1972; Ruchkin & Walter, 1975).

3. Wiener Filtering

The basic assumptions of this method are the presence of an invariant SDA and that SIA has zero mean is stationary. In Chapter 7, the detailed mathematical aspects of Wiener filtering were discussed. This method was first formulated for the estimation of the ERs by D. O. Walter (1968b) and applied by Nogawa, Katayama, Tabata, Kawahara, & Ohshio (1973). Later, Doyle (1975) made a correction for the application to averaged evoked responses, which was applied by Hartwell & Erwin (1976). The procedure is based on the calculation of the Wiener filter factor (Wiener, 1949). In it, the information at any frequency is weighted by the ratio of the power spectrum of the signal and of the background activity at the same frequency. Thus, information occurring at a frequency where there is a relatively little SIA will be virtually unaffected, as the filter is nearly unity. Information received at a frequency with much more SIA than SDA will be heavily discriminated against by the small filter value.

Strackee & Cerri (1977) have shown that application of Wiener filtering to individual ERs improves the signal-to-noise ratio, whereas when it is applied to the average signal, it does not lead to any improvement. Doyle (1977) proposed a method for comparing signal averaging and Wiener filtering for evoked potential estimation. Albrecht & Radil-Weiss (1976) have shown the dependence of Wiener filter estimation with respect to the interstimulus interval. Ungan & Basar (1976) demonstrated the drastic suppression of high-frequency components of the ERs by Wiener filtering, as is shown in Fig. 10.3. The recent demonstration provided by Valdés (1978) in relation with nonstationarity of the second order of the ER makes this procedure questionable for the estimation of the ERs.

4. Time-Varying Wiener Filtering (De Weerd, Martens & Colon, 1977).

This procedure considers an invariant SDA and an SIA with 0 mean that are not stationary. It has been developed to solve the problem of the estima-

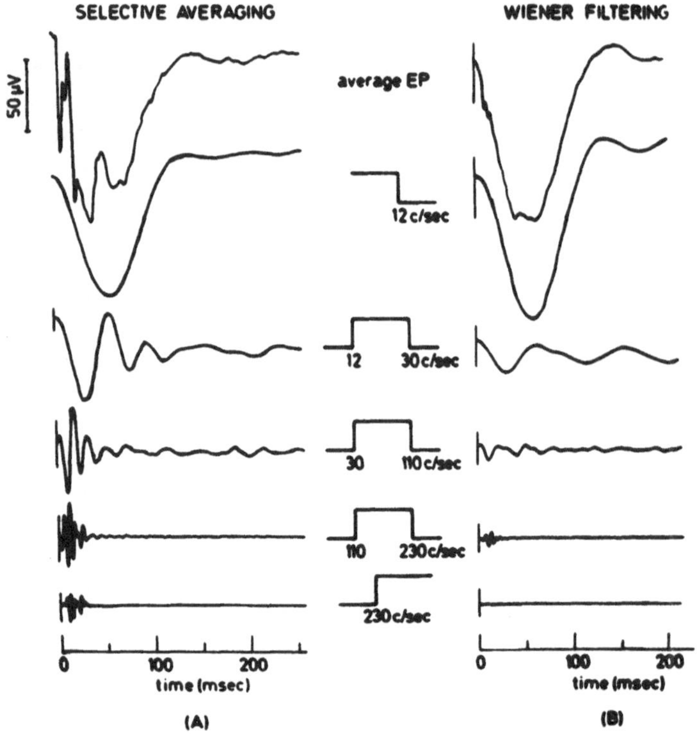

FIG. 10.3. Demonstration of the suppression of higher frequency AER components due to Wiener filtering process. Both AERs in (A) and (B) were obtained using the ER epoch recorded during the same experimental session from the cat inferior colliculus. AER components in different frequency bands were computed by means of a theoretical filtering method. (From Ungan & Basar, 1976.)

tion of the fast-amplitude variations by Wiener filtering. The theoretical basis for this method is given by the inverse relation of the spectral width of a bandpass filter and the time width of its impulse response. This implies that when ER is bandpass filtered with a set of octave filters, the output of these filters can be partitioned in time. For low frequency, there is only one time segment of large duration, whereas for high frequencies, there are many time segments of short duration. Each time segment defines a Wiener filter in a particular frequency band. The set of filters thus obtained is applied to the ER, which is then reconstructed by summation over all frequency bands and time segments. The inconvenience of the procedure is that, in improving the sensitivity for the high-frequency components, it also results in a higher sensitivity to noise.

B. Procedures That Assume That the Stimulus-Dependent Activity is Variable

1. Adaptive Filtering

For this type of ER estimation, it is assumed that the SDA is shifted in latency from trial to trial and that the SIA is stationary and with zero mean. The procedure was described by Woody (1967): The cross-correlation function for each ER is computed against a waveform template that is an estimate of the signal waveshape. The time lag at which the cross-correlation function is largest is taken as the latency of the signal. Each ER is then shifted in time to compensate for its latency. These latency-compensated waves are averaged together to obtain an improved estimate of the signal waveshape. The average replaces the original template or "stencil." The process is repeated until the stencil converges to an unchanging waveform, which serves as the latency-compensated average of the signal. The choice of the initial template may be a problem, depending on the signal-to-noise ratio. Woody reported that the waveshape of the initial stencil is not critical for rms signal-to-noise ratio greater than 0.2. Ruchkin, as described in John et al. (1978), applying the procedure to P300 waves, found that the method apparently works when the rms signal-to-noise ratio was above .4–.5. It is difficult to state at the moment whether reliable convergence to the signal will occur for lower ratios. Wastell (1977) studied not only the cross correlation between the template and the period of the EEG activity in which a stimulus was given, but also the cross correlation between the template and the period of EEG activity when no stimulation was given. His results showed that in both cases, as iterations proceeded, the values were higher. He recommended that if iterations beyond the first are to be pursued, it is desirable to include control trials and to define a suitable statistic to index the operating characteristics of the filter. He suggested a statistic defined as the distance between the mean of the "signal plus noise" and "noise only" distributions in noise standard-deviation units.

2. Minimum Mean-Square Error (MMSE) Filtering

In this procedure, the basic assumptions are that the SDA changes from trial to trial either in amplitude or latency or in both, and the SIA is considered as stationary with zero mean. According to Aunon & McGillem (1975), with this method, characterization of a single ER is possible (Fig. 10.4). The differences between the statistical properties of the SDA and the

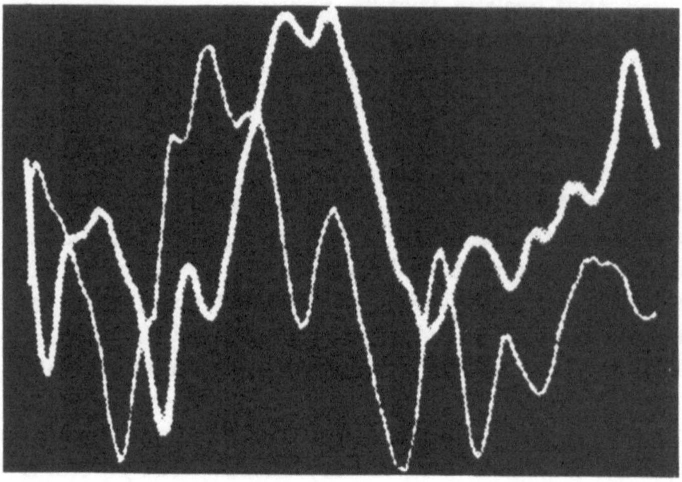

FIG. 10.4. Single evoked response of a subject (heavy line is filtered). Light line is average. Time interval is 500 msec. (From McGillem & Aunon, 1977.)

SIA are used to design a filter to provide an improved estimate of the ER waveform. The desired filter will have coefficients chosen to minimize the sum of the squared errors between the actual output (signal plus background activity) and desired output (signal). The analysis is made on the time domain. In this method, nonstationarities of the first order are eliminated, but those of the second order are not solved and, therefore, the same inconveniencies discussed in Wiener filtering are present. After estimation of single-trial VERs by MMSE filtering, McGillem & Aunon (1976, 1977) studied the individual components of the ERs by the automatic location and identification of the peaks. It was found that the occurrence of identifiable peaks was variable: Some of them were consistently present, whereas others were only observed for a small fraction of time. They computed a latency-corrected average by aligning the detected components in a defined interval, and averaging the waveforms over a 40 msec segment in the vicinity of the peaks.

3. Amplitude Sorting

This method was described by Ruchkin (1971). It assumes that a particular component of the SDA can vary with respect to amplitude or latency in a graded fashion, whereas other portions of the ER behave differently or are stable. These inhomogeneities of the SDA result because several types of ERs are being recorded; the purpose of the procedure is to decompose samples of

ERs into homogeneous subsets. Thus, it can be included within the procedures of cluster analysis. From the statistical point of view, it is a step-wise separation of Gaussian mixtures. It is also assumed that SIA is stationary, normally distributed, and with zero mean. The procedure consists of the computation of the variance for each time sample. At those latencies of the analysis epoch where the variance values are very high, the amplitude distribution is tested to establish whether it deviates from Gaussian. If so, amplitude values are specified that separate the observed distribution into different subgroups. The individual ERs are then classified one by one by comparing their amplitude at the critical latency with the selected voltage levels. This process is continued until the variance of the ERs classified similarly presents no deviant values. By this procedure, striking correlations between ER waveshape and behavior in animals have been described by John, Bartlett, Shimokochi, & Kleinman (1973). However, the following criticisms may be posed to this procedure: It is a univariate analysis; thus, it does not consider all the information contained in the ER, because only specific latencies (where the variances are too high) are used to classify the ERs, not taking into account intercorrelations between sampled values of the ERs.

4. *Multidimensional Scaling*

The SDA is assumed to be nonhomogeneous and the purpose is to classify the single ERs into clusters without a priori knowledge of how many different groups exist. Multidimensional scaling (Kruskal, 1964; Sammon, 1969) is a graphic technique that looks for the representation of each element (a vector in a multidimensional space) as a point in a low-dimensional space. Thus, if the final space obtained is two or three dimensional, it is possible to make a scatter plot of the final configuration of the points, each point being the representation of a single-trial ER. Visual inspection of the scatter plot may directly reveal the clusters obtained. In this procedure, the Euclidian distance between all pairs of single ERs is computed to obtain the distance or similarity matrix. The goal is to compute a new configuration of points in a reduced space with the property of distorting as little as possible the original distance matrix. Chapter 7 gave a more complete description of the procedure.

Although the method is computationally costly, it is considered to yield an especially accurate representation of data. Nevertheless, if the final space obtained has more than three dimensions, it is useless. The clusters obtained are defined by visual inspection, which may imply a subjective classification. The procedure has been applied with promising results to the estimation of ERs from electrodes chronically implanted in cats in a differential generalization paradigm (Ramos, Schwartz, & John 1974). The resulting clusters achieved an impressive separation of ER waveshapes elicited by the same indifferent stimulus in behavioral trials leading to performance of two different conditioned responses.

The method has also been used for discrimination between different groups of averaged evoked responses (see Chapter 13). In this case, the procedure does not provide a decision-making rule and further statistical inferences are not possible.

IV. HYPOTHESIS TESTING BETWEEN GROUPS OF EVOKED RESPONSES

The main question that is considered in these procedures is the validity of hypotheses about ERs—for example, whether significant differences between two or more groups of ERs exist. The groups are clearly identified before the analysis. All these procedures also have specific assumptions that should be examined before their use. In univariate procedures, each latency point is considered as an independent variable. Thus, the interrelationships between the different latency points are ignored, whereas in multivariate procedures, those interrelationships are taken into consideration.

A. *t* Test

This has been used by John (1977) and Shagass et al. (1977) to look for differences between averaged ERs. It assumes that the SDA is constant and that the SIA has a normal distribution with zero mean. For computing the *t* test, it is necessary to calculate not only the average, but the variance, at each latency point. Then, the *t* test (see Chapter 7) is computed for each latency point of the two averaged ERs, and the significance of the difference is evaluated using conventional statistical tables. This procedure has two main short comings: (1) the *t* tests are separately computed for each latency point and thus the alpha error is not controlled (because so many *t* tests are computed, some may be significant only by chance); and (2) the intercorrelations between each latency point are not taken into consideration. An example of the application of the *t* test is shown in Fig. 10.5.

B. Mann-Whitney *U* test

This is a nonparametric test that may be used for comparison of two groups of ERs. The single assumption is that the SDA is constant for each group. Kohn & Lifshitz (1976) used this procedure to compare responses to two dif-

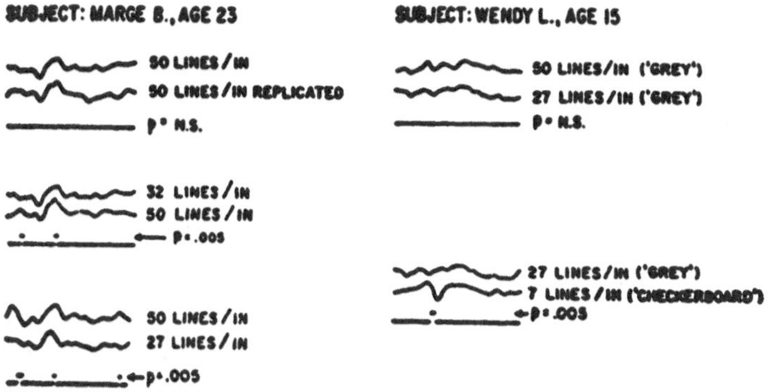

FIG. 10.5. Examples of the assessment of visual acuity by application of Student's *t* test to average visual evoked responses. Significant values as assessed by Student's *t* test are shown at the bottom of each pair of VERs. Grids with 50, 32, 27, and 7 lines/inch were used as visual stimuli. The grid with 27 lines/inch will be perceived as a checkerboard by a subject with 20/20 vision. Both subjects perceived 50 lines/inch as a gray field. The subject shown on the left reported that she perceived both 32- and 27-lines/inch stimuli as checkerboards. Significant differences were observed between 50 and 32 and 50 and 27 lines/inch. The subject shown on the right was tested without her glasses and perceived the 27-lines/inch stimulus as gray. No differences were found by the *t* tests between 50 and 27 lines/inch. However, she perceived the 7-lines/inch stimulus as a checkerboard, with the corresponding significant differences. (From John, 1977.)

ferent stimuli. The procedure consists of the computation of the *U* test for each latency point. This is done by taking the values at each latency for the two conditions to form a rank vector. The value of the *U* statistic is given by the sum of the number of times an element in the rank vector from the initial values to one stimulation precedes an element from the other stimulation. The sampling distribution of the *U* statistic is known, and with this knowledge, the probability at each point that two groups of ERs are from the same distribution can be determined. Thus, at each time point, a probability value is obtained, the same as for the calculation of the *t* test. This method has the same shortcomings as those discussed for the *t* test, plus lower power.

C. Linear Discriminant Analysis

This is a multivariate approach whose purpose is to compare different ensembles of single ERs. Other purposes, such as the decision whether a single ER belongs to one group or to another, are discussed later. The linear discriminant analysis assumes that the SDA is constant within each group, and that the SIA has a multinormal distribution with zero mean and that it has similar characteristics in all the groups of ERs; equivalently, it may be assumed that the Gaussianity of the ERs, as well as the homogeneity of the covariance matrices of the different groups of ERs, holds. The description of linear discriminant analysis was provided in Chapter 7. When only two groups of ERs are considered, the mean difference may be tested using Hotelling's T^2 statistic.

Sometimes, a reduction in the number of variables (latency points) is made before the determination of the discriminant equations by the step-wise discriminant analysis (Dixon, 1968). This proceeds as follows: A variable is selected that provides for the best possible discrimination among the groups. After all the information correlated with this variable is removed, a second variable is selected; a discriminant function is then determined for the space defined by these two variables. The second variable is added only if its addition provides an improvement over the discrimination based on one variable only. Additional variables are added similarly, the process terminating when no additional improvement in the classification procedure can be obtained with further inclusion of variables. The outcome of this procedure is a discriminant function (a classification rule) that utilizes the smallest number of variables that are required to provide the best discrimination.

Donchin (1966) used Hotelling's T^2 analysis for the discrimination of VERs to two different stimuli with good results. The step-wise linear discriminant analysis has been used by several authors, looking for differences between the ERs of different groups of subjects (Callaway, 1966), for differences between ERs produced by task relevant or irrelevant stimuli (Donchin & Cohen, 1967), or looking for differences between ERs produced by homophone words of different meanings (Brown, Marsh, & Smith, 1976).

D. Nonlinear Discriminant Analysis

This method assumes the multinormal distribution of the ERs, but the covariance matrices of the groups may be unequal. It can be used for hypothesis testing even if the mean vectors of the groups to be tested are equal, because it is also sensitive to the inhomogeneities of the covariance matrices (Victor, 1971). It has been described earlier in this chapter that Valdés (1978) demonstrated the inhomogeneities of the covariance matrices of the single-trial VERs to different interpretations of the same stimulus. Thus, in those circumstances, the linear discriminant analysis would not provide the best possible discrimination, and the nonlinear discriminant analysis should be used. In order to reduce the number of variables, Valdés & Baez (1977) developed the nonlinear step-wise discriminant analysis procedure. It is a generalization of the algorithms for the linear case, and it has been described in Chapter 7.

V. ANALYSIS OF THE STRUCTURE

Sometimes, the interest in the analysis of the ERs is to look for some latent features that are not easily observable in the voltage–time curve by some mathematical transformation, usually linear. Reduction of the number of variables provided by the series of voltage values in the ERs without a great loss in the amount of information is also desirable, and both goals may be fulfilled by finding underlying features (principal component analysis). It is also important to study the structure of a set of ERs and to analyze the similarities between them. This can be done by cluster analysis. We have mentioned cluster analysis in relation to the estimation of the ERs, but cluster analysis may also be used to classify the basic structure of a nonhomogeneous group of ERs.

A. Linear Transformations

The Fourier transform (see Chapter 7) has also been applied to the study of the ERs to obtain a frequency domain representation of them. The basic assumptions are that both the SDA and the SIA are stationary. If they have a multinormal distribution, the estimate will be more accurate. Davis (1973) made a spectral analysis of VERs to flashes and AERs to clicks recorded in the left and right visual and auditory areas. He found two major frequency groups of Fourier terms: Group I, from 0–5 Hz, occurred in a similar form in both sensory areas for both types of stimuli, being greater in auditory areas; Group II, from 6–12 Hz, were of shorter latency, were more variable than group I, and were greater in the primary projection area of the stimulus modality. Frequency analysis of VERs and AERs recorded in both hemispheres have also been performed for the study of hemispheric symmetry (Davis & Wada, 1974, 1977).

The Fourier analysis of the steady-state VERs to flickering light has shown that these responses fall into three different frequency ranges: high frequency (45–60 Hz), medium frequency (13–25 Hz), and low frequency (near 10 Hz) (Regan, 1972). Evidence from patients with known neurosurgical or cerebrovascular cortical damage indicates that VERs in these three frequency ranges are generated in different, though overlapping, cortical areas. This evidence is consistent with the observation that topographical distribution of these three types of responses are different in normal controls (Regan, 1977b). Childers (1977) reported great differences in the spectral analysis of VERs to the letters *b* and *d* between normal and dyslexic children.

The Walsh transform is somewhat similar to the Fourier transform, but the sinusoids are replaced by square waves of unit amplitudes. The computations are simplified and the resulting transform is comparable, although slightly less convenient than the Fourier transform (John et al., 1978). However, practical results applying the Walsh transform to large number of EEGs have been rather discouraging because of the pronounced sensitivity to shifts of the origin (Dumermuth et al., 1975; Künkel and EEG project group, 1975).

The Haar transform has its basic functions of 0th and 1st order, identical to those of the Walsh transform, but higher order functions are broken down along the time domain so that each contains only one square wave. For instance, there are two basis functions of order two, one for the first half epoch and one for the second half—that is, each spanning one-half second. Similarly, there are four basis Haar functions of order three, and so forth. Each basis function, therefore, has two indexes, one representing the order and the second one indicating the time location within the epoch. With increasing order, the time indexing becomes increasingly fine in a binary sequence. According to John et al. (1978), the Haar transform is extremely parsimonious and efficient with ER data. Haar transform is a nonstationary analysis and it also preserves the time ordering of the information. However, it is necessary to know its statistical properties in order to increase its use and applications.

B. Time-Varying Spectra

Aunon & McGillem (1977) designed a procedure to detect the changing character of the spectrum of the ER as a function of time relative to stimulus application. This was done by treating the data as an ensemble of sample functions from a nonstationary random process and computing estimates of the time-varying spectrum. The data to be analyzed were divided into a sequence of partially overlapping segments 250 msec long. The first segment started 250 msec before the stimulation and ended just before stimulus application. Succeeding segments were taken at 24-msec intervals with the last starting at 250 msec after stimulus application (Fig. 10.6). The power spectrum of each segment was computed to see how it varied with time, and the results plotted as three-dimensional graphs, as shown in Fig. 10.7. They observed the occurrence of high-frequency (16–17 Hz) and low-frequency (5–6 Hz) components immediately after the flash stimulation. They suggested that the two components are independent of one another, the low frequency corresponding to the primary response and the high frequency to a "monitoring" wave, related to the phenomenon of alpha blocking observed in the EEG when a stimulus is applied. They also concluded that the occurrence of these low-and-high frequency components is useful to improve the design of filters for the estimation of VERs.

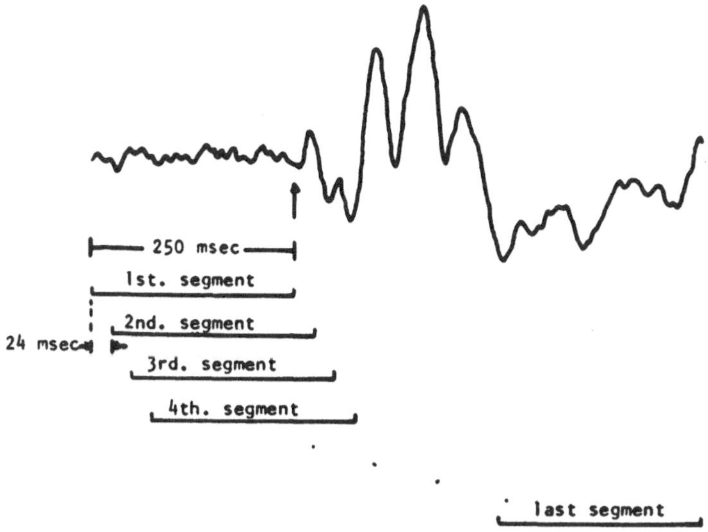

FIG. 10.6. Partitioning of data into overlapping segments for computation of time-varying spectra. (From Aunon & McGillem, 1977.)

C. Principal Component Analysis

This procedure has frequently been used for the analysis of averaged evoked responses. It is used to infer the structure of a set of data from correlations between all pairs of elements in the set (see Chapter 7). An adequate description of the structure of the data is provided if the relevant information is contained in the correlation or covariance matrices. Principal component analysis performs a reduction of the dimensionality of the original space by the selection of orthogonal functions to fit such a set of data. The first dimension accounts for the maximum possible variance of the data and the subsequent components are selected to account for additional portions of the residual variance. The dimensionality of the final signal space will be the number of factors required to account for a predetermined percentage of the variance of the original set of data. Considering a set of averaged evoked responses, principal component analysis may be performed in two basically different ways:

1. Taking into consideration the covariations between the waveshapes of the ERs; therefore, the variables will be the vectors formed by the amplitude values of the averaged ERs. In this case, as a result of the analysis, each ER may be described in terms of a common set of factors by a linear equation in

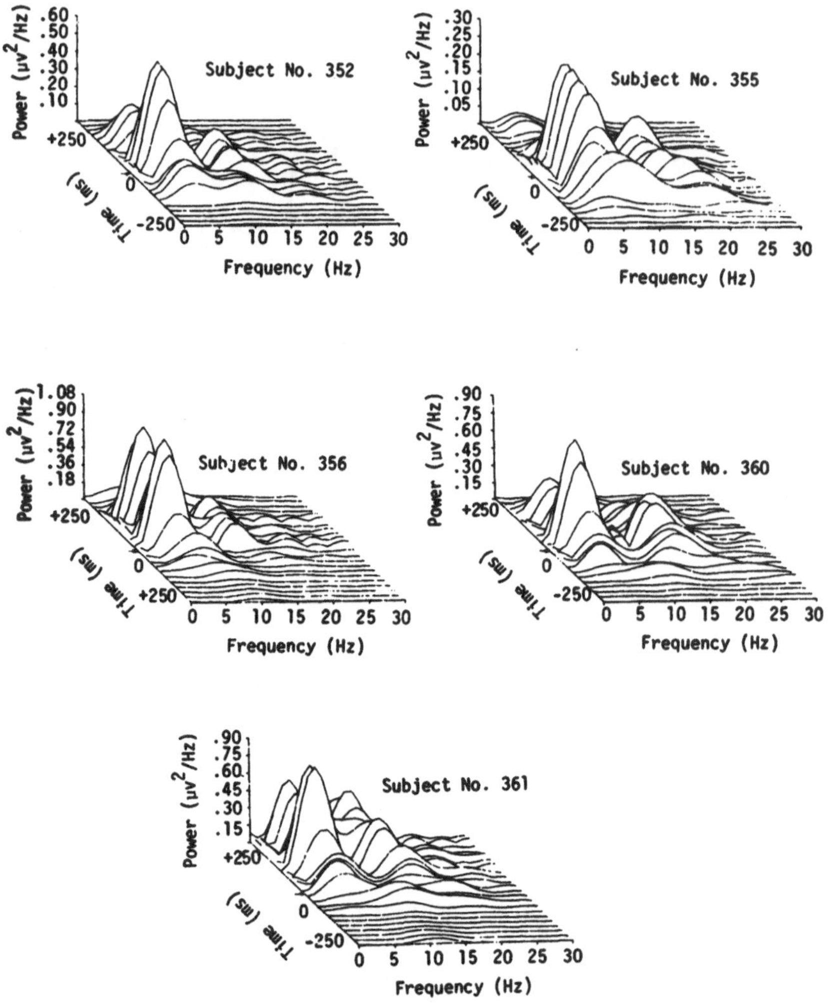

FIG. 10.7. Time-varying spectra of the averaged VERs in five different subjects. (From Aunon & McGillem, 1977.)

which the coefficients related to each factor (factor loadings) represent the contribution of such factors to the configuration of the ER (Fig. 10.8).

2. In the second variant, the covariations of activity at different latencies for the whole set of averaged ERs are computed; variables are the vectors formed at each latency (see Fig. 10.8). The factors obtained in this case may be related to different physiological events that occur at a particular moment or latency.

Selection of the procedure should be made according to the goals pursued. The questions that may be posed can be quite different: For a given subject, the set of ERs may correspond to recordings in the same place but during different conditions, or it may correspond to ERs from different derivations in a single condition; then, the factors obtained in the analysis must be interpreted in relation to the conditions or the locations. If the set of averaged ERs comes from several subjects, then each factor may be related to a peculiar group of subjects—for example, control and experimental groups (normals and neurological patients; see Chapter 13).

Another application of principal component analysis to a set of averaged ERs from different subjects is to reduce the dimensionality of the space for further processing by other methods such as cluster analysis (see Chapter 13). In all these circumstances, principal component analysis is used with the following assumptions: (1) noise is absent and the variabilities observed correspond to intrinsic variations of the SDA; (2) the relevant information is con-

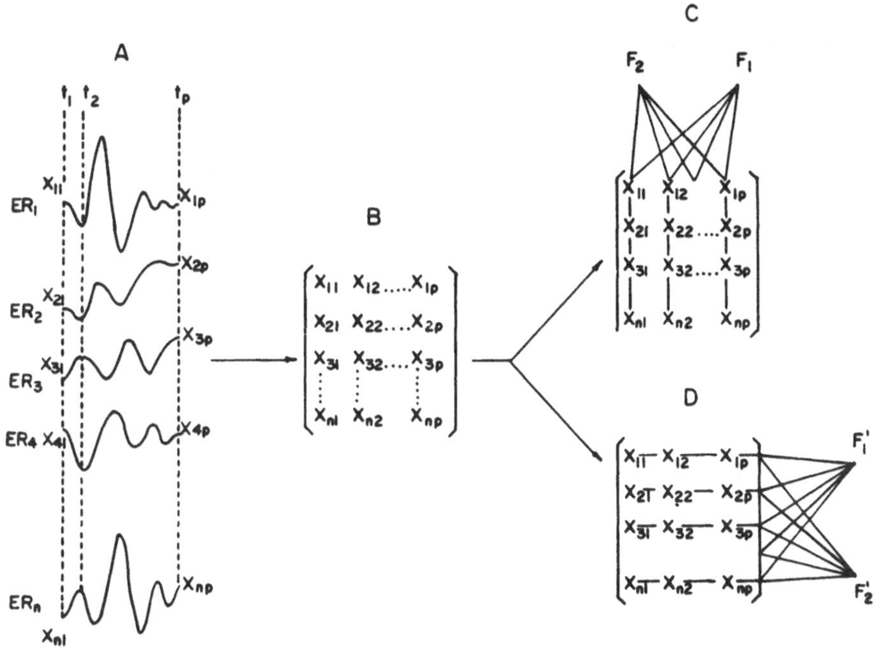

FIG. 10.8. Principal component analysis of a set of n ERs. Each ER is digitized in p equidistant values (A). In (B), a matrix of n rows and p columns is formed. With such a matrix, two different types of component analysis may be computed: taking p vectors, each one formed by the n values at a specific latency (columns), as is shown in (C); or taking n vectors, each one formed by the p values of an ER (rows), as is shown in (D). Two different solutions may be obtained: In (C), the covariations of activity at different latencies are considered for the calculation of the factors (F_1, F_2). In (D), the covariations of the ER waveforms are taken into account for the computation of the factors (F_1', F_2').

tained in the covariance matrix; and (3) the variables considered (time points in this case) are independent. The first assumption may be valid if the analysis is performed with averaged evoked responses and the assumptions for averaging are satisfied. The covariance matrix or the correlation matrix may contain the relevant information if they arise from a unimodal distribution. In case the data have a Gaussian distribution, further statistical inferences are also possible. It should also be remembered that the covariance matrix is inherently insensitive to high frequency–low energy components; thus, these types of waves are not taken into account well in principal component analysis. The third assumption is necessary for further statistical inferences, and is very difficult to justify because, obviously, each data point is correlated with the others; thus, the correlation coefficient between two ERs will be only a rough measure of similarity between them.

However, if the principal component analysis is made considering as variables the vectors formed by the values at a peculiar latency of the whole set of ERs, this third assumption is valid. In this manner, the covariance matrix will measure the degree to which activity at a given latency covaries with others at another specific latency. In this case, the variables are independent and, thus, the third assumption is valid.

It is sometimes difficult to find a meaningful physiological interpretation of the basic waveforms and weighting coefficients. According to John et al. (1978), the difficulty lies in the fact that the basis waveform set is a best mean-square fit to the data. The main principal component waveforms tend to resemble composites of the original data waveforms, and the weighting coefficients tend to emphasize similarities in the data. Consequently, differences between data waveforms may be obscured. When it is desirable to have a linear representation with a minimum number of basis waveforms necessary for a desired approximation accuracy, but which emphasizes rather than obscures waveform differences, application of a varimax rotation to the original principal component analysis may achieve this goal (see Chapter 7). A detailed description of the application of principal component analysis to the study of ERs may be found in John et al. (1964, 1978) and Donchin (1966). Its applications have been also reviewed in the second volume of this series (John, 1977); thus, we only briefly review some results obtained in the human.

Valdés (1974) performed a principal component analysis of the VERs to flashes recorded from central, occipital, temporal, and centro–occipital and occipito–temporal left and right derivations. He found that the waveshapes from all these derivations within a single subject could be described by three factors (97% of the variance). Later on, in a collaborative work with Dr. John from the New York University Medical Center, Valdés, Harmony and Ricardo (1974) computed a principal component analysis of the VERs recorded in the same set of 10 derivations of 10 normal subjects and found, also with three factors, that it was possible to span the space occupied by the full set of VERs (10 leads x 10 subjects). These results showed that interindividual variations, as well as the intraindividual waveshapes from various areas in a given subject, could be well described as combinations of few factors. These results were the basis for the application of principal component analysis to VERs of a larger number of normal subjects and neurological plain more than 91% of the variability for each condition and each subject, (1976) confirmed these results using 41 and 38 electrode placements in two subjects for recording the VERs to flashes to the left, right, and both eyes simultaneously. They found that with four factors it was possible to explain more than 91% of the variability for each condition and each subject, using waveshapes or sample times as elements for the computation of the correlation matrix.

D. Cluster Analysis

The purpose of clustering in ERs is to find sets or "clusters" of ERs such that members of each cluster are "similar" to each other and "different" from those belonging to other clusters. These procedures offer the enormous advantage that they permit the analysis of the structure of the data in the absence of any prior assumption about the nature of the structure. But, they have the disadvantage that statistical inferences are not possible (see Chapter 7). Cluster analysis may be applied directly to the amplitude sampled ERs or to such transformations of these ERs as the Fourier transform or the results of principal component analysis. In Cluster analysis, it is important to define the similarity measure, which is the basis for the construction of quantitative statements about the degree to which a given ER is "like" another. The similarity measures are used to construct a distance or similarity matrix describing the strength of all pairwise relationships among the ERs in the data set.

One class of cluster analysis methods operates on this matrix to construct a tree depicting specified relationships among the ERs (Fig. 10.9). In this tree, the branches represent the ERs, whereas the root represents the entire collection of ERs. There are methods that move down the tree from the branches toward the root, increasing aggregation of ERs into clusters, and others that begin at the root and work towards the branches. In the first case, when two ERs merge, they are joined together permanently; in the second case, when a group of ERs splits into two parts, the parts are separated permanently. Here lies the strength and weakness of this (hierarchical) type of method: By taking early decisions as permanent, the number of possibilities that can be examined is reduced greatly as compared with complete enumeration.

Other types of cluster analysis have been developed. This topic is too complex to review here. The interested reader should consult Anderberg (1973)

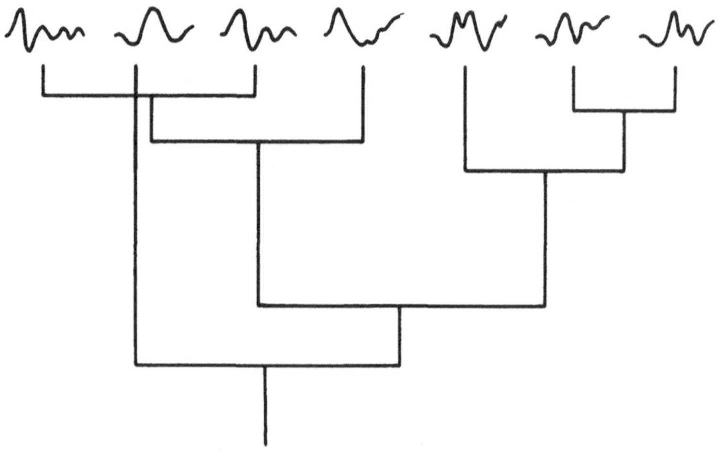

FIG. 10.9. Graphical display or dendogram of a cluster analysis of a set of ERs. The pairs of ERs with most similar waveshape are joined together. Later on, they are joined to the ER with the next most similar waveshape, and so on, until a single cluster is formed. At each step, the error committed is computed and graphically displayed by the dimension of the vertical segments.

for a more detailed treatment. The problem when applying most cluster analysis methods is that there are no objective statistical criteria to define the clusters. Thus, the analyst has to choose as many clusters as he or she considers real on the basis of experience (for example, in Fig. 10.9, once the tree is constructed for *n* ERs, the analyst may choose from many sets of clusters). There is an error in clustering. Thus, clusters can be identified as groups of elements that can be joined with minimum increase of the error. A measure of the error for one cluster may be considered as the sum of the squares of the distances of the members of the clusters to its centroid.

Valdés et al. (1974) analyzed the VERs to flashes obtained from left occipital monopolar leads in 30 healthy subjects with Lance and Williams' general algorithm used with Ward's criterion (Wishart, 1969), which consists of minimizing the total error in clustering. The total error is the sum of the errors for each cluster. The measure of the error for one cluster can be considered as the sum of the squares of the distances of the members to the centroids. The procedure is as follows:

1. Each ER starts out as a one-member cluster. The error in joining two one-member clusters into a larger cluster is simply the Euclidian distance between them. Those two ERs with smallest distance are thus joined.
2. The error that would result if one joined any two of the existing clusters is examined. Those two clusters whose fusion produces the smallest error in-

crease are joined. This second step is repeated until all ERs are joined into a single cluster.

Valdés et al. (1974) obtained five clusters of waveshapes. The groups formed by the analysis showed a high degree of correspondence with the subjective identification of "types" by trained technicians, and the groups also correspond to those previously described by Arnal et al. (1972) using correspondence factor analysis. These results were confirmed in a subsequent work with a larger group (Valdés, Ricardo, & Harmony, 1975), where comparisons with other clustering algorithms, such as single-link cluster analysis (Jardine, Jardine, & Sibson, 1967) and the *k*-means method (McQueen, 1967), were also made. In a more recent paper, Rodríguez, Garriga, Valdés, & Harmony (1977) compared five different hierarchical procedures of cluster analysis in a group of VERs to flash and to a flashed checkerboard pattern. The procedures used were: single-link cluster analysis (minimal spanning tree, the nearest neighbor), the furthest-neighbor method, the group-average method, the centroid method, and the Lance and Williams' algorithm. The best results were again obtained with the latter procedure, because, with the others, a great number of elements were not included in any cluster.

VI. PREDICTION METHODS

The problem here is to a assign, in some optimum fashion, a new ER to one of several known populations of ERs. Discriminant analysis uses the data obtained from members of different groups, whose group membership is known, to derive criteria for the classification of observations whose group membership is doubtful: The classification is achieved by partitioning the multidimensional space in which the observations are located into a number of mutually exclusive regions. Each region is identified with one of the classification groups. The classification of newly observed points then depends on the region on the space into which they fall. Thus, application of the functions obtained by the discriminant analysis of different groups of ERs to a new ER will yield an estimate of the probability of its belonging to the different groups. Squires & Donchin (1976) used the step-wise linear discriminant analysis for the classification of single auditory evoked responses. They recorded in three different electrode sites and computed the discriminant functions with single ERs from 16 subjects to whom trains of loud and soft tones were presented during three different performance tasks. An average of 84% correct classification was obtained using information from one electrode site and 89% when information of multiple electrodes was used. Then, they computed a subject-independent function with the information from all subjects and applied it to seven new subjects. This subject-independent function proved to be sufficiently generalized to classify correctly 81% of the trials.

Vidal (1975) has developed an extremely advanced procedure that classifies the single ERs in real time. The procedure is carried out in several steps: automatic rejection of electro-ocular and movement artifacts, estimation of the single ERs by Wiener filtering, and step-wise discriminant procedure. This step-wise method is used to solve the equation and select the best samples one by one into an ordered subset of predetermined size, somewhere between 5 and 10. After this reduction, a linear Bayesian decision rule is calculated for each class over the reduced vector. The rules are built on the assumption that the ERs population should distribute into the k stimulus classes. In addition, a $(k + 1)$th class is defined, an outlier class, containing those epochs for which, in the signal space, the Mahalanobis distance to the group mean exceeds a given threshold. By this test, it is possible to remove the outliers of the ERs used for the computation of the discriminant equation to obtain an updated selection and thus a correct decision rule. Once the initial decision rule has been established, real time classification can proceed with a minimum of computation between epoch acquisition. The only calculations involve the evaluation of the linear decision rules (one expression must be computed for each class) and a comparison of the results to identify the largest value. Under the experimental conditions tested so far, the rate of correct classification over small sets of stimuli (4 to 10) can exceed 90% with average subjects (John et al., 1978).

VII. TOPOGRAPHIC METHODS

As has been described in Chapter 9, topographic methods are very useful to study the distribution of the electrical brain properties. Contour-mapping methods in the time domain or the so-called spatio-temporal maps or cronotopograms were described by Rémond (1961). With this procedure, Rémond & Lesèvre (1967) and Rémond (1968) made important contributions to the study of the sources of the VERs (Fig. 10.10). Another method of contour mapping consists of recording the signal from a two-dimensional array of electrodes, measuring the amplitude at predetermined time instants, and constructing separate contour maps for each time at which the signal is sampled. This procedure (Fig. 10.11) has been used in the study of the topographical distribution of different components of the averaged evoked responses (Allison et al., 1977; G. D. Goff et al., 1977; W. R. Goff et al., 1969; Vaughan, 1969). Ragot & Rémond (1978), with plots of a chart every millisecond, have observed that generation of the different components of VERs to a checkerboard pattern appear to be of "saltatory" nature: Each component grows, culminates, and declines at the same region of the scalp, instead of rising, moving to another place, and declining.

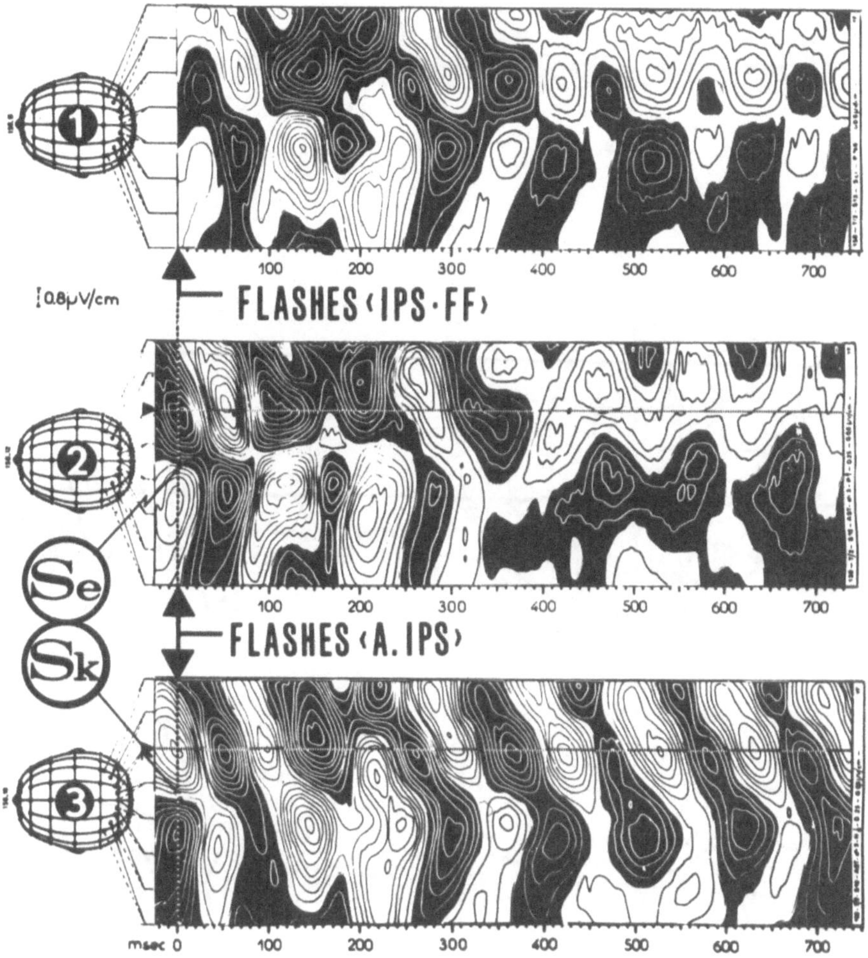

FIG. 10.10. Chronotopograms. (1) Activity evoked by flash at regular intervals. (2) Activity evoked by flash triggered when the third channel is in a "source phase." (3) The same for the "sink phase." (From Rémond & Lesèvre, 1967.)

VIII. SUMMARY

In this chapter, the stochastic properties of the evoked responses and the basic assumptions that underly every procedure of their quantitative analysis have been emphasized (see Table 10.1). These methods have been classified according to the specific statistical problems they tried to solve. Extraction of stimulus-dependent electrophysiological activity is a very important aspect of dealing with evoked responses, and different types of estima-

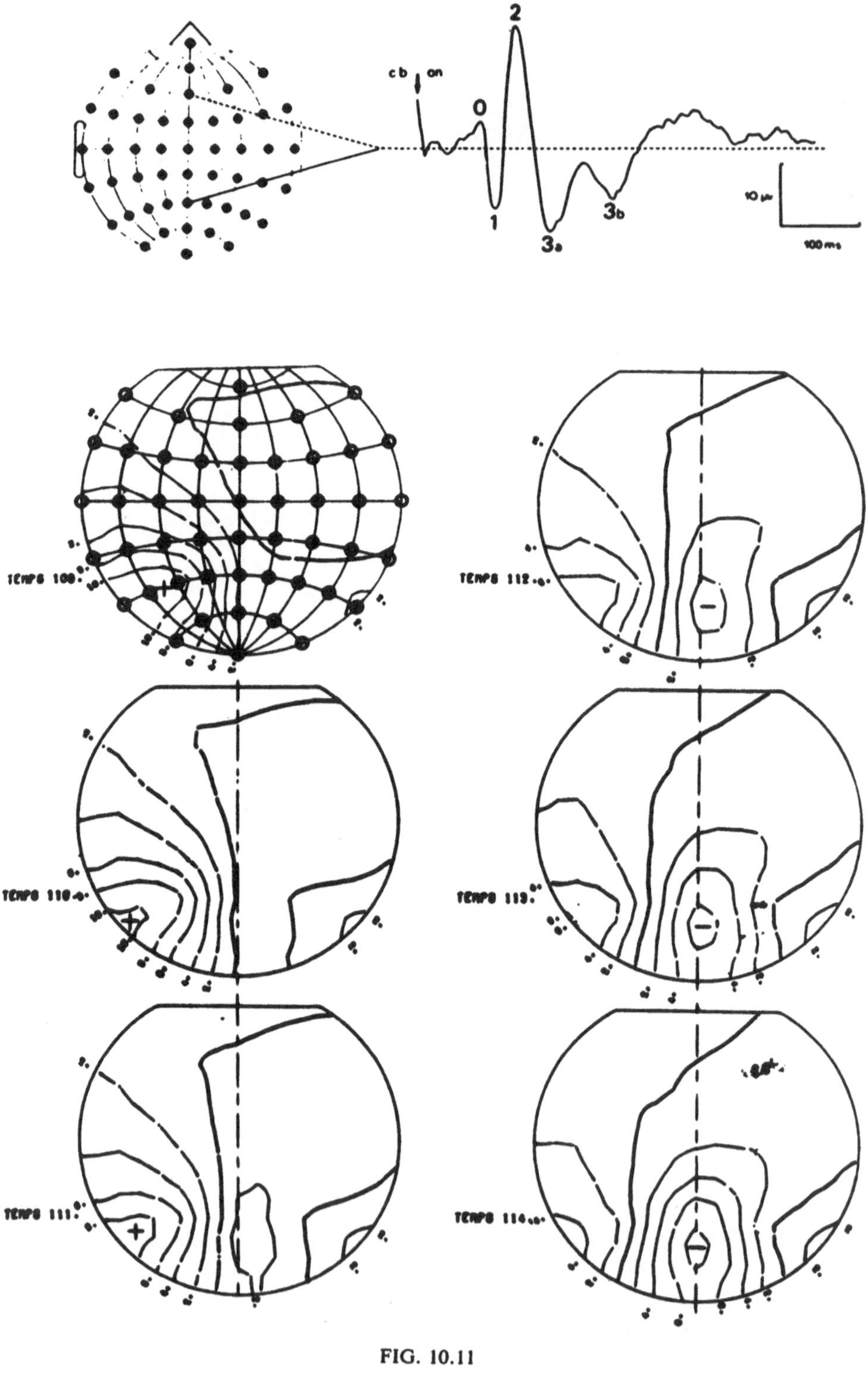

2
cb
on
0
1
3a
3b
10 µv
100 ms
TEMPS 109
TEMPS 110
TEMPS 111
TEMPS 112
TEMPS 113
TEMPS 114

FIG. 10.11

TABLE 10.1
Basic Assumptions Considered for the Stimulus-Dependent Activity (SDA) and the Stimulus-Independent Activity (SIA) in the Major Methods Used for Estimation and Hypothesis Testing of the Evoked Responses

Estimation		
SDA	*SIA*	*Method*
Constant	No assumption	Median evoked response
Constant	Symmetrical statistical distribution If Gaussian, estimates with confidence limits	Averaging
Constant[a]	Zero mean, stationary If Gaussian, precise estimates	Wiener filtering
Constant[a]	Zero mean, not stationary	Time-varying Wiener filtering
Shifted in latency[a]	Zero mean, stationary	Adaptive filtering
Variable in amplitude and latency[a]	Zero mean, stationary	Minimum mean–square error filtering
Variable in amplitude and latency[a]	Zero mean, Gaussian	Amplitude sorting
Hypothesis Testing		
SDA	*SIA*	*Method*
Constant	No assumption	Mann Whitney *U* Test
Constant	Zero mean, Gaussian	Student's *t* Test
Constant	Zero mean, Gaussian, homogeneity of the covariance matrices	Linear discriminant analysis
Constant	Zero mean, Gaussian, inhomogeneity of the covariance matrices	Nonlinear discriminant analysis

[a]For the application of these procedures, the mean of the SDA should be zero, but this is generally ignored.

FIG. 10.11. *(Opposite page) Top:* electrode position, and potential versus time representation of the VER recorded between two electrodes. *Bottom:* potential field distribution of the VER between peak 1 (positive) and peak 2 (negative), at 1-msec intervals. Sequence is from top to bottom, left to right. (From Ragot & Rémond, 1978.)

tion methods are now in use. Averaging has been the most widely applied procedure for the estimation of ERs, and the study of the effects of different types of brain lesions on them. Nevertheless, the assumption of the invariance of the stimulus-dependent activity may not hold in all circumstances. Future applications of other types of techniques of quantitative analysis of the ERs for the evaluation of brain damage seems desirable to improve our knowledge. The introduction of techniques for processing single-trial ERs has opened a new field of exploration in the study of sensory, perceptual, and cognitive mechanisms and their disturbances. It has been shown that with the application of multivariate statistical procedures to the analysis of the ERs, it is possible not only to discriminate adequately, but to predict, on the basis of the ER waveform, the quality of the given stimulus and even the behavior. Those results demonstrate that ERs are of great value in the study of the nervous system.

PART III:

NEUROMETRIC EVALUATION IN CLINICAL NEUROLOGY

11 EEG Background Activity

I. THE NEUROMETRIC APPROACH

In preceding chapters, we have reviewed the major methods of quantitative analysis of EEG background activity and we have also discussed the statistical basis for neurometric evaluation. As we have previously mentioned, neurometrics is the methodology, based on quantitative measurements of the brain electrical activity, for evaluating the anatomical integrity, developmental maturation, and the mediation of sensory, perceptual, and cognitive processes. Several steps may be distinguished in a neurometric procedure: the acquisition of accurate data sensitive to one or more of these brain functions, the extraction of relevant features of these data, and the establishment of a decision rule for assigning a given subject to one of a given number of sets on the basis of the previously extracted features.

The EEG background activity and the evoked responses contain diagnostically valuable information for the assessment of brain dysfunction in neurological patients, which can be made accessible by quantitative analysis. In this chapter, we refer only to those neurometric procedures that are based mainly on the analysis of EEG background activity. We have seen that computer methods permit quantification of many potentially diagnostic features of the EEG. Each method makes some specific mathematical assumptions and their violation may produce some inaccuracies in the subsequent stage of decision making and interpretation of the results. Thus, the selection of the procedure for EEG analysis is very important.

Another important problem that must be considered is the number of features to include in the procedure. Inclusion of as many features as can be extracted, in order to maximize the probability of an optimal decision rule, might appear reasonable during the development of a neurometric methodology, but it has several drawbacks. From the statistical point of view, in order to evaluate a large number of variables, one should have approximately a five-fold larger sample of subjects. Evidence has been provided that demonstrated great redundancy of the information content of many electrophysiological features. This problem may be solved by different statistical procedures in order to reduce the dimensionality of the space, but these procedures require large amounts of computation time.

A solution that should be explored is the creation of mathematical models and procedures in order to compress a great amount of information into a compound feature. Some work has been done in this direction with excellent results; the Age-Dependent Quotient is one example (see section IIC of this chapter). We consider this one of the most important and urgent problems to solve to obtain more powerful and practical neurometric procedures. Once the number of features has been reduced to those that are relevant for our specific goal, the procedure may have wider applications.

A decision rule may be obtained by the comparison of well-defined groups established a priori—that is the division of the population into two large groups of normality or abnormality, or into several groups according to the type of abnormality or the degree of abnormality. It may also be determined by the comparison of groups that emerge as a result of a classification procedure (cluster analysis) of the electrophysiological profiles of the different subjects. The decision rule thus obtained must be validated with new subjects, whose data were not used for the establishment of the decision rule. Once validated, the corresponding procedure will be ready for its introduction into clinical practice.

Although not all of the neurometric procedures discussed in this chapter for the assessment of EEG background activity in clinical neurology have completed the different stages just mentioned, they are each potentially capable of generating robust rules. They are described here to give the reader a realistic picture of the current state of this field. Although many procedures for the quantitative analysis of brain electrical activity have been described until now, relatively few contributions have provided solutions for the various aspects of the problem. This has been emphasized by Rémond and Storm van Leeuwen (1977):

> the fact that at first glance the electroencephalographer does not easily recognize his own preoccupation, in the often pin-point work carried out by machines in specialized laboratories, is due to there not yet existing a unique overall treatment of the EEG which should answer such questions; instead, we find a number of limited incomplete objectives located somewhere between data acquisition and decision making, e.g., at one of the following levels: automatic reading and realization of initial measurements, calculations of characteristic parameters, statistical analysis of parameters, classifying results.

Any partial solution limited to only one of these items soon turns out to be insufficient and unsatisfactory, if not supplemented by complementary means existing at other levels. Specialists in EEG data processing have progressively come to this conclusion, their work achieving full significance and operational efficiency only when they carried out as complete a treatment as possible [p. 2, 3].

II. FREQUENCY ANALYSIS

A. Canonograms

Gotman et al. (1973) developed a procedure to provide the electroencephalographer with simpler and more precise tools to supplement the paper record. The EEG given to the electroencephalographer for traditional EEG interpretation usually contains records from a bipolar antero–posterior montage, a coronal bipolar montage, a monopolar montage with cervical or average reference, and records from selected leads during hyperventilation and photic stimulation.

From a variety of such recordings, only two 40-second long samples were taken for computer analysis. These samples, as artifact free as possible, were selected from the data recorded from the bipolar antero–posterior and the monopolar montage. Each 40-second sample was then divided into eight 5-second segments, which were subjected to spectral analysis for the frequency range .7–30 Hz. The average power in the delta, theta, alpha, and beta bands across the eight spectra thus obtained were computed for 16 derivations in each montage. The 16 average spectra for each montage were then displayed on the computer terminal. The spectrum from each derivation was placed into array at a location corresponding to the position of that derivation on the scalp, relative to the other leads. Thus, the topography of the array was anatomically meaningful (see Fig. 11.1).

Next, two types of relations between the activities of different frequency bands were studied: intrachannel relations, in which the various activities within one given channel are compared, and interchannel relations, in which activities between different channels are compared. The intrachannel relations are computed as the ratios of the slow to the fast activity where a, b, c, and d are weighting constants:

$$\frac{(a \times \text{delta}) + (b \times \text{theta})}{(c \times \text{alpha}) + (d \times \text{delta})}$$

Using an empirical type of discriminant analysis, applied between a group of normal subjects and a group of patients with brain tumors and localized or lateralized nonintermittent EEG abnormalities of the type most likely to be

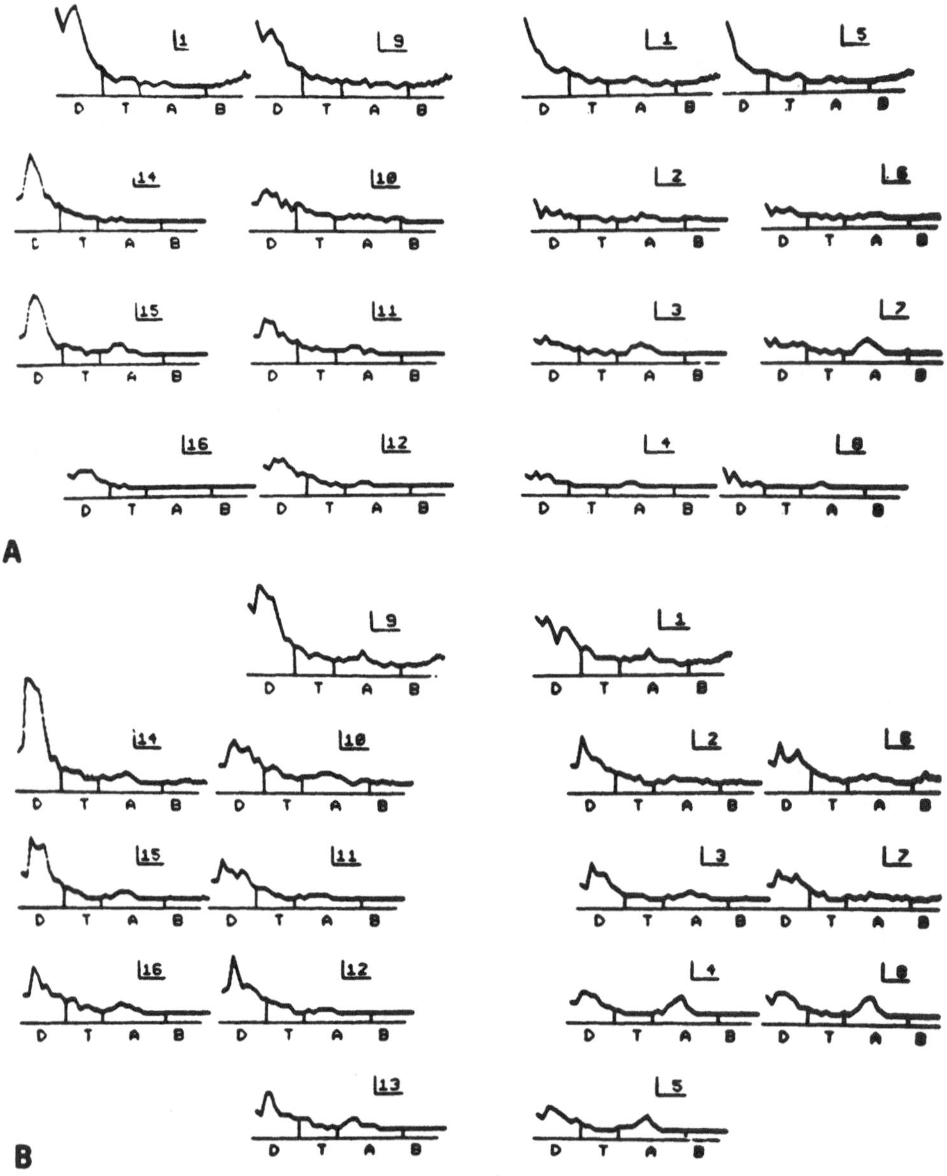

FIG. 11.1. Spectra from EEG of subject with large tumor (glioblastoma) in left posterior Sylvian region. (A) Antero-posterior bipolar montage covering parasagittal and temporal regions. (B) Monopolar montage with average reference. Frontal region at top of each Fig., occipital at bottom, temporal on outer right and left, centro-parietal in center. (From Gotman et al., 1975.)

seen in supratentorial brain lesions, Gotman et al. found that the best weighting coefficients *a*, *b*, *c*, and *d* for discriminating between the two groups were 2.0 for low delta (.7–1.1 Hz), 4.0 for high delta (1.5–3.9 Hz), 5.0 for low theta (4.3–6.3 Hz), 1.0 for high theta (6.7–7.1 Hz), 1.5 for alpha (7.5–12.5 Hz), and .5 for beta (13.1–29.9 Hz) for all but frontal electrodes. Different values were used there to compensate for artifacts due to slow movements.

These ratios were used to produce a *canonogram*, a display of these intrachannel ratios giving a rapid visual indication of the localization and importance of the abnormality (see Fig. 11.2). The diameter or number of concentric rings is proportional to the square root of the corresponding channel ratio; therefore, an increase in slow activity or a decrease in the faster normal rhythms will be shown as a larger polygon.

The interchannel relationships were evaluated by the asymmetry coefficient, defined as the ratio of the slow activity of the lead with more slow activity to that of the homologous lead on the other hemisphere. At the midline of the display in Fig. 11.2, there are arrows whose deviations from the midline are proportional to the asymmetry coefficient between left and right homologous areas.

This method was compared with visual EEG interpretation in 87 patients (50 had tumors, 31 had vascular lesions, and 6 had miscellaneous lesions), in order to define the accuracy of localization of the lesions (Gotman et al., 1975). Localization was evaluated by a structured EEG report. Lateralization, extent, and localization of maximal intrachannel ratios were the *abnormality descriptors*. An overall assessment of severity was made on a 3-point scale, using the terminology "mild, moderate, severe." In the "normal" cases, no further information was given. A first report was written by the EEGer reading the complete traditional examination with knowledge of the patient's clinical problem. A second report was written by another EEGer interpreting the two sets of spectra knowing only the age of the patient. Three more reports were written for the interpretation of canonograms by three interpreters (A, B, and C). Finally, a last report reflected the location of the lesion as known from unequivocal surgical, radiological, and clinical evidence, and was considered the "reference data."

For each subject, the difference between the three types of EEG evaluation and the reference data were then assessed: (1) traditional EEG and reference data; (2) spectra and reference data; (3) canonograms (from interpreters A, B, and C); and (4) reference data. In order to quantify these differences, the structures reports were transformed into eight numbers or scores, one for each of the anatomical regions (on both sides, frontal, centro-parietal, temporal, and occipital) in the following way: For each of the three abnormality

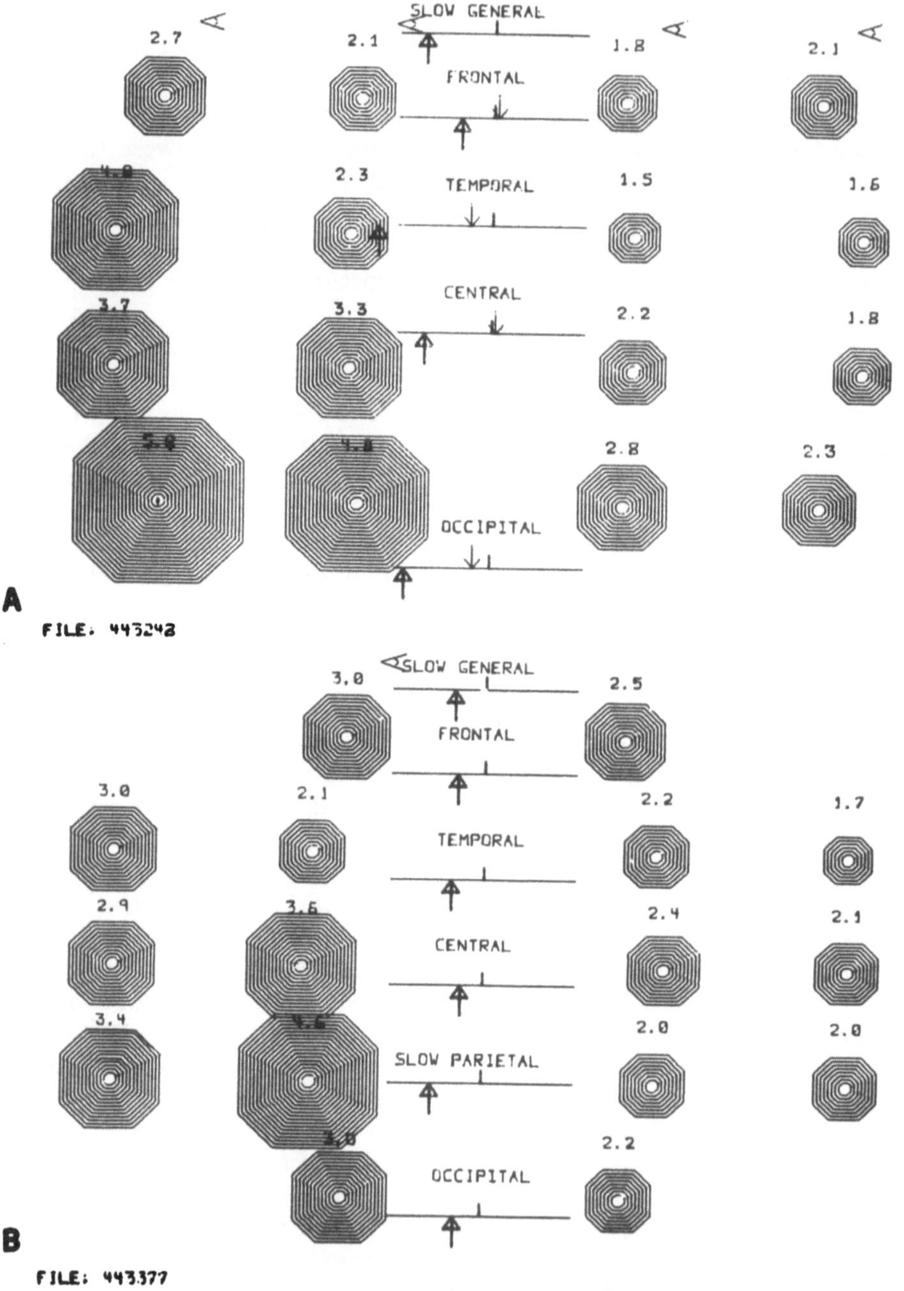

FIG. 11.2. Canonogram from the same subject as Fig. 11.1. Same montages. The arrows under the horizontal line indicate the asymmetry in slow activity. The arrows above the horizontal line (in the bipolar only) indicate the asymmetry in fast activity (alpha-beta). The arrows deviate toward the most abnormal side (more slow waves, fewer fast waves). (From Gotman et al., 1975.)

descriptors, points were distributed over the anatomical regions, according to the following rules:

1. Lateralization: If symmetrical, one point for each of the eight regions of the head; if right or left, one point for each region on that side.
2. Extent: If generalized, one point added to each of the regions of the head; if lateralized diffuse, one point added to each region of the side chosen; if localized, one point over the regions chosen under the "localization of maximum" entry.
3. Localization of maximum: One point over the regions selected in this entry, on one side if lateralization is right or left, on both sides if it is symmetrical. The score finally allocated to each anatomical region is equal to the sum of amounts successively allocated to this region by the foregoing evaluation rules. In each region, the difference between the scores of one source and the scores of the reference data is called the error of that source. Table 11.1 shows the errors committed using each different procedure.

The results varied according to the anatomical region: Whereas in frontal and occipital regions, the EEG was slightly more accurate than the canonograms, both methods were similar in the temporal areas and the canonogram seemed more accurate in the centro-parietal regions. Consistent interpretations were obtained by the three interpreters of the canonograms. One of them had no formal training in EEG. With a brief, 45-minutes explanation, he was able to encode and interpret the canonograms of 87 patients in 4 hours. Overall accuracy was best for the EEGer reading the conventional examination, slightly less for the average canonogram reader, and least, but still quite good, for the EEGer reading the power spectra. The computer evaluations were of sufficient accuracy to be useful supplementary information for an EEGer or to give a nonspecialist the basis for a tentative conclusion that definite neuropathology was present. These results show the reliability and value of this simple computer display for the EEG interpretation. Although the intention of the authors of this volume has not been to develop a procedure for the automatic assessment of the EEG, but to provide a simpler and better tool than the paper record for the electroencephalographer, this procedure can be considered to have completed some stages in the construction of a neurometric technique. One such stage is the extraction and selection of some features that permit the construction of a display that is easily interpreted and clinically accurate. Such features may be used as the basis for the establishment of a decision rule for completely automatic assessment of the EEG.

TABLE 11.1
Number and Percentage of Subjects Erroneously Declared Normal and with Erroneous Lateralization[a]

	EEG		*Canon. A*		*Canon. B*		*Canon. C*		*Spectra*	
	n	%	*n*	%	*n*	%	*n*	%	*n*	%
Within normal limits:	4	4.6	9	10	6	6.8	8	9.1	12	13.7
Erroneous lateralization including "symmetrical":	6	6.8	6	6.8	7	8.0	12	13.7	9	10.0
Erroneous lateralization excluding "symmetrical":	2	2.3	4	4.6	3	3.4	1	1.1	4	4.6

[a]From Gotman et al., 1975.

B. The "Deviance" Measure: A Comparison of Power Spectral Features, Normalized Slope Descriptors, and Visual EEG Interpretation

Binnie, Batchelow, Bowring, Darby, Herbert, Lloyd, Smith, Smith, and Smith (1978) compared visual EEG interpretation of EEG records with two procedures of quantitative analysis—power spectrum and normalized slope descriptors—in 63 patients with established pathology and 140 control subjects. The EEG was recorded in 24 bipolar derivations, 12 for each hemisphere. Sixteen artifact-free 8-sec epochs were chosen for analysis, eight with eyes opened and eight with eyes closed. The values obtained from spectral and slope descriptor analysis were averaged across these epochs for each derivation. Arithmetic means were calculated for each channel under eyes open and eyes closed. Spectral analysis was submitted to feature compression of six different types of combinations of frequencies, banding spectral values into delta (1–4 Hz), theta (4–8 Hz), alpha (8–14 Hz), and beta (more than 14 Hz) bands, or banding into seven frequency ranges (1–2 Hz, 2–4 Hz, 4–6 Hz, 6–8 Hz, 8–11 Hz, 11–14 Hz, and over 14 Hz) for each channel, or grouping the values from sets of three channels corresponding to anatomical regions, and by the addition of right/left quotients for each four frequency bands. Slope descriptors were also computed for the 24 derivations during eyes closed and eyes opened. All features were submitted to a logarithmic transformation and the mean and S/D were then calculated from 140 control subjects. The values of both patients and controls were then normalized by subtracting the mean and dividing by the SD of each feature of the control group. This is equivalent to Z-transforming all features, yielding measures reflecting relative probability, as used by John et al. (1977). This also ensured that in the control group, each feature had a zero mean and a S/D of 1. For each feature-compression strategy, derivation, and condition, the "deviance" (mean distance in the feature space from the point representing the EEG under analysis to the 10 nearest neighboring points from the control population) was calculated both for each normal subject and each patient. The 95th and 99th percentile values of the deviance were estimated, and were used to assess normality. Every EEG was classified as abnormal if two or more values deviated beyond the 99th percentile or if three exceeded the 95th. With this approach, no more than 5% of the controls were classified as abnormal using any of the feature-compression strategies.

Information about the percentage correct identification in the group of patients is not provided by Binnie et al. (1978). They present the results as mean, standard deviation, modulus mean, and median of error scores obtained by comparison of structured reports (like those previously described by Gotman et al., 1975) of various methods of EEG assessment with reference data. Table 11.2 shows these results. All methods based on power spectral analysis were more accurate than visual analysis (significant at .01 level for all strategies). Error rates obtained from slope descriptors were similar to those from visual analysis. There was no significant difference between the various strategies to compress spectral features: When compared to reference data, all tended to overestimate EEG abnormalities. The procedure was also compared with the results obtained by computation of canonograms. Significant lower ($P<.01$) errors were observed by the computation of deviance from spectral features. Table 11.2 shows the mean variance of signal error scores obtained by the different procedures. The lower the mean variance, the more constant (less variable) the error. Deviance computations of features derived from power spectral analysis have lower values than canonograms, visual inspection, and slope descriptors. Fig. 11.3 is a graphical display of deviance values in a patient with a right centro-parietal glioma.

We consider the results presented up to now as very promising. Nevertheless, it is extremely important to know the overall accuracy of the procedure in relation to the correct discrimination of patients and control subjects, as well as for localization of the lesion. We hope that as further development and evaluation of this technique progresses, the authors will provide, in the near future, more complete information.

C. Age-Dependent EEG Quotient (ADQ)

The group headed by Petersén in Göteborg, has developed a completely automatic procedure for the evaluation of the EEG background activity by means of frequency analysis. The similarities between abnormal EEGs with increased slow activity and normal EEGs in younger subjects were used as the basis for such a procedure (Matousek & Petersén, 1973b). The development of the method was made possible by the availability of a vast body of normative data. EEG recordings were made from fronto–temporal (F_7T_3 / F_8T_4), central (C_3C_z/ C_4C_z) temporal (T_3T_5 / T_4T_6), and parieto-occipital (P_3O_1 / P_4O_2) derivations of 560 normal subjects from 1 to 21 years old (Matousek & Petersén, 1973a). Epochs 60 seconds in duration stored on analog magnetic tape were chosen from these resting records and subjected to frequency analysis. This frequency analysis was performed by an analog device that divided the activity into six frequency bands (delta 1.5-3.5 Hz, theta 3.-7.5 Hz, $alpha_1$ 7.5-9.5 Hz, $alpha_2$ 9.5-12.5 Hz, $beta_1$ 12.5-17.5 Hz, and $beta_2$ 17.5-25 Hz). The primary output values were further processed by means of a digital computer, in which 20 variables were calculated: amplitude of activity in six frequency bands; the sum of these values; the relative quantity or percent of activity in six frequency bands; and 7 quotients ($alpha_1/alpha_2$, theta/ ($alpha_1$ + $alpha_2$ + 8), theta/ ($alpha_2$ + 8), $beta_1$/ ($alpha_1$ + $alpha_2$), $beta_2$/ ($alpha_1$ + $alpha_2$), delta/theta, $beta_1$/ $beta_2$.

Next, using these 20 variables, Matousek and Petersén (1971) obtained the

TABLE 11.2[a]
Mean and Standard Deviation of Error Scores[b]

Feature Extraction	Strategy	Error Scores X	SD	Modulus Mean	Error Median
Power spectral density	d[c]	.48	3.38	2.70	1
	e[d]	1.50	3.55	2.88	0
	f[e]	.14	3.03	2.95	4
Slope	h[f]	2.29	3.88	4.20	4
Visual		.35	5.12	4.04	4

Mean variance of signed errors of structured reports of various methods of EEG assessment with reference data (to permit comparison with results of Gotman et al., 1975).

Feature extraction	*Feature compression and decision-making*	*Mean of variances of signed errors for eight regions*
Power spectral density	Strategy (d)[c] + Deviance	.61[h]
	Strategy (e)[d] + Deviance	.40[hi]
	Strategy (f)[e] + Deviance	.49[hi]
	Canonograms + Visual[g] (best of three observes)	.95
	Visual inspection of raw spectral values	.97
Slope descriptors	Strategy (h)[f] + Deviance	.75
Visual (present study)	Subjective	.97
Visual (Gotman et al.)	Subjective	.73

[a] From Binnie et al., 1978.

[b] These scores were obtained by comparison of structured reports of various methods of EEG assessment with reference data. The means of signed errors are positive in all cases, reflecting a tendency to overestimate cerebral abnormality. Modulus errors indicate reliability; both mean and median values are given because the modulus scores are not normally distributed.

[c]Strategy (d): Banding spectral values into delta, theta, alpha, and beta and grouping (without summation or averaging) the values from sets of three channels corresponding to anatomical regions for eyes closed, together with eyes open/eyes closed quotients, for all four frequencies for groups of three channels. This gave 24 features for each of eight regions.

[d]Strategy (e): Banding spectral values into four frequency ranges and grouping the values from sets of three channels with eyes open and closed, but with the addition of right/left quotients for each of four frequencies from three channels per region. This gave 24 features on eight regions during eyes open/closed.

[e]Strategy (f): Banding spectral values into four frequency ranges and grouping the values from sets of three channels with eyes open or closed, and with mean quotients for each region of alpha and theta, eyes open/eyes closed, and alpha, theta and beta, right/left. This gave 17 features for eight regions.

[f]Strategy (h): Activity, mobility, and complexity, in 24 derivations (eyes open/closed).

[g] From Gotman et al., 1975.

[h] Differs from values both for visual analysis and for canonograms at 1% level (*F* test).

[i]Differs from lowest values for slope descriptor analysis (strategy h) at 1% level.

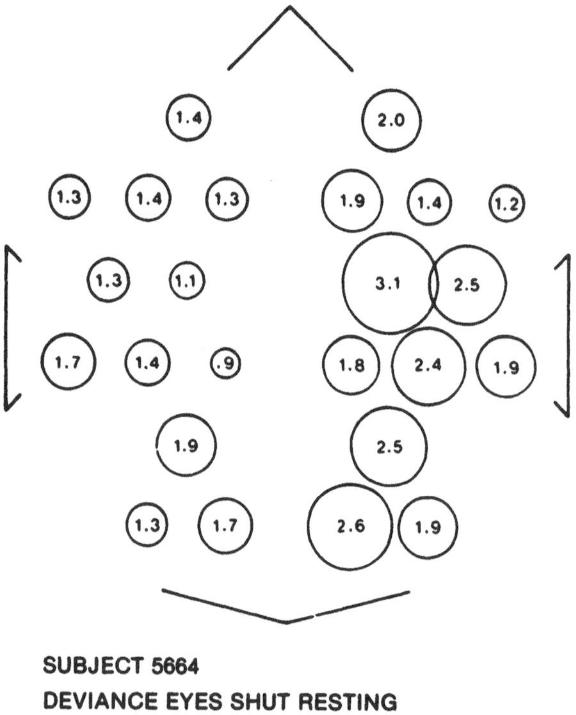

FIG. 11.3. Topographic display of deviance. Each circle is centered on the midpoint of the straight line joining the two electrodes contributing to the underlying bipolar derivation; radius is proportional to the corresponding deviance value. Patient with right centro-parietal glioma. (From Binnie et al., 1978.)

linear equations for calculating age (in months) for each derivation in any EEG for the total 560 EEGs, by a multiple regression analysis, in order to reach the highest possible correlation with age (Fig. 11.4). These equations could then be subsequently applied to any other EEG record and the hypothetical age calculated. The ratios obtained by dividing the age calculated from the EEG frequency distribution by the actual age of the patient were called Age-Dependent Quotients. They provided a powerful data-reduction method for the evaluation of EEG background activity, because the most important features of the EEG spectrum could be expressed in terms of single figures.

In normals EEGs, the computed values came close to 100 (the ratio expressed in percent) independently of the EEG derivation used and the age of the subject examined. If low frequencies contribute greater energy than normal to the spectrum from particular head regions, the hypothetical age calculated will be lower than the real age, and the ADQ will become less than

100. In general, the more abnormal the activity of a focal region, the lower the ADQ. The computer also evaluates symmetry between the quotients obtained in each pair of symmetrical EEG derivations. The numerical results are printed, together with identification data for the patient. A series of programs has been developed to present the results in verbal form. The global assessment is expressed by the computer using an 8-point scale from normal to very severe abnormality, taking into account differences between various EEG derivations, suppressing the less-pronounced changes, and combining the final information in a grammatically correct text.

To obtain an automatic assessment in a form similar to conventional formulation, some additional information is printed. For example, such findings as low-amplitude background activity or abundant fast rhythms may also appear in the conclusions. When the automatic assessment is completed, a series of additional programs check possible sources of error. An increased variability of the EEG signal during the 60 seconds of registration may cause some errors. For example, a pronounced fluctuation of alpha activity is

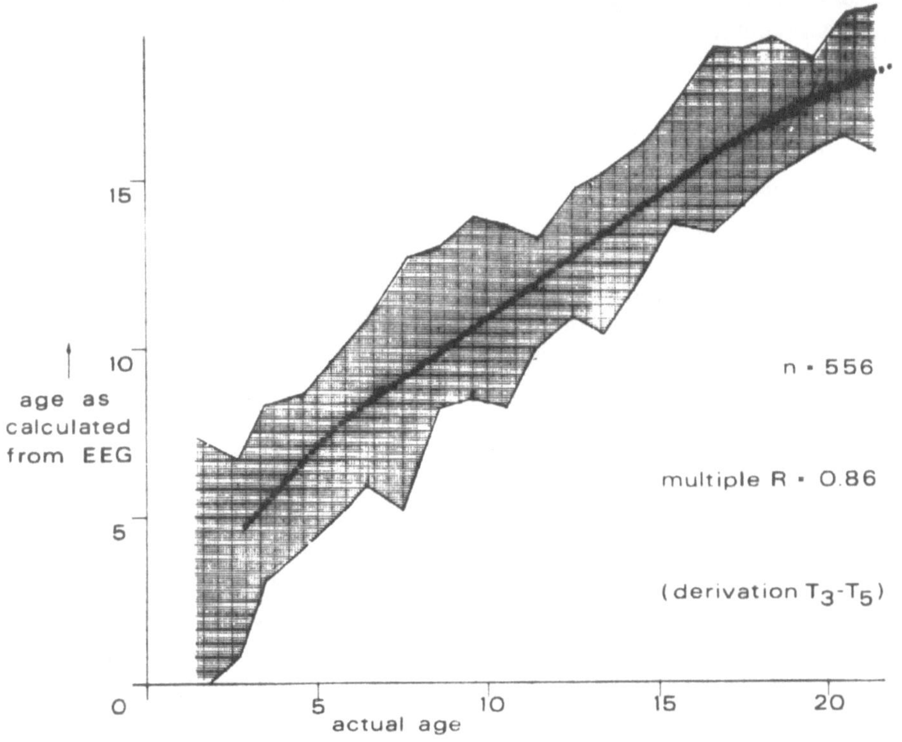

FIG. 11.4. Multiple regression analysis. It is possible to observe a strong correlation between real age and age as calculated from 20 variables of the EEG. The analysis was performed in 556 subjects 1 to 20 years old. Derivation: T_3 - T_5. (From Petersén & Matousek, 1975.)

related to drowsiness in many subjects. The appearance of sleep activity could be erroneously interpreted as EEG abnormality in these cases. The computer therefore prints a special notice about this. Some typical deviations in the spectrum and/or increased variability within the delta frequency bands serve to detect artifacts. In addition to an explanatory text, the computer tries to compensate for some of these disturbances. Thus, the appearance of diffuse slow activity in drowsy patients does not influence the final description of the EEG abnormality as much as do other types of slow activity. In records with suspected artifacts, the computer prints two alternatives to the final assessment; in the second one, the influence of very slow activity is partially supressed. Muscle artifacts are recognized by a disproportional increase of high-frequency activity (Friberg et al., 1976).

As a result, after 3 or 4 minutes of computation, an automatic assessment is printed with both numerical values and a written text, resembling conventional assessment. Fig. 11.5 shows an EEG from a patient with a right-sided brain disorder. The corresponding computer assessment starts with identification of the subject and the date of the examination. Then, a symbolic head containing the ADQs for the different derivations follows. Low values imply severe abnormality and 100 corresponds to complete normal. The assessment ends with a verbal description of the different activities and with a verbal conclusion. This print-out is obtained in a completely automatic way, the only inputs being the date of birth of the subject and one minute of that subject's EEG.

The method has been applied in more than 500 routine EEGs (Matousek, Petersén, & Friberg, 1975; Petersén & Matousek, 1975). Clinical evaluation of the method showed that 80% of the cases were in good agreement with the traditional EEG diagnosis based on the whole EEG record, whereas computer diagnosis was based on six 10-second epochs of the recording. More than one-half of the automatic print-outs could be used directly, without any change, as substitute for conventional EEG evaluation. The laterality of the actual cerebral involvement correlated to a high degree with laterality as determined by automatic EEG analysis (correlation coefficient = .98), whereas the correlation between clinical findings and the visual EEG assessment was significantly lower (correlation coefficient = .93). When the computer and the EEG technician agreed about the degree of abnormality, then the supervising electroencephalographer was of the same opinion.

The procedure has been also used as an objective measurement in the comparison of various EEGs taken from the same patient during clinical follow-up. In a progressive disease, a parallel increase in the ADQ is observed, whereas in subjects with an episodic abnormality of the EEG, the ADQ is similar during repeated observations (Fig. 11.6). Thus, a small series of short EEG examinations may be effective in solving the diagnostic problem of slight nonspecific abnormalities of the EEGs that may occur in normals, but that can also be the first step of some progressive brain disease.

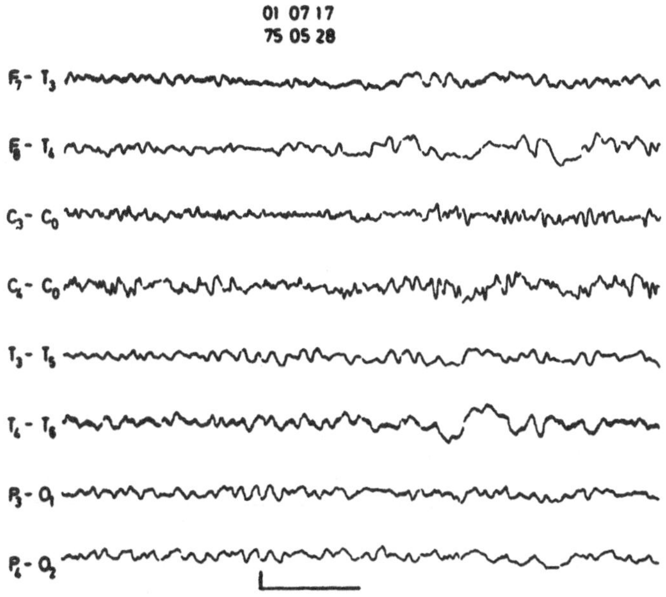


```
                                                   PATIENT:       01.07.17.
------------------------          *********        DATE:          75.05.28.
                                 *  47  29 *       EXAM. NO.:     01
                                 *  73  56 *
                                 *  11   4 *
                                 *  59  58 *     (MEAN  42)
                                  *********

THETA ACTIVITY WITH AN AMPLITUDE OF ABOUT 30 UV IS PROMINENT .
THE BACKGROUND ACTIVITY OCCURS WITH SOMEWHAT HIGHER AMPLITUDES
IN THE CENTRAL AND IN THE FRONTO-TEMPORAL REGION ON THE RIGHT
SIDE . MODERATE AMOUNT OF DELTA AND ALPHA ACTIVITY . THE
FIRST ACTIVITY IS MORE PRONOUNCED IN THE TEMPORAL REGION
WHERE IT OCCURS WITH RIGHT-SIDED PREPONDERANCE .

CONCLUSION:
VERY SEVERE ABNORMALITY IN THE FRONTO-TEMPORAL AND TEMPORAL
REGION ON THE RIGHT SIDE .
```

FIG. 11.5. An example of an EEG from a 74-year-old patient with a right-sided brain disorder. Calibrations are 50 μV and 1 second. The print-out from the automatic assessment program is very similar to the statement based on visual evaluation. (From Friberg et al., 1976.)

Bosaeus, Matousek, and Petersén (1977) correlated the ADQ with so-called tests of organicity (Bender–Gestalt test and the Bender Visual Retention test) and intelligence tests (Wechsler Intelligence Scale for Children) in 138 children, between 5 and 16 years of age, who had no pathological antecedents and no neurological signs. A detailed psychiatric examination showed that 13 children of the 138 had slight symptoms of cerebral dysfunction. They differed in their EEG frequency pattern from the rest of the group, being characterized by lower ADQs. In the whole sample, ADQ of

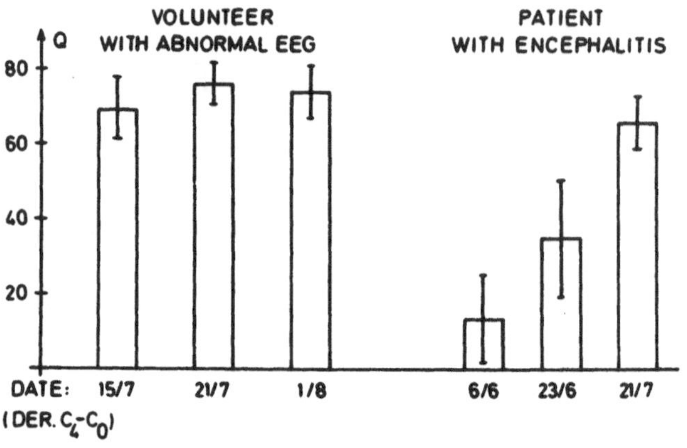

FIG. 11.6. Comparison of EEGs taken in two subjects at different time intervals. A volunteer with an abnormal EEG (left) displays similar results during repeated examinations. A patient with encephalitis (right) shows a considerable tendency to improvement of the EEG, and the quantitative information on variability makes the comparisons and evaluations of differences easier that it would be with access to the original tracing only. (From Friberg et al., 1976.)

temporal and parieto-occipital derivations showed a significant correlation with IQ values. Also, ADQ of temporal regions showed a significant correlation with the Bender–Gestalt test. Although significant correlations were also obtained between visual assessment of the EEG and the psychometric tests, the quantified data gave more pronounced results (higher correlation coefficients). This study confirms the sensitivity of the ADQ in the assessment of subtle brain abnormalities.

It can be concluded that the method described may be employed for fast EEG screening, in which only questionable results would have to be subjected to further supervision by an electroencephalographer. Theoretically, at least half of all routine EEGs could be assessed without this qualified help. Normal EEGs would be clearly identified, and, because the method provides a very sensitive and objective measurement, it seems to be extremely useful in the follow-up of neurological patients.

D. EEG Pattern Discrimination Using Autoregressive Analysis

On the basis of a time-series description of the EEG by a linear difference equation with constant coefficients, Sato, Ono, Chiba, and Fukata (1977) computed 15 autoregressive coefficients of the EEG in F_z–P_z derivation from 90 normal subjects in the resting state (standard group) and during hyperventilation. The distance between the average AR coefficient vector from a group of EEGs and the AR coefficients from an individual time series follows the F distribution. Thus, by this computation, it is possible to test if an EEG belongs to the standard group, with a critical level of significance ($P < .05$). All distance in the 90 EEGs during resting condition compared with the average vector of the standard group were below the critical level, whereas during hyperventilation, 7 (8%) were outside the critical limits. In 14 EEGs from epileptic-patients, 100% of the distances were outside the critical limit, suggesting an abnormal spectral pattern. Fig. 11.7 shows the differences between the 15 average coefficients of the standard EEG group and those during hyperventilation and those of epileptic patients. Marked difference of the third, fourth, and fifth coefficients between the standard group and the epileptic patients are observed.

In this procedure, the features used for the derivation of a decision-making rule were the 15 AR coefficients of the EEG segments. The decision-making rule was established on the basis of the definition of a multidimensional (15-dimension) normal space. Any subject whose EEG fell beyond this space with $P < .05$ was considered abnormal. The results suggest that with this procedure, it is possible to obtain an objective and accurate discrimination between normals and epileptics. Results from other types of neurological diseases will permit a more complete and definite evaluation of the method.

Crowell, Jones, Kapuniai, and Leung (1977) computed the AR coefficients of the EEG of three different groups of babies: low birth weight with gestational age lower or equal to 35 weeks; full-term babies 2 days old, and full-term babies from 6 weeks to 3 months old. They observed clear statistical differences between the three groups in occipital derivations. The AR coefficients of the EEG of the three groups were used as references for the classification of the EEG of two more babies. The first baby, with a gestational age of 24 weeks at birth, was recorded at 84 days after birth. He later died of sudden infant death syndrome. The record from his occipital regions

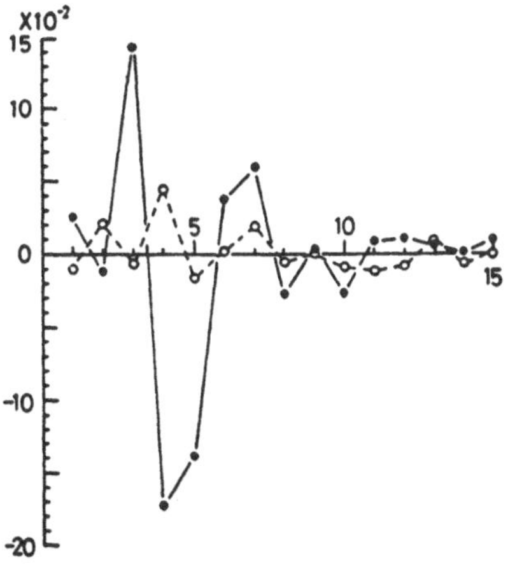

FIG. 11.7. Differences between the average AR coefficients of the standard group of 90 normal adults and those during hyperventilation (empty circles and broken line) and those between the former group and those of an epileptic group (filled circles and continuous line). *Abscissa*: order of AR coefficient. *Ordinate*: differences in the average AR coefficients. (From Sato et al., 1977.)

was classified in the low birth-weight group, and the EEG recorded from the central regions as belonging to the full-term babies 2 days old. The second baby was premature with a Cornelia de Lange syndrome, which was recorded 60 days of age and expired at 14 months. His central and left occipital EEG were classified in the 2-day-old group and the right occipital in the group 6 weeks to 3 months old.

III. INTERVAL-AMPLITUDE ANALYSIS: NEUROMETRIC APPROACH

Yamamoto, Shimazono, and Miyasaka (1977) recorded, from F_{p1}, C_3, and O_1, the EEG of 306 normal subjects and computed several parameters: (1) the average frequency; (2) the percent time in each frequency band; (3) the average amplitude in each frequency band; and (4) continuity or number of consecutive waves within the alpha and theta bands. Mean and standard deviation values for every measure in each location were obtained (see Table 11.3). These authors found that values under mean − 1.65 SD of the percent time alpha and the values over mean + 1.65 SD of the average amplitude of theta, the percent time theta, the continuity of theta, and the percent time delta were highly correlated with the EEGs judged as abnormal by visual inspection. This study is intended to establish a diagnostic logic for the automatic assessment of the EEG. Interval-amplitude analysis provides a high degree of data reduction and may be performed extremely fast, which allows implementation of on-line, real-time, multichannel analysis.

Yamamoto et al. have accomplished the first stages of a neurometric

TABLE 11.3
Interval-Amplitude Analysis: Normal Mean and Standard Deviations[a]

	F_{P1}		C_3		O_1	
	X	*SD*	*X*	*SD*	*X*	*SD*
Mean Frequency (Hz)	10.1	1.2	10.3	1.1	10.3	1.0
Delta % time[b]	2.9	4.1	1.4	1.5	1.1	1.0
Theta % time[b]	22.3	7.4	21.0	7.7	18.1	7.1
Alpha % time[c]	55.0	14.0	60.0	13.5	63.9	14.2
Beta % time	14.9	9.0	15.5	8.9	14.3	8.5
Maximal continuity of alpha	14.2	8.8	16.4	11.9	18.4	11.0
Maximal continuity of theta[b]	2.9	1.1	2.7	1.1	2.4	1.0
Delta average amplitude	-	-	-	-	18.0	13.7
Theta average amplitude	-	-	-	-	19.1	6.8
Alpha average amplitude	-	-	-	-	21.7	8.7
Beta average amplitude	-	-	-	-	13.8	4.1

[a] From Yamamoto et al. (1977).
[b] Values from X + 1.65 SD were correlated with EEG abnormality.
[c] Values under X - 1.65 SD were correlated with EEG abnormality.

method, because they have extracted more features that correlated with EEG abnormality. We hope that multivariate statistical analysis of such features will yield a good procedure for automatic EEG assessment.

IV. SYMMETRY ANALYSIS: POLARITY COINCIDENCE CORRELATION COEFFICIENT (PCC) AND SIGNAL ENERGY RATIO (SER)

On the basis that, in clinical EEG interpretation, asymmetries between both hemispheres are very important, a simple and rapid procedure has been used by Harmony, Otero, Ricardo, and Fernández (1973a); Otero, Harmony, and Ricardo (1975a, 1975b, 1975c), and Otero, Harmony, Ricardo, Llorente, Penalver, Estévez, and Roche (1974) for quantification of such asymmetries. They used two measures: the polarity coincidence correlation coefficient (PCC) and the signal energy ratio (SER). The basis for computation of PCC has been previously discussed in Chapter 9. It was considered particularly appropriate for quantification of the similarity between two electrophysiological signals because it emphasizes polarity and phase relationship, which intuitively seem physiologically relevant. Amplitude differences were assessed by computing the SER, which is the ratio between the squares of the amplitudes of the two signals. If the two signals have the same energy, SER is unity. For signals of different energy, SER values are expressed as the ratio of the larger to the small square, yielding values higher than unity, with a left or a right dominance.

Measures were done directly on-line with a Symmetry Analyzer (Neuro Data Model 2200) connected directly to the output of the electroencephalograph. All data appear as direct meter readings: from -1 to + 1, full scale for PCC and from 1 to 10 left/right and 1 to 10 right/left, full scale for SER measurements. PCC and SER were computed successively for homologous derivations. Measurements were obtained between left and right frontal, central, occipital, and temporal monopolar leads using linked ears as reference, and between left and right fronto-central, centro-occipital, occipito-temporal, temporo-frontal, and centro-temporal bipolar derivations.

A. PCC and SER in Adults

In a study of 92 normal subjects, PCC and SER appeared to be highly stable individual measures at time intervals of several weeks (Harmony et al., 1973a). Their relative frequency distribution showed low dispersion. No zero or negative values of PCC were found, which shows a high interhemispheric waveshape symmetry. PCC values from temporal derivations were found to be significantly lower than in other regions. Flicker stimulation produced a significant increase in the individual PCC values for all derivations except centro–temporal. When normal subjects were grouped into those with dominant alpha rhythm and those characterized by low-voltage activity, PCC values were found higher in the former group during rest and flicker stimulation, except in temporo–frontal and frontal derivations. These results showed that PCC was a sensitive measure, presenting regional differences, higher values during a stimulation that synchronized the EEG, and showing significantly different values in low-voltage EEGs. SER values were similar for all derivations and were not affected by flicker. A comparison of the percentage of subjects with left- or right- SER dominance showed a slight right dominance in frontal and fronto–central derivations, both with and without flicker. Although some subjects showed left-dominant and others right-dominant SERs, there were usually not significant differences in the absolute value of SER between left-dominant and right-dominant groups for the same derivation. This supported the utility of the absolute value of the SER for the detection of lateralized lesions, no matter which hemisphere is affected. Table 11.4 shows the mean and standard deviation values for each derivation in 144 healthy subjects. The Fischer z transform was used for computation of mean PCC values. Absolute SER values were used for calculation of means and standard deviations.

Otero et al. (1975a) studied 35 patients with intracranial tumors (six pituitary adenomas, three from brain stem, two from the cerebello–pontine angle, one thalamic, one from corpus callosum, and 22 from the hemispheres). Because no significant differences between left- and right-SER values were observed in normals, only absolute values of the SER measure

TABLE 11.4
Means and Standard Deviations for PCC and SER Measures from the Control Group, at Rest and During Visual Stimulation

Derivation	*Rest*				*Flicker*			
	PCC[a]		*SER*[b]		*PCC*[a]		*SER*[b]	
	X	*SD*	*X*	*SD*	*X*	*SD*	*X*	*SD*
Frontal	.53	.18	1.23	.12	.54	.18	1.24	.13
Central	.55	.18	1.21	.11	.57	.16	1.22	.06
Occipital	.52	.18	1.22	.09	.53	.18	1.23	.10
Temporal	.37	.13	1.25	.12	.39	.14	1.26	.11
Fronto–Central	.56	.15	1.23	.10	.58	.14	1.22	.10
Centro–Occipital	.59	.15	1.21	.11	.60	.15	1.22	.11
Occipito–Temporal	.48	.15	1.27	.11	.51	.16	1.25	.11
Temporo–Frontal	.45	.15	1.24	.10	.49	.18	1.24	.13
Centro–Temporal	.39	.12	1.26	.11	.40	.13	1.26	.12

[a]The Fisher z transform was used for computation of PCC values.
[b]Absolute SER values were used for computation.

were used. Mean PCC and SER values of this group are shown in Table 11.5. As expected, significant lower PCC values and higher SER values were observed in patients with brain tumors than in the control group, reflecting greater asymmetries in waveshape and amplitude. Of the 35 tumor cases, 10 had a normal EEG. In view of the locations of these tumors, the incidence of normal EEGs in this sample was comparable to that provided by other authors (Gibbs & Gibbs, 1964; Velasco, Lopez, Zenteno-Alanis, & Velasco, 1970).

In a group of 65 patients with cerebrovascular lesions, which included 38 cases of arterial occlusion, 12 cases with transitory vascular insufficiency, 5 subarachnoidal hemorrhages, 6 aneurysms, and 4 intraparenchymal hemorrhages, significant differences in PCC and SER values were also found (Otero et al., 1975b; see Table 11.6). Of the 65 patients, 26 had a normal EEG; considering the different kinds of lesions studied, this accuracy in the detection of abnormal EEGs was within the accepted criterion of Gibbs and Gibbs (1964) and other authors (see Chapter 2).

Twenty-five patients with a generalized epilepsy and 36 with focal epilepsy were also studied (Otero et al., 1974). Lower values of the PCC in FC and CT derivations during rest and in CO, OT, and CT derivations during visual stimulation were observed. Significantly higher values of the SER were obtained in temporal, CO and TF derivations in rest, and in temporal during flicker stimulation. A discriminate analysis with 36 variables showed no significant differences between this group of patients and the control group. The epileptics studied were characterized in their EEG by the presence of

TABLE 11.5
Means and Standard Deviations for PCC and SER measurements From the Group of Brain Tumor Patients, at Rest and During Visual Stimulation

Derivation	*Rest*				*Flicker*			
	PCC[a]		*SER*[b]		*PCC*[a]		*SER*[b]	
	X	*SD*	*X*	*SD*	*X*	*SD*	*X*	*SD*
Frontal	.55	.16	1.28[c]	.17	.53	.14	1.28	.22
Central	.53	.15	1.31	.28	.56	.14	1.30	.20
Occipital	.49	.13	1.31[c]	.17	.49[c]	.11	1.34[c]	.21
Temporal	.36	.13	1.31	.22	.36	.16	1.35	.25
Fronto-Central	.50[c]	.16	1.29[c]	.16	.51[c]	.19	1.31	.20
Centro-Occipital	.51[c]	.11	1.31[c]	.20	.50[c]	.13	1.34[c]	.10
Occipito Temporal	39[c]	.15	1.33	.18	.31[c]	.13	1.39[c]	.21
Temporo-Frontal	.42	.19	1.38[c]	.23	.41[c]	.16	1.34[c]	.22
Centro-Temporal	.34[c]	.10	1.39	.30	.35[c]	.13	1.45[c]	.33

[c]Significant different values from the control group ($P < .05$).
[a]The Fisher *z* transform was used for computation of PCC values.
[b]Absolute SER values were used for computation.

TABLE 11.6
Means and Standard Deviations for PCC and SER Measurements from the Group of Cerebrovascular Disease Patients, at Rest and During Visual Stimulation

Derivation	*Rest*				*Flicker*			
	PCC[a]		*SER*[b]		*PCC*[a]		*SER*[b]	
	X	*SD*	*X*	*SD*	*X*	*SD*	*X*	*SD*
Frontal	.51	.18	1.27[c]	.17	.52	.12	1.28[c]	.17
Central	.51[c]	.14	1.27	.26	.53[c]	.16	1.24	.12
Occipital	.47[c]	.17	1.29[c]	.17	.49[c]	.15	1.28[c]	.14
Temporal	.36	.14	1.31[c]	.17	.35[c]	.13	1.33[c]	.18
Fronto-Central	.49[c]	.14	1.27[c]	.17	.50[c]	.15	1.27[c]	.16
Centro-Temporal	.52[c]	.13	1.28[c]	.20	.52[c]	.14	1.26[c]	.15
Occipito-Temporal	.40[c]	.13	1.32[c]	.18	.43[c]	.12	1.30[c]	.17
Temporo-Frontal	.40[c]	.11	1.28[c]	.15	.41[c]	.18	1.28[c]	.14
Centro-Temporal	.34[c]	.11	1.31[c]	.17	.35[c]	.11	1.34[c]	.17

[c]Significant different values from the control group ($P < .05$).
[a]The Fisher *z* transform was used for computation of PCC values.
[b]Absolute SER values were used for computation.

isolated spikes in 52%, or short paroxysmal discharges of spikes and slow wave complexes (17%). The remaining cases showed a normal EEG (15%) or generalized slow waves (16%). It is clear that paroxysmal activity, unless it appears frequently, is difficult to detect with a procedure that only measures the average symmetry during long periods. Therefore, it was concluded that the method was not useful in detecting those pathologies in which a paroxysmal EEG activity is suspected.

1. Discrimination of Normal Subjects from Patients with Brain Tumors and Cerebovascular lesions.

For the computation of a multiple discriminant equation between these three groups, those variables with the highest significant differences between normals and the other two groups were selected (Otero et al., 1975c). The following variables used were : PCC values during rest in FC, CO, OT, and CT; PCC values during flicker stimulation in FC, CO, OT, and TF; and SER values during photic stimulation in CT. Two canonic variables (see Chapter 7) were obtained. The first one explained 85% of the total covariance and the second one the remaining 15%. The centroids of the corresponding groups are shown in Fig. 11.8. It is clear that the first canonical variable defines the limits between normality and abnormality, and the second one the differences between tumors and cerebrovascular lesions. Assignment of the different subjects to the group in which the Mahalanobis distance to the cen-

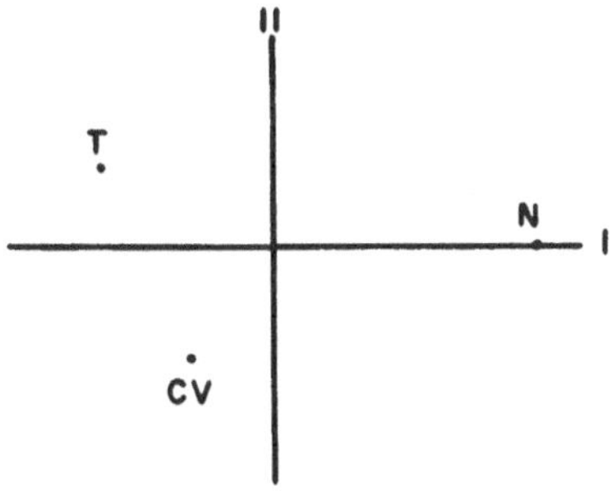

FIG. 11.8. EEG symmetry analysis: I and II, the two canonical variables resulting from the multiple discriminant analysis between the normal group (N), the group of cerebrovascular diseased patients (CV), and the group of patients with brain tumors (T). The centroid of each group has been plotted. It is possible to observe larger distances from T and CV to N than from CV to T. (From Otero et al., 1975c.)

troid was smallest produced the results shown in Table 11.7. Of the 100 patients with cerebrovascular and tumor lesions, 75 were correctly defined as abnormals, with 25 false negatives (25%). Of the 75 patients classified as abnormals, the differential diagnosis was correct in 50 cases (67%). These results show that this method defines the boundary between normal and abnormal subjects relatively well, but is somewhat less accurate in discriminating between different types of lesions. Patients with slight but numerous deviant values tended to be classified as cerebrovascular lesions, and patients with localized and higher deviant values as tumors. This agrees with what should be expected by their EEG alterations. No significant differences were found in the age distributions of the 38 (26%) misclassified normal subjects. However, the number of false positives that present a low-voltage EEG activity in their EEG was highly significant (15 out of 19 subjects with low-voltage EEG were classified as abnormal). In such cases, desynchronization of the EEG activity produces lower PCC values (Harmony et al., 1973a) and this may be the reason why they were classified as pathological. Further studies on this type of subject are in progress.

If we compare the number of patients with cerebrovascular lesions and normal EEG ($n = 26$) with the number of such patients that were assigned to the normal group by symmetry analysis ($n = 17$), it is clear that discriminant analysis of symmetry data provided a higher discriminatory accuracy than the visual examination of the EEG. Similar results were observed in the brain tumor group: 10 cases had a normal EEG, whereas eight were considered normal by symmetry analysis. Both methods, visual inspection of the EEG and symmetry analysis, yield a higher percentage of discrimination when used as complementary to each other: Of 100 patients, only 10 were considered normal. This indicates that their routine combination in clinical practice is highly desirable. Their combination with some other measures of evoked activity is discussed in a subsequent chapter. Apparently, the major drawback that this procedure presents is the high rate of false positives.

In selecting the members of the control group, our definition of "normali-

TABLE 11.7
Number and Percentage of Subjects Classified as Normal (N), Tumor (T), or Cerebrovascular Disease (CV)[a]

	Discriminant Analysis of Symmetry Measures								*EEG*				*EEG + Discriminant Analysis of Symmetry Measures*			
	N		*T*		*CV*		*A*[b]		*N*		*A*		*N*		*A*	
	n	%	*n*	%	*n*	%	*n*	%	*n*	%	*n*	%	*n*	%	*n*	%
Normals	106	74	14	9	24	17	38	26	144	100	0	0	106	74	38	26
Tumors	8	23	14	40	13	37	27	77	10	29	25	71	2	6	33	94
CV	17	26	12	18	36	55	48	73	26	40	39	60	8	12	57	88

[a]These were classified by discriminant analysis of EEG symmetry measures, such as normal (N) or abnormal (A), by EEG routine examination, and using both methods as complementary.

[b]Subjects who were assigned to the tumor or CV groups were consigned here.

ty'' took into consideration a negative neurological history, no clinical symptoms or signs of any disease and a normal EEG. A pilot study with a psychological test battery (Wechsler Adult Intelligence Scale, Bender-Gestalt, Machover, and Rorschach) was carried out in 30 subjects, selected from the normal group so as to maintain in a distribution of age and educational achievement levels similar to the whole sample. In 11 subjects, these tests revealed some type of abnormality—for example, signs of organic lesion, low IQ, or a very neurotic personality. Seven out of these 11 subjects had been classified as abnormal by the symmetry analysis and were among the false positives. This result suggests that this procedure may even be sensitive to subtle brain abnormalities not detected by medical or EEG examination. Because the procedure can be performed by an EEG technician and evaluated numerically without the presence of a specialist, it seems very useful as an item to be included into a mass-screening neurometric battery for the assessment of brain dysfunction in neurological patients.

B. PCC and SER in Children: Discriminating Normal Children From Children with Neurological Diseases

Using PCC and SER, a group of 110 children, consisting of 56 males and 54 females from 5 to 12 years old, was studied, (Figueredo, Pascual, Pozo, & Harmony, 1978). They were considered normal by clinical and electroencephalographic examinations. Table 11.8 shows the mean values and standard deviations of PCC for each year of age in five different bipolar derivations, during rest and flicker conditions. In normal children, the absolute SER values did not have a normal distribution; the most frequent value was 1.0, with a consequent extremely skewed distribution. For this reason, the logarithm of the SER values was used, being positive in the case of a left dominance and negative otherwise. Normative data from these children are presented in Table 11.10.

Correlation coefficients between each of the 20 variables and age were also computed. No significant correlation with age was found, with the exception of the PCC values from the OT derivation during rest, which only reached significance at the $p = .05$ level. This result makes possible the computation of the means and standard deviation values from the whole sample, making the comparison with other groups of similar age simpler.

With respect to normal adults, children were characterized by lower PCC and SER values. Thus, children present greater asymmetries in waveform than adults, but greater symmetry in amplitude. PCC values were also increased by flicker stimulation and maintained a similar distribution pattern, but still with lower values than that observed in adults: The highest values were observed in FC and CO derivations, both in rest and during flicker, and

TABLE 11.8
Means and Standard Deviations of PCC Values in Normal Children[a]

Age	*n*	*FC* *X*	*FC* *SD*	*OT* *X*	*OT* *SD*	*TF* *X*	*TF* *SD*	*CO* *X*	*CO* *SD*	*CT* *X*	*CT* *SD*
Rest Condition											
5	23	.41	.15	.34	.11	.32	.10	.43	.16	.32	.11
6	10	.45	.08	.35	.11	.31	.10	.42	.09	.38	.07
7	20	.42	.13	.35	.09	.32	.09	.42	.14	.28	.18
8	10	.41	.13	.34	.09	.33	.08	.41	.08	.35	.16
9	15	.47	.12	.42	.12	.39	.12	.51	.16	.34	.07
10	12	.41	.13	.35	.10	.35	.11	.46	.13	.34	.12
11	10	.41	.14	.41	.14	.32	.09	.41	.12	.31	.07
12	10	.45	.16	.41	.12	.35	.12	.49	.12	.40	.14
T[b]	110	.43	.14	.37	.12	.34	.11	.45	.14	.33	.13
During Flicker											
5	23	.43	.14	.41	.11	.35	.09	.47	.15	.39	.11
6	10	.49	.15	.42	.10	.35	.08	.43	.12	.40	.09
7	20	.44	.13	.40	.10	.35	.11	.45	.15	.33	.15
8	10	.42	.13	.42	.09	.40	.13	.49	.14	.41	.15
9	15	.52	.15	.46	.13	.45	.15	.52	.15	.39	.10
10	12	.48	.12	.43	.14	.40	.12	.54	.11	.37	.14
11	10	.45	.13	.45	.12	.35	.11	.46	.17	.33	.07
12	10	.51	.20	.47	.08	.35	.14	.51	.11	.40	.14
T[b]	110	.46	.15	.43	.12	.37	.12	.48	.15	.37	.13

[a]Fisher z transform of PCC values was used for computation.
[b]Total

lower values were found in temporal areas. These results suggest that children from 5 to 12 years old have not yet fully developed the synchronizing mechanisms that determine the interhemispheric coherence observed in the adult.

In relation to the greater symmetry in children, these results are in accord with those of Varner, Ellingson, Danahy, and Nelson (1977). They reported, also based on quantitative analysis of the EEG, that newborns were characterized by a great interhemispheric amplitude symmetry. The asymmetry in amplitude observed in normal adults has been related to hemispheric dominance. If this is so, higher amplitude symmetry in children may reflect that the complex mechanisms involved in hemispheric dominance are not yet completely developed. This has been suggested by Giannitrapani (1967) who reported that EEG activity in anterior temporal regions becomes asymmetrical with maturation, apparently reflecting the lateralization of neural process related to language acquisition.

A group of 150 5 to 12-year-old children with neurological diseases were also studied using these measures. This group was composed of 93 epileptic children, 30 with "minimal brain dysfunction," and 27 children with "miscellaneous other diseases" (eight cerebral palsy, five mentally retarded, four brain tumors, four meningoencephalitis, and six with other diseases). Minimal brain dysfunction (MBD) is a term that has been criticized by several authors. The group thus labeled consisted of children from 7 to 12 years old, who presented learning difficulties and/or hyperquinesis, with a normal IQ. These patients had all been sent to the EEG department of the William Soler Children's Hospital in Havana, where EEG and symmetry analyses were performed. Thus, the distribution of these patients according to different types of diseases is fairly representative of the more common disorders observed in an EEG department of a children's hospital.

Table 11.9 shows the means and standard deviations of PCC values for each group and for the whole sample of patients. Significant different values ($p \leq .05$) from the control group, as assessed by the t test, are also shown. It is possible to observe lower PCC values in the epileptic and miscellaneous group in several derivations. Table 11.10 shows the means and standard deviations of the absolute values and logarithmic transforms of the SER. We present the SER absolute values to give the reader a point of comparison with the values described in adults subjects. Student's tests were only computed using logarithmic values. Significant differences between the groups of patients and the normal group were again found.

A step-wise nonlinear discriminant analysis (see Chapter 7) was computed between the 110 control children and the 150 patients, using the Fisher z transform for the PCC values and the logarithmic transform for the SER values. The following variables were selected: (1) SER in FC during rest; (2) PCC in FC during flicker; (3) SER in CO during rest; (4) SER in OT during flicker; and (5) SER in TF during flicker. Of these five variables, only the first, second, and fourth appeared as significant in the univariate analysis. With these five variables, a nonlinear discriminant analysis (Victor, 1971) between the two groups was computed, considering equal a priori probabilities. The accuracy of classification of these children by the application of the equation is shown in Table 11.11. Table 11.11 also shows the number of subjects who displayed a normal (N) or abnormal (A) EEG, and the benefit of utilizing PCC and SER measures as complementary to the EEG.

Visual EEG examination yielded a total of 67% abnormal EEGs. Considering the different diseases studied, this result is similar to the figures reported by Forssman and Frey (1953), Ellingson (1955), and Gibbs and Gibbs (1964). Symmetry analysis achieved a higher level of detection (81%) in patients, but introduced 17% false positives, which were randomly distributed with respect to age. When both procedures were used as complementary, the detection of abnormalities increased to 93% of the total pa-

TABLE 11.9
Means and Standard Deviations of PCC Values in Different Groups of Children

Rest Condition		*FC*		*OT*		*TF*		*CO*		*CT*	
Group	*n*	*X*	*SD*	*X*	*SD*	*X*	*SD*	*X*	*SD*	*X*	*SD*
Epilepsy	93	.35[a]	.11	.37	.10	.29[a]	.09	.37[a]	.10	.33	.09
MBD	30	.45	.13	.39	.10	.38[a]	.10	.45	.13	.35	.09
Miscellaneous	27	.35[a]	.08	.35	.13	.31	.07	.36[a]	.14	.34	.07
TOTAL	150	.36[a]	.12	.37	.10	.31[a]	.10	.38[a]	.12	.34	.09
Normals	110	.43	.14	.37	.12	.34	.11	.45	.14	.33	.13
Flicker Condition											
Epilepsy	93	.36[a]	.11	.40[a]	.10	.34[a]	.10	.40[a]	.10	.35	.10
MBD	30	.49	.16	.42	.11	.40	.11	.49	.12	.39	.11
Miscellaneous	27	.35[a]	.10	.38[a]	.14	.33[a]	.10	.39[a]	.15	.35	.08
TOTAL	150	.39[a]	.14	.40[a]	.11	.35[a]	.10	.41[a]	.12	.35	.10
Normals	110	.46	.15	.43	.12	.37	.12	.48	.15	.37	.13

[a]Significant different values from the normal group ($P < .05$).

TABLE 11.10
Means and Standard Deviations of Absolute Values and Logarithmic Transformations of SER in Different Groups of Children

Group	n	FC X	FC SD	OT X	OT SD	TF X	TF SD	CO X	CO SD	OT X	OT SD
Rest Condition											
Epilepsy	93	1.17	.10	1.18	.14	1.15	.10	1.19	.12	1.17	.10
		.19[a]	.080	−.006	.080	−.021[a]	.080	−.013	.080	−.010[a]	.080
MBD	30	1.16	.14	1.15	.11	1.11	.11	1.13	.11	1.13	.20
		.009	.080	−.002	.100	−.005	.100	−.015	.070	.005	.080
Miscellaneous	27	1.18	.08	1.20	.10	1.16	.11	1.18	.10	1.15	.10
		−.054	.095	.017	.070	−.004	.075	.003	.080	.13	.070
Total	150	1.17	.10	1.18	.12	1.14	.11	1.17	.11	1.16	.11
		−.020[a]	.080	−.004	.080	−.010[a]	.070	−.010	.080	−.010[a]	.080
Normals	110	1.09	.12	1.11	.12	1.08	.09	1.09	.10	1.11	.11
		.015	.050	−.002	.070	−.005	.050	−.018	.050	.012	.060
Flicker Condition											
Epilepsy	93	1.17	.10	1.19	.14	1.17	.12	1.20	.11	1.20	.11
		−.001	.080	.006[a]	.085	−.002	.113	−.002[a]	.090	−.014[a]	.090
MBD	30	1.12	.12	1.13	.10	1.12	.11	1.12	.12	1.15	.18
		.011	.070	.015[a]	.070	.007	.060	−.005	.070	−.007	.080
Miscellaneous	27	1.15	.12	1.19	.11	1.17	.12	1.15	.10	1.20	.12
		−.017	.100	−.020	.080	.003	.080	.009	.070	−.001	.090
Total	150	1.15	.12	1.18	.12	1.16	.12	1.16	.12	1.19	.12
		−.005	.070	.006[a]	.080	−.010	.080	−.003	.080	−.006	.090
Normals	110	1.08	.14	1.11	.13	1.08	.10	1.10	.11	1.12	.13
		−.003	.050	−.015	.060	−.005	.050	−.013	.070	.011	.060

[a]Significantly different values from the normal group ($P < .05$).

TABLE 11.11
Number and Percentage of Children Classified as Normal (N) or Abnormal (A) by EEG Routine Examination, Discriminant Analysis and Using Both Methods as Complementary.

Group	EEG				Discriminant analysis of Symmetry Measures				EEG + Disc. analysis of Symmetry Measures			
	N		A		N		A		N		A	
	n	%	n	%	n	%	n	%	n	%	n	%
Normal	110	100	0	0	91	83	19	17	91	83	19	17
Epilepsy	28	30	65	70	13	14	80	86	4	4	89	96
M B D	14	46	16	54	13	43	17	57	6	20	24	80
Miscellaneous	8	29	19	71	3	11	24	89	1	3	26	97
Total Patients	50	33	100	67	29	19	121	81	11	7	139	93

tients. An interesting finding was that 86% of the epileptic children were detected with symmetry analysis. This is a very different result compared to that observed in adults. Because the miscellaneous group was mainly composed of children with severe brain damage, it was not unexpected to find a high percentage of abnormals. In the minimal brain dysfunction group, the discrimination was only 57% by symmetry analysis, similar to what was observed in the routine EEG examination (54%). However, if both procedures were used complementary, 80% were classified as abnormal. Within this group, 11 patients had slow waves and five paroxysmal activity; eight who had a normal EEG were classified as abnormal by the symmetry analysis.

The results just described using PCC and SER measures suggest that these variables are useful in the assessment of brain dysfunction in neurological patients. However, we consider this information as preliminary. More accurate results may be obtained by combining these variables with other variables of the EEG and the evoked responses. Our group at the CENIC is working in this direction with the hope of achieving optimal levels of detection of brain dysfunctions with a minimum incidence of false positives.

V. THE Z VECTOR: SPECTRAL PLUS SYMMETRY ANALYSIS

John et al. (1977) described the application of the z transform to each variable computed during a powerful neurometric battery that analyzed the spontaneous background activity and the evoked responses of the subject (see Volume II of this series, John, 1977). The z value was obtained by the difference between the individual index and the group mean value, divided by the standard deviation of the whole sample. In this way, every individual index was transformed from its original units to a common metric, reflecting the relative probability of that value within a healthy normal reference group. "Abnormality" was defined statistically as improbably values, exceeding those expected randomly allowing for the large size of the measure set.

The "abnormal profile" of any individual can now be represented as a z vector (or $\mathbf{z}$). The $\mathbf{z}$ of the perfectly normal individual only randomly leaves the normal domain defined by a hypersphere with radius $\mathbf{z} = 2$ ($P < .05$ on each dimension independently) centered at the origin of this space. The distance matrix, D_{ij}, can how be computed between $\mathbf{z}$ representing each individual and $\mathbf{z}$ of every other relevant individual, yielding interindividual distances in probabilistic terms. However, the following criticisms are valid for this procedure: For computation of the $\mathbf{z}$ vector, it was assumed that each variable is independent, which is very difficult to ensure without a statistical test; the interrelationships between the different variables were not taken into account; the Type I error was not controlled and a signficant value may be observed, when making comparisons, that is not due to real differences.

Thus, treatment of data in such a way should be considered as preliminary. A more correct final approach, following the same idea, would be the computation of the "normal space" in a multivariate form and the evaluation of a given individual with respect to that person's position in such space.

The EEG features computed by John et al. (1977) for the comparison between learning-disabled children and normal children were:

1. Absolute power in low delta (.5-1.5 Hz), high delta (1.5-3 Hz), theta (3–7 Hz), alpha (7–13 Hz), low beta (13–19 Hz), high beta (19–25 Hz), gamma (25–40 Hz), and total (.5–40 Hz) frequency bands.
2. Relative power (percentage) in each frequency band;
3. Ratio of delta plus theta to alpha power.
4. Power symmetry within each frequency band and between each pair of homologous derivations.
5. Waveshape symmetry as assessed by cross correlation of the total signals and by coherence within each frequency band between each homologous pair.

The following features extracted from the VERs to blank flashes and spatial grids with 27 and 7 lines per inch were also computed:

1. Difference in signal power between homologous pairs.
2. Normalized difference in signal power between homologous pairs, broken down into one term representing waveshape asymmetry and one term representing power asymmetry.
3. Cross correlation coefficients between homologous pairs.

As a first step, a polynomial regression was computed to fit the set of values for power in the various EEG bands as a function of age and electrode derivation obtained from normal children by Matousek and Petersén (1973a). For each frequency band and electrode derivation, this procedure yielded a smoothed regression function based on 561 subjects. The regression function offers the further advantage of allowing interpolation of values corresponding to the actual age of any child, whereas the original data were quantized into yearly increments. These polynomial functions agreed very well with comparable data obtained from 85 children considered normal by John, and only minor adjustments were made to compensate for interlaboratory differences.

Means and standard deviations for EEG and VER symmetry were computed in a group of 118 control children. Using these normative data, the EEG and VER indices from 533 learning-disabled and 50 normal children (randomly selected from the initial normal sample) were subjected to z transformations. Indices with z transform values equal to or larger than 1.96

($p < .05$) were defined as "dysfunctional" and tallied separately for bilateral parieto–occipital (PO), central (C), and temporal (T) derivations. The VER indices were only considered dysfunctional if the same index was deviant in the same region for at least two out of three of the visual stimulus conditions (blank, 27, and 7 lines per inch). Table 12.12 presents the results obtained, expressed as percentage of cases shown with "dysfunctional values" in normal (*N*) and learning-disabled (*LD*) children according to anatomical locations (columns) and "types" of neurometric dysfunction (rows).

For computation of the percentage of cases that show "dysfunctional values," the LD were divided into two groups of 265 and 268 children each. The correlation between the distribution of abnormal z values in both groups was highly significant ($r = .99$). Data from both groups were then combined to give the figures presented in Table 11.12. Thus, the two groups of LD children, evaluated independently, showed the same results.

If all possible locations and types of neurometrics abnormalities are considered, 92.6% of the LD group and 20% of the normal group showed "dysfunctional values." The unusual values in the normal group were always restricted to one anatomical location (PO or T) and consisted of dysfunction on only a single type of neurometric measure (EEG frequency or EEG symmetry). This pattern of dysfunction was rarely observed in LD children (7%). A high percentage of LD children were characterized by displaying more than one type of neurometric dysfunction in more than one anatomical derivation. These results demonstrate the possibility of discrimination by neurometric procedures of LD from normal children with high accuracy, and they suggest the existence of different subgroups of LD children. Extensive retrospective, longitudinal, and behavioral studies of these children are now in progress and will be presented in a later volume of this series.

VI. FACTOR SCORES DERIVED FROM EEG AND VERS PARAMETERS FOR THE CLASSIFICATION OF ALCOHOLIC AND SCHIZOPHRENIC PATIENTS

This procedure shows the possibility of feature extraction by the application of principal component analysis (see Chapter 7) to a set of measures of the EEG and VERs. This approach has also been used by John (1977) for the discrimination of learning-disabled children and was described in Volume II of this series (John, 1977).

Coger, Dymond, and Serafetinides (1976) recorded the EEG and VERs to flashes in left and right centro–occipital derivations in different groups of patients: 22 male alcoholic patients who had been withdrawn from alcohol (stabilized alcoholics); 18 male alcoholics undergoing alcoholic withdrawal one week after cessation of drinking (withdrawal alcoholics), and 17 male

TABLE 11.12
Z Vector: Percentage of Cases with Dysfunctional Values Accordings to Anatomical Location and Types of Neurometric Dysfunction in Normal (*N*) and Learning-Disabled (*LD*) Children[a]

PO		*C*		*T*		*PO + C*		*PO + T*		*C + T*		*PO + C + T*		*Total*	
N	*LD*	*N*	*LD*	*N*	*LD*	*N*	*LD*	*N*	*LD*	*N*	*LD*	*N*	*LD*	*N*	*LD*
EEG Frequency															
6.0	.4	0	1.1	6.0	.6	0	.4	0	.2	0	.9	0	1.5	12.0	5.1
EEG Asymmetry															
4.0	.6	0	0	4.0	3.9	0	0	0	.4	0	0	0	.4	8.0	5.3
EEG Frequency and EEG Asymmetry															
0	0	0	.4	0	.6	0	0	0	4.5	0	.9	0	4.7	0	11.1
VER Asymmetry															
0	3.0	0	1.7	0	1.5	0	3.4	0	.8	0	.9	0	3.0	0	14.3
EEG Frequency and VER Asymmetry															
0	0	0	.4	0	0	0	.9	0	.8	0	.6	0	7.3	0	9.9
EEG Asymmetry and VER Asymmetry															
0	0	0	.2	0	.4	0	1.1	0	1.7	0	1.7	0	7.1	0	12.2
EEG Frequency and EEG Asymmetry and VER Asymmetry															
0	0	0	0	0	.6	0	.9	0	4.5	0	1.9	0	26.8	0	34.7
Total															
10.0	4.0	0	3.8	10.0	7.6	0	6.8	0	12.9	0	6.9	0	50.8	20.0	92.6

[a]From John et al. (1977).

schizophrenics who had been stabilized for four weeks on the antipsychotic drug, Penfloridel. They then computed the log EEG power for every 2 Hz band from 0–30 Hz, the P100–N140 amplitude and latency of VERs, the least-squares slope for amplitude as a function of four intensity flash values, and the asymmetry score for all the EEG and VER variables using the formula (L-R)/L + R). Using the 56 variables so obtained in the three groups, a principal component analysis was performed.

A total of 10 factors accounted for approximately 84% of the variance. Power, asymmetry, and evoked potential variables showed different factor loadings, indicating relative independence between these measures. A preliminary comparison of the factor scores for each group was made by the Behrens–Fisher *t* test. The factors that were found to differentiate the two alcoholic groups ($P < .05$) included the asymmetry of the ER amplitude and the asymmetry of the power between 2 and 14 Hz. The results indicate that the withdrawal group tended to have significantly higher amplitude on the right side, whereas the stabilized alcoholics tended to have higher left-side values. The schizophrenics differed from both alcoholic groups in the high-frequency power band factor as well as the evoked-response slope and amplitude factors. They were distinguished from the stabilized alcoholic group on the basis of 2–14 Hz asymmetry in addition to high-frequency power.

Step-wise linear discriminant analysis was performed, using the factor scores as input variables for one-half of the subjects. The remainder of the subjects were later classified on the basis of the resulting equation. A total of four factors entered into the discrimination formula: slope and evoked potential amplitude, asymmetry of the 2–14 Hz power, 10–30 Hz power, and 6–12 Hz power as a final step. The percentage of correct discrimination of the group of subjects used for computation of the equation was 100% for schizophrenics, 73% for stabilized alcoholics, and 78% for withdrawal alcoholics. Replication of the equation on those subjects who had not been included in the initial calculation showed a correct classification of 100% for schizophrenics, 82% for stabilized alcoholics, and 67% for withdrawal alcoholics.

As has been discussed in Chapter 7, many complex multivariate predictors perform well for the sample used to construct the equation, but do not predict well in replication studies. The similarity of the correct classification obtained in this study with both groups supports the conclusion that the factors obtained by principal component analysis may well describe real differences between the three groups. These results seem very promising, although the small size of the same compels us to regard them as only preliminary. Further, one must remember that the factors were obtained by principal component analysis of the whole sample. This might introduce a bias on the results of the replication study, because the factors that were obtained reflected most of the variance of the individual measures not only of the group used for the initial computation of the linear-discriminant equation, but also of the remaining subjects used to validate the equation. We look forward to a truly independent replication of this interesting study, which will permit evaluation of the effect of this potential technical flaw.

VII. CONCLUSIONS

In the development of automatic procedures for the assessment of the EEG background activity, the intention of many authors has been basically to provide more simple and objective tools to the electroencephalographer than the standard paper records. Whether it is possible to supplant traditional EEG by automatic procedures has long been discussed. One major purpose of this book is to show that this is possible by neurometric methods. In order to be of practical value, these new methods must be at least as accurate as visual EEG interpretation for the assessment of brain dysfunction.

By the comparative study of neurometric procedures based on the analysis of brief time periods of the EEG versus EEG routine traditional interpretation of long records, the following conclusions may be reached to date:

1. In patients with well-defined brain lesions, deviance computations based on spectral features and the Age-Dependent Quotient (ADQ) have achieved significant greater accuracy than routine visual interpretation. The results obtained with canonograms varied according to the anatomical region of the lesion, being more accurate than the routine EEG in frontal and occipital areas.
2. Evaluating a large amount of unselected material consisting of 500 cases referred to an EEG department, ADQ showed 80% agreement with traditional EEG diagnosis.
3. In subtle brain abnormalities—for example, in children with cerebral dysfunction—lower ADQs were observed. ADQs have higher correlation coefficients with psychometric tests than visual EEG interpretation in a group of healthy children.
4. Symmetry analysis by PCC and SER measurements discriminate more brain tumors and cerebrovascular lesions, but fewer cases of epilepsy in adults than the routine EEG. In children, more cases of epileptics and other neurological lesions were discriminated by symmetry analysis than by EEG visual assessment, whereas the accuracy of the two methods was similar for children with MBD. Nevertheless, this procedure yields approximately 20% false positives, which is an important inconvenience that must be taken into account and rectified.

Two more facts should be considered:

1. Neurometric procedures provide an objective measurement in the comparison of various EEGs recorded from the same patient during clinical follow-up.
2. If a neurometric procedure is designed not only to evaluate the EEG background activity, but to utilize spike detection and the analysis of evoked responses as well, it is possible to increase the level of accuracy (as we see in Chapter 13). Even subtle brain abnormalities can be detected, as already described with the computation of the **Z** vector in learning-disabled children.

These results clearly establish that objective, sensitive, and accurate procedures for the automatic assessment of brain dysfunction are now available using neurometric evaluation of EEG background activity. These procedures already exceed the accuracy of the EEG for detection of certain kinds of brain diseases and dysfunction. They offer the possibility of serving as extremely useful supplements to the routine EEG examination for other purposes in which neurometric plus routine methods yield much greater accuracy than either alone. For the electroencephalographer who has more patients requiring attention than he or she can examine, and for those many regions where electroencephalography is effectively not available, neurometric evaluation of the background EEG offers an immediate and practical way to improve the diagnosis of the patient with brain disease or dysfunctions.

12 Automatic Spike Detection and Seizure Monitoring

I. INTRODUCTION

The traditional EEG interpretation is of great value in diagnosing various types of epilepsy, as we have seen in Chapter 2. Diagnosis is often made during interictal activity, and it is rare to record a seizure. In the last few years, continuous monitoring of the EEG activity has been a valuable tool in the study of epileptic patients in many ways: providing a reliable means of recording the patient's spontaneous seizures; aiding the study of the relationships between seizures and interictal spike activity and the development of warning devices for prediction of onset of seizures; yielding a better definition of the localization of the foci for subsequent surgery; providing an objective measurement of the effect of different treatments, enabling studies of the effects of various environmental and/or psychological factors, either positive or negative, on the frequency of seizures; and facilitating study of the ultradian characteristics of epileptic activity. For continuous monitoring of the EEG activity, telemetric systems or small portable cassette recorders have been used. These procedures allow the patient to maintain a normal routine, without restricting activity and without reduction in the quality of the EEG obtained compared with conventional recording methods. Emphasis has been also made on the simultaneous video and EEG recording of seizures in order to study clinical and electroencephalographic interrelationships (see Kellaway & Petersén, 1976).

The visual evaluation of these long-term recordings is obviously laborious and time consuming. Thus, it seems desirable to obtain a more efficient procedure that, by the automatic recognition of spikes and related epileptogenic activity, may provide a quantitative evaluation of the type, frequency, localization, and so on, of such activity. In some cases, such as in the development of warning devices for the prediction of onset of seizure activity, it is necessary to establish decision rules, based on the analysis of the interictal spike activity, in order to emit a warning signal to the patient so that the patient or the medical personnel may act in time to control the imminent seizure. For the automatic assessment of EEG activity for diagnostic purposes, the inclusion of spike-detection procedures is also necessary to obtain an integrated system that can be applied to any patient.

Recognition of spike foci has proved to be a difficult field for EEG automation, and although many methods have been described, progress has been slow. This may be related to the lack of an adequate theoretical model as the basis for the design of many procedures of spike detection. With the exception of inverse filtering, which is based on the AR model of the EEG and has proved to be a very powerful method, in general, the strategy used has been to try to simulate the criteria used by the electroencephalographers to identify the spikes and related epileptogenic activity. We want to direct the attention of the reader to three fundamental interrelated difficulties that have retarded the successful development of automatic spike detection: (1) the lack of an objective reference for the evaluation of the accuracy of spike detection methods; (2) the absence in the EEG literature of a precise characterization of spike activity and related epileptogenic patterns, which would permit their differentiation from the remaining EEG activity; and (3) the great apparent variability of the patterns proposed. The three factors are directly related to the present state of knowledge about the physiological mechanisms involved in the generation of epileptogenic activity and its propagation. Many years of intense research in this field have provided much valuable information, but many facts still have not been clarified. Progress in basic research will enhance the creation of theoretical models and more efficient procedures for the identification of different patterns of epileptogenic activity. On the other hand, clinical applications of automatic detection will provide quantitative information that might be useful in the explanation of some basic mechanisms of epilepsy.

The great variation observed in the spikes and spike-like waves, as well as the lack of precise definitions of their characteristics, is also revealed in routine visual EEG interpretation. It is well known in electroencephalography that there are some types of spikes that any specialist would no doubt declare as epileptic spikes by visual inspection, but there are also some types of waves that different specialists would interpret differently. Chiappa et al. (1976) constructed test sheets containing spikes, artifacts, and other transients and polled experienced electroencephalographers to mark the components that they would regard as spikes. These studies showed that electroencephalographers were inconsistent when retested in spike-data displays and that they had difficulty in deciding how many spikes were present in a test sheet. This creates another problem for the evaluation of automatic spike detection procedures, because the reference for evaluation will be the report of a human scorer, and this reference is not absolutely certain. From a theoretical point of view, this might be seen as an unsolvable problem, but in practice this can be overcome by comparing the accuracy of the automatic detection with that of various experts. If the computer detection is within the range of the interexpert variability, we can accept it as an adequate procedure. Thus, to seek for 100% precision in an automatic spike detection procedure is meaningless at this stage of our knowledge.

Following are the characterization of spike activity: some definitions concerning Jasper and Kershman (1949) divided focal epileptiform activity into spikes (10-50 msec duration) and sharp waves (50-500 msec); Chatrian et al. (1974) considered that spikes have a duration from 20-70 msec and sharp waves from 70-200 msec; Celesia and Chen (1976), in a study of 600 spikes of 100 epileptics, found that the range of duration varied from 9-200 msec with a mean of 45.06 msec, and that no evidence exists for the differentiation of sharp waves and spikes. These definitions are obviously unsatisfactory for computer usage. Gloor (1977) proposed different criteria that may help to distinguish spike and sharp waves of epileptogenic origin from those that are not epileptogenic. According to this author, EEG transients that must mot be regarded as epileptiform waves are sharp waves and spikes that are simply distortions of the ongoing background activity, 6 and 14 positive spikes during sleep, the 6 cps spike-and-wave pattern, the so-called small, sharp spikes, the lambdoid waves of sleep, and frontal sharp transients in newborn babies.

He proposes the following criteria:

1. Symmetry versus asymmetry of the waveform: Epileptic sharp waves and spikes have a sharply rising wave front and a more slowly decaying second phase, whereas nonepileptiform sharp waves are symmetrical with respect to time.
2. Epileptiform spikes and sharp waves are frequently followed by a slow afterwave, either of the same or of the opposite polarity as the main epileptiform transient. Nonepileptiform sharp waves and spikes are not followed by such slow afterwaves.
3. Epileptiform spikes and spikes and sharp waves are bi- or triphasic. Nonepileptiform sharp waves are monophasic.
4. Epileptiform sharp waves or spikes have a different duration than that of the ongoing EEG background activity—they are slower or faster. The duration of nonepileptiform sharp waves is often approximately the same as that of the waves contributing the ongoing background activity from which they emerge.

5. The background activity surrounding epileptiform sharp waves and spikes is disturbed by the presence of slow waves of a frequency range below that of the predominant or normal background activity. Nonepileptiform spikes and sharp waves are not associated with such abnormal slow activity.

In automatic spike detection, two main approaches may be defined: One is to recognize a spike according to different, fixed parameters that are not related to characteristics of the background activity. This is termed a deterministic approach. The features that are commonly taken into account are the amplitude, duration, slope, and sharpness of the wave. Some procedures have considered only one of these attributes; others consider several of them at the same time to make a decision. Within this line of thought, it is also possible to construct a model of a spike (a template) and then to compare the waves of the EEG with this model, classifying them as spikes if very similar.

The second approach is a statistical one. The normal EEG activity is considered a realization of a stochastic process with specified parameters. Transient deviations from these statistical parameters are identified as spikes. In this model, the features of the spikes cannot be specified in absolute terms. They can be only defined in relation to the overall characteristics of the signal from where the transient abnormality arises. Different statistical criteria may be taken into account: the mean amplitude, the mean frequency, the mean measures of sharpness, etc. Some procedures exist that also combine those statistical criteria to reach a conclusion about the presence of a spike. To this statistical approach belong the procedures that consider the EEG activity as a stationary process. From this viewpoint, transient deviations from stationarity or nonstationarities will be candidates to be spikes.

Because the electroencephalographer not only considers what is happening in one channel to make a decision about the presence of a spike, but takes into account the interrelationships between channels, there are also automatic procedures that analyze such interrelationships to reach conclusions about the presence and source of spike activity.

In this chapter, we present a review of the major methods used for spike detection. We include not only those procedures that have been implemented and tested, for which parameters are stated and accuracy given, but also those reports that propose procedures that seem to be useful, even if their accuracy has not yet been provided by the authors. In order to simplify the presentation, we have classified the different methods according to the main features of the spikes that are taken into consideration. The reader should be aware that this is a tentative division only valid for a didactic presentation. A large number of possibilities arise when combinations of different criteria are used. Even when similar approaches have been used, the methods sometimes present slight technical or logical differences. Although classifying spike-detection methods is undoubtedly less difficult than classifying spikes, nonetheless, we admit there may be possible inaccuracies in our decisions, about which a group of EEGers might not unanimously concur.

II. DETECTION PROCEDURES BASED ON WAVE AMPLITUDE

One of the main characteristics of spikes or seizure discharges is that they have a large amplitude. In deterministic models, detection is made according to a certain threshold, which can be fixed as a priori value, or according to previous observations on spikes in the specific patient. Amplitude per se is not enough for the detection of spikes or seizures, because one might possibly pick up larger slow waves with this criterion alone. Absolute amplitude is only used in combination with other measures. It has the great inconvenience of not taking into account the interindividual variability. It is only valuable if the threshold values are set for each patient on the basis of previous recordings, thus limiting its use to seizure monitoring.

In the statistical approach, computation of the mean and standard deviation of the amplitude values of the EEG activity from a sample early in the record permits inferences about the probability that a given value observed later does or does not belong to the EEG background activity. Because EEG amplitude distributions are Gaussian, the usual univariate approach to identify events that are probably not members of the normal distribution can be used. If, for example, deviations greater than 2 SD of the mean are selected, waves with those amplitude values that exceed that confidence limit have a probability of 0.05 of belonging to the normal amplitude distribution of that background activity. This criterion has been useful for labeling those epochs that are suspect of containing spikes (MacGillivray & Wadbrook, 1975). Some authors have used the criterion for the inclusion of waves as suspect of being spikes if they have twice the mean amplitude value (Ives, Thompson, & Woods, 1973). Harner (1977, Chapter 9), makes an estimate of "average peak amplitude" by using a measure that increases by one count when it is exceeded by wave amplitude, but requires 20 smaller waves in order to decrease by the same amount. Values above twice the "average peak amplitude" are considered as spikes. Further statistical treatment provides a display with the number of paroxysmal events detected for the delta, alpha, and beta, as well as for a high-frequency band that contains muscle artifacts and other high-frequency noise. In the computed EEG topography display, paroxysmal events are represented as vertical lines to distinguish them from background activity, with the height of the line proportional to the amplitude of the paroxysmal event (Fig. 12.1).

III. DETECTION PROCEDURES BASED ON THE MEASUREMENT OF SLOPE

Spikes are characterized by presenting a sharply rising wave front and a decaying second phase, which can be measured by the slope.

The ratio of amplitude (y) to time (x) is an indicator of the slope, as can be seen in Fig. 12.2. This ratio is the tangent of the angle α, and can be measured in standard units of μV/msec. Geometrically, computation of

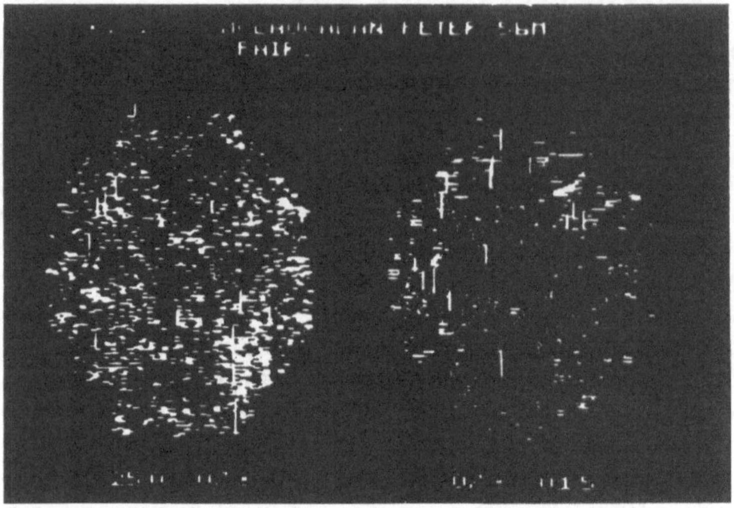

FIG. 12.1. CET with paroxysmal activity. Each paroxysmal wave is displayed as a vertical line proportional to its amplitude. Fast and slow paroxysmal activity is bilateral, but maximal in the left fronto-temporal region. (From Harner, 1977.)

the first derivative of the EEG signal at the point a, $[f'(a)]$, with respect to time (x) will be the tangent of the angle α, formed by the positive direction of the X axis and the positive direction of the tangent to the curve at the point a (Fig. 12.2). The derivative function will be positive in the interval in which the function is increasing, and negative in the interval in which the function decreases. A sharp transient will show a relatively high maximal value of the first derivative of the EEG signal with respect to time, when compared with the EEG background activity.

Kooi (1966) considered that spikes could be well categorized by slopes greater than 2 μV/msec.. Considering that spikes have a triangular form with a relatively large and smooth slope quickly followed by a relatively large and smooth slope of opposite polarity, and that, although the two sides may be of unequal length, there will be an identifiable base of between 20-80 msec, Smith (1974) developed a system in a digital computer and implemented the hardware of a special-purpose circuit for detection of spikes. He combined the criterion of a first derivative that must exceed a slope threshold with the idea that the sharp wave must reach a peak and return to the baseline with a high first derivative of opposite sign. The slope was defined by setting a threshold (2μV/msec) and an interval (20–80 msec) during which the first derivative must pass across the threshold. These criteria detected 85% of clearly abnormal spikes in three 15-minute long abnormal records. The system also detects EMG spikes. Using average EEG frequency in 2-second epochs, it is possible to reject those periods that include EMG frequencies. Smith also observed that the EEG signal could be low filtered with a cut-off frequency of 30 Hz without destroying the spike characteristics. Blume and Vera (1977) used similar criteria: A spike is identified when the first derivative of the ongoing EEG signal exceeds a predefined level twice in 80 msec, one derivative being opposite in polarity to the other. They have achieved an accuracy of 80-90% when compared with visual EEG interpretation.

Although these procedures are easy to implement, they have the disadvantage that the definition of the threshold level is arbitrary, and the whole procedure relies on these values. Nevertheless, many workers agree that approximately 2μV/msec is a pretty good value of slope to get a reasonable detection level.

IV. DETECTION PROCEDURES BASED ON SHARPNESS

In a spike or sharp wave, the first derivative of the voltage signal with respect to time changes rapidly at the peak of the wave. This suggests that the most sensitive measurement of sharpness in a waveform would be the second derivative of the signal with respect to time, which measures the rate of rate of voltage change. The procedure developed by Carrie (1973) consists of the computation of the moving average of the amplitude of the second derivative of 256 waves, in which waves are defined by zero crossings. At the end of each wave, a check is made to see whether the magnitude of the second derivative is two or three times greater than the moving average of the preceding 256 waves. If this is so, a pulse is generated by the computer and a rectangular pulse appears in the output of the machine (Fig. 12.3). In this method, differentiation of pathological activity from artifacts is made, indicating the occurrence of an abnormality only when it detects an abnormally sharp waveform together with a following wave or waves of

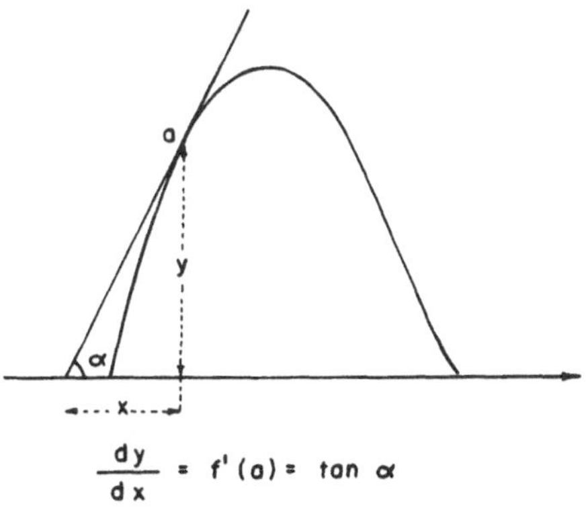

FIG. 12.2. Geometrically, computation of the first derivative of the EEG signal at the point *a*, with respect to time (*x*) will be the tangent of the angle α, formed by the positive direction of the *X* axis and the positive direction of the tangent to the curve at the point *a*. A sharp transient will show a relative high maximal value of the first derivative of the EEG signal with respect to time when compared with the EEG background activity.

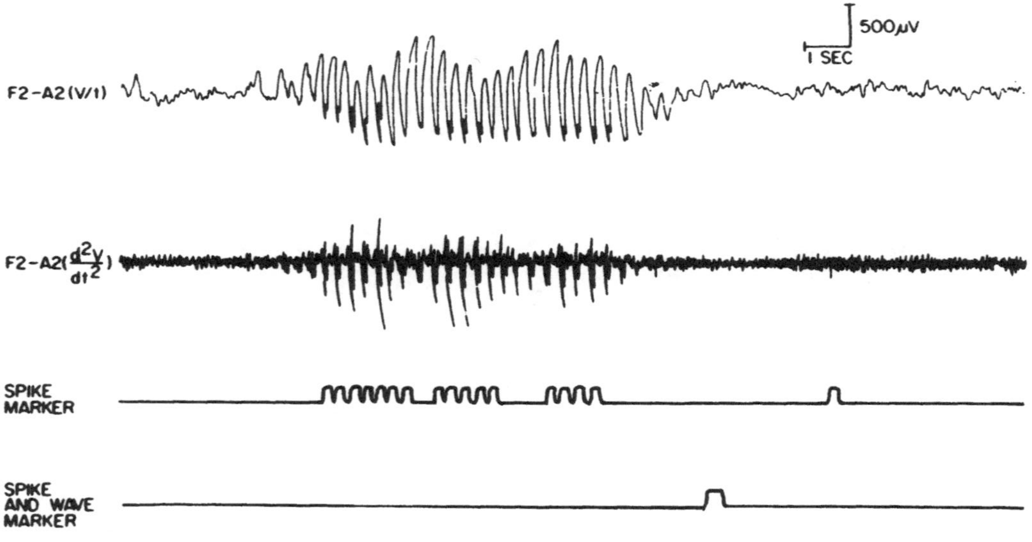

FIG. 12.3. Channel 1: EEG signal that includes burst of spike and wave. Channel 2: filtered second derivative of the EEG signal with respect to time, showing selective amplification of sharply contoured waves. Channel 3: output from digital computer marking the occurrence of waves three or more times as sharp as the average sharpness of the preceding 256 waves. Channel 4: output from digital computer marking the end of the preceding burst of spike and wave when the computer was programmed to respond specifically to spike and wave pattern. There is one pulse at the end of the burst of spike and wave, but the sharp transient occurring approximately 3 sec later is not rated abnormal. (From Carrie, 1973.)

specified slowness. This method is useful only for the detection of episodic, transient abnormalities, because, in EEGs with continuously abnormal and sharply contourned waves, as in hypsarhythmic records, the comparison with the preceding 256 waves does not detect any difference. The same author (Carrie, 1976) used this procedure in the detection and quantification of spike activity during overnight recordings in an epileptic patient. The outputs of the computer were compared with the results of independent visual analysis of the same records by two electroencephalographers. It was found that in 86.9% of the 1122 computer counts, both electroencephalographers indicated a paroxysmal event, in 9.8% only one specialist did, and 3.3% were false positives. In addition, there were 114 cases (10%) in which one electroencephalographer signaled a paroxysmal event and 58 (5%) false negatives (both specialists indicated a paroxysmal event with no computer response).

The procedure of successive differentiation of the EEG enhances the high-frequency noise present in the data. Carrie (1973) proposed solving the problem by analog filtering before and after successive differentiation, resulting in a substantial attenuation of components between 30 and 100 Hz, and rejecting, by software, those waves of less than the specified duration.

Lieb, Woods, Siccardi, Crandall, Walter, and Leake (1978) used an automatic spike-detection system (COUNTR) based on the second derivative technique. The incoming EEG is prefiltered (3 dB down at 40 Hz) and the second derivative is computed. The absolute value of the differences between each sample and each of the preceding 11 samples are computed. The maximum of these 11 absolute values is defined as the peak-to-peak (PTP) of the second derivative of the EEG signal. COUNTR compares the current PTP with a previously determined "checking level" to determine whether or not the PTP represents background activity. The checking level is set at 2.5 SD above the mean amplitude value of EEG background activity. Independently, the PTP is compared with the current threshold level for spike detection. This threshold level was selected in order that correct spike detection should be twice as desirable as the avoidance of false spike identification (9 SD above the mean amplitude). At this optimum threshold level for patients, correct spike identification was between 80-90% with 18-30% false positive detections. This system has been used for the quantitative analysis of depth spiking in relation to seizure foci in patients with temporal epilepsy. They found a clear relation between depth spike occurrence and the apparent origin of seizure episodes, but a relation between depth spike occurrence and time of onset seizure was not so evident.

Chik, Sokol, and Rosen (1977) have developed a method for sharp wave detection in fetal EEG to assess the electrical status of the fetal brain and provide a procedure for early detection of aberrant neurological development. The procedure is based on the computation of the first and second derivatives of the EEG. When the first derivative changes sign, a sharp wave is considered probable if the absolute value of the second derivative exceeds a minimum threshold determined empirically. In the presence of this probable sharp wave, four additional parameters of the first derivative, which characterize the sharp wave prior to the maxima and minima detected, are also computed. With these five variables, they compute a discriminant equation between visually detected sharp waves and not acceptable sharp-wave patterns. The resulting equation produced classifications from 85-89% consistent with visual identification. As a final step, the number of sharp waves automatically identified was used as a variable along and in combination with other variables from fetal EEG (the relative frequency of four dominant patterns: low-voltage irregular, mixed, high-voltage slow, and *tracé alternant*), and with Apgar scores and results of neonatal neurological examination, for the classification of infants for neurological outcome at 1 year of age. Using the five variables from EEG, 74% of the infants could be correctly classified for neurological outcome at 1 year of age. Adding the other data, 80% of the outcomes were correctly classified. These findings imply that some forms of brain damage are present before birth and can be detected using fetal EEG.

Another measurement of the sharpness of a wave is the curvature in a wave's peak region. Gevins, Yeager, Diamond, Zeitlin, Spire, and Gevins (1976) used curvature for isolating waves that are sharp with respect to background activity. They described a simple relation to set a threshold (T) for curvature that distinguishes reasonably well between a set of records containing significant sharp transients from a set without them: $T = 25\ (\bar{C}^{1/2} + \log_2 \bar{C})$. The threshold T is determined for each patient by computing the average curvature ($\bar{C}$) during the first part of the record to be analyzed. Candidate waves are then subjected to a sequential series of tests modeling the methods of clinical EEG: number of peaks making up the sharp transient complex, similar events occurring in adjacent channels, slow waves associated with a transient, first component surface negative in monopolar recordings, and phase reversal found in bipolar derivations. Evaluation of the method was made in 28 1-minute eight-channel EEG recordings. From a total of 139 events marked by two or more scorers, 53 were adequately classified by the computer with 24 false detections. With minimal modifications in average sharpness, 84 or 139 events were detected, with 28 false positives. If it is considered that interexpert variability was high, because only 11 of the transients were found by all five experts, and 83 were identified by three or more, the performance obtained by this algorithm, although subject to error, may be adequate for detection of sharp transients.

V. DETECTION PROCEDURES BASED ON COMBINED CRITERIA OF AMPLITUDE AND DURATION

We have seen that absolute amplitude values are not useful for spike detection, because larger slow waves may also be detected. If the EEG is filtered within a frequency range that includes the presence of spike discharges but excludes the slow waves, then the probability of correct detection of epileptic activity increases. There are typical epileptic patterns, for example petit mal, that are characterized by the high amplitude and frequency of the appearance of spikes and waves. Bickford (1959) described a system that detected waveforms of specified frequency whose amplitude exceeded a preset threshold, useful in patients showing petit mal. Ehrenberg and Penry (1976) described a procedure for detection of paroxysmal events in patients with absence seizures, using a telemetric system for four EEG channels, which included preprocessing equipment with a voltage summator and an electronic filter to detect periods with 2-33 Hz. Each 250 msec epoch for each channel was continuously compared to a fixed amplitude threshold, and series of EEG waves that were simultaneously greater than the threshold for at least 750 msec were classified as paroxysms. From 609 paroxysms detected by three different electroencephalographers in seven different patients, the computer recognized 516 (85%). The computer accuracy raised 92% when portions of the EEG segments recorded during sleep were discounted.

Marchesi, Tascini, Angeleri, Quattrini, and Scarpino (1976) and Von Albert (1977) used an electronic device that detects spikes, waves, or spike-wave combinations, taking into account amplitude, rising or falling times, and polarity. Amplitudes greater than 1.2-3.0 times the averaged foregoing EEG lasting 15-55 msec indicate the presence of spikes. Waves are detected and counted if the amplitude of the foregoing EEG is lower in a proportion of 3:1 to 1.5:1 and if it has a frequency under 6 Hz. Spike-wave combinations are counted if within 300 msec after detection of a spike, a wave is detected. By this procedure, differences between visual counts of three experts and automatic recognition were between 10-20%, and the most frequent error was false positive counts by the computer. Marchesi et al. (1976) used this spike detector for evaluation of the independence of two foci, evolution of the spike discharges during wakefulness and sleep, and the possible modification of discharge patterns by pharmacotherapy. Von Albert (1977) used it successfully to study prolonged EEG recordings, increasing the probability of detecting spikes in epileptic patients and as an objective measurement for the indication of therapy.

For seizure detection in long-term recordings, Stevens, Kodamo, Lonsbury, and Mills (1971) combined rise time or duration of the ascending branch of the wave with a frequency of 6-10 Hz and a voltage trigger. These three parameters are set empirically to recognize indisputable spikes for each individual record and to exclude muscle and movement artifacts. After this has been done, a tape recording of the entire 24 hours/day/patient was processed, according to the parameters determined from the patient's own seizure discharges. They observed proportional relationships between seizure length and pre- and postseizure intervals in patients with different types of epilepsy. Babb, Manani, and Crandall (1974) described an analog-digital circuit that accepts one or more EEG channels as input. The EEG of any number of channels is summed together to produce a composite signal. This signal is passed through an RC high-pass filter that allows reliable triggering by a comparator whenever a sufficiently high amplitude and high frequency input occurs. The output pulses are integrated and used to feed a second comparator that can be triggered if the input continues at a high voltage. If the reference level of this comparator is set low, a single paroxysm may trigger it, but as the reference level is increased, the criterion for seizure detection is raised. The performance of the seizure detector was superior to nurses' reports in making correct detections (46 to 26), but was inferior in avoiding false positive detections (18 to 2). These false positive alarms were never of biological origin and they served as early warnings of system failure in data transmission (mistakes during battery or tape changes).

Other approaches combining amplitude and wave duration have been those of Kaiser (1976) and Goldberg, Samson-Dollfus, and Grémy (1973). The first author has developed a multichannel spike-wave detector that is based on amplitude detection by a threshold level selected by the operator, a maximum of 36 msec for spike duration and a presence of a larger slow wave after the spike. Goldberg et al. (1973) filtered the EEG signal above 7 Hz (7-point moving average, 70 Hz sampling rate) and detected short duration paroxysmal events that exceeded thresholds based on average amplitude.

VI. DETECTION PROCEDURES BASED ON COMBINED CRITERIA OF AMPLITUDE, DURATION, SLOPE, AND SHARPNESS

Jacob (1976) studied 15 features of spikes (see Fig. 12.4), including duration of different intervals from the original and first derivative functions, the amplitude values of the rising and falling phase of the spike, and maximal values of the positive and negative phases of its first derivative. On the basis of visual inspection, spikes and spike-like waves were classified in the following categories: (1) definitive or clear spikes; (2) doubtful spikes; and

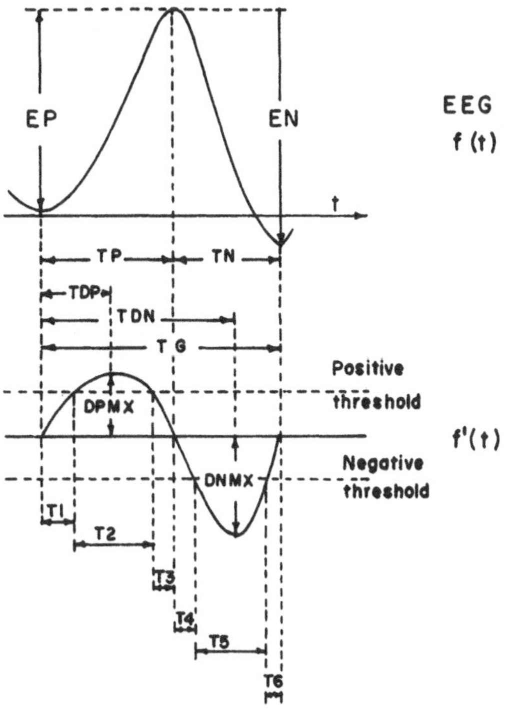

FIG. 12.4. The EEG signal, its first and second derivatives are shown. The 15 features studied by Jacob (1976) are illustrated. (From Jacob, 1976.)

(3) suspicious spike-like waves that coincide with a clear spike in another derivation. Table 12.1 shows the mean and standard deviation values of the 15 features of these groups. To reduce the number of features, Jacob combined different sets of features and thresholds for spike recognition, and calculated correlations between wave features. The following criteria were the optimal for spike detection:

1. Threshold values from 200-300 μV/0.1 sec for the positive phase of the first derivative (DPMX).
2. Threshold values from 250-350 μV/0.1 sec for the negative phase of the first derivative (DNMX).
3. A duration from 7-12 msec of the rising phase of the original wave (*T2*).
4. In the first derivative, a threshold of plus or minus 150 μV/0.1 sec. Criteria for spike detection were met if the negative phase of the first derivative exceeded this threshold from 12-20 msec (*T5*).
5. Duration of the original wave should be between 60-90 msec (*T6*). With these five parameters, Jacob was able to adequately classify 75% of the spikes.

TABLE 12.1[a]

	Definitive Spikes		*Doubtful Spikes*		*Suspicious Spikelike Waves*	
	X	*SD*	*X*	*SD*	*X*	*SD*
EP[b]	73	39.0	43	22.9	40	18.6
EN[b]	110	46.2	67	28.8	62	39.1
DPMX[c]	470	247.9	268	121.0	236	93.5
DNMX[c]	621	289.3	371	162.8	331	180.8
TP[d]	23	7.3	23	10.2	25	7.9
TN	29	8.8	28	8.9	27	8.2
TG	52	12.6	51	14.9	53	12.1
T1	4	4.6	5	4.9	7	5.3
T2	16	5.7	11	5.6	11	5.5
T3	3	4.6	6	7.3	6	7.1
T4	2	1.4	3	2.0	3	1.7
T5	21	5.5	17	6.2	16	5.7
T6	5	6.6	6	6.7	7	6.3
TDP	11	4.9	9	4.8	10	4.9
TDN	33	7.9	33	10.7	34	8.9

[b]EP and EN are given in μV.
[c]DPMX and DNMX are given in μV/0.1 sec.
[d]From TP to TDN, values are given in milliseconds.
[a]From Jacob, 1976. A description of each parameter is given in Fig. 12.4.

MacGillivray and Wadbrook (1975) described a system for computing a diagnosis from the routine clinical EEG. In this system, data acquisition of 16 channels is under the control of the person recording, who is responsible for marking the artifacts as the record passes. These markers are used for data handling and editing by program. The raw EEG signal (free from artifacts) is filtered with center frequencies at 1.25, 2.5, 5.0, 10.0, and 20.0 Hz. Means and standard deviations of the amplitude values for each band are computed. Those values that exceed a threshold of 2 SD above the mean are labeled, and all the information is stored. The spike-detection program operates in the following way: The recalled labeled epoch (1 second) of the raw EEG, together with the immediately preceding and succeeding epochs, are scanned for maxima, and the slopes of the rising and falling edges are checked to determine if they exceeded some threshold value (greater than 2 μV/msec). If a possible spike is detected, the next procedure is to perform a Fourier transform of the data with the coefficients up to 120 Hz. Pure EMG treated in this way produces a flat spectrum. If the sum of the 60-120 Hz coefficients exceeds some value, then EMG is present and the spike detected is invalidated. With this procedure, it is possible to detect paroxysmal events, the channels affected, and the dominant frequency.

Therefore, the procedure is useful not only for the detection of short spike-and-wave episodes, but longer episodes of focal activity or generalized paroxysmal activity. The performance is about 80% compared to clinical assessment, the errors being omissions rather than false positives (MacGillivray, 1977).

Nagypol, Tomka, and Bodó (1976) have designed an automatic spike-detection procedure based on the coincidence of the three following conditions: EEG amplitude three times greater than the mean value of the absolute amplitude of the background activity within a 1-second data window; the first derivative with respect to time must exceed 2.5 μV/ msec in absolute value within a 40-msec data window, and 90% of the instantaneous power density spectra must be contributed by the 20-40 Hz frequency domain within a 40-msec data window.

Gotman and Gloor (1976) have developed a procedure with a minicomputer that accomplishes the following: The system is able to process 16 channels in real time, is not disturbed by eye movements, and gives as a final result the spatial distribution and the type of epileptiform activity. It is a sequential pattern-recognition technique, in which the EEG is broken down into half-waves. A half-wave is characterized by its duration and its amplitude, relative to the background activity. A wave is characterized by the duration and amplitudes of its two component half-waves, by the second derivative at its apex, measured relative to the background activity, and by duration and amplitude of the following half-wave. The channels are first processed independently of each other. For each half-wave, the following operations take place sequentially (if the answer to any question is no, analysis proceeds to the next half-wave): first, it is determined whether the relative amplitude of the current half-wave and of the preceding one are above present thresholds; in the second stage, whether the durations of the half-waves are below appropriate limits is checked; in the third stage, it is determined whether the relative amplitude is large enough according to the relative sharpness of the wave, and the last step analyzes whether the total duration of the wave is equal to or larger than 35 msec.

Although not frequently, it happens that a wave detected using the previously mentioned method is not a spike, but muscle activity, rapid eye blinks, or onset of sharp alpha activity. It is necessary to do further processing to reject the waves corresponding to these three possibilities. If a wave's immediate surroundings (1/3 sec) have a large number of higher amplitude segments, it is rejected as muscle activity. If this is not sufficient, the autocorrelation function is then computed, using 1/3 sec centered at the apex of the detected wave. This autocorrelation function decreases faster for muscle activity than for genuine spikes. Eye blinks may present the characteristics of a sharp wave. Thus, a detected spike is rejected if it occurs in a frontal channel, if it is of positive polarity, and if it has a duration longer than 150 msec. A suddenly appearing alpha burst may contain waves having the characteristics of spikes, particularly when then alpha is sharp. Such waves can be rejected by computing the aut orrelation functions of 1/3 sec centered at the apex of the detected wave, and 1/3 sec centered 100 msec before and after the apex over a lag of 60 msec; a high correlation indicates the presence of alpha activity.

In a second stage, assuming that the selected wave is a spike, the interrelationships with other channels are analyzed for the localization of the epileptic focus. In the display, the spikes detected on the EEG are marked, and the number of locations of the spikes, as well as phase reversal, are given (Fig. 12.5). This method was evaluated by determining the unequivocal errors in 30 normal subjects and in 30 nonepileptic patients. Sections of 2 minutes of EEG were analyzed. No false detections were observed in normal subjects, and a very low detection rate of .18 spikes or sharp waves/min/16 channels was observed in nonepileptic patients.

In order to make a comparison between visual EEG interpretation and computer detection in 50 epileptics, two electroencephalographers interpreted the data independently. The EEGers first interpreted the paper records of 2 to 3 minutes used in the analysis, filling a first form encoding their findings regarding the localization of the focus and the extent of the abnormality, for every EEG (Fig. 12.6A). They also interpreted the set of computer displays from the same patients, filling a second form for every EEG (Fig. 12.6B). The interpretations of the paper records and of the computer displays were done independently, so that the results of one interpretation were not available when the other was done. Names of patients were not available to the EEGers. The correlation coefficients between two interpretations were computed for each electrode position. This was possible by attributing to each electrode the value 0, 1, 2, or 3, depending on whether that electrode was interpreted respectively as being normal, mildly abnormal, moderately abnormal, or above the focus. The correlation coefficients of the 16 channels were then averaged to obtain a general measure of correlation between interpretations.

The correlation coefficients (expressed as percentages) between the filled forms of paper records and computer displays for EEGers A and B were 58 and 61 respectively; the correlation between filled forms of paper records of EEGer A and B was 72%; and the correlation between filled forms of computer displays between both EEGers was of 84%. In relation to the localization of the focus, a high level of agreement (above 70%) was found for all comparisons. There were few waves erroneously rejected as artifacts. The proportion was somewhat higher for eye blinks (14%), because they are extremely similar to bilateral frontal sharp waves in their morphology and mode of occurrence.

VII. DETECTION OF SPIKES BY THEIR COMPARISON WITH A TEMPLATE WAVEFORM

This technique is based on detecting a transient for which the waveform is known (i.e., a template), but whose time of occurrence is not known. Obviously, the success of the method depends entirely on the adequate selection of the template. Saltzberg, Lustick, and Heath (1971) solved the problem by using as the template the waveform of the EEG signal at the scalp when subcortical spikes occur simultaneously. After they obtained the template, they then compared the EEG signal with the template by cross correlation. Ninety-five percent of 130 spikes were adequately detected in an animal experiment. For clinical purposes, this procedure is of limited value.

The problem has been also tackled by collecting a massive amount of EEG data for the description and classification of different patterns of epileptic activity, according to some criteria (Cinca, Apostol, Pestroiu, Serbanescu, & Florescu, 1977a; Jacob, 1976; Viglione, Ordon, & Risch, 1970). The EEG activity of a given subject is then continuously compared with those patterns for the recognition of epileptic activity. Cinca, Florescu, Pestroiu, Serbanescu, and Apostol (1977b) have used this technique for detection of petit mal epilepsy. Viglione et al. (1970) developed a pattern-recognition algorithm based on preclassified preseizure and nonpreseizure data for each different patient. Using these results, they designed seizure warning devices for prediction of onset of seizures in different patients. The results have been excellent; in the majority of epileptic patients, generalized seizures or other type of seizures experienced by the subject were predicted with ample time to take a remedial action. Some false positive warnings were also found in some patients, but these were not observed in normal subjects (Viglione, Ordon, & Risch, 1974; Viglione & Walsh, 1976). These warning devices are of low weight and patients carried them continuously. This approach opens a new field in the care of epileptic patients.

Zetterberg (1973a) has proposed another procedure for the detection of spikes, once the pulse form is known. He assumes that the spike is added to the normal EEG activity and that a detection of a pulse in noise is possible by constructing an appropriate filter, according to the spike characteristics, and passing the incoming EEG signal through this filter (detector or matched filter). If the output exceeds a certain threshold, the presence of a pulse is announced. The method consists of supressing the alpha and delta components of the EEG and introducing the residual signal to the detector filter. Using a logic algorithm based on coincidence of spikes and phase reversals in two channels, decisions on the presence of a spike are made.

Template procedures are only useful if the characteristics of the patterns

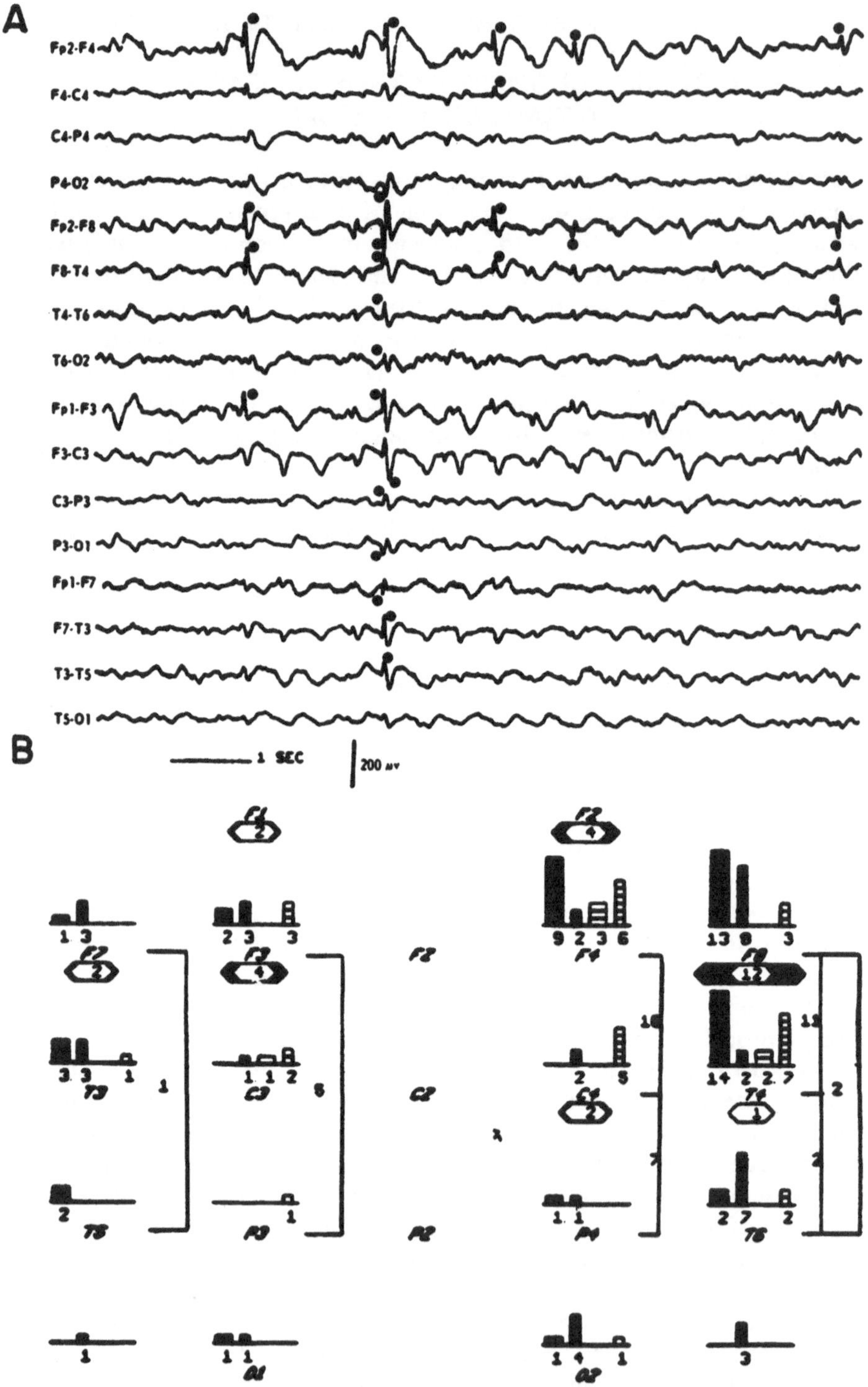
A
Fp2-F4
F4-C4
C4-P4
P4-O2
Fp2-F8
F8-T4
T4-T6
T6-O2
Fp1-F3
F3-C3
C3-P3
P3-O1
Fp1-F7
F7-T3
T3-T5
T5-O1
B
1 SEC
200 µv

FIG. 12.5.

of interest are well established. This is a difficult task, because there is a wide range of variation of spikes and related patterns, and spikes can change quite markedly in the course of a trace. The development of an automatic system for the detection and statistical analysis of EEG transients, such as that developed by Lüders, Daube, Taylor, and Klass (1976), may provide important information that will facilitate the identification of different types of epileptogenic patterns and the implementation of more accurate spike-detection algorithms.

VIII. DETECTION OF NONSTATIONARITIES IN THE EEG USING THE AUTOREGRESSIVE MODEL

Lopes da Silva et al. (1975, 1976) and Lopes da Silva, Van Hulten, Lommen, Storm Van Leeuwen, Van Vellen, and Viegenthart (1977) introduced another interesting approach for the detection of epileptic spikes with an automatic spike-detection program (ASD). The basic assumption in this method is that the EEG background activity is a stationary process and, therefore, it can be described by means of a linear difference equation with constant coefficients. In this way, the EEG is considered as the output of an autoregressive (AR) filter, having stationary input noise with normal distribution. If the inverse AR filter is applied to a stationary EEG, the result would be an uncorrelated, normally distributed random series (white noise). However, when an EEG contains transients, such as spikes or spike-and-wave complexes, the assumption of stationarity does not hold. It is conceivable that those EEGs are composed of the superposition of two processes: a stationary filtered noise and a series of transients. Deviations from stationarity are found at those time samples where transients occur (this holds, of course, as long as the power due to the spikes forms a negligible part of the total signal power). In such a case, the application of the inverse AR filter to the EEG will show samples in which the estimated noise deviates from a normal distribution at a certain probability level, which corresponds with nonstationarities.

FIG. 12.5. (*Opposite page*) Example of results from automatic recognition of spikes. (A) Dots indicate spikes detected by the system. (B) Results of analysis of 2 min of EEG. The names of the electrodes of the 10–20 system are in their usual location. The number of spikes found in a channel is displayed between the corresponding electrodes, in the form of four columns. From left to right: the number of spikes sharp–large, sharp–small, less sharp–large, less sharp–small (for instance, there are 14, 2, 2, 7 spikes of the corresponding categories in channel F8–T4). The number of phase reversals at one electrode is indicated just under the electrode (four phase reversals at F3). Connecting lines indicate equipotential zones between two electrodes (11 equipotential zones between F8 and T6). (From Gotman et al., 1978.)

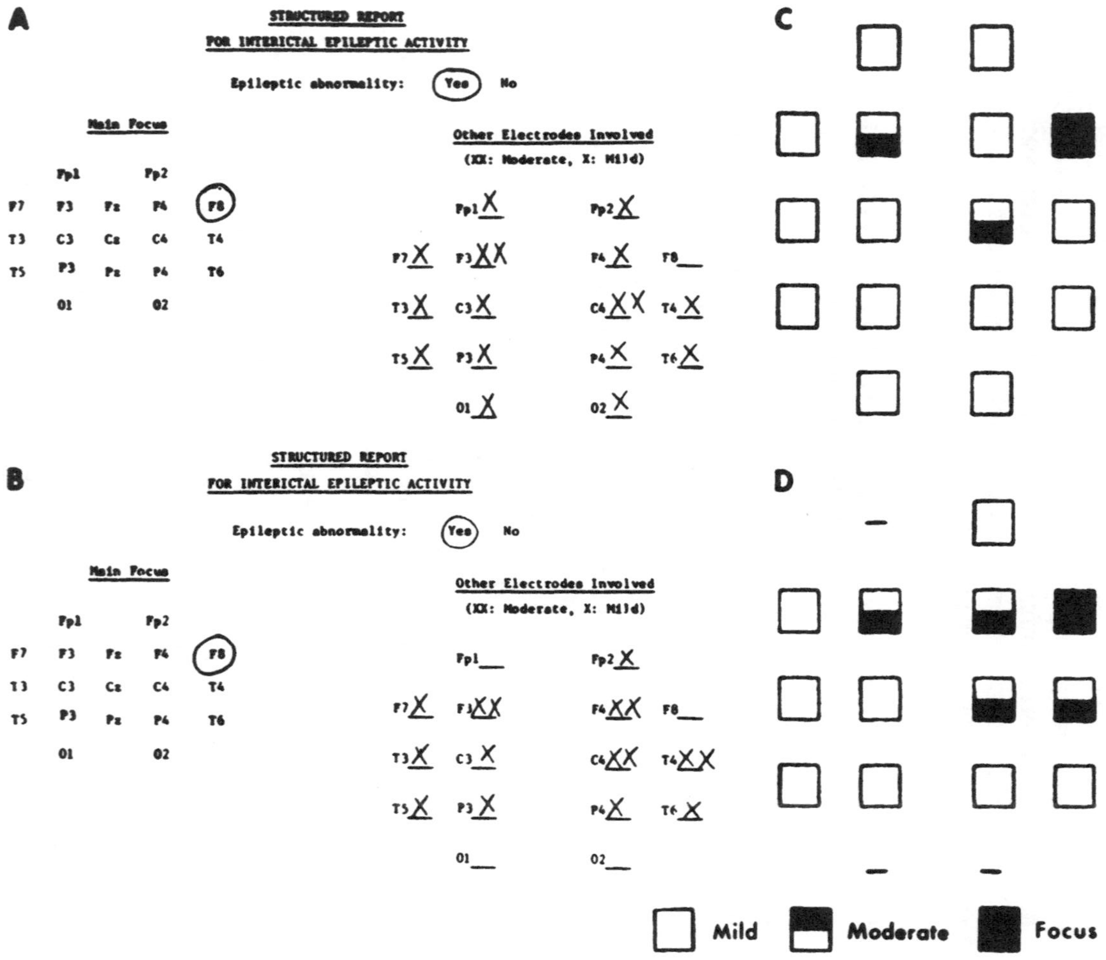
A
STRUCTURED REPORT
FOR INTERICTAL EPILEPTIC ACTIVITY
Epileptic abnormality: Yes No
Main Focus
Fp1 Fp2
F7 F3 Fz F4 F8
T3 C3 Cz C4 T4
T5 P3 Pz P4 T6
O1 O2
Other Electrodes Involved
(XX: Moderate, X: Mild)
Fp1 X Fp2 X
F7 X F3 XX F4 X F8
T3 X C3 X C4 XX T4 X
T5 X P3 X P4 X T6 X
O1 X O2 X
B
STRUCTURED REPORT
FOR INTERICTAL EPILEPTIC ACTIVITY
Epileptic abnormality: Yes No
Main Focus
Fp1 Fp2
F7 F3 Fz F4 F8
T3 C3 Cz C4 T4
T5 P3 Pz P4 T6
O1 O2
Other Electrodes Involved
(XX: Moderate, X: Mild)
Fp1 Fp2 X
F7 X F3 XX F4 XX F8
T3 X C3 X C4 XX T4 XX
T5 X P3 X P4 X T6 X
O1 O2
C
D
Mild
Moderate
Focus

FIG. 12.6.

From the technical point of view, the inverse filtering of the signal might be done in the time domain (Lopes da Silva et al., 1975) or in the frequency domain (Etévenon, Rioux, Pidoux, & Verdeaux, 1976). A comparison between both procedures showed that the two gave approximately the same result, with few exceptions (Lopes da Silva et al., 1976). For a more detailed mathematical description of the procedure, consult Chapter 7.

Once the nonstationarities have been detected within each EEG channel, the ASD program continues, forming clusters of those nonstationarities that were related to each other. A single-channel cluster is defined as a collection of successive sample points, which exceeded the threshold (this was set at a value corresponding to a probability of .005). A cluster was also accepted if two sample points, which exceeded the threshold, were separated by only one sample below the threshold. In order to avoid false positives as much as possible, the criterion for acceptance of a single-channel cluster for further classification was that, within a cluster, there should exist at least one sample at which the detection signal reached a threshold corresponding to $p < .001$. The analysis between channels is carried out by considering as related clusters those that occur at the same time. In those cases in which a cluster found in one channel coincided in time with nonstationarities in other channels that lay below the .005 level and above the .001 level, the latter was also accepted in a table of related clusters. A summary table for all channels in one epoch of EEG is made, including the total number of clusters per channel, the number of clusters in one channel only, and the number of maxima scored by channel (a maximum was defined in that channel in which the largest amplitude was found of those clusters occurring in several channels). Finally, a graphic display with a spatial map containing the summary information for the whole set of EEG channels is provided.

Application of the ASD program has shown that it is able to detect: (1) changes in the statistical characteristics of the ongoing EEG activity; (2) the presence of spikes and spike-and-wave complexes that are also evident by visual inspection; and (3) the most important aspect, the presence of irritative phenomena that lie below the recognition capability of most electroencephalographers. This has been shown in simultaneous recordings of scalp and subdural EEG. A number of transient nonstationarities, detected in the scalp by the program, coincided with clear paroxysmal patterns in subdural derivations and were not identified by visual inspection of the scalp recordings (Fig. 12.7). In this way, conventional definitions of the

---

FIG. 12.6. *(Opposite page)* The structured report for the representation of the localization and extent of interictal epileptic activity. (A) and (B) are the original structured reports filled out for the paper record (A) and for the computer display (B); (C) and (D) are their diagrammatic representations. (From Gotman and Gloor, 1976.)

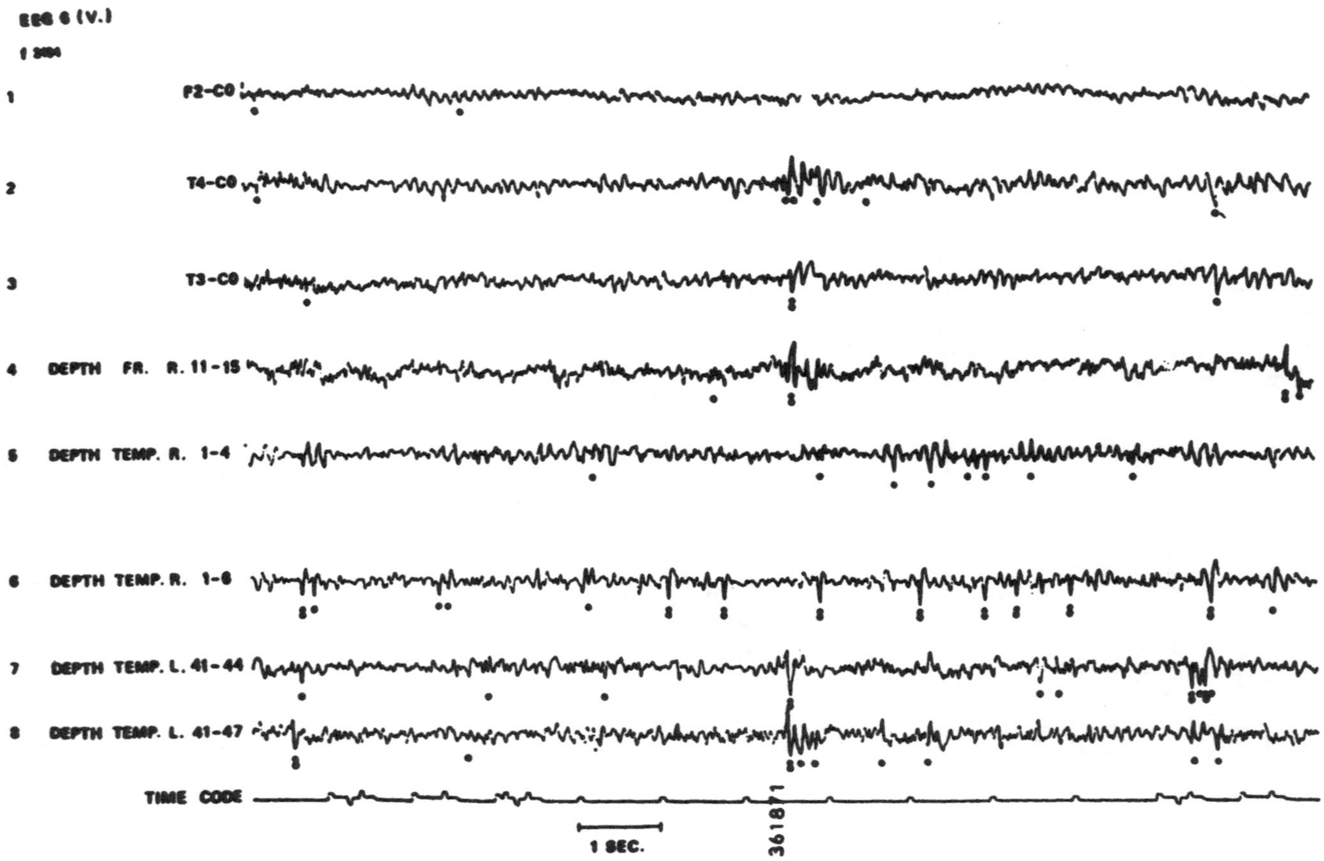

FIG. 12.7. An epoch of an EEG recorded from scalp and depth derivations. The first three channels are from scalp electrodes. The others are from depth. One circle indicates the points at which the computer detected nonstationarities ($P < .005$). Two circles indicate those events that were also classified as of irritative nature by one electroencephalographer. (From Lopes da Silva et al., 1975.)

characteristic paroxysmal patterns at the scalp are put in question. The ASD program has been also useful in determining spatial and temporal relationships between several EEG derivations and in displaying the results in a compact form with a remarkable amount of data reduction. Identical conclusions regarding the localization of an epileptogenic zone in four patients were obtained, either using the conventional methods of recording electroclinical seizures in EEGs of long duration or applying the ASD method to short epochs (100 secs at most).

A comparison between this method and the detection by the second derivative (Fig. 12.8) showed, in most cases, a coincidence in the detection of the spikes. However, there were usually other samples having a second

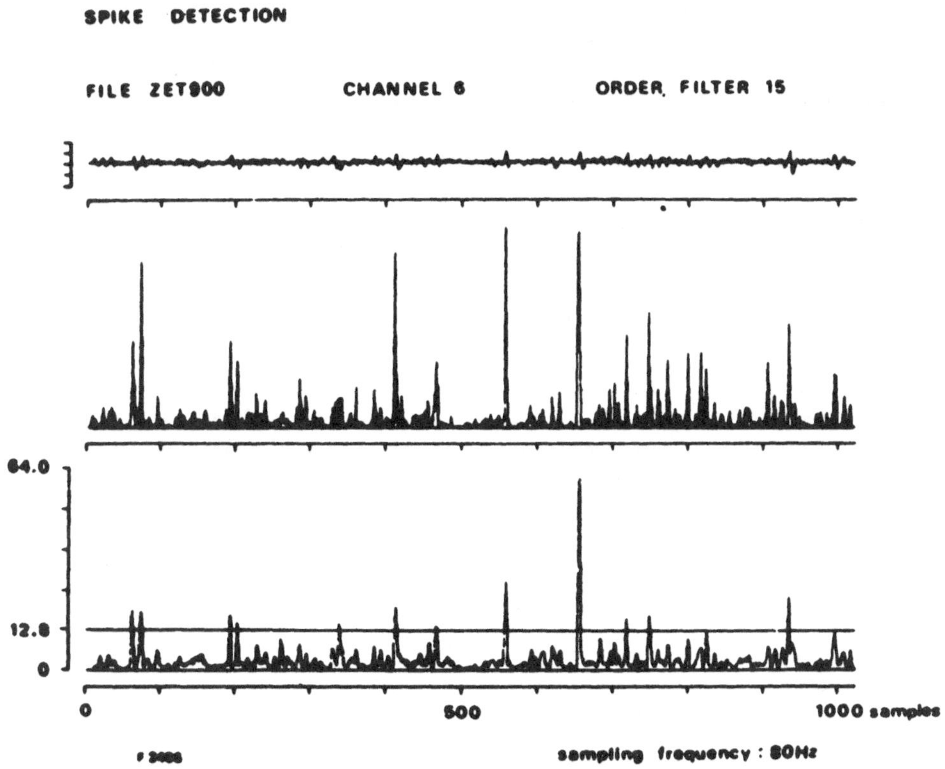

FIG. 12.8. The first signal is the EEG epoch. The second trace gives the rectified second derivative. The third gives the detection signal obtained using the AR method. The probability level $P < .005$ is indicated. Note that there are several sample points that exceed that level. It can also be a certain threshold. However, there were usually an extra number of samples having a second derivative value exceeding the same threshold, but that were not found according to the method based on the AR model and also not classified by the electroencephalographer. (From Lopes da Silva et al., 1975.)

derivative value exceeding criterion, but not found positive by the method based on inverse filtering, nor classified as positive by the electroencephalographer (Lopes da Silva et al., 1975). Birkemeier, Fontaine, Celesia, and Ma (1978) compared the second derivative and autoregressive predictive methods for the automatic detection of epileptic transients. They observed that the two procedures provide about equal discrimination. The second derivative and the method of linear prediction use independent sources of information, one making use of the sharpness of the waves and the other of the difference in predictability of stationarity of the spikes and the background EEG. These authors combined both methods, taking the second derivative of the residual signal resultant from the difference between the original and predicted EEG (cascade method). The threshold was set above three times the value of the ongoing EEG rms amplitude for a 2-second period. Application of this procedure to the EEG of six patients, in comparison with electroencephalographers' judgments, showed correct classification of 187 (87%) out of 215 epileptogenic spikes, with 63 false alarms.

Pfurtscheller and Fischer (1978) have combined inverse and matched filter techniques. As a first step, they used the same inverse filter process described by Lopes da Silva for the detection of the spikes, followed by the matched filters for the classification of spike events, in accordance with the assumed spike templates. In the analysis of the EEG of one patient, more spike events were detected by the combined procedure than with only the inverse filter technique, even though the same error probability was chosen. Another advantage of this method is the possibility of making a classification of the detected spikes in accordance with the assumed spike templates. However, more experience is needed in order to give a final evaluation of the method.

In general, the main disadvantage of inverse filtering procedures is the excessive processing time required.

IX. SUMMARY

Numerous spike- and seizure-detection procedures have been described. Table 12.2 summarizes the most relevant results obtained with different criteria. Those procedures that are based on the recognition of spikes according to their different characteristics with fixed a priori parameters, although very economic, suffer from one great disadvantage. At the present time, it is not possible to select those thresholds in an entirely satisfactory way, because spikes show a wide range of variation. Another type of approach is to consider the spikes as a deviation from certain statistical characteristics of the EEG background activity. Here, interindividual differences are taken into account, and it is possible to make statistical inferences.

Sharpness, the most relevant characteristic for the detection of spikes, can be measured in very different ways. Calculation of the first and second derivatives appears to be an economic procedure, with a detection of 80-90% of the spikes. However, it enhances the high-frequency noise present in the data and results in a high number of false detections.

Combinations of several parameters, such as amplitude, duration, and sharpness, maintain the same level of accurate detection, but decrease the number of false positives. Inverse autoregressive filtering of the EEG is an extremely advanced procedure, making possible the detection of spikes at the scalp even when they were not apparent upon visual inspection. Nevertheless, it requires a large amount of computation.

Template-matching methods depend entirely on the adequate selection of the template. This is a difficult task. It might be overcome by studies of the different features of the spikes, such as those that are now in progress, which will permit not only the design of different types of templates, but the automatic classification of spikes detected even by other procedures.

Applications of spike-detection procedures have proved useful for increasing our knowledge of epilepsy and its medical care. The results obtained demonstrate that effective spike-detection algorithms exist and should be included as part of the neurometric assessment of brain dysfunctions in neurological patients.

TABLE 12.2
Major Procedures of Spike and Seizure Detection

Criteria	Results	Observations	Reference
Slope: 1st derivative (fixed thresholds)	85% of spikes detected	False detections of EEG and of large amplitude slow waves.	Smith (1974)
Slope and sharpness: deviations from the mean (1st and 2nd derivative) followed by a wave of specified slowness.	87% of spikes detected	Only useful for episodic, transient abnormalities. It enhances the high frequence noise present in the data, which can be diminished by attenuation of components from 30-100 Hz. False detections.	Carrie (1973, 1976)
Slope and sharpness: 1st derivative measurements and second derivative preset thresholds. Discriminant analysis.	85-89% of sharp waves detected	Very few false positives. Useful to predict neurological outcome, together with other features of fetal EGG.	Chik et al. (1977)
Sharpness: curvature in a wave's peak region and a subsequent logic modeling the methods of EGG.	60% of detection of events marked by two or more experts.	False positive detections. Performance of the computer within the variability range of 5 EGG experts.	Gevins et al (1976)
Amplitude and duration (fixed thresholds)	85% detections in patients with absences.	The computer raised to 92% when portions of the EEG during sleep were discounted.	Ehrenburg and Penry (1976)
Amplitude deviations from the mean, duration of rising and falling edges of waves, polarity.	80-90% of spikes detected	False positive detections are the most frequent error.	Marchesi et al. (1976) Von Albert (1977)
Amplitude, duration and slope (1st derivative)	75% of spike detections		Jacob (1976)

Amplitude, deviations from the mean and slope (greater than 2 microvolts/msec).	80% of spike detections	Presence of EMG is also analyzed and rejected. Detects short spikes and wave episodes as well as long episodes of focal or generalized activity. Errors being omissions rather than false positives.	MacGillivray and Wadbrook (1975) MacGillivray (1977)
Amplitude, duration, sharpness (2nd derivative) deviations. Sequential pattern recognition techniques. Interchannel relationships.	Production of computer displays encoding the localization and extent of the abnormality. Correlation of 60% between visual and computer encoded interpretations.	The procedure includes rejection of EMG, eye blink or onset of sharp alpha bursts. Very few false positives. It requires a large amount of computation.	Gotman and Gloor (1976) Gotman et al (1978)
Templates based on pre-seizure and non pre-seizure data from each patient.	Construction of warning seizure devices. Some false positive alarms were observed in epileptices but no alarms were observed in normal subjects.	Opens a new field in the medical care of epileptic patients.	Viglione et al (1970, 1974) Viglione and Walsh (1976)
Detection of nonstationarities by inverse AR filter process. Interchannel relationships.	Detection of events at the scalp even not classified as spikes by visual inspection, but coincident with clear paroxysmal patterns in subdural derivations. Identical conclusions regarding the identification of the epileptic zone were obtained by using conventional methods of long recording of electroclinical seizures as with 100 secs of automatically analyzed EGG.	The single drawback is the excessive processing time required.	Lopes da Silva et al (1975, 1976, 1977)

13 Neurometric Evaluation of Evoked Responses in Clinical Neurology

I. INTRODUCTION

Chapters 3 to 5 described the alterations of the ERs most frequently encountered in different types of brain lesions or dysfunctions. From those data, it was evident that the ERs reflect the anatomical and functional integrity of different subsystems within the nervous system. However, the studies that were discussed only provided descriptions of the main abnormalities seen in relation to peak latencies, amplitudes, and interhemispheric symmetry. In those works, little or no attempt was made to use those parameters to establish decision rules or to classify the subjects into categories. In Chapter 11 we described the basic stages in the development of a neurometric procedure for the assessment of alterations in nervous-system functions. Three essential steps were defined: (1) *identification and extraction* of those electrophysiological features that are most directly related to the anatomical and functional integrity of the nervous system; (2) the establishment of a *decision rule* for assigning a given subject to one of a given number of sets (known a priori or as a result of the analysis); and (3) the *validation* of such a decision rule with new subjects.

The most important features of the ERs that have been taken into account for the construction of neurometric procedures are: the peak latencies of well-defined waves of the ERs, amplitude of different waves of the ERs, the amplitude excursion from the most positive to the most negative value in a defined epoch of the ER, the waveshape of the ER defined by the amplitude values at certain time intervals, the energy of the ER in a defined epoch, the frequency characteristics of the ER, the waveform symmetry in homologous left and right derivations as measured by the correlation coefficient or by the Student's t test, the amplitude symmetry measured by amplitude ratios or energy ratios, the appearance of a defined wave within a specified latency range as a result of changed stimulus characteristics, and so on. These features may be extracted from the ERs yielded by different estimation procedures, which were described in Chapter 10. In that chapter, the following were also discussed: different procedures for hypothesis testing, and procedures such as discriminant analysis that make it possible to predict, with good accuracy, that a given ER is a member of a particular group of ERs. Because an essential step in neurometric assessment consists of the quantitative analysis of the ERs, it is necessary to bear in mind the assumptions that were pointed out as underlying the different analysis procedures in order to make an adequate interpretation of the results.

The simplest approach to the establishment of a decision rule has been the computation of the means and standard deviations of some features of the ERs in normal subjects and the definition of confidence limits, considering "abnormal" all the values beyond this limit. I want to comment on two aspects of this approach:

1. Multiple comparisons of means can increase the possibility of committing a Type I or alpha error—that is, rejecting the null hypothesis when in fact it is true. Thus, if more than one variable is considered, the Type I error is not controlled if intercorrelations between variables are not taken into account.
2. The confidence limits are defined by the results obtained in a sample of control subjects and not in the whole population of normal subjects. Thus, with a confidence limit of .05, for example, in theory a 5% incidence of "false positives" (control values beyond the 5% limit) is expected. However, it is essential to verify this in the control sample and highly desirable to replicate it in an independent normal sample. Information about the number of false positives is very rarely published, but it is extremely important for a complete evaluation of the validity, as well as accuracy, of a procedure. A related important point is that the probability distribution of extracted features used in decision rules is also too often ignored.

Some comments may be worthwhile about those procedures that are based on the measurement of peak amplitudes and latencies or other characteristics of the waves of the ERs. When working with ERs, we deal with electrophysiological events, some of which we know to be related to sensory, perceptual, and cognitive processes. We also know that some of the waves or ERs are related to the activation of well-defined anatomical structures. However, we do not yet know the physiological meaning of all the waves. We know the consequences of many different types of brain dysfunctions of the ERs, but we are not able to relate those consequences to specific pathophysiological mechanisms in all the cases. Further, some similar consequences can be produced by different physiological mechanisms; for example, small amplitudes of averaged evoked responses may be caused by a decrease in the amount of receptors or pathways activated, or by an asynchronous activation of the structures from which we are recording. Although some waves have been shown to be very reliable in normal subjects, such as wave V of the BAERs or P100 of pattern-reversal VERs, this is not the rule for many neurological patients. In the department of Neurophysiology at CENIC (Havana), in collaboration with Pedro Valdés, Guido Fernández, Josefina Richardo and Gloria Otero, I have been searching for ER features that might be useful for clinical purposes, for quite a few years. We started by measuring latencies and amplitudes of the waves of the averaged ERs. Even in groups of normal, healthy subjects, it is extremely difficult to definitely identify all the positive and negative components that one often finds described in the literature as if they occurred invariantly. In fact, even for flash-evoked VERs, numerous exceptions to the presumed rules of "normal" morphology become apparent after even the most casual examination of real data. As stimuli become more complex and as stimulation conditions change, the attempt to define some "typical" normal morphology becomes more and more contrived. A dynamic process does not lend itself well to a static description. We found that identification of such "typical" waves was especially difficult in many cases in which, as a consequence of the brain lesion, the ER waveshape was distorted.

For example, suppose that we are trying to identify a wave on the basis of the specifications of the statistical limits of confidence for its peak latency. If we look at an ER with fewer components than those normally observed [see Fig. 13.1], how can we be sure that some particular wave, $w2(t_2) = x$ corresponds to the wave $w1(t_2) = c$ of the same polarity usually found within the confidence limits of peak latency t_2 in healthy subjects? Or, does it represent what would normally be an earlier wave, $w1(t_1) = a$, defined in the healthy subjects, but that, in this individual appears with a delayed latency? Or, is it a new wave, $x(t_2)$, that appears as a consequence of the lesion? Thus, it is very difficult to reach a firm decision based on the evaluation of such bizarre ER waveshapes. Our group CENIC has preferred, therefore, to direct our attention to other features, which can be analyzed in every patient and which take into account aspects of the ER across the whole latency domain.

In this chapter, there are review the principal neurometric approaches that have been used for the assessment of neurological patients. After the foregoing discussion, the reader might be surprised by the presentation of procedures that use latency and amplitude measurements. We admit that

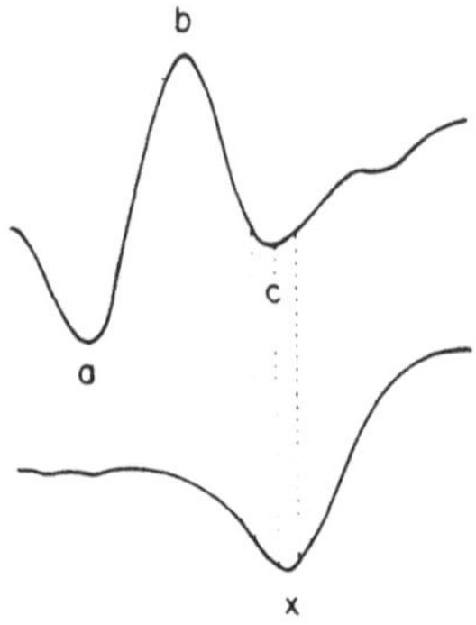

FIG. 13.1. Drawing of two imaginary evoked responses. *Top*: Normal ER with peaks *a*, *b*, and *c*. The confidence limits of the peak latency of wave *c* are also shown. *Bottom*: ER of a patient, in which component *x* is observed. Identification of the wave *x* on the basis of the specifications of the statistical limits of confidence for its peak latency requires that wave *x* corresponds to wave *c* of the normal subjects. It is difficult to ascertain that this is so, or that it represents what would normally be an earlier wave (*a*) but with a delayed latency, or that it is a new wave, which appears as a consequence of the lesion.

these features have been extremely useful in some patients, such as MS patients, in whom the basic waveform is conserved and only delayed responses are observed. Nonetheless, they cannot be considered as optimal general procedures to be applied in all neurological patients. This conclusion has also been stressed by Halliday et al. (1976) in the study of pattern-reversal VERs in compression of the visual pathway, and by Jonkman (1967) in the study of VERs in different types of neurological patients.

II. TRANSIENT VISUAL EVOKED RESPONSES TO FLASHES

A. Symmetry Analysis

1. Discrimination of Normal Subjects from Neurological Patients

Although considerable interindividual variability in the waveform of VERs to flashes exists in normal subjects, the waveforms obtained from bilateral symmetrical or homologous derivations are basically similar—that is, they are electrically symmetrical. On the other hand, patients with brain damage often display marked VER asymmetries. In order to establish the diagnostic utility of VER symmetry, it seemed necessary to evaluate various measures of VER symmetry. The measures used by Harmony, Ricardo, Otero, Fernández, and Valdés (1973b) were: peak latency differences measured in milliseconds, amplitude differences expressed as a percentage of the maximal VER in the pair, and two general measurements of similarity—the Pearson correlation coefficient, *R*, as a measure of waveform similarity and the Signal Energy Ratio (SER) as a measure of amplitude symmetry. *R* was computed as the correlation coefficient between the two sets of numbers representing the two homologous ERs after digitizing each 2.5 msec. For computation of the SER, the amplitude values of the VERs, digitized each 2.5 msec, were squared and summed. This sum of squares is a measure of the "energy" of the VER. The ratio of the larger to the smaller value of the sum of squares was computed for homologous pairs of ERs. This SER was positive if the right hemisphere value exceeded the left hemisphere value, and the negative if vice versa. Recordings were obtained from monopolar left and right central, occipital, and temporal leads and from left and right centro-occipital and occipito-temporal derivations. The results showed a remarkable interhemispheric symmetry in a healthy population: High correlation coefficients (80% were greater than .85) for all derivations; very slight differences in peak latencies (5 msec or less for 85% of the sample of peaks studied), and SER absolute values lower than 2.0 for 80% of the VERs in all derivations.

The same measurements were made in VERs obtained from several groups of patients: 34 brain tumor cases, 50 patients with cerebrovascular lesions, 55 epileptics, 38 patients with different types of lesions (miscellaneous group), and 20 cases with Parkinson's disease (Ricardo, Harmony, and Otero, 1975). All the patients were clinically studied, with diagnosis confirmed in many of them by angiography, pneumoencephalography, electroencephalography, and, in some cases, during subsequent surgery or necropsy. In only a few cases in the miscellaneous group was a definitive diagnosis not obtained, but because these patients presented severe symptoms of brain lesions, they were also included in the study.

In order to know which measures were more useful, a derivation-by-derivation comparison was carried out for every measure between the normal group and each of the first three groups of patients. Cumulative frequency curves for every group were constructed for each measure in each derivation and compared with corresponding curves in normals, using the Kolmogorov-Smirnov test. The point of maximum separation between the curves from the normal and pathological groups was identified. The percentage separation between the two goups at that value (*D*) was determined to test levels of significance ($P < .05$): Table 13.1 shows the maximum separation obtained and the values of the parameters that best separated normals and tumor patients, cerebrovascular disease cases, and epileptics. It is important to indicate that latency differences were considered for all derivations only in 22 tumor patients and 37 cerebrovascular disease cases. The remaining 23 patients had VERs in one or several derivations that were extremely asymmetrical and could not be compared. From the analysis in Table 13.1, it became evident that the most powerful and efficient measure

TABLE 13.1[a]
Comparison of Different Measures of VER Symmetry

	R[c]		*SER*[d]		*AD*[e]		*ML*[f]	
Derivations	M. Sep	Value	M. Sep	Value	M. Sep	Value	M. Sep	Value
Tumors								
Central	29%	.95	14%	2.1	14%	18	18%	5
Occipital	43%	.94	29%	1.6	38%	26	21%	10
Temporal	42%	.83	14%	2.1	16%	15	24%	5
Centro–Occipital	46%	.89	53%	1.6	45%	21	21%	5
Occipito–Temporal	46%	.89	44%	2.2	28%	29	34%	7.5
Vascular								
Central	44%	.93	10%	1.4	8%	31	8%	0
Occipital	48%	.92	25%	1.7	33%	24	19%	5
Temporal	40%	.88	14%	1.3	25%	12	23%	5
Centro–Occipital	38%	.88	25%	1.7	30%	24	15%	5
Occipito–Temporal	41%	.89	34%	1.7	27%	21	20%	7.5
Epileptics								
Central	11%	.90	13%	1.5	14%	5	27%	5
Occipital	28%	.93	24%	1.6	34%	23	36%	7.5
Temporal	31%	.73	20%	1.7	23%	18	38%	5
Centro–Occipital	24%	.93	16%	1.7	19%	19	26%	10
Occipito–Temporal	26%	.93	27%	1.6	23%	18	31%	5

[a]From Ricardo et al., 1975. Maximum separation (M Sep) obtained between cumulative frequency curves of normals and each group of patients, and parameter values (value) at points of maximum separation.

[b]A 23% separation was significant at $P = .05$.

[c]R = correlation coefficients.

[d]SER = signal energy ratio (absolute value).

[e]AD = amplitude difference (%).

[f]ML = the greatest of the latencies discrepancies observed across the whole analysis epoch (msec).

was the correlation coefficient. Amplitude differences and SER values have a similar power for statistical discrimination, but SER reflects modifications along the whole duration of the VER better. Therefore, correlation coefficients and SER values were selected for discriminant analysis.

A multiple linear discriminant analysis was carried out between the six different groups (five patient groups and one control), using the Fisher z transforms of the correlation coefficients and SER values. Computation of Mahalanobis distance showed no significant differences between the centroids of the groups of patients. However, a rather significant difference was found between the centroid of the normal group and the centroids of the different groups of patients. Therefore, the data of the different patient groups were pooled together and compared with the values of the normal group by a Hotelling T^2 test. A highly significant difference was found between the control and the patient groups ($P < .01$). Discriminant scores were calculated for each subject. Table 13.2 shows the results obtained by classification according to the scores obtained by the application of the discriminant equation, and the comparison with the EEG routine examination.

Inspection of this table shows that VER symmetry increases the number of subjects considered abnormal, both in the group of patients and in the control group. Although the majority of the patients had asymmetric VERs, only 12 had visual field defects. The asymmetries were not exclusively confined to the occipital regions, but were often present in central and temporal regions. Another striking finding is that no correlation was found between the localization of the lesion and the major VER asymmetry. Fur-

TABLE 13.2
Classification of Subjects According to the VER Symmetry Scores and The Routine EEG Examination[a]

	VER Symmetry		*EEG*		*VER Symmetry* + EEG	
	P[b]	N[c]	P	N	P	N
Tumors	28	6	23	11	29	5
Vascular	41	9	34	16	43	7
Epilepsy	35	20	47	8	49	6
Miscellaneous	28	10	23	15	31	7
Parkinson	8	12	8	12	12	8
Control	21	71	0	92	21	71

[a]From Ricardo et al., 1975.
[b]P means pathologic.
[c]N means normal.

ther, in some subjects it was found that the larger VERs were on the side of the lesion, whereas the contrary was found in others. These findings emphasize the difficulty in deciding which VER was abnormal. These various considerations, together with the fact that no significant differences were found between different types of pathologies, suggest that VER asymmetry is a very unspecific sign of brain dysfunction.

2. Complementary Use of EEG Symmetry and VER Symmetry

As a subgroup of these patients in which VER symmetry was studied had also been subject to the analysis of their EEG symmetry, it was of interest to compare the accuracy of both methods with conventional EEG examination of the same patients. Because epileptics are not well discriminated by EEG symmetry, we only present the results for the groups of brain tumor patients and cerebrovascular disease cases. Table 13.3 shows the number of subjects that were classified as abnormal: (1) by discriminant analysis of EEG symmetry values; (2) by discriminant analysis of VER symmetry values; and (3) on the basis of routine EEG examination. A high percentage of cases were considered abnormal by one or both of the symmetry methods. Only one patient with a brain tumor and another patient of the cerebrovascular group had an abnormal EEG with normal values of both EEG and ER symmetries. This suggests that a combination of quantitative parameters in an electrophysiological diagnostic battery may accomplish a good screening

TABLE 13.3
Classification of Patients According to the VER Symmetry Scores, the EEG Symmetry Scores, and the Routine EEG Examination

Discriminant Scores for EEG Symmetry	*Discriminant Scores for VER Symmetry*	*Visual EEG*	*Tumor Patients*		*Cerebrovasvular Patients*	
			N	*%*	*N*	*%*
0[a]	0	0	2	6.5	3	6
1[b]	0	0	3	9.7	4	8
0	1	0	1	3.2	3	6
0	0	1	1	3.2	1	2
1	1	0	4	12.9	11	22
0	1	1	5	16.1	6	12
1	0	1	1	3.2	3	6
1	1	1	14	45.2	19	38

[a]0 means classified as normal.
[b]1 means classified as pathologic.

method in clinical neurology. In relation to epilepsy, a separate section is dedicated to this approach later in this chapter.

B. Waveform Analysis

1. *Utility of Peak Latency of VER Waves for the Discrimination of MS Patients.*

In a study of 50 control subjects, Ellenberg and Ziegler (1977) found that the most reliable wave of the VERs to monocular flash stimulation, recording over the contralateral occipital cortex and using vertex as reference, was the first major upward deflection, which has a mean latency of 52.8 ± 4 msec. Considering 60 msec as the upper limit, only 4% of the control subjects were beyond this limit. Analyzing each eye separately, 97% of the eyes with a previous history of optic neuritis and 56% of the asymptomatic eyes in a group of 24 MS patients with a history of at least one attack of optic neuritis were found. These figures were higher than the percentages obtained using quantitative perimetry (56 and 14% respectively). In a group of 25 MS patients who had never suffered from visual symptoms, 16 subjects (64%) presented delayed VERs from at least one eye. However, this finding should not be considered as a specific sign of MS, because in ischemic optic neuropathies, six out of 15 eyes showed delayed VERs.

2. *Amplitude and Latency Values of the Different Waves: Discriminant Analysis Between Normal Subjects and Patients with Ophthalmic and Neuro-Ophthalmic Lesions.*

Maccolini, Meduri, Cavicchi, and Cristini (1977) found certain similarities between the VERs obtained from patients with the same ophthalmic or neuro-ophthalmic lesions. On this basis, they made a univariate and multivariate statistical comparison between four groups: (1) 100 normal individuals between 2 and 71 years old; (2) 22 patients with detachment of the retina; (3) 42 patients suffering deficient optic nerve conduction due to different lesions; and (4) 42 patients with strabismic amblyopia, 34 of whom had esotropic and eight exotropic amblyopia. In group 4, the comparison was made against 18 normals of the same age. The deflections of each VER, identified by visual inspection and adopting Cigánek's (1961) nomenclature, were subjected to the following measurements: The amplitude of wave I was calculated measuring the voltage difference between the onset of the curve and the wave apex. The amplitude of the subsequent waves was measured as the difference between the peak of the examined wave and that of the previous wave. The other measure, called bases (milliseconds), corresponds to the difference between the latency of the examined wave and the latency of the previous wave. For wave I, the bases were not determinable and were replaced by the latency of the apex. Thus, each VER was defined by the value of 10 parameters: amplitude and latency of wave I, and amplitude and bases of waves II, III, IV, and V. VERs were recorded from a monopolar sagittal derivation with the active electrode 3 cm above the inion and the reference on the right auricular lobe. In normal subjects, the responses obtained by monocular stimulation were utilized for the analysis; in patients, only those responses obtained through the stimulation of the affected eye were used.

With respect to distinctions between normal subjects, cases of retinal detachment, and optic nerve conduction deficiency, significant differences were found for the amplitudes of the different waves between the pathological groups and the normal subjects. However, no differences existed between the two groups of patients on the basis of univariate analysis. The latency of wave I and the bases of the subsequent waves did not allow differentiation between the three groups. No significant differences were found between amblyopics and normals of the same age.

The multivariate approach to the discrimination between normals, cases of retinal detachment, and conduction defects revealed highly significant differences. Two canonical variables were obtained: The first one explained 91.5% of the total covariance and the second one the remaining 8.5%. Fig. 13.2 shows the relative position of the centroids of the three groups, with

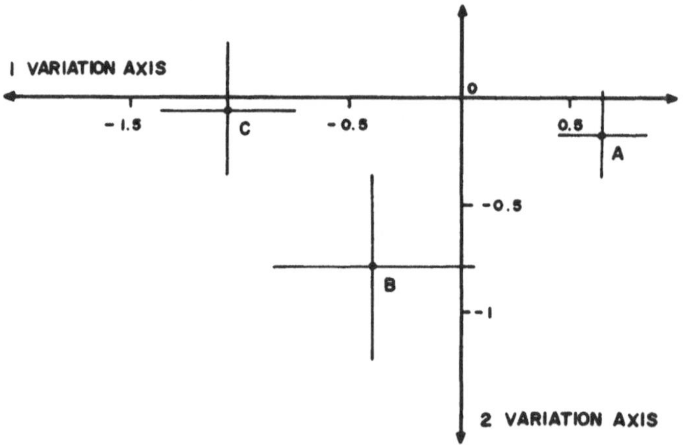

FIG. 13.2. Graphic representation of the results of the canonical analysis of variance: relative position of the three groups (A = normal individuals; B = retinal detachments; C = conduction defects of optic nerve) with their 95% confidence limits. The groups are clearly discriminated. (From Maccolini et al., 1977.)

their 95% confidence limits projected on the two-dimensional space defined by the canonical variables. Maccolini et al. (1977) also published a graphic representation of the relative position of each individual after calculating the individual values of the discriminant function. On the basis of these graphs, I calculated the Euclidean distance from every individual to each centroid. Considering equal a priori probabilities, approximately 80% of the normals were adequately classified and approximately 75% of the patients were located in one or another pathological group. However, the discrimination between retinal detachment and conduction deficiency was not so high. Note that these results should be considered as only approximate, because I did not have access to the original data. Thus, the canonical analysis of variance between the healthy subjects, the amblyopic esotropic patients, and the amblyopic exotropic patients yielded highly significant differences. These results clearly demonstrate the advantages of using multivariate procedures, because with the univariate analysis, no significant differences were observed.

3. Cluster Analysis

Valdés et al. (1975) submitted to principal component analysis the VERs from left and right central, occipital, and temporal regions of 54 normal subjects and 109 neurological patients. This analysis was made to reduce the dimensionality of the space. It was found that, for every region, seven factors could account for more than 94% of the variance of the data, and three factors explained more than 69%. For each individual VER, factor scores were computed on these last three factors and were used in a subsequent cluster analysis. Results obtained from left and right occipital leads are shown in Table 13.4. These data show that two (groups I and V) of the seven resulting groups were almost exclusively comprised of VERs from patients with neurological diseases. Fig. 13.3 shows the left and right occipital

TABLE 13.4[a]
Clusters Obtained from Left and Right Occipital VERs in a Group of Normal Subjects and Neurological Patients

	Cluster						
	I	*II*	*III*	*IV*	*V*	*VI*	*VII*
Number of VERs	33	65	39	18	54	70	46
% from normals	6	44	46	33	19	43	43
% from patients	94	56	54	67	81	57	57

[a]From Valdés et al. (1975). Cluster analysis was computed with the first three factor scores obtained by principal component analysis.

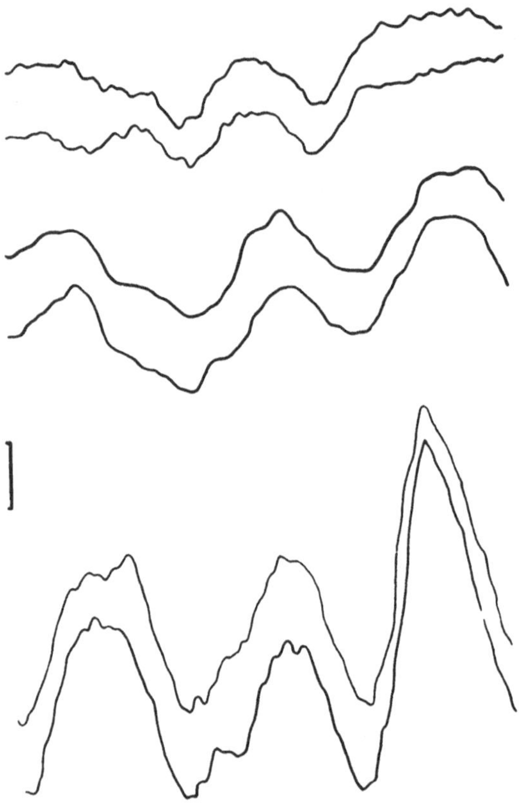

FIG. 13.3. Left and right occipital VERs from three different patients of one of the "abnormal" groups; these were obtained by cluster analysis. The VERs are highly symmetric, but with an abnormal waveshape. (From Valdés et al., 1975.)

VERs from three different patients of one of these "abnormal" groups. The VERs are highly symmetric, but with an abnormal waveshape. In this study, it was not possible to establish a correspondence between the groups obtained by cluster analysis and the different diseases, which emphasizes the fact that VER waveshapes may only be useful for discriminating between normality and abnormality.

4. Step Wise Principal Component Analysis: A Simulated Screening Procedure

In a collaborative study between Dr. E. R. John of New York University and our laboratory at CENIC, the utility of regression principal component analysis for the discrimination between VERs waveshapes from normal subjects and from patients with various neurological disorders was investigated (John et al. 1977). The basic idea of this analysis was to provide the definition of the normal signal space for VERs, as a step toward development of a screening procedure for patients at risk for brain diseases. In principle, individuals whose responses do not lie within this space could be tentatively identified as "not normal". Using data from 10 derivations in 50 normal subjects, a principal component factor analysis was computed on this set of 500 normal VERs. A Varimax rotation was carried out and a set of factors identified that accounted for 93% of the variance in the signal space. Using these Varimax factors and the 500 VERs from this group of normal subjects, three indices were computed:

1. The correlation coefficients between VERs from bilateral symmetrical derivations.
2. Percent regression: The percentage of each individual VER that could be accounted for by the set of Varimax factors that accounted for 93% of the energy in the "normal signal space" containing those 500 VERs (10 derivations/subject x 50 normal subjects).
3. The regression asymmetry, or RA: For each pair of symmetrical electrodes, the individual factor loading asymmetry, ΔF, was obtained by calculating the absolute difference in loading coefficients representing the relative contribution of each factor to the two VER waveshapes. The total factor loading asymmetry, $\Sigma\Delta F$, for the pair was obtained by adding the individual factor loading asymmetries for all the factors required to construct the two waveforms. The RA was obtained by summing the total loading asymmetries across the five derivations for each normal subject. Thus, RA constituted a single measure for the *cumulative asymmetry* of the VERs from the entire head of the subject.

With these values, first approximations for the criteria of "normality" were established for the three indices just defined. Next, the data from four different groups were evaluated using the same criteria. Each of these four groups was a subsample of neurological patients that included the most difficult cases of those previously analyzed by symmetry analysis: group (1) 25 normal controls; group (2) 25 patients with brain tumors; group (3) 25 patients with cerebrovascular lesions; and group (4) 25 patients with epilepsy.

The overall accuracy of the method was good. If any single computer index was found to be positive (1 +), the patient was considered "at risk of brain damage." If any two computer indices were positive (2 +), the subject was classified as "abnormal." For resolving the classification of 1 + patients "at risk," the EEG examination was taken into consideration. If he had an abnormal EEG, he or she was classified as "abnormal." If all computer indices were normal, the EEG evaluation was not taken into account. This procedure simulated a three-class screening procedure:

1. Patients classified as "abnormal" on the basis of 2+ computer evaluation would be referred to the neurologist.

2. Patients evaluated as "at risk" (1 +) would be referred for a conventional EEG examination.
3. Patients found normal by the computer would not be further examined.

The results are presented in Table 13.5. It is obvious that the discrimination by the computer procedure was better for the brain tumors and cerebrovascular disease patients than the EEG conventional evaluation, but for the group of epileptics, the EEG still provided much more information.

5. Multidimensional Scaling

In a preliminary study, Schwartz and John (1976) used the *multidimensional scaling procedure* (see Chapters 7 and 10) for separation of VERs from occipito-temporal derivations in 20 normal subjects and 20 patients with brain tumors. An impressive separation of the two groups were obtained. Three control subjects lay in the "abnormal" domain and three patients in the "normal" domain. If we consider that the accuracy obtained with a single derivation was similar to that obtained with the discriminant analysis of multilead EEG or VER symmetry, the results are quite promising. However, the procedure does not provide a decision rule, and no predictive statistical tests are possible; thus, its use is limited to a particular sample.

TABLE 13.5
Classification of Subjects According to the Step-Wise Principal Component Analysis of VERs and the Routine EEG Examination, Using a Stimulated Screeing Procedure[a]

Groups	*Computer Indices*		*EEG*		*Computer (1 +) and EEG*	
	Abnormal (2 +)	0	Abnormal	0	Abnormal	0
Normal	Risk (1 +)	5	Normal	25	Normal	25
	Normal	20				
Tumors	Abnormal (2 +)	20	Abnormal	15	Abnormal	22
	Risk (1 +)	2	Normal	10	Normal	3
	Normal	3				
Vascular	Abnormal (2 +)	15	Abnormal	15	Abnormal	20
	Risk (1 +)	6	Normal	10	Normal	5
	Normal	4				
Epilepsy	Abnormal (2 +)	7	Abnormal	20	Abnormal	18
	Risk (1 +)	13	Normal	5	Normal	7
	Normal	5				

[a] Adapted from John et al. (1977).

These shortcomings will hopefully be overcome as this type of analytical procedure is further developed.

6. Prognostic Value of VER Waveform in Functional Amblyopia

Arnal et al. (1971) studied the VERs of 56 children with unilateral functional amblyopia. They observed that the averaged VERs of the amblyopic eyes displayed longer latencies for the earliest component, remained smaller, and ended earlier than VERs from normal eyes. They performed several discriminant analyses and evaluated the performance according to the accuracy obtained in the prediction of the results of functional remediation. The first discriminant analysis was performed on the basis of clinical parameters, with 82% accuracy in the prognosis. The second one was based on the amplitude values of the VERs at 80 and 100 msec of latency, with a correct prediction in 86% of the cases. The combination of clinical findings and VER parameters gave a correct prognosis in 96% of the cases.

III. TRANSIENT VISUAL EVOKED RESPONSES TO PATTERN-REVERSAL STIMULI

In Chapter 3, we referred to the great value of VERs to pattern reversal in the assessment of neurological lesions. The evaluation has been mainly based on measuring the delay of the major positive component, which has a latency of 80-100 msec in normal subjects, depending on the method for stimulus generation. For similar conditions of stimulation, the interindividual variability of this latency is so small that it can be used for the discrimination of abnormalities in the retina and in the optic nerve with high accuracy. But, what appears more remarkable is the possibility of detecting electrophysiological abnormalities due to optic neuritis in the absence of clinical signs, a fact that has been used as a test to aid in the clinical diagnosis of MS. In a patient with damage to the central nervous system, other than in the optic nerves, the finding of delayed VER establishes the presence of multiple lesions in the central nervous system, thus suggesting the diagnosis of MS when the history has been of intermittent episodes with relapse and remissions. The test is of interest in patients with definite MS, but its real value is for those in whom the diagnosis is doubtful. However, the finding of a delayed VER in a patient with a spinal-cord lesion, for example, occurs not only in MS, but also in other progressive diseases such as spinocerebellar degeneration or tropical spastic neuropathy.

Table 13.6 shows the values of the mean peak latency of the major

TABLE 13.6
VERs to Pattern-Reversal Stimuli

	X	*SD*	*L*	*MS Patients Discriminated*			
Reference	*msec*	*msec*	*msec*	*With ophthalmic Signs %*	*Without %*	*Total %*	*n*
Halliday et al., 1973a	103.8	4.3	115	100	92	96	51
Asselman et al., 1975	90.5	4.3	104	100	47	67	51
Lowitzch et al., 1976	103.8	4.3	112	87	33	73	135
Bynke et al., 1977	90.3	11.3	110	100	63	76	25
Hennerici et al., 1977	102.5	2.92	112	100	-	61	57
Celesia and Daly, 1977b	97.8	-	-	96	52	71	52
Celesia, 1978	97.8	-	-	94	55	74	74
Shahrokhi et al., 1978	102.3	5.1	116	87	36	57	149

[a]Peak of major positive wave (X, SD), maximal acceptable normal value (*L*), and incidence of delayed VERs in multiple sclerosis.

positive component and the standard deviations obtained by different authors. The maximum acceptable value defined by each laboratory is also shown. This value has been obtained as the mean plus 2, 2.5, or 3 SD. The incidence of delayed VERs in MS is highest for those cases with a history of visual symptoms. Delayed VERs are found in practically all cases with convincing history of a previous episode of optic neuritis. These responses remained abnormal for months or years after a complete recovery of clinical function following optic neuritis. A higher percentage of delayed VERs is also observed in patients with definite than with probable or possible MS. An overall estimate of 69% of delayed VERs in patients with MS is obtained, considering different publications.

Delayed VERs are not exclusive of MS. Halliday et al. (1973a) and Asselman et al. (1975) have also found delayed VERs in ischemic optic neuropathy, optic nerve compression, tropical amblyopia, tropical spastic neuropathy, and spinocerebellar degeneration. We described in Chapter 3 that delayed VERs have been also reported in other diseases of the nervous system, such as cerebrovascular diseases, migraine, and Parkinson's disease. Thus, the interpretation of delayed VERs depends on the clinical history. According to Duwaer and Spekreijse (1978), one should be cautious in attributing a longer latency to an increased conduction time. They have found that, contrary to the good correspondence between apparent (see section IV of this chapter, Steady-State VERs) and peak latencies in healthy subjects, in some MS patients, the apparent latency is much longer than the peak latency. This cannot be ascribed to an increase of the peak latency of the first positive component, on which the criterion is based, but to the absence of this component or to the presence of displaced components on these records. Displaced components are also observed in the presence of scotomata, as well as in demyelination. Furthermore, latency increase may be also due to a lower mean luminance (A. M. Haliday, 1977), or to optical imperfections: in normal subjects, the VERs obtained during blurring the horizontal edges of the checks with cylindrical lens of +3D, although very similar in shape to those obtained without lens, have a latency increase of about 25 msec. Duwaer and Spekreijse also point out that because demyelination may have a patchy character, the final VER may be built up by components with normal and increased latencies. Thus, contrast VERs can be expected with either a multipeaked or a sluggish appearance. They found in a MS patient that, comparing the VERs to the left and right eyes separately when the stimulus was an appearing-disappearing checkerboard of 55′ checks, the VERs were rather similar. However, stimulation with 20′ checks showed that the VER of the right eye seemed to consist of two components. These results clearly indicate that an increased latency may have several causes, only one of these being an increased conduction time due to demyelination.

Hennerici, Wenzel, and Freund (1977) compared the VERs to a pattern-reversal checkerboard and to a small, bright rectangle in the assessment of MS patients. They found delayed VERs to both types of stimuli in 100% of the patients who had a history of optic neuritis and/or optic nerve atrophy. However, responses to the small rectangle were delayed in a higher percentage of cases in MS patients without optic neuritis. Delayed VERs to both types of stimuli were also observed in patients without lesions of the visual pathway (i.e., congenital nystagmus, tumors of the posterior fossa).

Celesia and Daly (1977a, 1977b) studied the pattern-reversal responses and the driving responses to flicker in four groups of subjects: 72 healthy subjects, 36 neurological patients without lesions of the visual pathway, 39 patients with lesions of the visual pathway, and 53 MS patients. In the control group, they computed the regression line of *N*74 and *P*100 latencies according to age. The abnormal limit was set above 2.5 SD of the regression line. Ninety-nine percent of the healthy subjects were below this line. The driving responses were computed for several frequencies of stimulation and the following parameters were measured: peak latencies of the major negative and positive deflections and the critical frequency of photic driving. Combination of pattern VERs and driving measurements formed the VECA profile. This profile was normal in all neurological patients without lesions of the visual pathway and in patients with retrochiasmatic visual pathway lesions. VECA was abnormal in all patients with optic lesions and in 77% of MS patients (of which 71% had delayed VERs). These results led the authors to suggest this test for the specific diagnosis of optic nerve lesions. However, their results contradict those of other authors who report abnormality of the driving responses in cases with lesions outside of the visual pathway. Although the great majority of patients in this group were epileptics, we describe in the next section that photic driving responses are altered in many neurological patients, including epileptics. As discussed earlier, delayed pattern reversal VERs are found in different types of patients.

IV. STEADY-STATE VISUAL EVOKED RESPONSES

A. "Driving Curve" for the Evaluation of Brain Damage

Ricardo et al. (1974), Harmony (1975), and Harmony et al. (1975) have studied the "driving curves" in groups of normal subjects and different types of neurological patients. The procedure consists of using a CAT 400 C computer as a digital filter and averaging the EEG activity during successive epochs of time, corresponding precisely to the period of the particular frequency under study. This was accomplished by controlling the address advance of the computer by a pulse produced by an oscillator at a frequency equal to the product of the frequency of stimulation by the number of addresses. A pulse obtained from the CAT computer triggered the photic stimuli each time the first address in the memory was reached. Flicker stimuli were delivered at several frequencies: 1, 2, 4, 7, 10, 12, and 15 Hz and recording electrodes were situated in bilateral frontal, central, occipital, and temporal regions. The same procedure was repeated for all subjects removing the stroboscope lamp to study the amount of phase-locked spontaneous activity at each frequency, which was of very low amplitude. For every frequency, the ERs were averaged during 30 secs, depending the epoch of the frequency of stimulation. Thus, for example, at 1 Hz, 30 responses with an analysis time of 1 second were averaged, and at 10 Hz, the average of 300 responses with an analysis time of 100 msec was obtained. To have a graphic representation for the analysis of each subject, "driving curves" were obtained for all derivations. These graphs described the energy of the driving response as a function of the frequency of stimulation; in other words, the total energies of the driving responses were plotted for every frequency explored. A continuous line was drawn between the different points to make visual inspection and interpretation easier, but without intending a faithful interpolation. The correlation coefficient (R) between the homologous left and right pairs of filtered evoked responses were computed as a measure of waveform similarity. These R values were written below each frequency in the axis (see Fig. 13.4). Thus, in the driving curve, all the information is summarized: the symmetry of the driving responses (by the R values and the differences in shape of the driving curves of each hemisphere) and the behavior of the responses as a function of the frequency of stimulation.

Table 13.7 presents the mean R values for the four derivations in the seven frequencies used in a group of 20 normal subjects. Higher values were observed in frontal and central derivations when compared with occipital and temporal regions. The analysis of the "driving curves" showed that the energy of the responses in temporal, and in some cases in frontal, was lower than the energy of the central and occipital responses. The energy distribution of the driving curves of the central and occipital derivations showed a clear differentiation of two groups of normal subjects: one group with a great amount of energy at 10 or 12 Hz in occipital regions, the other with highest energy at these frequencies in central areas. Normal subjects were characterized by a clear response to photic stimulation in the alpha frequency band either in occipital or central regions (see Fig. 13.5).

The result of the application of this method to a preliminary group of 25 neurological patients with different types of brain lesions (10 cerebrovascular lesions, 6 tumors, 2 MS, and 7 with various other diseases) showed a great variability in the responses, which suggested that this was

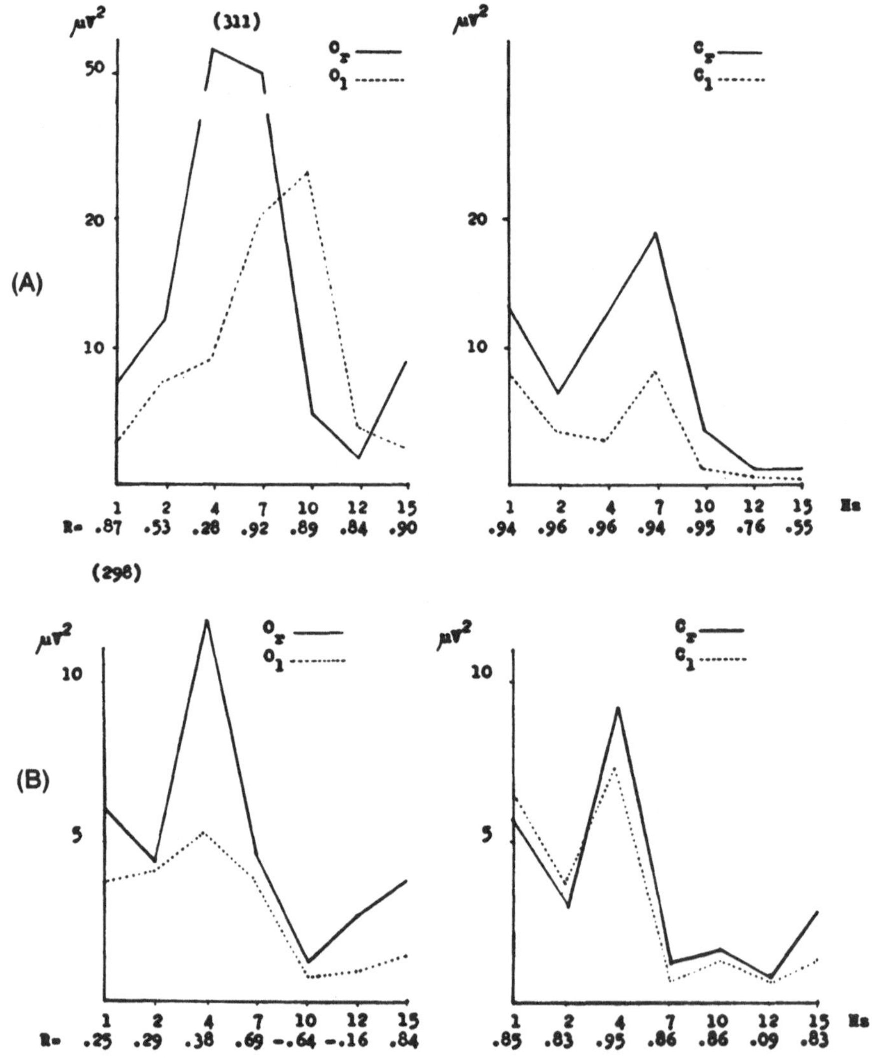

FIG. 13.4. (A) Driving curves of case 311, a patient 63 years old with a right middle cerebral artery occlusion and a normal EEG. The driving curves show the energy (μV^2) of the responses as a function of the frequency of stimulation (Hz) in right and left occipital (O_r, O_l) and right and left central (C_r, C_l) leads. The correlation coefficient (*R*) between left and right homologous evoked responses at each frequency of stimulation is also shown. The *R* values were abnormal in 2 and 4 Hz in occipital regions and in 12 and 15 Hz in central regions. Great asymmetry of the driving curves in both derivations is evident. In the right side, energy of the slow frequencies is predominant and a very small response to 10 Hz is observed. In the left side, a normal response to 10 Hz is present. It can be concluded that the lesion was in the right hemisphere. (B) Driving curves of case 298, a patient 43 years old with an optochiasmatic tumor. The EEG was normal. Same abbreviations as in (A). *R* values are extremely low in the occipital regions. A dominance of the energy of the responses to low frequencies may be observed. (From Harmony, 1975.)

TABLE 13.7[a]

Driving Responses: Mean and Critical Values of Correlation Coefficients[b]

Derivations	*1 Hz*		*2 Hz*		*4 Hz*		*7 Hz*		*10 Hz*		*12 Hz*		*15 Hz*	
	X	*X - 3S*	*X*	*X - 3S*	*X*	*X - 3S*	*X*	*X - 3S*	*X*	*X - 3S*	*X*	*X - 3S*	*X*	*X - 3S*
Frontal	.96	.84	.96	.85	.98	.90	.97	.85	.97	.88	.94	.75	.88	.56
Central	.96	.82	.97	.87	.96	.83	.95	.80	.97	.86	.93	.76	.88	.57
Occipital	.87	.56	.93	.74	.90	.63	.91	.65	.92	.69	.86	.52	.81	.39
Temporal	.83	.45	.86	.51	.83	.44	.79	.35	.80	.37	.71	.17	.65	.05

[a]From Harmony et al. (1975).

[b]Mean values were calculated using Fisher z transformation of R values.

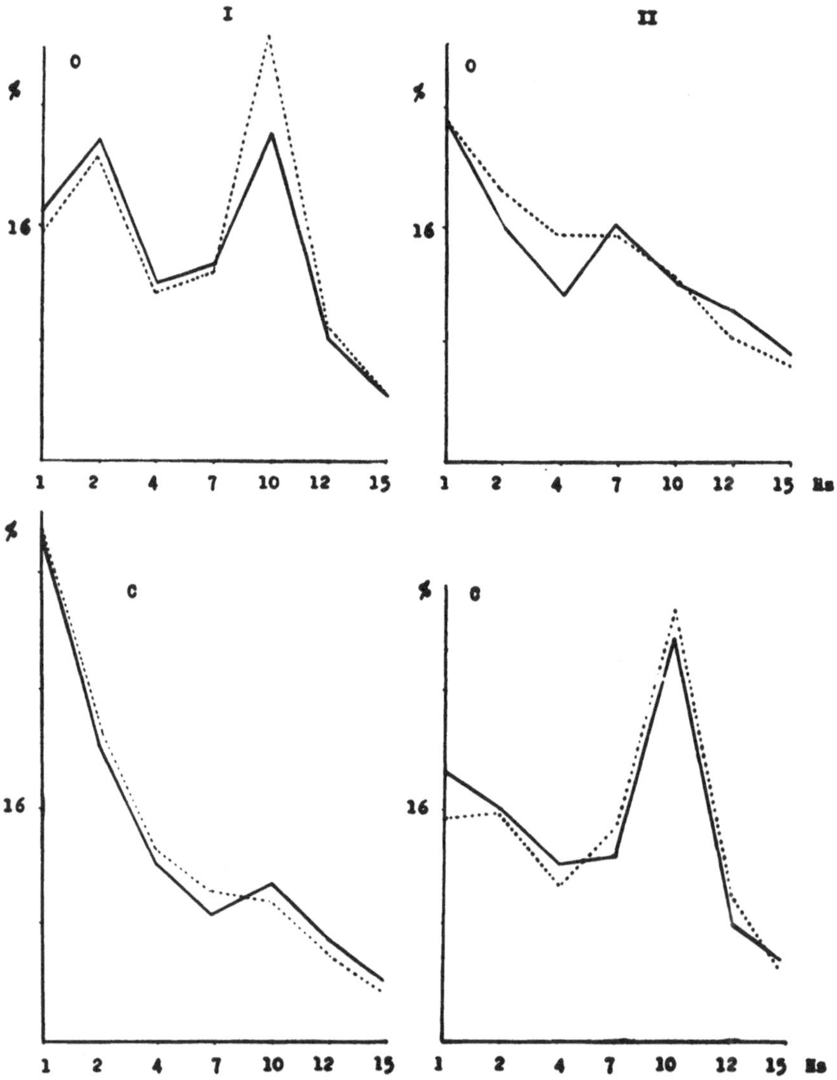

FIG. 13.5. Mean driving curves in normal subjects. Two groups of subjects may be observed: I, those with clear response to 10 Hz in occipital (O) regions; and II, those with prominent response to 10 Hz in central (C) regions. *Continuous lines*: driving curves from right leads. *Discontinuous curves*: left leads. Great interindividual variations in the energy of the responses exist. For this reason, computation of mean values was performed taking into account the percent energy of the responses at each frequency of stimulation, considering as 100% the sum of the energies of the ERs to the seven frequencies used. (From Harmony et al., 1975.)

caused by the heterogeneity of the group. For this reason, each R value was compared with the normal values and was considered "abnormal" when it was lower than 3 SD from the mean of the control group (Table 13.7 also shows these "critical values"). Only central and occipital leads were considered for the analysis. In the normal group, seven R values out of a total of 280 were abnormal, corresponding to seven different subjects. Of the 25 patients, 14 had a normal EEG. In 23, it was possible to observe several abnormal values. One case, although symmetry measures were normal, showed predominance of lower frequencies with no response at 10 Hz. The single case in which the procedure failed was a MS patient with a normal EEG. Some examples of driving curves and the R values reflecting asymmetry of the filtered visual evoked potential at each frequency are shown in Fig. 13.4 A and B.

Later, a group of 44 epileptics (30 with temporal epilepsy, 5 with an occipital focus, and 9 generalized epileptics) were also studied. Using the Student's t test, significant differences ($P < .05$) with lower R values in the group of epileptic patients were found in frontal at 10 and 12 Hz and in occipital regions at 2, 10, 12, and 15 Hz. However, the analysis of all the epileptic patients showed that many of them had very low R values in some frequencies for which the comparison between normals and epileptics showed no significant differences. Thus, the epileptics also showed great heterogeneity in their driving curves. Following the criterion of considering abnormal those values lower than 3 SD from the normal mean, 48% of the epileptics showed several abnormal R values. In 17 (39%) of the epileptics, no dominant peak at 10 Hz in central or occipital derivations was observed, which was also considered an abnormal response. Eight of these cases were not previously classified as abnormals by the criterion followed in the analysis of the R values. Thus, the overall accuracy was 67%. After anticonvulsant treatment, great improvement in the driving responses of epileptics has been observed (Fernández & Harmony, 1978; see Fig. 13.6).

The driving curves were also studied in nine patients with probable and six patients with possible MS. In six cases, great asymmetries of the waveform of the evoked responses and the absence of a dominant peak at 10 or 12 Hz in one patient were observed (Fernández, Pérez, & Harmony, 1977).

The torementioned results showed that in patients with brain lesions, the most frequently observed disturbances in their driving curves were the great asymmetry of the filtered evoked responses (as expressed by very low values of the correlation coefficients to different frequencies and in different locations) and a lack of a clear response at 10 Hz in central or occipital areas. It was not possible to relate any specific pattern of abnormality according to a

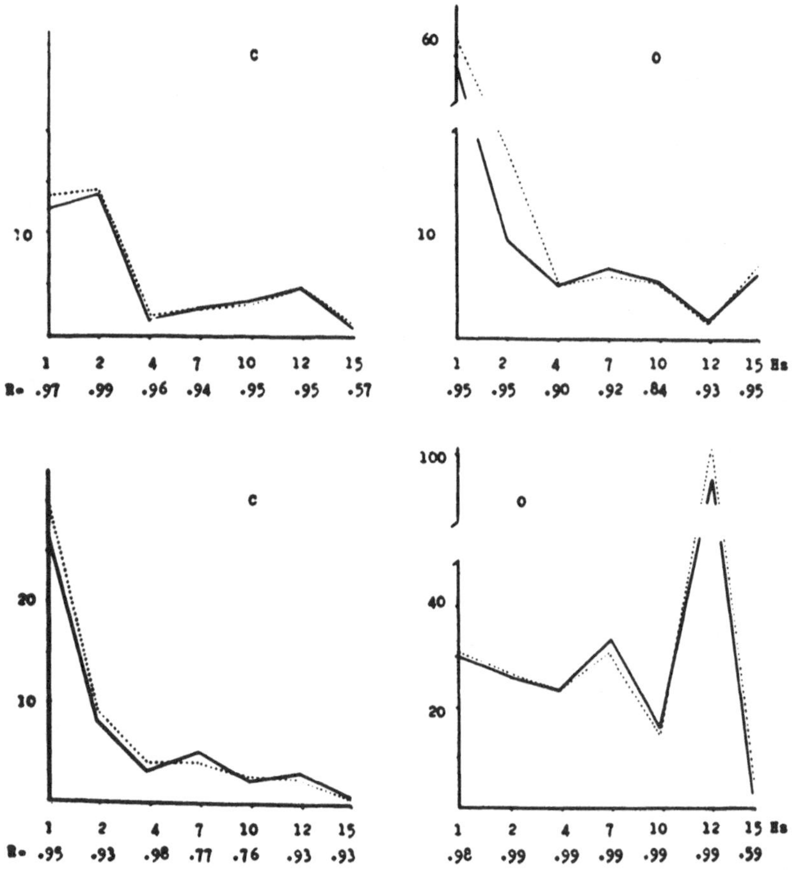

FIG. 13.6. Driving curves of a patient with temporal epilepsy without treatment (*top*) and during treatment (*bottom*). Before treatment, no response to frequencies within the alpha range may be observed. During treatment, a clear response to 12 Hz appeared in occipital regions. *R* values were within normal limits in both conditions (From Fernández & Harmony, 1978a.)

peculiar disease or location of the lesion. Thus, the procedure is only useful as an unspecific index of brain damage or dysfunction.

B. Discrimination of MS Patients

Regan et al. (1976) studied the steady-state ERs to flicker and to pattern reversal in normal subjects and in MS patients. For a stimulus of repetition frequency *F*, the sine wave component of the same frequency was extracted from the steady-state responses and its amplitude and phase were measured.

The phase lag was plotted versus stimulus-repetition frequency. This approximates a straight line, so that ER latency could be estimated from the slope of the line, which the authors called *apparent latency*. Amplitude provided little useful information: response attenuation when visual acuity was markedly depressed. Thus, apparent latency and the difference in latency between left and right eyes were used for the discrimination between normal and MS patients. In all MS patients who had suffered an attack of unilateral retrobulbar neuritis, delayed responses to both types of stimuli were found. More interesting are the results obtained in patients with spinal MS who had never experienced an attack of retrobulbar neuritis. Of the 13 patients studied, only two had experienced any visual symptoms at any time. Taking the results provided by Regan et al. (1976) from the exploration of both eyes, we have constructed Table 13.8. For the total positive cases (column 3), we considered as abnormal every patient who had either an abnormal value for the apparent latency or interocular difference for flicker and pattern stimulation. In the third row, we have placed every patient with a deviant value either to flicker or to pattern responses. From the table, it is clear that both types of stimuli and both types of measures are useful in the detection of MS patient, and that using them as complementary, a higher percentage of cases were detected. From the 12 patients with some type of abnormality, two present only a slight increase of the interocular difference for flicker, however, the remaining 10 had severe alterations. These results are very suggestive of the potential utility of the procedure and they should be extended to a larger sample.

Duwaer and Spekreijse (1978) recorded the pattern-reversal responses to various check sizes and repetition rates and luminance ERs to stimulation with noise modulated light (0-60 Hz) in a group of 11 healthy subjects and 18 MS patients. They measured the latency of the first major positive com-

TABLE 13.8
Spinal Multiple Sclerosis: Cases above Normal Limits of Apparent Latency and Interocular Differences of Steady-State VERs[a]

	Apparent Latency		*Interocular Difference*		*Total*	
	n	%	*n*	%	*n*	%
Flicker	5	38	5	38	8	62
Pattern	5	38	7	54	7	54
Total (flicker pattern)	9	63	10	77	12	92

[a]Modified from Regan et al. (1976). Upper normal values are: 148 msec for apparent latency, both for flicker and pattern; 10 msec of interocular difference for flicker, and 12 msec for pattern responses.

ponent of transient pattern-reversal responses, the apparent latency of VERs to repetition rates exceeding 5 Hz to pattern reversal and of VERs to modulated light, and the interocular latency difference in all cases. The normal mean values for transient reversal VERs given to a frequency of 2 Hz was of 101 ± 8 msec and 102 ± 7 msec for checks of 55 feet and 20 feet respectively, with interocular latency differences of 4 and 5 msec. With repetition each 180 msec, the latency was of 102 ± 6 msec and interocular differences of 4.5 msec. The apparent latency to repetition rates exceeding 5 Hz was of 105 ± 7 msec with 6 msec of interocular difference. On the basis of the normal values, VERs in MS patients were classified as abnormal when latency exceeded 3 SD from the normal mean, or when the interocular difference exceeded 3.5 times the average difference found in normal subjects. On the basis of these two criteria, 12 (67%) out of the 18 patients had abnormal reversal VERs. The failure rate was found to be least for high-frequency pattern reversal (5-20 Hz). With Gaussian noise modulated light, on the basis of a 3 SD criterion, only three out of 13 patients showed an abnormal apparent latency. However, two of these three patients were not discriminated by pattern-reversal evoked responses. Thus, it appears that using both as complementary, a high accuracy is obtained (78%).

V. AUDITORY EVOKED RESPONSES

A. Brain-Stem Responses

1. Discrimination of MS Patients

Robinson and Rudge (1977a) studied the BAERs in a group of normal subjects and in a group of MS patients. Wave V was the largest and also had the least relative variation both in amplitude and latency. Therefore, it was selected to classify the records.

In normal subjects, wave V has a mean latency of 6.0 ± .24 msec and a mean amplitude of .97 + .23 μV. Fig. 13.7 shows the amplitude and latency values of wave V in 88 MS patients. The dotted contour indicates the 95% confidence limit based on the 45 control subjects. Four percent of the normals and 65% of the MS patients lie beyond these limits. The peak-to-peak amplitudes and peak latencies of middle and long latency AER components were also studied. The middle components in the normal group had the following peak latencies: P_a (30.26 + 3.58 msec), N_b (40.76 + 4.82 msec), and P_1 (52.53 + 4.67 msec). The normal limit was set on 2 SD above the normal mean. Forty-five percent of the MS patients had delayed middle components, although no amplitude differences were observed. Of this 45% of MS patients, 12% had normal early brain-stem responses. Thus, if

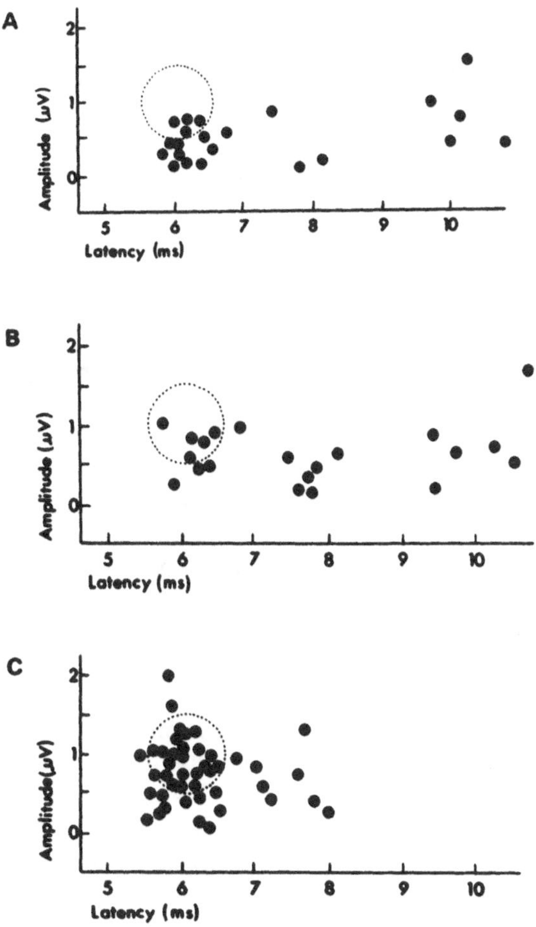

FIG. 13.7. Distribution of amplitude and latency of component V in patients with multiple sclerosis. (A) Patients with definite clinical evidence of brain-stem lesion. (B) Patients with nystagmus. (C) Patients with no clinical evidence of brain-stem lesion. *Broken circle*: 95% confidence limits for normal subjects. *Horizontal axis*: time in msec. *Vertical axis:* amplitude in μV. (From Robinson & Rudge, 1977a.)

either early or middle components were considered, 77% of the MS patients were detected by the AERs. The late components were delayed only in three cases, who also showed delayed middle components.

In an attempt to increase the sensitivity of the method, the auditory pathways were stressed by presenting paired clicks, because it is known that demyelinated fibers fail to conduct trains of pairs of impulses as well as normal fibers. Pairs of clicks, 5 msec apart, were given at a rate of 20 Hz to 17 control subjects and 24 MS patients, 12 of whom have shown abnormalities to one click (Robinson & Rudge, 1977b). The mean latency of the V component to the second click was 6.22 ± .4 msec and the mean amplitude .384 ± 153 μV in normal subjects. Using the paired clicks, the percentage of abnormalities of component V in MS patients increased from 50 to 63%. In relation to the clinical findings, from those patients with unequivocal evidence of a brain stem plaque, 92% had abnormalities of component V to the paired stimulus. In those patients with nystagmus and, therefore, probable brain-stem lesions, 84% had abnormal responses. Of particular interest was the group of patients in whom no clinical signs of brain-stem lesion were found. Of these patients, 42% presented abnormalities of wave V. These results are similar to those observed in MS patients without visual symptoms and abnormal VERs. It appears that early and middle-latency AERs components will be an important part of a battery of evoked responses in the assessment of patients with MS.

2. Brain-Stem Evoked Responses in Acoustic Neuromas

In the search for methods to diagnose acoustic neuromas at an early stage, Thomsen, Terkildsen, and Osterhammel (1978) studied the BAERs in 27 patients with surgically verified acoustic neuromas. The records were performed from vertex referred to neck, with a bandpass extending from 200 Hz to 4 KHz. The stimuli used were a 2 KHz tone burst with a rise-fall time of .3 msec and a plateau of 1 msec, and with an intensity of 98 dB p.e. SPL. The comparative study of this group of patients with another group of 70 patients with Menière's syndrome confirmed that the main indicator of retrochloclear versus cochlear disease was the interaural latency difference of the V wave, or IT_5. In Menière's syndrome, the IT_5 range was from 0 to 1 msec. In the group of acoustic neuromas, only one patient was within this range. In 20 patients, the IT_5 was greater, and in six, no response was found in the side of the tumor. Most of the responses from the ears of the same side of the tumor were a good deal smaller than those from the normal ears—roughly, about half of the amplitude, as an average. From 23 patients in whom computerized tomography was also performed, 13 were negative for tumor. The authors considered that, for the time being, among the functional audiological tests, the auditory brain-stem response examination is the most reliable indicator for the presence of retrocochlear lesions.

B. Cortical Auditory Evoked Responses

Peronnet and Michel (1977) studied the AERs to 1000 Hz delivered monoaurally in control subjects and in patients with possible lesion of the Heschl gyrus or of the auditory radiation in one side. Recordings were made from 13 electrodes along a coronal chain from the right mastoid to the left one, referred to nose. The asymmetry of each individual record was estimated by an asymmetry index (*C*) computed on the basis of the peak-to-peak amplitude of the responses. This asymmetry index was independently obtained from the responses recorded to the stimulation of the left and right ears.

$$C = \frac{1}{\text{integer}(\frac{n}{2})} \sum_{i=1}^{\text{integer}(\frac{n}{2})} \left[\frac{X_i}{X_{n-i}} - \frac{X_{n-i}}{X_i} \right]$$

where n is the number of electrodes and x_i is the peak-to-peak amplitude of the response in the ith electrode. A C value higher than zero means that the responses on the right hemisphere are predominant. If C is lower than zero, it means that the left responses are predominant; and C equal to zero means a lack of asymmetry. In normal subjects, the asymmetry index showed a significant contralateral predominance to the stimulation of both ears. Mean C values to left and right stimulation are: 1.85 ± .62 and −.83 ± .66. In Fig. 13.8, each individual record is represented by a point in a two-dimensional space. The abscissa and the ordinate are the asymmetry indices

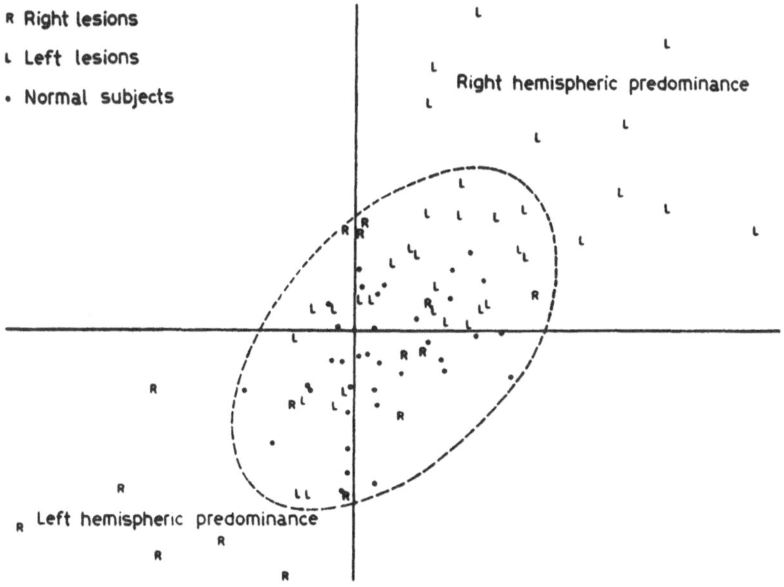

FIG. 13.8. Two-dimensional representation of the AER asymmetry of normal and pathological subjects. The abscissa and ordinate are the asymmetry index when the left and right ears, respectively, were stimulated. Some pathological AERs are clearly out of the range of the normal subjects (circled by interrupted line). A clear correlation, in this case, may be reported between right lesions and a left hemispheric predominance of the AERs and between left lesions and a right hemispheric predominance of the AERs. (From Peronnet & Michel, 1977.)

obtained by the stimulation of the left and right ears respectively. Some pathological values are clearly out of the range of the normal subjects (circled by the interrupted line). A clear correlation between right lesions and left hemisphere predominance of the AERs and between left lesions and a right hemispheric dominance of the AERs may be observed. Although many patients were within the normal region, the authors considered that the index was useful as supplementary information in patients with speech disorders. When the AERs are poor or even absent in one side (hemiawoacusia), there may be supposed that the underlying hemisphere is deaf. Peronnet and Michel (1977) proposed to define this deficit by the term *hemianoacusia*. When the AERs are poor or even absent in one side (hemiamoacusia), there is always an extinction of hearing to the contralateral ear stimulation in the dichotic test, but the inverse is not true. A unilateral extinction in the dichotic test does not imply a hemianoacusia. This probably means that the lesion involves gnostic areas outside the sensory areas. Thus, AERs may help to differentiate various clinical syndromes because, in the case of the left temporal lobe lesions, the patient is aphasic and cannot succeed in a task such as the dichotic listening test.

VI. SOMATOSENSORY EVOKED RESPONSES

A. Far-Field Potentials in Patients with MS

Anziska, Cracco, Cook, and Feld (1978) studied the somatosensory far-field potential to the stimulation of the left and right median nerve in 15 normal subjects and 26 patients with definite MS. Recordings were made from C_z, C_3 and C_4. The dorsum of the hand contralateral to the stimulated median nerve usually served as the reference electrode site. The shoulder or knee contralateral to the side of stimulation was substituted for the hand whenever reference location failed to yield technically satisfactory recordings. P_1, P_3, and N_1 were consistently recorded in all normal subjects. The absolute peak latencies varied considerably and were directly related to the length of the subject's arm; thus, peak latency differences were used, because they were unrelated to arm length and were consistent from subject to subject. Table 13.9 shows the mean and standard deviation of peak latency differences in normal subjects.

Recordings in patients with MS were judged abnormal if they met one or more of the following criteria: (1) absence of P_1, P_3, or N_1; (2) peak latency differences between components evoked by left and right median nerve stimulation that deviated from control values by at least 2.5 SD; and (3) differences in the amplitude of the P_3 and N_1 potential to left versus right median nerve stimulation that deviate from control values more than 2.5 SD.

TABLE 13.9
Somatosensory Evoked Responses: Component Peak Latency Differences in Normal Subjects[a]

Components	*Left Median Nerve Stimulation* *X*	*SD*	*Right Median Nerve Stimulation* *X*	*SD*
P_1-P_2	2.2	.3	2.1	.4
P_1-P_3	4.6	.4	4.4	.5
P_1-N_1	9.3	.9	9.6	.8
P_2-P_1	2.3	.4	2.3	.4
P_2-N_1	7.2	.9	7.5	.8
P_3-N_1	4.7	1.0	5.2	1.0

[a]From Anziska et al. (1978).

This difference was greater than 70% for P_3 and greater than 44% for N_1, comparing left to right median nerve stimulation. On this basis, abnormal results were obtained in 25 out of 26 patients. The most frequent alteration seen was the absence of P_3 and of N_1 (65%). Abnormal peak latency differences were present in 50% of the cases. Differences in the amplitude of the P_3 and N_1 potential to left versus right median nerve stimulation were abnormal in 12% of the cases. No patient fulfilled all three criteria of abnormality, but seven patients satisfied two and 18 patients satisfied one of the criteria. All 12 of the MS patients with normal sensory examination were considered abnormal by the SSERs. Even though five of the 26 patients had no evidence of brain-stem or cerebellar dysfunction on examination, abnormalities in the ERs were observed in all of them (Fig. 13.9). The P_1 potential was observed in all patients with both left and right median

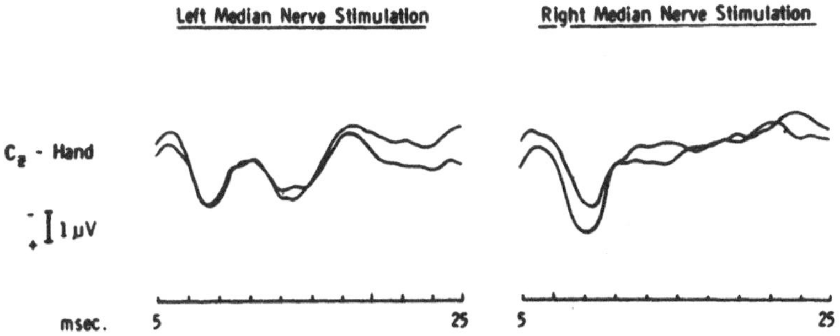

FIG. 13.9. Somatosensory far-field potential to the stimulation of the left and right median nerve in a MS patient. Recordings were made from C_Z, using the dorsum of the hand contralateral to the stimulated nerve as reference. Absence of components to the stimulation of the right median nerve may be observed. (From Anziska et al., 1978.)

nerve stimulation. It has been suggested that this potential is a volume-conducted event that arises primarily in peripheral nerve fibers; the result obtained in MS patients is consistent with this interpretation.

The forementioned results suggest that the recording of the far-field potential may have clinical applications in patients with neurological disorders. It would obviously be important to record these potentials in patients with possible or probable MS to see if the method is useful in the evaluation of these patients whose clinical diagnosis is less certain.

B. Amplitude and Period of Cortical SSER Components in Brain Lesions

Shibasaki et al. (1977a), on the basis of the measurement of the amplitude and the period of waves *N*20, *N*33, and *N*62 of the SSERs to the left and right median nerve stimulation, have described some indices for discriminating between normal subjects and patients with brain lesions of different types (Fig. 13.10). Recordings were made with electrodes located 2 cm posterior and 7 cm lateral to the vertex on each side, the amplitude of the three negative components was defined as the height from the preceding positive peak to the negative peak in question(a_1, a_2, and a_3 in Fig. 13.11). The period was defined as the time interval between the preceding and the following positive peak (p_1, p_2 and p_3). Two indices were calculated for each of the components:

Index I $= \log (a/p \times 100)$ and

Index II $= \log (ap \times ½)$

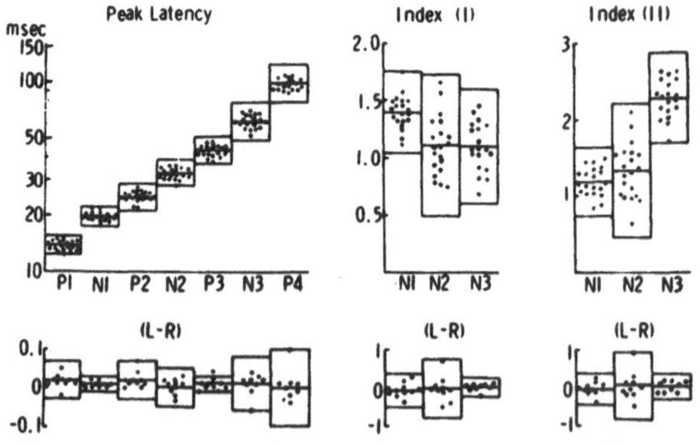

FIG. 13.10. Distribution of peak latencies of the first seven components and two indices of the first three negative components in the control group. Left and right differences are shown at the bottom of each graph. Also, 2.38 SD from the mean value are illustrated. (From Shibasaki et al., 1977a.)

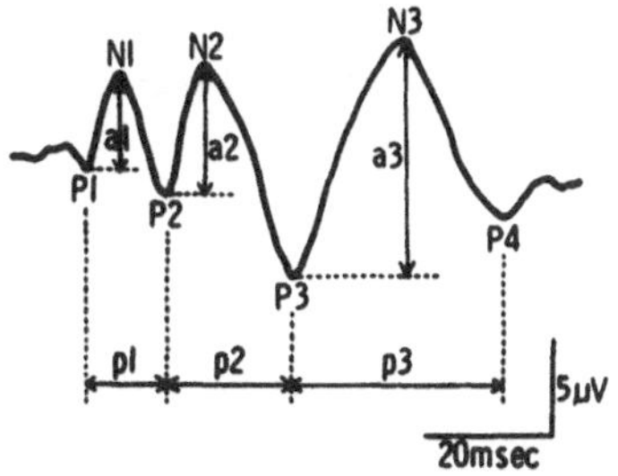

FIG. 13.11. Normal SSER on median nerve stimulation at wrist. N and P indicate the negative and positive peaks respectively. Amplitude (*a*) and duration (*p*) of each negative component are defined as shown here. The upward deflection indicates negativity. (From Shibasaki et al., 1977a.)

For each of the three negative waves, the following eight parameters were considered: (1) onset peak latency, which corresponds to the peak latency of the preceding positive wave; (2) peak latency; (3) Index I; (4) Index II. The four remaining parameters were symmetry measures between the left cortical response to the stimulation of the right median nerve, and the right cortical response to the stimulation of the left median nerve. Such measures were: (5) the onset peak latency differences; (6) the peak latency difference; (7) the Index I difference; and (8) the Index II differences. Fig. 13.10 shows the distributions of such parameters for each component in normal subjects. Mean and 2.38 SD from the mean value are illustrated. As can be seen, all values were included within these limits. The SSER was considered abnormal when any of these parameters was beyond 2.38 SD from the mean value of the control group. Abnormal SSERs were found in 61 out of 65 patients (94%). Among 56 patients with unilateral cerebral lesions, 53 (95%) showed SSER abnormalities; these were exclusively over the affected hemisphere in 36 patients and over both hemispheres in 17 patients. Among 9 patients with diffuse cerebral lesions or dysfunctions, the SSERs were abnormal in 8 patients (89%). The SSER was abnormal in 20 of 21 patients with cerebrovascular accidents, in all 5 patients with arteriovenous malformations, in 19 of 20 patients with brain tumors, in 6 of 7 patients with anoxic encephalopathy, and in 11 of 12 patients with other types of lesions. Thus, there was not significant difference in the incidence of SSER abnormalities among these diseases. The rates of abnormalities localized over the affected hemisphere were shown to be significantly greater in the SSER as compared with the routine EEG.

The results obtained by Shibasaki et al. (1977a) are extremely impressive from the point of view of the accuracy obtained. However, from the description of the procedure, it appears necessary to identify the waves studied. According to previous descriptions in literature, from my own experience, and even from some of the Shibasaki et al. recordings, in some cases, the response is markedly depressed on the side of the lesion, making identification of such components very difficult and sometimes impossible. In these cases, it would be preferable to consider the absence of response as a sign of abnormality.

C. Interhemispheric Latency and Amplitude Differences of SSERs to Simultaneous Bilateral Median Nerve Stimulation in Patients with Brain Lesions

Yamada et al. (1978) studied the SSERs to bilateral median nerve stimulation in a group of 28 healthy subjects and in 20 patients with cerebral lesions. The interhemispheric latency difference for the early (up to P40) and later components never exceeded ranges of 4.5 msec and 8.5 msec, respectively, in normal subjects. Amplitude difference for each component was expressed as a ratio of left to right. Individual and interhemispheric differences were greater in amplitude than in latency. However, in the control group, no two successive components showed a consistent asymmetry above 50 percent. Based on the normative data, latency differences greater than 5 msec for early components and 10 msec for late components (greater than 3 SD from normal), and an amplitude difference of two consecutive components greater than 50%, were arbitrarily considered abnormal. The group of patients was composed by 10 brain infarcts, eight tumors, and two MS patients. Seven patients had a normal EEG, brain scanning, and computerized axial tomography, whereas all patients presented at least one abnormal value. The most frequent alterations observed were in the long latency components (P93 and N135), which were either depressed, delayed, or unidentified. Although age differences existed between the two groups, the patient group was older than the control group. The results obtained suggest that bilateral median nerve stimulation is a promising technique for detecting SSER abnormalities caused by relatively small cerebral or brainstem lesions that may not be demonstrated by any other routine complementary study.

The procedures described in this section clearly demonstrate the discriminant power of SSERs in neurological patients. However, we think that they are liable to further improvement by the application of multivariate techniques to the same features considered.

D. Somatosensory Evoked Response Train (SSERT): Discrimination of Normal Subjects from MS Patients

A similar procedure to that described by Ricardo et al. (1974) for the study of photic driving responses has been used by Namerow, Sclabassi, and Enns (1974) and Sclabassi, Namerow, and Enns (1974) for the analysis of the steady-state responses to trains of electrical pulses of different frequencies applied to the median nerve. The SSERT are filtered by a narrow band filter centered at the stimulating frequency and then averaged to obtain the "single-cycle average response." The frequencies used were: 12, 20, 40, 60, 80, 100, 160, and 200 Hz. In a comparative study between a control group and a group of patients with MS, these authors observed significant differences in the single-cycle average amplitude values (Fig. 13.12). A stepwise discriminant analysis showed that with the peak-to-peak amplitude values of the single-cycle average response to four different frequencies (40, 60, 100, and 160 Hz), 100% discrimination was obtained. Further application of the equation to 27 unknown new subjects (11 normals and 16 MS) also gave 100% discrimination. The authors also observed that the distributions of the single-cycle average amplitudes were related to the severity of the clinical symptoms. The sensitivity of the method is illustrated by the results in one patient who had normal SSERs to single electrical shocks, but who, by the application of the discriminant equation, was classified as having MS. The technique is also highly specific: Demyelination must be present in the pathway under study for the observation of abnormal responses.

E. Somatosensory Conduction Velocity in MS

Dorfman (1977) described a technique for an indirect estimation of spinal-cord conduction velocity in man. The latency to onset of the SSER elicited by stimulation of the posterior tibial nerve at the ankle ($SSER_L$) is considered to be the sum of three components: T_L, which is the time for impulse transmission from the site of stimulation to the lumbar spinal cord; T_0, the time for impulse transmission from the lumbar to the cervical spinal cord; and T_B, the impulse transmission time from the cervical cord to the recording scalp electrodes. Similarly, the SSER to median nerve stimulation ($SSER_A$) at the wrist is considered to have two elements: T_A, impulse transmission time from the wrist to the cervical cord; and T_B. In order to derive estimates of the conduction delays in the spinal cord and supraspinal segments of the somatosensory pathway, it is necessary to have independent measures of the peripheral conduction times T_L and T_A. These times may be calculated on the basis that the stimulation of the nerves evoked a direct muscular response (M) and a reflex muscular response (F). The peripheral conduction time will be the difference between the F and M responses minus the central delay:

$$T_L = (F_L - M_L - 1) / 2\ (s/m)$$

$$T_A = (F_A - N_A - 1) / 2\ (s/m).$$

One millisecond is allowed for central delay of the *F* wave. The term s/m, a correction factor that adjusts the *F*-wave latency to reflect sensory rather than motor conduction, is derived from the ratio of the maximal conduction velocity (CV) to the maximal motor CV in the median nerves of each

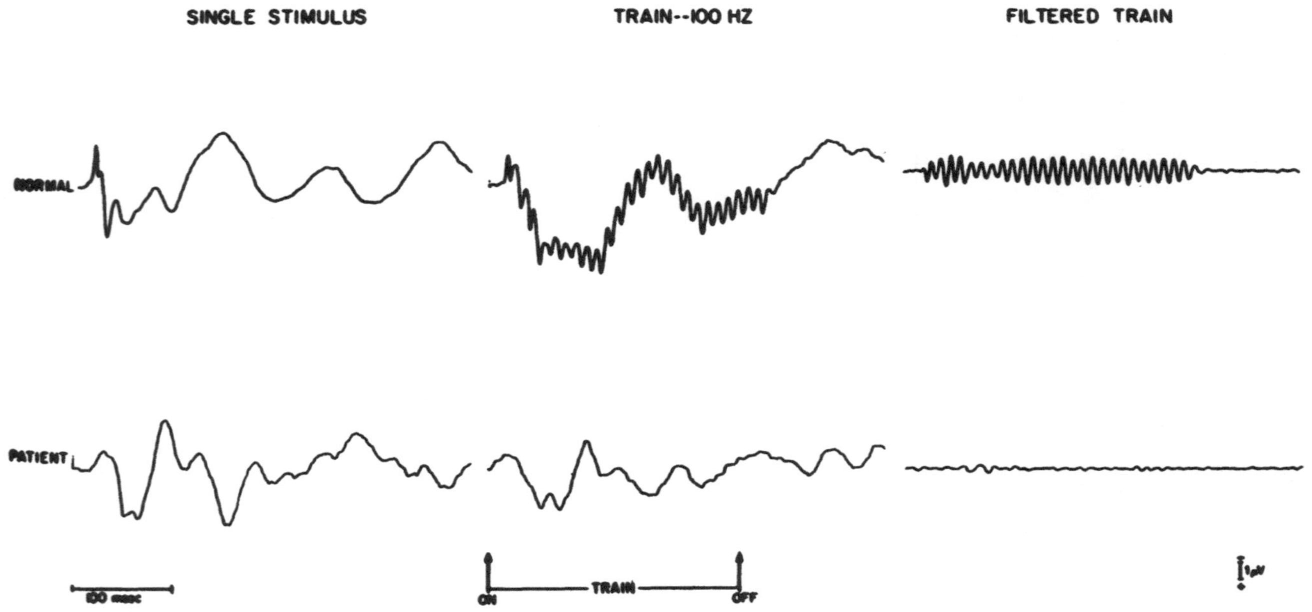

FIG. 13.12. *Upper series*: a single stimulus SSER from a normal subject followed by the same subject's SSERT at 100 Hz and, in the last column, the filtered SSERT for 64 presentations of the stimulus train. *Lower series*: data from an MS patient with moderate symptoms. The first response is the SSER in a single stimulus. The middle response is to a train of stimuli at 100 Hz. The lack of cortical activity at this frequency is evident. This is further demonstrated in the last column where the filtered SSERT shows virtually no 100 Hz activity. (From Sclabassi et al., 1974.)

subject. Because the latency to onset of the SSER and the peripheral conduction times are independent measures, T_C may be calculated and used—together with a measure of spinal cord length (DC)—to derive an indirect estimate of spinal-cord sensory conduction velocity:

$$CV_C = D_C / T_C$$

where $T_C = SSER_L - T_C - T_B$

and $T_B = SSER_A = T_A$

A diagrammatic illustration of the technique is shown in Fig. 13.13. Table 13.10 shows the mean and standard deviation of the measurement obtained in a group of 15 normal subjects and 30 MS patients (Dorfman, Bosley, & Cummins, 1978). Abnormally slow CV_C was defined as a value more than 2 SDs below the mean of the normal population (33 m/seg), and prolonged T_B as greater than 2 SDs above the normal mean (7.5 msec). Twenty-two of the 30 MS patients had abnormally slow CV_C on one or both sides, and 24 had at least one abnormal CV_C or T_B value; thus, only six MS patients had normal examinations and five of these had never experienced any form of sensory disturbance. In three patients with probable MS, the CV_C estimate offered electrophysiological evidence of an additional (spinal) lesion that could not be confirmed by clinical examination alone. One normal control showed a prolonged unilateral T_B measurement.

Dorfman et al. (1978) suggest that the attempt to localize a somatosensory disturbance should begin with the measurement of $SSER_L$. If this potential has normal onset latency (within 2 SDs of the normal mean), there may be little profit in carrying out the test, because none of their 60 procedures gave abnormal CV_C results when $SSER_L$ was normal. If $SSER_L$ is prolonged, the additional measurement and calculations will aid in localization of the lesion. If a supraspinal lesion is suspected, it may be reasonable to begin with the measurement of $SSER_A$ or T_A.

According to the authors, with this method, it is possible to make a crude localization of the level of the sensory lesion to either the spinal or the supraspinal segment of the somatosensory pathway, while simultaneously confirming that the peripheral nerves are intact. The method is quite sensitive even to mild degrees of sensory disturbance, particularly of joint position or vibration, and, as such, could probably also serve in a negative sense to identify psychogenic sensory symptoms, or in the evaluation of patients with other neurological diseases that affect the central somatosensory system.

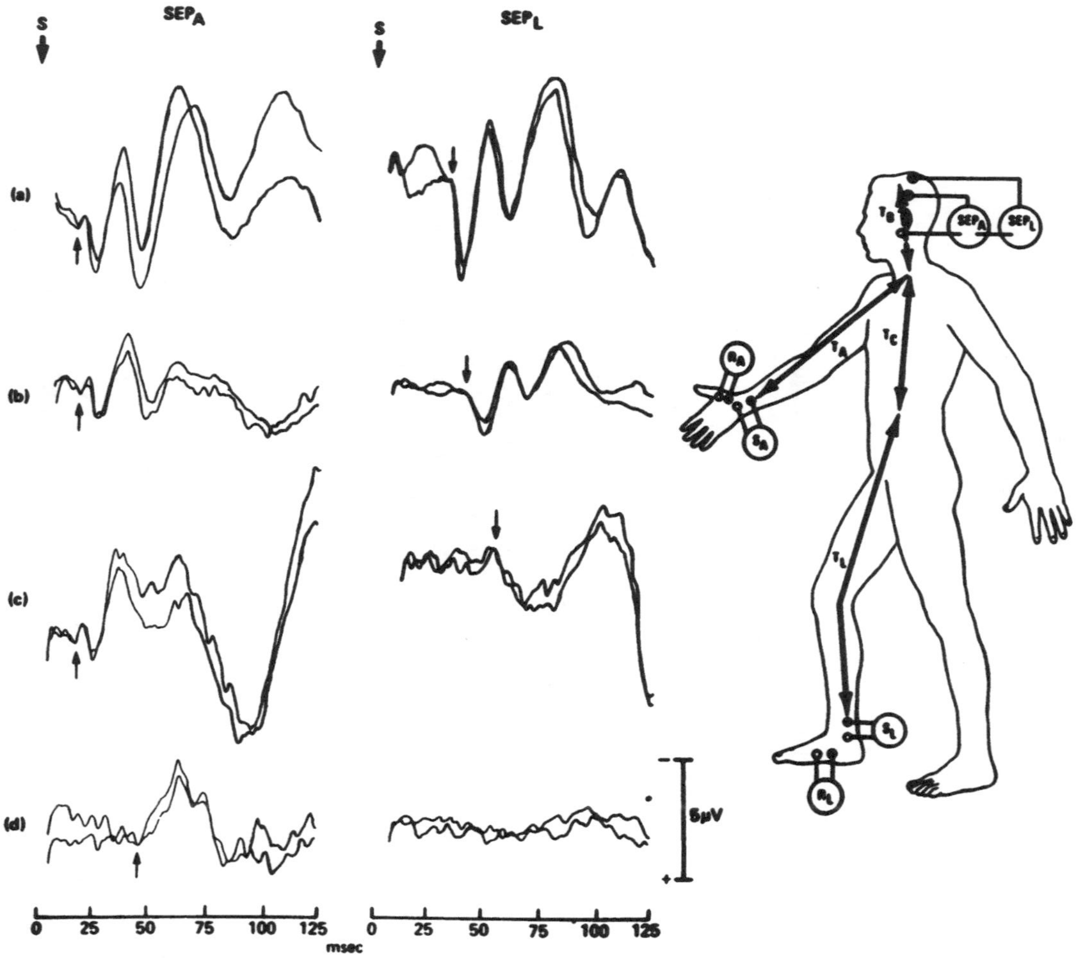
S
SEP_A
S
SEP_L
(a)
(b)
(c)
(d)
0
25
50
75
100
125
msec
0
25
50
75
100
125
5μV
SEP_A
SEP_L
T_B
T_A
T_C
T_L
R_A
S_A
S_L
R_L

FIG. 13.13.

TABLE 13.10
Mean and Standard Deviation Values of Somatosensory Conduction Time[a]

Measure	*Normals*		*MS*	
	X	*SD*	*X*	*SD*
T_A	10.5	.9	10.7	1.0
T_L	20.3	2.1	20.9	2.7
$SSER_A$	16.0	1.4	18.7[b]	5.4
$SSER_L$	34.4	2.7	45.6[b]	9.1
T_B	5.5	.9	8.0[b]	5.3
T_C	8.5	1.6	16.0[b]	6.7
CV_C	55.8	11.0	33.5[b]	18.5

[a]From Dorfman et al. (1978).
[b]Significant differences between the two groups ($P<.001$).

VII. METHODS THAT USE COMBINATIONS OF AVERAGED EVOKED RESPONSES TO DIFFERENT SENSORY MODALITIES

A. Amplitude and Latency Values of Pattern-Reversal VERs and Spinal Cord Evoked Responses (SCERs) in Diagnosis of MS

Mastaglia, Black, and Collins (1976) recorded the VERs to pattern reversal at O_zP_z and the SCERs to stimulation of median nerves over C2 and using P_z as reference in a group of 23 definite, nine probable, and 36 possible cases of MS. VERs were regarded as abnormal if the latency of the major surface positive potential exceeded 118 msec (normal mean + 2.5 SD), or if the latency difference between the responses of the two eyes exceeded 6 msec. SCERs were regarded as abnormal if the latency of the major

FIG. 13.13. (*Opposite page*) Diagrammatic illustration of the technique and examples of cortical ERs in normal subjects and in patients. Stimulation of the median nerve at the wrist (SA) elicits a cortical evoked potential (SEP_A) as well as *M* and *F* responses in the abductor pollicis brevis muscle (R_A). Stimulation of the posterior tibial nerve at the ankle (S_L) evokes a cortical potential (SEP_L) and *M* and *F* responses in the abductor hallucis brevis muscle (R_L). From the time relationship of these responses, it is possible to estimate the temporal delays corresponding to the segments of the somatosensory pathway indicated by T_A, T_L, T_B, and T_C, as described in the text. The four pairs of SEPs represent corresponding arm and leg ERs in a normal subject (a) and in three MS patients (b)–(d). The arrow indicates the onset of each potential except for SEP_L in (d), which exhibits no discernible response. The indirect estimate of spinal conduction velocity (CV_L) in each case are: (a) 67.2 m/sec; (b) 36.8 m/sec; (c) 25.9 m/sec; (d) indeterminate. (From Dorfman et al., 1978.)

negative surface peak exceeded 15.8 msec (normal mean + 2.5 SD) or if the amplitude was less than 1.1 μV. In the definite MS group, 19 of the 23 patients (83%) had an abnormal VER, and 16 out of 17 (94%), an abnormal SCER; three patients with normal VER had abnormal SCERs. In the probable MS group, three of the nine patients (33%) had an abnormal VER and four out of eight (50%) (two with normal VERs), an abnormal SCER. Of the 36 possible cases, 12 patients had an abnormal VER (33%) and 10 out of 27 (37%), an abnormal SCER. Of the 27 possible cases in which both VERs and SCERs were recorded, 16 patients (59%) gave an abnormal result with one or the other or both techniques; six patients with normal VERs had abnormal SCERs, and four with normal SCERs had abnormal VERs. Of the cases with abnormal VERs, five (22%) of the definite, two (22%) of the probable, and eight (22%) of the possible cases had no clinical evidence of optic neuropathy. Of the patients with abnormal SCERs, three (13%) of the definite, one (11%) of the probable, and eight (22%) of the possible cases had no sensory symptoms or signs.

The increased yield of abnormal results in the possible MS group when both techniques were applied suggest that they have a complementary role in investigating suspected MS. The ability to detect subclinical abnormalities with these techniques emphasizes their diagnostic potential in MS.

B. Visual, Auditory, and Somatosensory Evoked Responses in the Discrimination of Different Types of Aphasia

Morley and Liedtke (1976) studied the evoked responses to flashes, tones, and to the electrical stimulation of the median nerves in eight control subjects, four cases with Wernicke's aphasia, four patients with alexia and agraphia, and four patients with Broca's aphasia. The aim of the study was to demonstrate that evoked potentials can be used to localize brain lesions. The AERs to left, right, and both ears stimulation were obtained from electrodes located in areas 22 (Wernicke's), 39 (visual and auditory association), 44 (Broca's), 4 (motor), and 41 (primary auditory) of both hemispheres, according to Brodal's classification. VERs to the stimulation of left and right visual fields were recorded from areas 39, 44, 41, 22, and occipital regions. SSERs to left and right median nerve stimulation were recorded in areas 39, 44, 41, 22, occipital, and the hand area. Thus, 37 evoked responses in each hemisphere were obtained in every patient. In each ER, 20 measurements were derived from the amplitude and latencies of significant peaks. Two types of analysis were performed:

1. In order to enhance the differences between left and right, the right measurements were subtracted from the left. Using 14 features, 67% accuracy was obtained.

2. By the analysis of the left side only, using the best features of all stimuli, 78% correct classification was reached.

Because these results were obtained by a manual procedure of selection of significant peaks and measurements, which took several days, and because any manual procedure tends to become inconsistent and subjective over long periods of time, an algorithm for the automation of the measurement extraction was developed (Morley & Liedtke, 1977). The algorithm consists of three major steps:

1. Preprocessing: removal of artifact spikes, base-line correction, and noise by digital pass low filtering.
2. Recognition of significant peaks by two main criteria: The highest amplitude in a portion that is entirely above or below the baseline is a significant peak when it exceeds an absolute threshold and when, compared with the neighboring significant peaks, the peaks show an amplitude difference greater than a given threshold.
3. Calculation of measurements: After the significant peaks were marked, 20 measurements were extracted from each ER. They were based on the amplitude differences and latencies of significant peaks, and contained the sum of the amplitudes, area, and hypotenuse of the triangle subtended by a positive-to-negative or negative-to-positive amplitude shift, maximum peaks, sum of maximum peaks, etc.

For each type of stimuli, the best measurements from the left hemisphere were found by a step-wise regression technique. The "best" measurements from each of the subgroups were combined in a composite run in which a final selection was made. Because the number of subjects per class was already very small, the following approach was used for the evaluation of the classification rule: From the total sample, one subject was removed and the remainder of the subjects were used to derive the decision rule, which was then tested on the isolated subject (leave-one-out technique; see Chapter 7). The process was then repeated by removing each subject in turn, deriving a decision rule from the rest and finally classifying the total sample. With 18 variables, which included seven measures of SSERs, seven of AERs, and four of VERs, the percentage correct classification obtained was of 87.5% in the control group, 62.5% in Broca's aphasia, 87.5% in Wernicke's aphasia, and 62.5% in alexia and agraphia, for an overall accuracy of 75%. A comparative evaluation of the classification rule, both for manual and automated procedures, showed the same slope and tends to converge at the same level, about 73% correct classification. In analyzing the "best" measurements that have been selected from the set of normally extracted and the automatically extracted, it turns out that the latter were much more consistent with expected results, which suggests that inconsistency based on subjective judgment was removed. The time for manual processing, over a week per subject, was reduced to half an hour, which justifies the application of the method both from the cost and time consumption standpoints.

C. Visual, Auditory, and Somatosensory Evoked Responses in the Discrimination of Different Neurological Diseases

In the search for a diagnostic evoked-response battery, we have conducted a series of studies in different groups of neurological patients. In all subjects, the same experimental procedure was followed. Averaged evoked responses to a flash, to a checkerboard pattern situated in front of the stroboscope lamp, to three different tones (250, 1000, and 6000 Hz) delivered binaurally, and to the left, right, and simultaneous bilateral electrical stimulation of the median nerves were recorded in C_3, C_4, O_1, O_2, T_3, and T_4, with linked ear lobes as reference. The ERs to 150 stimuli were obtained in a 250 msec time analysis and were digitized by an AD converter at 100 equally spaced points. The baseline was adjusted to the mean value of the 100 points.

In the averaged ERs, three different parameters were computed:

1. Peak-to-peak amplitude of the ERs were defined as the voltage difference between the most negative and the most positive voltages within the 250 msec.
2. The Pearson product moment correlation coefficient (R) between the value of the left and right pairs of ERs, as a measure of waveform similarity.
3. The signal energy ratio (SER) as the ratio of the larger to the smaller value of the sum of the squares of the 100 digitized values. If the left side had more energy than the right side, the ratio was considered positive, negative otherwise.

These measures were selected according to previous results in literature, as had been referred to in Chapters 4 to 6. All these computations and the graphs of the ERs, as well as the subsequent analysis that is described in the next section, were performed in a minicomputer CID 201-B.

1. Univariate Statistical Analysis

a. Normative Data. The control group was composed of 36 subjects, 23 males and 13 females between 15 and 65 years of age (X = 29), who were considered normal by clinical and electroencephalographic standards. For each derivation and type of stimuli, means and standard deviations of peak-to-peak amplitudes, Fisher *z* transform of *R* values, and *ln* SER values were computed (to ensure a normal distribution). Results are shown in Tables 13.11 to 13.13.

The means and standard deviations are slightly different from those previously published by Fernández and Harmony (1977a, 1977b), because the sample is larger.

b. Epileptic Patients. Selection of the cases was performed according to their EEG characteristics. Because previous studies in our laboratory with EEG and VER symmetry analysis (Otero et al., 1974; Ricardo et al., 1975) had failed in the discrimination of epileptic patients with a normal EEG background activity and isolated paroxysmal discharges, the authors decided to study this type of patient to search for new methods for their adequate discrimination. In a previous paper, Fernández, Harmony, and Rodríguez applied the ER battery to a group of 44 epileptics of different types—30 with temporal epilepsy, five with an occipital focus, and nine with a generalized epilepsy—who were or had remained without treatment for several months before the investigation. No significant differences between the three groups of epileptics were observed when Student's *t* tests comparisons were made. Later on, Fernández and Harmony (1980) computed a stepwise nonlinear discriminant analysis between a group of 20 patients with temporal epilepsy and 20 normal subjects matched by age and

TABLE 13.11
VERs in Normal Subjects: Means and Standard Deviations of Amplitude, Correlation Coefficients, and Signal Energy Ratio Values

Derivation	*Amplitude*[a]		*Correlation Coefficient*[b]			*SER*[c]	
			z		*R*		
	X	*SD*	*X*	*SD*	*X*	*X*	*SD*
			Flash				
Left central	11.98	6.35	2.52	.57	.99	-.069	.239
Right central	12.75	6.10					
Left occipital	11.15	4.43	1.50	.43	.91	.090	.462
Right occipital	10.50	3.35					
			Checkerboard				
Left central	9.68	5.30	2.28	.58	.98	-.045	.299
Right central	9.95	5.55					
Left occipital	12.58	6.80	1.94	.43	.96	.145	.511
Right occipital	11.48	5.23					

[a]Amplitude values are given in μV.

[b] Mean and SD were calculated using the Fisher *z* transform of *R* values. Both means (*z* and *R*) are shown.

[c] Mean and SD of ln transform of SER values are shown.

TABLE 13.12
AERs in Normal Subjects: Means and Standard Deviations of Amplitude, Correlation Coefficients, and Signal Energy Ratio Values

Derivation	Amplitude[a] X	Amplitude[a] SD	Correlation Coefficient[b] z X	Correlation Coefficient[b] z SD	Correlation Coefficient[b] R X	SER[c] X	SER[c] SD
			250 Hz				
Left central	7.50	3.70	2.32	.45	.98	-.022	.269
Right central	7.33	2.85					
Left temporal	4.78	2.35	1.32	.55	.87	.039	.620
Right temporal	4.70	2.38					
			1,000 Hz				
Left central	6.23	2.85	2.14	.52	.97	.027	.628
Right central	6.10	2.75					
Left temporal	3.98	1.90	1.15	.52	.82	-.023	.300
Right temporal	3.98	2.03					
			6,000 Hz				
Left central	5.55	3.13	1.94	.53	.96	.035	.271
Right central	5.33	2.50					
Left temporal	3.43	1.55	1.03	.41	.77	.109	.546
Right temporal	3.25	1.28					

[a]Amplitude values are given in μV.
[b] Mean and SD were calculated using Fisher *z* transform of *R* values. Both means (*z* and *R*) are shown.
[c]Mean and SD of *ln* transform of SER values are shown.

sex. Variables used were the amplitude and the correlation coefficient of the ERs in frontal, central, occipital and temporal leads, to a flash, to a checkerboard pattern, to three different tones and to the bilateral median nerve stimulation. Results showed 95% correct discrimination of epileptic patients with no false positives. Application of the discriminant equation already obtained to a new group of epileptic subjects showed that 100% of temporal epileptics were adequately classified, while patients with generalized epilepsy were randomly discriminated from normals. These results strongly suggest that different electrophysiological profiles of the ERs exist among different types of epileptics.

For our presentation here we have selected 31 patients with temporal epilepsy. Selection was based on those patients which had the same variables as those measured in tumor and cerebrovascular diseased patients. From 31 patients with temporal epilepsy, 14 were males and 17 females, between 15 and 57 years of age (X = 27). In six of them, epileptogenic activity was only observed during sleep recordings. Mean and SD values are shown in Tables 13.14 to 13.16. In these tables, significant ($P < .05$) different values with respect to the control group, as assessed by Student's *t* test, are

TABLE 13.13
SSERs in Normal Subjects: Means and Standard Deviations of Amplitude, Correlation Coefficients, and Signal Energy Ratio Values

	Left Median Nerve Stimulation						
Derivation	*Amplitude*[a]		*Correlation Coefficient*[b]			*SER*[c]	
			z		*R*		
	X	*SD*	*X*	*SD*	*X*	*X*	*SD*
Left central	6.93	3.13	1.52	.45	.91	-.089	.462
Right central	7.45	3.73					
Left occipital	3.80	1.45	.87	.38	.70	-.279	.604
Right occipital	4.33	1.68					
	Right Median Nerve Stimulation						
Left central	9.48	6.15	1.73	.50	.94	.120	.340
Right central	8.53	5.00					
Left occipital	4.50	1.73	1.12	.52	.81	.210	.590
Right occipital	4.27	2.05					
	Bilateral Median Nerve Stimulation						
Left central	9.43	4.93	1.99	.53	.96	-.038	.379
Right central	9.75	5.78					
Left occipital	4.80	1.73	1.34	.37	.87	-.058	.463
Right occipital	4.79	1.75					

[a]Amplitude values are given in μV.
[b]Mean and SD were calculated using Fisher *z* transform of *R* values. Both means (*z* and *R*) are shown.
[c]Mean and SD of *ln* transform of SER values are shown.

also shown, In the group of epileptic patients, lower correlation coefficients in central regions to flash and in occipital leads to a checkerboard pattern were observed. Lower symmetry of VERs to flash has also been described by Ricardo et al. (1975). Although a huge literature exists on VERs to patterned stimuli, no reference was found related to the study of epilepsy. The patients also have higher amplitude values in occipital regions to unilateral median nerve stimulation and in central and occipital regions to the simultaneous bilateral median nerve stimulation. These results were in accord with those previously described by other authors (Broughton et al., 1969; Dawson, 1947b; A. M. Halliday, 1965; Hrbkova, 1969; Lüders et al., 1972; Vitová & Faladová, 1975b).

c. Cerebrovascular Occlusions. Harmony, Fernández, Alvarez, and Roche (1978a) described the results obtained by the comparison of a group of patients with cerebrovascular diseases and a control group. In this section, we present the results obtained in a group of 26 patients with cerebrovascular thrombosis; included were 19 males and 7 females between 25 and 70 years of age (X = 59). Four patients had normal EEGs. Tables 13.17 to 13.19 present the results obtained. Patients were characterized by

TABLE 13.14
VERs in Temporal Epileptics: Means and Standard Deviations of Amplitude, Correlation Coefficients, and Signal Energy Ratio Values

			Flash				
Derivations	*Amplitude*[a]		*Correlation Coefficients*[b]			*SER*[c]	
			z		*R*		
	X	*SD*	*X*	*SD*	*X*	*X*	*SD*
Left central	12.00	4.88	2.26[d]	.36	.98[d]	-.075	.270
Right central	12.85	5.15					
Left occipital	12.05	6.33	1.36	.46	.88	-.058	.648
Right occipital	12.25	5.93					
			Checkerboard				
Left central	9.60	4.10	2.17	.47	.97	-.057	.252
Right central	9.78	3.70					
Left occipital	10.78	6.78	1.53[d]	.64	.91[d]	-.102	.759
Right occipital	11.03	6.13					

[a]Amplitude values are given in μV.

[b]Mean and SD were calculated using Fisher *z* transform of *R* values. Both means (*z* and *R*) are shown.

[c]Mean and SD of *ln* transform of SER values are shown.

[d]Significant different values ($P < .05$) when compared with normal subjects.

lower amplitude values than the control group of all the ERs in all derivations with the exception of the occipital SSERs to bilateral median nerve stimulation. Because this result may be due to a selective depression of the ERs in the side of the lesion, amplitudes of the ERs of patients with left ($n = 16$) and with right ($n = 10$) thrombosis were separately computed. Amplitudes lower than normal were observed in both hemispheres independently of the side of the lesion.

Because the mean age of the group of patients was higher than the mean age of the control group, an aging factor should be analyzed. Dustman et al. (1977) studied life-span ER changes. Amplitude of ERs to flash appears to fall and stabilize at about age 16. Attenuation of late and potentiation of early (0-100 msec) components characterize the electrical pattern of the aging brain. These changes were more clearly seen in occipital recordings. Although some changes im amplitude were seen in central regions, these changes were minimal when compared to those recorded in the occiput. They also reported a decrease in amplitude of SSERs after 40 years of age, but the amplitude of central AERs does not change with age. These changes with senescence cannot explain per se the results obtained in patients with cerebrovascular thrombosis, because they were characterized by small amplitude of the evoked responses to all sensory modalities explored, including the AERs, and in all derivations studied. Thus, another factor must

TABLE 13.15
AERs in Temporal Epileptics: Means and Standard Deviations of Amplitude, Correlation Coefficients, and Signal Energy Ratio Values

Derivations	*Amplitude*[a]		*Correlation Coefficient*[b]			*SER*[c]	
			z		*R*		
	X	*SD*	*X*	*SD*	*X*	*X*	*SD*
			250 Hz				
Left central	7.43	4.88	2.11	.41	.97	-.135	.258
Right central	7.88	5.70					
Left temporal	4.45	1.93	1.16	.48	.82	-.323	.645
Right temporal	5.08	2.45					
			1,000 Hz				
Left central	6.55	2.83	2.10	.56	.97	-.016	.206
Right central	6.57	2.98					
Left temporal	4.03	1.88	.94	.60	.74	-.059	.780
Right temporal	4.13	1.93					
			6,000 Hz				
Left central	5.20	2.23	1.89	.52	.96	-.079	.301
Right central	5.33	.28					
Left temporal	4.05	1.88	.91	.43	.72	-.138	.550
Right temporal	4.15	1.73					

[a]Amplitude values are given in μV.

[b]Mean and SD were calculated using Fisher *z* transform of *R* values. Both means (*z* and *R*) are shown.

[c]Mean and SD *ln* transform of SER values are shown.

be involved in the amplitude reduction of the ERs observed in these patients. Ischemic changes may explain them. Branston and Symon (1974) described a linear relationship between the rate of depression of the SSERs and the residual blood flow in baboons. Patients with cerebrovascular thrombosis generally present atherosclerosis of several brain vessels, although the clinical symptoms correspond with the site in which the nervous system has been most severly affected. These atherosclerotic lesions may produce a degree of ischemia of the whole cortex, not intense enough to produce neurological symptoms, but sufficient to produce a reduction of the amplitude of the ERs. Two of the patients had senile dementia, but it is unlikely that this is a factor to take into account, because Visser et al (1976) observed an amplitude increase of components III and VI of VERs in this pathology.

Another important characteristic of the ERs in the patients with cerebrovascular thrombosis was the waveform asymmetry expressed by the low correlation coefficient values observed in almost all leads and to all types of stimuli used. This finding is in accord with previous results in the

TABLE 13.16
SSERs in Temporal Epileptics: Means and Standard Deviations of Amplitude, Correlation Coefficients, and Signal Energy Ratio Values

Derivations	*Amplitude*[a]		*Correlation Coefficient*[b]			*SER*[c]	
			z		*R*		
	X	*SD*	*X*	*SD*	*X*	*X*	*SD*
Left Median Nerve Stimulation							
Left central	9.13	2.50	1.53	.65	.91	-.207	.608
Right central	9.65	6.23					
Left occipital	4.85[d]	1.88	1.06	.42	.79	-.242	.590
Right occipital	5.58[d]	2.70					
Right Median Nerve Stimulation							
Left central	11.85	10.30	1.61	.52	.92	.236	.603
Right central	9.98	6.60					
Left occipital	5.98[d]	2.80	1.17	.49	.82	.279	.619
Right occipital	5.33	2.83					
Bilateral Median Nerve Stimulation							
Left central	12.85[d]	7.43	2.00	.72	.96	-.136	.300
Right central	13.53[d]	7.48					
Left occipital	6.73[d]	3.33	1.45	.44	.90	.107	.486
Right occipital	6.85[d]	3.33					

[a]Amplitude values are given in μV.
[b]Mean and SD were calculated using Fisher *z* transform of *R* values. Both means (*z* and *R*) are shown.
[c]Mean and SD of *ln* transform of SER values are shown.
[d]Significant different values ($P < .05$) when compared with normal subjects.

literature, as has been discussed earlier in this chapter and in Chapters 3 to 6. Although the correlation coefficient does not give an idea of the side of the lesion, it is an important sign of abnormality of the ERs.

Harmony et al. (1978a) made a study of the ER characteristics for the definition of the lateralization of the lesion. VERs were indistinctly enlarged or decreased in the side of the lesion. Alterations of the AERs in temporal regions were more frequently seen than in central areas, the AERs being absent or depressed over the side of the lesion. Three factors were taken into account for the analysis of the SSERs:

1. Absence, amplitude reduction, or increased latencies of the primary components were considered a sign of abnormality. Criterion for amplitude reduction or increased latency was reached by comparing left and right contralateral responses in each subject.
2. *R* values lower than 2 SD of the normal mean.
3. SER absolute values higher than 2.0. In the condition of unilateral

TABLE 13.17
VERs in Cerebrovascular Patients: Means and Standard Deviations of Amplitude, Correlation Coefficients, and Signal Energy Ratio Values

Derivations	Amplitude[a]		Correlation Coefficient[b]			SER[c]	
			z		R		
	X	SD	X	SD	X	X	SD
Flash							
Left central	7.30[d]	3.00	1.89[d]	.72	.96[d]	.044	.315
Right central	7.18[d]	2.98					
Left occipital	8.20[d]	3.20	1.55	.58	.91	.280	.697
Right occipital	7.13[d]	1.98					
Checkerboard							
Left central	5.03[d]	2.15	1.77[d]	.54	.94[d]	-.015	.598
Right central	4.95[d]	2.20					
Left occipital	6.43[d]	4.03	1.37[d]	.70	.88[d]	.152	.853
Right occipital	5.48[d]	2.73					

[a]Amplitude values are given in μV.
[b]Mean and SD were calculated using Fisher *z* transform of *R* values. Both means (*z* and *R*) are shown.
[c]Mean and SD of *ln* transform of SER values are shown.
[d]Significant different values ($P < .05$) when compared with normal subjects.

stimulation, the result was considered abnormal if the ipsilateral response was greater than the contralateral response in the same range (SER = 2).

The SSERs were useful for the detection of the injured side in 85% of the cases. Fig. 13.14 and 13.15 show the ERs of two different cases to illustrate the forementioned results.

The battery of ERs to different types of stimuli and sensory modalities provides a sensitive method for the evaluation of patients with cerebrovascular thrombosis. This conclusion is supported by the preliminary results obtained by Fernández-Bouzas and Harmony (1979). They recorded the ERs in a group of patients with severe peripheral atherosclerosis, which required surgical intervention, but were asymptomatic from the neurological point of view. In a group of patients, the ERs presented the same alterations previously described. In these patients, a cerebral angiography was performed; 80% of such patients had occlusion of a cerebral artery.

d. Intracranial Tumors. Twenty-three patients, 11 males and 12 females from 15 to 70 years of age (X = 42), were studied (Alvarez & Harmony, 1978). Seventeen cases had hemispheric tumors, four had hypophyseal adenomas, one case had a cerebellar tumor, and one patient had

TABLE 13.18
AERs in Cerebrovascular Patients: Means and Standard Deviations of Amplitude, Correlation Coefficients, and Signal Energy Ratio Values

Derivations	*Amplitude*[a]		*Correlation Coefficient*[b]			*SER*[c]	
			z		*R*		
	X	*SD*	*X*	*SD*	*X*	*X*	*SD*
250 Hz							
Left central	3.92[d]	1.33	1.85[d]	.55	.95[d]	−.140	.377
Right central	4.13[d]	1.23					
Left temporal	3.23[d]	1.15	.77[d]	.56	.65[d]	.165	.911
Right temporal	3.05[d]	1.43					
1000 Hz							
Left central	3.98[d]	1.60	1.77[d]	.58	.94[d]	−.026	.463
Right central	3.93[d]	1.43					
Left temporal	3.18[d]	1.20	.86[d]	.47	.70[d]	.224	.860
Right temporal	2.70[d]	1.00					
6000 Hz							
Left central	2.78[d]	1.05	1.46[d]	.56	.90[d]	−.066	.407
Right central	3.03[d]	1.23					
Left temporal	2.40[d]	.83	.54[d]	.36	.49[d]	.185	.733
Right temporal	2.63[d]	2.30					

[a]Amplitude values are given in μV.
[b]Mean and SD were calculated using Fisher *z* transform of *R* values. Both means (*z* and *R*) are shown.
[c]Mean and SD of *ln* transform of SER values are shown.
[d]Significant different values ($P < .05$) when compared with normal subjects.

a right chemodectoma that compressed the brain stem. In six cases, the EEG was normal. The results obtained are shown in Tables 13.20 to 13.22. In these tables, it is possible to observe lower amplitude values than in normal subjects of the VERs and AERs in central regions and of the SSERs to unilateral median nerve stimulation on the ipsilateral central region. Smaller amplitudes were independent of the hemisphere affected. Lower correlation coefficients were also found in different regions to different types of stimuli. These results are in accord with those previously described in the literature, as we have mentioned in Chapter 3 to 6 and previously in this chapter. Examples are shown in Figs. 13.16 and 13.17.

e. Multiple Sclerosis. Nine patients with probable and six with possible MS, six male and nine female with a mean age of 30 years, were studied (Fernández et al., 1977). The EEG was normal in six cases. In these patients, AERs in temporal regions were so small that they were difficult to differentiate from background activity and therefore, were discarded. Lower amplitude values than those observed in the central group were

TABLE 13.19
SSERs in Cerebrovascular Patients: Means and Standard Deviations of Amplitude, Correlation Coefficients, and Signal Energy Ratio Values

Derivations	*Amplitude*[a]		*Correlation Coefficient*[b]			*SER*[c]	
			z		*R*		
	X	*SD*	*X*	*SD*	*X*	*X*	*SD*
	Left Median Nerve Stimulation						
Left central	3.63[d]	1.48	1.05[d]	.39	.78[d]	-.221	.811
Right central	4.50[d]	2.25					
Left occipital	2.88[d]	1.05	1.12	.47	.81	-.070	.507
Right occipital	3.08[d]	1.40					
	Right Median Nerve Stimulation						
Left central	5.32[d]	2.50	1.04[d]	.46	.78[d]	.684[d]	.710
Right central	3.53[d]	1.35					
Left occipital	3.38[d]	1.08	1.35	.59	.87	.332	.574
Right occipital	3.00[d]	1.15					
	Bilateral Median Nerve Stimulation						
Left central	5.80[d]	3.08	1.28[d]	.51	.86[d]	.057	.695
Right central	5.53[d]	2.35					
Left occipital	4.45	4.00	1.25	.51	.85	.184	.538
Right occipital	3.88	2.00					

[a]Amplitude values are given in μV.
[b]Mean and SD were calculated using Fisher *z* transform of *R* values. Both means (*z* and *R*) are shown.
[c]Mean and SD of *ln* transform of SER values are shown.
[d]Significant different values ($P < .05$) when compared with normal subjects.

found in the central region for all types of stimuli used, and in the right occipital lead for VERs to a checkerboard pattern. This finding is consistent with what should be expected in a demyelinating illnes: Some fibers will present a lower conduction velocity and an increased threshold, thus reducing the number of synchronic impulses that arrive to the cerebral cortex with lower ER amplitudes as a result. There was also a good clinical and electrophysiological correlation. Those cases in which the main alteration was in the VERs had visual defects before or after the study. The cases in which an abnormal SSER was observed had a joint position sense impairment in the upper extremities at the moment of the study.

2. *Multivariate Statistical Analysis*

In previous papers, we have demonstrated that it is possible to discriminate normal subjects from epileptics (Fernández & Harmony, 1977, 1978b), normal subjects from MS patients (Fernández, et al., 1977), normal subjects from epileptics and MS patients (Harmony & Fernández, 1977),

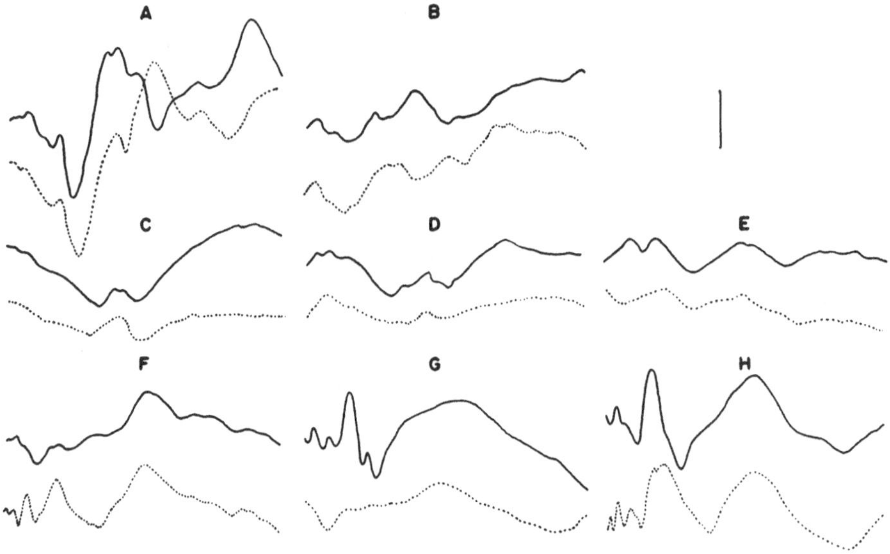

FIG. 13.14. Left (*continuous line*) and right (*discontinuous line*) averaged evoked responses of a patient with a right carotid artery occlusion. Generalized slow waves were observed in the EEG. (A) Occipital VERs to flash (R = .67). (B) VERs to a checkerboard pattern in occipital regions (R = .83). (C) Temporal AERs to 250 Hz (R = .79). (D) Temporal AERs to 1000 Hz (R = .89). (E) Temporal AERs to 6000 Hz (R = .46). (F) Central SSERs to left median nerve stimulation (R = .50). (G) Central SSERs to right median nerve stimulation (R = .71). (H) Central SSERs to bilateral median nerve stimulation (R = .74). This patient showed alterations in the evoked responses to different types of sensory modalities. Note waveshape asymmetries of VERs; VERs to a checkerboard pattern were of smaller amplitude than VERs to flash. The AERs in the right temporal region were very poor. Stimulation of the left median nerve produced SSERs of smaller amplitude and longer latencies in right central area than stimulation of the right median nerve in left central area. SSERs to bilateral median nerve stimulation were also very asymmetric. Calibration: 2.5 μV, 250 msec analysis time. (From Harmony et al., 1978a.)

normal subjects from patients with cerebrovascular disorders (Harmony et al., 1978a), and normal subjects from patients with intracranial tumors (Alvarez & Harmony, 1978), on the basis of amplitude of the ERs and correlation coefficients between pairs of ERs of homologous regions, using the previously mentioned ER battery.

In such papers, the first steps considered in a neurometric methodology were accomplished, but validation of decision rules was not considered. Our purpose has been to develop a procedure that may serve as a mass screening test and as a diagnostic tool for the discrimination of different types of neurological patients. The latter objective is a rather difficult task, because there is a great variety of brain lesions and individual differences. Only with the collection of a huge amount of data will it be possible to define the type, and in some cases, the site of the lesion. We have not yet such a great amount of information. However, we think it was important to define, with the data already collected, the usefulness of such simple measures as amplitude, correlation coefficients, and SER values or the ERs for the assessment of brain damage. We have been interested not only in the selection of the best features and the obtainment of a decision rule, but in the validation of such a decision rule. It has been emphasized (Chapter 7) that the drawback of discriminant analysis is that even if it is possible to obtain a quasiperfect classification of the subjects from which the equation is derived, later replication of the same equation with new subjects may result in a very poor discrimination.

Discriminant Analysis. Application of discriminant analysis assumes

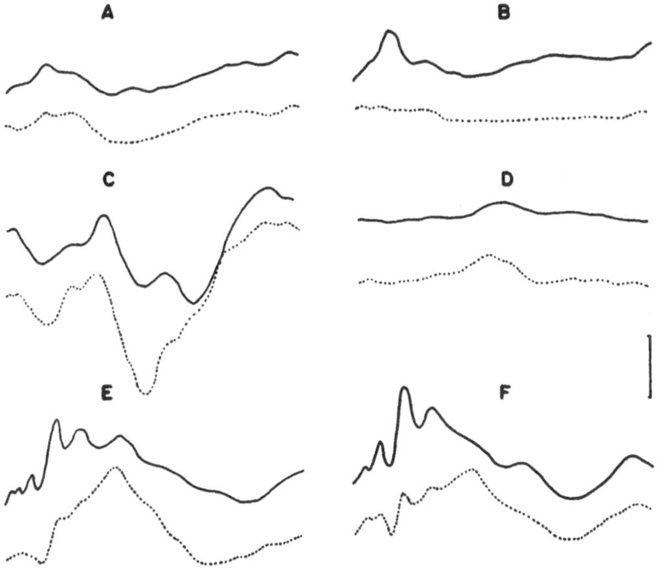

FIG. 13.15. Left (*continuous line*) and right (*discontinuous line*) averaged evoked responses in a patient with a right middle cerebral artery thrombosis. The EEG has slow waves in right centro-occipital derivation. (A) Central AERs to 6000 Hz (R = .92). (B) Temporal AERs to 6000 Hz (R = .24; SER = 2.87). (C) Occipital VERs to a checkerboard pattern (R = .68). (D) Central SSERs to left median nerve stimulation (R = .78; no response). (E) Central SSERs to right median nerve stimulation (R = .84). (F) Central SSERs to bilateral median nerve stimulation (R = .78). Note the absence of response in right temporal areas (B) and of SSER in right central area (D). Calibration: 2.5 μV, 250 msec analysis time. (From Harmony et al., 1978a.)

TABLE 13.20
VERs in Intracranial Tumors: Means and Standard Deviations of Amplitude, Correlation Coefficients, and Signal Energy Ratio Values

Derivations	*Amplitude*[a]		*Correlation Coefficient*[b]			*SER*[c]	
			z		*R*		
	X	*SD*	*X*	*SD*	*X*	*X*	*SD*
			Flash				
Left central	7.65[d]	3.40	1.84[d]	.72	.95[d]	-.075	.420
Right central	7.95[d]	3.15					
Left occipital	10.08	4.58	1.38	.58	.88	.091	.600
Right occipital	10.23	5.13					
			Checkerboard				
Left central	5.60[d]	2.85	1.82[d]	.72	.95[d]	.0170	.305
Right central	5.53[d]	2.73					
Left occipital	9.00[d]	6.40	1.56[d]	.52	.92[d]	-.020	.453
Right occipital	8.78	5.24					

[a]Amplitude values are given in μV.
[b]Mean and SD were calculated using Fisher z transform of R values. Both means (z and R) are shown.
[c]Mean and SD of *ln* transform of SER values are shown.
[d]Significant different values ($P < .05$) when compared with normal subjects.

that multinormality of the data holds. Using probability plots, it is possible to analyze multinormality of the data. If the data are multivariate normal, the empirical cumulative distance of each subject to the centroid of the group will approximate the theoretical function. If Mahalanobis distances are used, then they have approximately a chi-squared distribution with p (number of variables) degrees of freedom if multinormality holds. Each subject will be represented by a point defined by the theoretical and estimated distances. Consequently, the sample order statistics against suitable estimates of the corresponding quantities of the theoretical distribution will tend to yield a set of approximately collinear points. Departures from multinormality will be indicated by departures from linearity in the plot. Such deviations from multinormality may be due to the presence of outliers or several mixed distributions (Everitt, 1978). Mahalanobis plots of the data from each group of subjects or patients showed that they seemed to have a multinormal distribution.

The second question that must be solved before the selection of the type of discriminant analysis to be performed is whether the homogeneity of the covariance matrices holds. In our case, it was found that for the group of temporal epileptics, the group of cerebrovascular disease patients, and the group of intracranial tumor patients did not hold. Thus, it was indicated to use a nonlinear discriminant analysis.

TABLE 13.21
AERs in Intracranial Tumors: Means and Standard Deviations of Amplitude, Correlation Coefficiencies, and Signal Energy Ratio Values

Derivations	Amplitude[a]		Correlation Coefficient[b]			SER[c]	
			z		R		
	X	SD	X	SD	X	X	SD
			250 Hz				
Left central	5.15[d]	2.20	1.94[d]	.52	.96[d]	.060	.459
Right central	5.10[d]	2.05					
Left temporal	4.38	2.55	.82[d]	.82	.68[d]	.319	.680
Right temporal	3.95	2.28					
			1000 Hz				
Left central	4.50[d]	2.40	1.89[d]	.51	.96[d]	.082	.355
Right central	4.43[d]	2.10					
Left temporal	3.85	2.23	.69[d]	.67	.59[d]	-.083	.783
Right temporal	3.85	2.10					
			6000 Hz				
Left central	3.83[d]	1.78	1.61[d]	.52	.92[d]	.006	.401
Right central	3.95[d]	1.68					
Left temporal	3.45	2.10	.59[d]	.65	.53[d]	-.046	.951
Right temporal	3.63	3.05					

[a]Amplitude values are given in μV.
[b]Mean and SD were calculated using Fisher *z* transform of *R* values. Both means (*z* and *R*) are shown.
[c]Mean and SD of *ln* transform of SER values are shown.
[d]Significant different values ($P < .05$) when compared with normal subjects.

The analysis was performed on the basis of the 64 variables per subject (32 amplitude values of VERs to flash and to a checkerboard pattern, AERs to three tones, and SSERs to left, right, and bilateral median nerve stimulation, the *z* transform of 16 correlation coefficients, and 16 logarithmic SER values). Selection of variables was made by the step-wise nonlinear discriminant analysis (Valdés & Baez, 1977; see Chapter 7). The assignment of the individuals to a particular group was made by predictive discriminant analysis based on likelihood criteria (see Chapter 7) for the case in which differences between mean vectors and covariance matrices are considered. Each subject was classified twice: (1) including the subject in the computation of the decision rule that was then applied to him or her; and (2) leaving the subject out of the calculation of such a decision rule (replication).

Comparisons were performed between the normal group and each of the groups of patients. Only the first 10 variables selected by the step-wise nonlinear discriminant analysis were taken into account for the classification of the subjects. Table 13.23 shows the variables and the order in which they were selected in each comparison. In this table, it is possible to observe

TABLE 13.22
SSERs in Intracranial Tumors: Means and Standard Deviations of Amplitude, Correlation Coefficients, and Signal Energy Ratio Values

Derivations	*Amplitude*[a]		*Correlation Coefficient*[b]			*SER*[c]	
			z		*R*		
	X	*SD*	*X*	*SD*	*X*	*X*	*SD*
	Left Median Nerve Stimulation						
Left central	5.32[d]	2.65	1.12[d]	.59	.81[d]	-.390	.796
Right central	7.00	2.85					
Left occipital	3.75	2.43	.99	.68	.76	-.080	.860
Right occipital	4.58	3.80					
	Right Median Nerve Stimulation						
Left central	7.03	4.00	1.29[d]	.61	.86[d]	.391	.371
Right central	5.50[d]	2.98					
Left occipital	4.25	2.75	1.33	.52	.87	.136[d]	.411
Right occipital	4.45	2.80					
	Bilateral Median Nerve Stimulation						
Left central	8.73	6.58	1.32[d]	.70	.87[d]	.176	.516
Right central	8.28	6.03					
Left occipital	5.28	5.00	1.16	.63	.82	.050	.679
Right occipital	5.35	5.75					

[a]Amplitude values are given in μV.
[b]Mean and SD were calculated using Fisher *z* transform of *R* values. Both means (*z* and *R*) are shown.
[c]Mean and SD of *ln* transform of SER values are shown.
[d]Significant different values (P < .05) when compared with normal subjects.

that in all comparisons, variables of ERs to different types of stimulation were primarily selected. These results supported the conclusion that an ER battery may be more powerful than the study of a single type of ER for discriminating among normal subjects and neurological patients.

Table 13.24 presents the results of the classification obtained for each comparison. Results obtained when including the subject for the computation of the decision rule, as well as when the subject was excluded from such computation (replication) are shown. In all cases, the accuracy was higher for the first case than for replication, as could be expected. Such results may be explained by the fact that the groups were not absolutely homogeneous. In the group of intracranial tumors, different types and localization of the lesions were present; the procedure for the selection of the variables takes into account those that produced a greater differentiation between the two samples. Thus, it is possible that, for a given patient, the variables selected may not be the best for detecting the lesion. Our group is working to improve the procedure for the selection of variables, in order to increase its robustness by taking into account such individual differences. The accuracy was good for the comparison between the control group and the groups of patients with cerebrovascular occlusions and the intracranial tumors, but it was not so good for the detection of temporal epileptics. This might be because only 10 variables were taken into account in the analysis, because, with a higher number of variables, much better discriminations were previously reported (Fernández & Harmony, 1977b, 1980). Therefore, a new nonlinear discriminant analysis was computed with 16 variables between the normal group and the group of temporal epileptics. These 16 variables were the first 10 already obtained by the step-wise discriminant analysis and six more: SER value in occipital regions of VERs to a checkerboard pattern, and the amplitudes of the left central and right temporal AERs to 250 Hz, the left temporal AERs to 6000 Hz, the right occipital SSERs to median left stimulation, and the left occipital SSERs to right median nerve stimulation. The results of classification are shown in Table

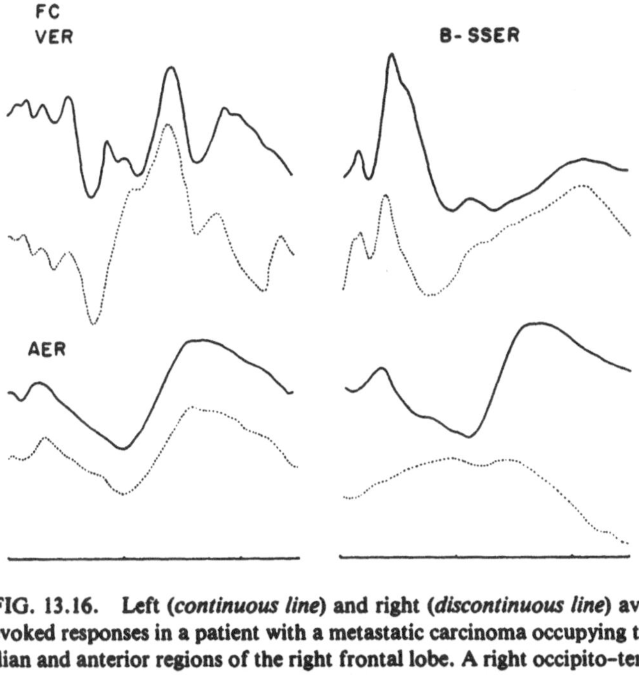

FIG. 13.16. Left (*continuous line*) and right (*discontinuous line*) averaged evoked responses in a patient with a metastatic carcinoma occupying the median and anterior regions of the right frontal lobe. A right occipito-temporal slow-wave focus was observed in the EEG. *Top*: VERs to flash in occipital areas (R = .44). *B-SSER*: central SSERs to bilateral median nerve stimulation (R = .17). *Bottom*: AERs to 6000 Hz tones in central (left) and temporal (right) areas; R values were .98 and -.41 respectively. Note the great asymmetry of the VERs, the smaller amplitude of the SSER in the right central area, and the absence of AER in the right temporal region. Calibration: 2.5 μV, 250 msec time analysis. (From Alvarez & Harmony, 1978).

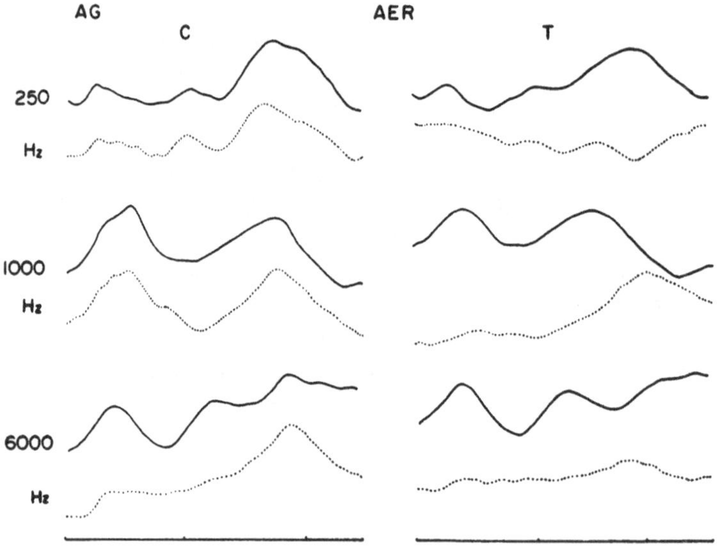

FIG. 13.17. Left (*continuous line*) and right (*discontinuous line*) AERs in central (C) and temporal (T) regions to 250, 1000, and 6000 Hz tones, in a patient with a metastatic carcinoma occupying the right parieto-temporal cortical area. The EEG showed a slow-wave focus in the right temporal area, with diffuse paroxysmal activity. It is possible to observe that although AERs in central areas are slightly asymmetric (R = .96; .87, and .85 respectively), the main alterations are in the temporal responses, with absence of AERs in the right side (R = .57, -.43, .15 respectively). Calibration: 2.5 μV, 250 msec analysis time. (From Alvarez & Harmony, 1978.)

14.24. Higher accuracy was obtained when considering the subjects for the calculation of the decision rule with the 16 variables (93%) than with the first 10. However, replication was even worse (75%) when more variables were included. Differences between these results and those previously published by Fernández and Harmony (1980), may be explained by the inclusion of more leads (as frontal recordings) in the first study.

Comparing the results obtained by the replication and those obtained by the visual inspection of the EEG, the accuracy was similar for the groups of patients with intracranial tumors and cerebrovascular thrombosis. When both procedures were used as complementary, only two patients (90%) with intracranial tumors (a pituitary adenoma and meningioma of the left wing of the sphenoid) and one patient (4%) with an occlusion of the left carotid artery were normal in both examinations. However, patients with temporal epilepsy were better discriminated by the EEG than by the ER battery.

TABLE 13.23
Variables Selected by the Stepwise Nonlinear Analysis[a]

Stimuli	*N vs. E*	*N vs. CV*	*N vs. T*
Flash	Amplitude in 0_2 (4)	—	—
Checkerboard	Amplitude in C_4 (7) R in 0 (5)	SER in 0 (7)	R in 0 (3)
250 Hz	—	Amplitude in T_3 (9) R in T (4)	—
1000 Hz	Amplitude in T_3 (9)	—	Amplitude in C_4 (6)
6000 Hz	Amplitude in C_4 (8)	Amplitude C_3 (5) Amplitude T_4 (10)	Amplitude in C_3 (5) Amplitude in T_3 (7) R in T (10)
Left Median nerve stimulation	Amplitude in C_3 (1) Amplitude in C_4 (3)	SER in C (8)	Amplitude in 0_2 (4) SER in C (9)
Right Median nerve stimulation	Amplitude in C_4 (6)	Amplitude in C_4 (1) SER in C (3)	Amplitude in C_4 (2)
Bilateral median nerve stimulation	Amplitude in 0_1 (10) Amplitude in 0_2 (2)	Amplitude in 0_1 (2) SER in C (6)	Amplitude in 0_2 (1) SER in C (8)

[a]From Harmony et al. (1978c). Numbers within parenthesis indicate the order in which the variables were selected. N: normals. E: epileptics. CV: cerebrovascular. T: tumors.

We would like to make some additional comments on our experience with the ER battery. We have been using it for five years in the routine examination of the patients in the Carlos J. Finlay Hospital. Taking into account not only the amplitude and symmetry measures of the ERs, but visual analysis of the waveform of the AERs and SSERs, we have achieved fairly good accuracy in the detection of some types of brain damge. In cerebrovascular disorders and brain tumors, conclusions regarding the localization of the lesion may also be reached on the basis of the waveform of the SSERs and AERs, as has been illustrated in Figs. 14.14 to 14.17. Thus, it seems obvious that automatic analysis of the waveform of the ERs may increase the accuracy of the procedure. Work in this direction is now in progress. We have also used the ER battery in the follow-up of patients with minor cranial traumas and have found that it is much more sensitive and reliable for the prognosis of the patients than is the visual inspection of the EEG (Harmony and Alvarez, 1981). It is also very useful for the assessment of some types of treatments, such as transcatheter embolization of large arteriovenous malformations in patients who have poor neurological symptoms, or who are even asymptomatic. One example is shown in Fig. 13.18.

TABLE 13.24[a]
Classification Obtained by the Stepwise Nonlinear Discriminant Analysis[b]

	First Classification				Replication			
Normal Subjects vs. Temporal Epileptics (10 Variables)								
	N		E		N		E	
	n	%	*n*	%	*n*	%	*n*	%
Normals	34	94	2	6	31	86	5	14
Epileptics	8	25	23	75	10	32	21	68
Overall Accuracy:	85%				78%			
Normal Subjects vs. Temporal Epileptics (16 Variables)								
	N		E		N		E	
Normals	36	100	0	0	31	86	5	4
Epileptics	5	16	26	84	12	39	19	61
Overall Accuracy:	93%				75%			
Normal Subjects vs. Cerebrovascular Patients								
	N		CV		N		CV	
Normals	32	89	4	11	32	89	4	11
CV	2	8	24	92	5	18	21	81
Overall Accuracy:	90%				85%			
Normal Subjects vs. Intracranial Tumor Patients								
	N		T		N		T	
Normals	33	92	3	8	33	92	3	8
Tumors	0	0	23	100	7	30	16	70
Overall Accuracy:	95%				83%			

[a]From Harmony et al. (1978c).
[b]Results are shown including the individual to be classified for the Computation of the Predictive Criteria (*First classification*) and excluding the subject from this computation (*Replication*).

VIII. CONCLUSIONS

Neurometric procedures based on the quantitative analysis of averaged ERs are a valuable tool in clinical neurology. Although important contributions have been made by the analysis of ERs to a single type of stimulus, it is obvious that the study of ERs to different types of sensory modalities increased the probability of detection of neurological diseases. As we have seen in this chapter, neurometric assessment of ERs is not only much more sensitive than the visual interpretation of the EEG in some types of patients, but, in some cases, it is even better than computerized axial tomography.

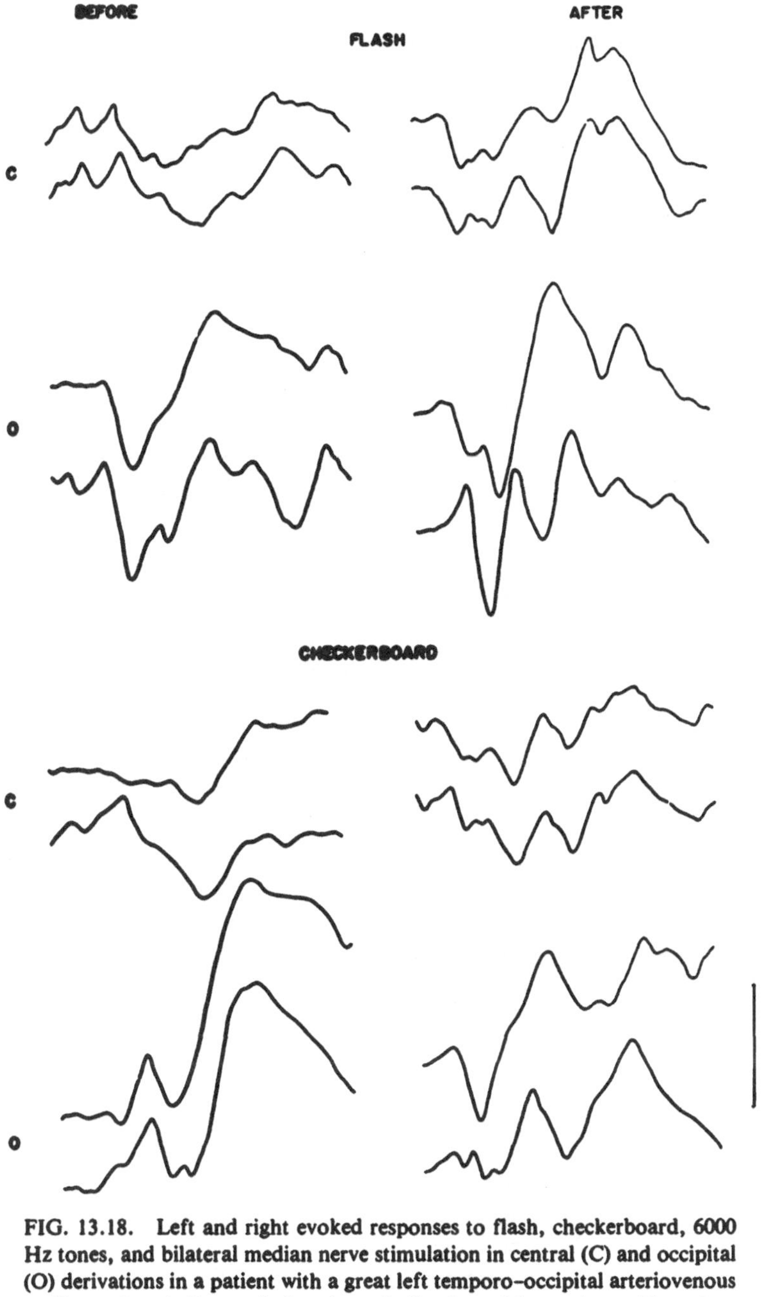

FIG. 13.18. Left and right evoked responses to flash, checkerboard, 6000 Hz tones, and bilateral median nerve stimulation in central (C) and occipital (O) derivations in a patient with a great left temporo–occipital arteriovenous malformation, before and after the embolization of the angioma. Note that, after treatment, the VERs to flash became of higher amplitude and more symmetric. The symmetry of the VERs to a checkerboard pattern also increased after embolization. The AERs increased in amplitude, and the SSERs to bilateral median nerve stimulation were much more symmetric, with a clear primary response in both central regions. Calibration: 2.5μV, 250 msec analysis time. (From Fernández-Bouzas et al., 1977.)

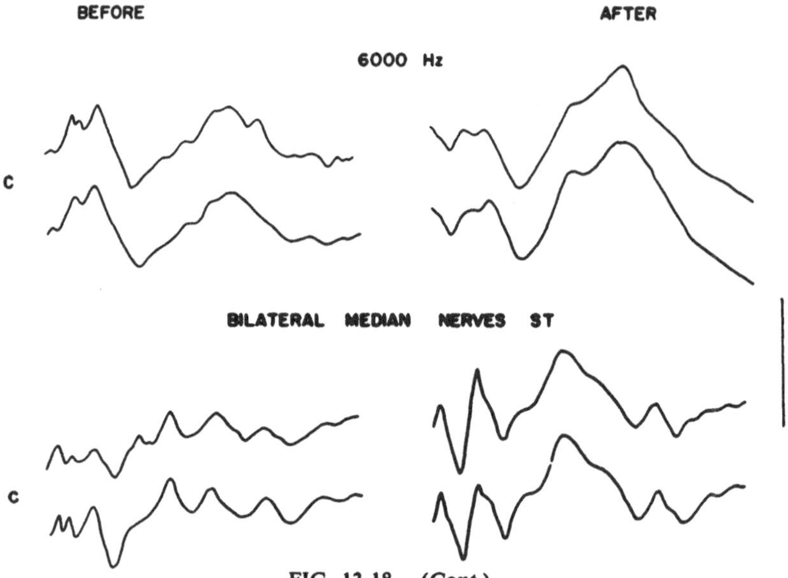

FIG. 13.18. (*Cont.*)

Nonetheless, we consider that there are several aspects of the neurometric assessment of ERs that should be improved and on which intense efforts must be devoted:

1. Waveform analysis of the ERs. Several procedures have been based on the measurements of peak latencies and amplitudes of the averaged ERs. It has been emphasized that identification of "typical" waves was especially difficult in many cases, in which, as a consequence of the brain lesion, the ERs were distorted. Step-wise principal component analysis and cluster analysis are examples of procedures that analyze the ER in the whole latency domain, and that reveal clear waveform differences between the normal subjects and different types of neurological patients.
2. Development of neurometric procedures based on the estimation of the ERs by other procedures that take into account the intraindividual variability of the stimulus-dependent activity. Averaging has shown to be useful, but other procedures of estimation might yield a better discrimination of subtle brain dysfunctions.
3. The inclusion of the ERs obtained during different conditions in the experimental design of comparisons. As ERs reflect not only sensorial, but perceptual and cognitive processes as well, great insight may be obtained in the physiopathology of different diseases by the neurometric assessment of ERs recorded during performance of different tasks.
4. Research in statistical theory, in order to propose new models that take into account the specific problems that are posed in clinical neurophysiology.

PART IV:

SUMMARY

14 A Summarized Review on the Principal Electrophysiological Findings in the Major Neurological Diseases

In this chapter, I try to concentrate the information contained in previous chapters concerning the most relevant neurological diseases, in order to offer the clinical neuroscientist a summarized picture of our present knowledge in this field. From this brief review, those aspects that have not yet been investigated, but that seem promising for the improvement of the neurometric diagnosis, are brought into focus.

I. CEREBROVASCULAR DISORDERS (see Table 14.1)

A. EEG

1. Visual Interpretation

The main types of EEG abnormalities that can be observed are: asymmetry, with depression of voltage on the damaged area, the presence of a slow wave focus, and/or the presence of spikes. Cortical lesions produce more abnormalities than noncortical vascular accidents. According to different studies, the percentage of patients with cerebrovascular occlusions exhibiting abnormal EEG ranges from 40 to 87% (see Chapter 2).

2. Neurometric Assessment of EEG Background Activity

a. Frequency Analysis. Neurometric procedures based on frequency analysis of the EEG have been shown to be very useful in the evaluation of

TABLE 14.1
Accuracy of EEG and Different Neurometric Procedures in the Assessment of Cerebrovascular Disorders

Procedure	*Finding*	*Accuracy*	*Observations*	*Reference*
EEG Visual Interpretation	Depression of Voltage; Presence of slow wave focus; Epileptogenic activity	40-87%	Subjective component in interpretation	Birchfield et al. (1959) Gibbs and Gibbs (1964) Lavy et al. (1964)
Canonograms	Based on frequency analysis of the EEG; detection of slow focus and asymmetries	Less than EEG	Display simple to interpret	Gotman et al. (1975)
Deviance Computation	Based on features derived from power spectral analysis; detection of slow frequencies and asymmetries	Higher than EEG	Display simple to interpret	Binnie et al. (1978)
Age-Dependent Quotient	Computes theoretical age according to EEG frequency characteristics	80% agreement with EEG	Provides a single value per derivation; written text with automatic EEG interpretation	Matousek and Petersén (1973b); Petersén and Matousek (1975)
EEG symmetry analysis	Detects amplitude and wave-form asymmetries	86% detections 80% overall accuracy	25% false positives	Otero et al. (1975b)

VER symmetry analysis	Detects waveform and amplitude VER asymmetries	82%	Incidence of false positives	Ricardo et al. (1975)
EEG + Symmetry		95%	Incidence of false positives	John et al. (1977) Harmony (1977)
Step-Wise Principal Component Analysis of VERs	Definition of a normal signal space and analysis of waveform symmetry	60% detections 24% "At risk"		John et al. (1977)
Step-Wise Principal Component Analysis of VERs and EEG of Patients "At Risk"	A simulated screening procedure	80%	No false positives	John et al. (1977)
Amplitude and Duration of SSER Components	Detects alterations of amplitude or duration of the components of the first 100 msec	95%	Difficulties in the identification of SSER components in all patients	Shibasaki et al. (1977a)
Amplitude of Readiness Potential	Depression of the RP	75% midbrain lesions		Shibasaki (1975)
ER Battery	Discrimination based on amplitude and symmetry of VERs, AERs, and SSERs	Overall accuracy: 90% Discrimination 85% Replication	Simple measures to be computed	Harmony et al. (1978c)

cerebrovascular disorders. Canonograms are more accurate than visual EEG interpretation in centro–parietal lesions, both methods are similar in temporal lesions, and the EEG is slightly more accurate than the canonograms when the lesion is localized in frontal or occipital regions (Gotman et al., 1975). The deviance computations based on features derived from power spectral analysis have higher accuracy than canonograms, visual inspection of the EEG, or deviance measures derived from slope descriptors (Binnie et al., 1978). The age-dependent quotient (ADQ), based on six 10-second epochs of recordings, shows 80% agreement with the traditional EEG diagnosis based on the whole EEG record. ADQ also provides objective information in the follow-up of patients (Friberg et al., 1976; Matousek & Petersén, 1973b).

b. Symmetry Analysis. Using PCC and SER measures between left and right homologous derivations, the discriminant analysis between a group of patients with cerebrovascular disorders and a control group showed an overall accuracy of 80% (Otero et al., 1975b). There is a remarkable difference between EEG visual evaluation and quantitative symmetry analysis: With the first technique, a high percentage of patients were considered normal (35%), when compared with symmetry analysis (14%), whereas 25% of control subjects were considered abnormal by symmetry analysis. For screening purposes, it seems that the latter error might be less dangerous than the former one. The discriminant equation obtained by the comparison of a control group, a group of patients with cerebrovascular diseases, and a group of tumor patients showed that this procedure defines the boundary between normal and abnormal subjects relatively well (75%), but yields somewhat less accuracy in discriminating between different types of lesions (67%) (Otero et al., 1975c).

B. Averaged Evoked Responses

1. VERs

VERs to flashes and to a checkerboard pattern are characterized by asymmetries between left and right homologous derivations. It is very difficult to identify the side of the lesion, because larger or smaller amplitudes or latencies may be detected on either side, although there is a tendency to find the smaller VER, as well as a slower afterdischarge, on the side of the lesion. We think that such individual differences may be related to circulatory compensatory changes that occurred after the stroke and the time elapsed between onset of stroke and recording. Another general characteristic of VERs in cerebrovascular patients is the reduction in amplitude of the responses recorded in all derivations. VER amplitude and asymmetry are directly related to the severity of the clinical findings, and they may be used as indices in the follow-up of patients with strokes (Chapter 3). The steady-state VERs to flicker stimulation are characteized by enhanced responses to low frequencies and reduction of the responses in the alpha range in the affected hemisphere (Harmony, 1975).

a. Symmetry Analysis. By the application of an equation obtained as a result of a discriminant analysis between a group of neurological patients and a control group, 82% of the cases with cerebrovascular diseases were detected, whereas only 68% had abnormal EEGs (Ricardo et al. 1975). However, this procedure did not permit discrimination between different types of diseases. Complementary use of EEG and VER symmetry showed that 95% of cerebrovascular patients had either EEG or VER asymmetry.

b. Step-Wise Principal Component Analysis. By this procedure, it was possible to discriminate 60% of the patients as abnormal, in need of referral to the neurologists. Twenty-four percent were considered "at risk" and 16% as "normal." Following the idea of a simulated screening procedure, if those patients at risk were then submitted to a conventional EEG examination, more cases were identified as abnormal, for a final accuracy of 80%.

2. *AERs*

Cerebrovascular lesions of the brain stem may be detected and localized by the recording of brain-stem auditory evoked responses (BAERs). Absence, amplitude depression, increased latencies, and increased interpeak latencies of the BAER components may be observed (Stockard & Rossiter, 1977). Middle and long latency AER components are severely affected in patients with lesions of the temporal areas (Michel & Peronnet, 1974). Patients with sensory aphasia are more likely to present amplitude reduction of the AER on the hemisphere affected than those with motor aphasia (Barat et al., 1974). In cerebrovascular occlusions, the amplitude of the AERs in all areas is smaller than in control subjects (Harmony et al., 1978a).

3. *SSERs to Electrical Stimulation of the Peripheral Nerves*

SSERs are a very powerful tool for the localization of the hemisphere affected. Absence, amplitude reduction, and/or increased latencies of SSER components are frequently observed in the side of the lesion in patients with cerebrovascular lesions. In cases with brain-stem lesions, the *N*15 component to median nerve stimulation is absent (Nakanishi et al., 1978). If the VPL thalamic nucleus is affected, *N*19 and *P*24 are particularly altered, although all components may be reduced if the lesion is large (Domino et al., 1965). Lesions of the VL thalamic nucleus produce a selective decrease in amplitude of *P*180 (Velasco et al., 1975). Cortical lesions also produce great alterations of SSERs even in the absence of joint position and vibration sense impairment (A. M. Halliday, 1975c). A general reduction in amplitude of SSERs, probably due to ischemic factors, has been reported (Harmony et al., 1978a).

With the definition of confidence limits for the measurements of amplitude and duration of different waves of the SSERs to the stimulation of the median nerve, it is possible to detect 95% of the patients with cerebrovascular diseases (Shibasaki et al., 1977a). This procedure has the drawback that in patients with brain lesions, the identification of the components of the SSERs is very difficult and sometimes impossible.

4. Other Event-Related Potentials

Reduction of CNV on the affected side in 80% of the patients with vascular diseases has been described (J. Cohen, 1975). CNV has been also used as a proof of concept discrimination in aphasic patients (objective speech audiometry). The readiness potential (RP) is frequently decreased in amplitude on the side of the lesion. These abnormalities of the RP have been observed in patients without weakness of the hand, and with or without pyramidal signs. In midbrain cerebrovascular lesions, it has been reported that 75% of the cases showed depression of the RP (Shibasaki, 1975; Shibasaki & Kuroiwa, 1977).

5. Evoked-Response Battery

The application of discriminant equations using amplitude values and correlation coefficients between homologous left and right leads of the VERs to flashes and to a checkerboard pattern, AERs to three different tones, and SSERs to the left, right, and simultaneous bilateral median nerve stimulation yields an accuracy of detections of 92%, with 11% false positives. The replication study yields an overall accuracy of 85%. The number of patients detected in the replication study was similar to the number of patients with an abnormal EEG. Considering both procedures as complementary, only 4% of patients were normal in both examinations (Harmony, Valdes, Fernández, Alvarez, & Solis, 1978c).

The side of the lesion was correctly identified by the analysis of the AERs and SSERs in 95% of the patients (Harmony et al., 1978a).

C. Conclusions

At present, there are some neurometric procedures based on the analysis of the EEG and the ERs that seem to have greater accuracy in the detection of cerebrovascular lesions than EEG visual interpretation. These studies have been conducted in patients with proved cerebrovascular lesions, in whom the clinical diagnosis is generally not very difficult. Nevertheless, because cerebrovascular occlusion is the most frequent cause of a cerebrovascular disease, and it is observed in atherosclerotic patients, what is more important is that these procedures offer a unique opportunity for the investigation of cerebrovascular occulsions in neurologically asymptomatic patients with atherosclerosis, because detection of brain dysfunction prior to the appearance of clinical symptoms gives the possibility of preventive intervention in such cases, with a much more favorable prognosis in relation to life expectancy and future neurological status. My group at CENIC is working in this direction, and the results, although preliminary, show that the ER battery is sensitive enough to detect such types of lesions (Fernández-Bouzas & Harmony, 1979).

II. INTRACRANIAL TUMORS (see Table 14.2)

A. EEG

1. Visual Interpretation

A slow wave focus is the most significant finding and nearly characteristic abnormality in brain tumors. Paroxysmal activity is also frequently observed. The accuracy of detection varies with the size and location of the tumor: Abnormal EEGs are found in 96% of cortical tumors and in 43% of tumors of the optic chiasm, brain stem, and cerebellopontine angle (Gibbs & Gibbs, 1964).

2. Neurometric Assessment of EEG Background Activity

a. Frequency Analysis. As in cerebrovascular disorders, the deviance computation based on features derived from power spectral analysis have

TABLE 14.2
Accuracy of EEG and Different Neurometric Procedures in the Assessment of Intracranial Tumors

Procedure	*Finding*	*Accuracy*	*Observations*	*Reference*
EEG Visual Interpretation	Slow wave focus	96% Cortical 43% Others	Subjective component in interpretation	Gibbs and Gibbs (1964)
Canonograms	Based on EEG frequency analysis; detects slow wave focus and asymmetries	Less than EEG	Display simple to interpret	Gotman et al. (1973, 1975)
Deviance Computation	Based on features derived from power spectral analysis; detection of slow frequencies and asymmetries	Higher than EEG	Display simple to interpret	Binnie et al. (1978)
Age-Dependent Quotient	Computes theoretical age according to EEG frequency characteristics	Higher accuracy than EEG in localization	Provides a single value per derivation; automatic written text with interpretation	Matousek and Petersén (1973b)
EEG symmetry analysis	Detects waveform and amplitude asymmetries	71%	13% false positives	Otero et al. (1975a)
EEG Symmetry and EEG Visual Assessment		94%	13% false positives	Otero et al. (1975a)

VER Symmetry Analysis	Detects waveform and amplitude asymmetries	82%	Incidence of false positives	Ricardo et al. (1975)
EEG + Symmetry		97%	Incidence of false positives	Harmony (1977) John et al. (1977)
Step-Wise Principal Component Analysis of VERs	Definition of a normal signal space; waveform symmetry analysis	80% Detections 8% At risk		John et al. (1977)
Step-Wise principal Component Analysis of VERs and EEG of Patients "At Risk"	A simulated screening procedure	88%	No false positives	John et al (1977)
Multidimensional Scaling of VERs	Graphic procedure that reduces to two the original space dimensions	85%	15% false positives	Schwartz and John (1976)
BAERs	Interaural latency difference of wave	97% Acoustic neuromas	Higher accuracy than CAT	Thomsen et al. (1978)
Amplitude and Duration of SSER Components	Detects alterations of the waves in the first 100 msec	95%	Difficulties in identification of SSER components in all patients	Shibasaki et al. (1977a)
ER Battery	Discrimination based on amplitude and symmetry of VERs, AERs, and SSERs	Overall accuracy: 95% discrimination 83% Replication	Simple measures to be computed	Alvarez & Harmony (1978)

higher accuracy than canonograms, visual inspection, and deviance measures derived from slope descriptors (Binnie et al., 1978). The laterality of the actual cerebral involvement correlated to a high degree with laterality as determined by the ADQ, whereas the correlation between clinical findings and the visual EEG assessment was significantly lower (Petersén & Matousek, 1975). ADQ is also very useful as an objective measurement in the follow-up of neurological patients (Matousek, 1977).

b. Symmetry Analysis. Using PCC and SER measures between left and right homologous derivations, discriminant analysis between a group of patients with brain tumors and a control group showed an overall accuracy of 87%. Comparing EEG visual evaluation and discrimination by symmetry analysis, similar results were obtained (71% detection). However, if both methods were used as complementary, 94% accuracy was obtained, with 13% false positives (Otero et al., 1975a).

B. Averaged Evoked Responses

1. VERs

VERs to flashes and to patterned stimuli are more likely to be altered if the tumors are located along the visual pathway (A. M. Halliday, 1975a; R. Halliday et al., 1976). Nevertheless, other tumor locations also produced VER asymmetries, the definition of the injured side being difficult (Jonkman, 1967; Ricardo et al., 1975).

a. Symmetry Analysis. Computation of a discriminant equation, taking into consideration the correlation coefficients and the SER values between VERs to flashes in left and right homologous derivations, has shown that 82% of patients with brain tumors were considered abnormal, whereas only 59% had an abnormal EEG. However, by symmetry analysis of VERs, a higher incidence of false positives is observed. If EEG symmetry and VER symmetry are used as complementary, 97% of patients were detected.

b. Step-Wise Principal Component Analysis. With this procedure, 80% of patients with brain tumors were considered definitively "abnormal," 8% "at risk," and 12% as "normal." In this particular group of patients, 40% had a normal EEG. However, if, in those patients considered at risk, the EEG was also taken into account, the accuracy of the procedure increased to 88% (John et al., 1977).

c. Multidimensional Scaling. This procedure yields 85% accuracy with the analysis of VERs in occipito-temporal derivations (Schwartz & John, 1976).

2. AERs

The early auditory evoked response components are very useful in the detection of acoustic neuromas or brain tumors (Daly et al., 1977; Stockard & Rossiter, 1977). In a study of a group of patients with surgically verified acoustic neuromas, 75% of the patients presented an interaural latency difference of wave V larger than the confidence interval; in 22%, no response was found in the side of the lesion (Thomsen, Terkildsen, & Osterhammer, 1978). The accuracy of the procedure was even higher than computerized axial tomography, in which only 43% of the patients had a positive CAT examination.

Middle and long latency components may be absent or depressed in cortical temporal lesions (Michel & Peronnet, 1974). A general amplitude reduction, as well as an asymmetry between left and right homologous derivations, have also been reported (Alvarez & Harmony, 1978).

3. SSERs to Electrical Stimulation of the Peripheral Nerves

As with cerebrovascular lesions, SSERs are frequently abnormal in patients with brain tumors. Far-field potentials may be very useful for the detection of spinal-cord and brain-stem tumors. Most authors considered that absence, amplitude depression, and increased latencies are generally found in the side of the tumor. Nevertheless, in some cases, characterized by a Jacksonian epilepsy, SSERs may be of higher amplitude on the side of the lesion (Düsseldorf, 1975).

Measuring amplitude and duration of the SSER components in the first 100 msec, Shibasaki et al. (1977a) reported 95% detections in patients with brain tumors of different locations.

4. Evoked-Response Battery

With the computation of a discriminant analysis, based on amplitude measures, correlation coefficients, and SER values between left and right VERs to flashes, to a checkerboard pattern, AERs to three different tones and SSERs to left, right, and bilateral median nerve stimulation between a group of patients with intracranial tumors and a control group, an accuracy of 95% was obtained when the subject was included for the computation of the predictive criteria, and of 83% when the subject was excluded from this computation (leave-one-out replication). The number of patients detected in the replication study was similar to the number of patients that had an abnormal EEG. If both procedures were used as complementary, only 9% of the patients were normal in both examinations.

C. Conclusions

Early detection and treatment of brain tumors is highly correlated with prolonged life expectancy; thus, mass screening procedures play an extremely important role in the medical care of the population. Several neurometric procedures with higher accuracy than EEG visual assessment in well-known samples of patients with brain tumors have been described. Such methods should be applied in larger samples in order to define their utility. Diagnosis of brain tumors depends mainly on their size and location, which account for a wide range of electrophysiological abnormalities. thus, a more powerful neurometric battery will be obtained by the combination of different types of procedures.

III. EPILEPSY (see Table 14.3)

A. EEG

1. Visual Interpretation

The EEG is characterized by the presence of abnormal paroxysmal activity. During routine EEG examinations epileptic patients present different percentages of abnormal EEGs, according to the type of epilepsy. In patients with grand mal, 70% of the records are abnormal; in psychomotor epilepsy, 50%; in focal epilepsy, 70%, and in petit mal 90% of the EEGs are abnormal (Gastaut & Tassinari, 1975).

2. Automatic Spike Detection

In Chapter 12, several procedures for automatic spike recognition were reviewed. Those based on amplitude, slope, and sharpness criteria yielded approximately 80% correct detections. Procedures based on inverse AR filter-

TABLE 14.3

Accuracy of EEG and Different Neurometric Procedures in the Assessment of Epilepsy

Procedure	*Finding*	*Accuracy*	*Observations*	*Reference*
EEG Visual Interpretation	Spikes, sharp waves, etc.	70% Grand mal 50% Psychomotor 70% Focal 90% Petit mal	Subjective component in interpretation	Gastaut and Tassinari (1975)
Automatic Spike Detection	Different types of criteria used; amplitude, slope, and sharpness of EEG waves most frequently used; detection of nonstationarities by inverse AR filtering	Dependent on procedure used (see Table 13.2); similar or better than EEG	Quantitative, objective evaluation	See Chapter 12
EEG Symmetry	Detects amplitude and waveform asymmetries	Not useful in adult patients; 86% in children	Incidence of false positives	Figueredo et al. (1978)
VER Symmetry	Detects amplitude and waveform asymmetries	64% (lower than EEG)		Ricardo et al. (1975)
Driving Curves	VER waveform asymmetry and amplitude as a function of frequency	67% (lower than EEG)		Harmony et al. (1978c)
Step-Wise principal Component Analysis of VERs	Definition of a normal signal space; waveform symmetry analysis	Lower than EEG		John et al. (1977)
ER Battery	Discrimination based on amplitude and symmetry of VERs, AERs, and SSERs	Overall accuracy: 85% Discrimination 78% Replication	Simple measures to compute	Harmony et al. (1978)

ing are able to detect events at the scalp not classified as spikes by visual inspection, but coincident with clear paroxysmal patterns in subdural derivations. Conclusions regarding the identification of the epileptogenic zone, obtained with 100 secs of automatically analyzed EEG by inverse AR filtering were identical with those obtained using conventional methods.

3. Symmetry Analysis

In adult subjects, no discrimination was obtained between a control group and a group of epileptic patients (Otero et al., 1974). However, in children 5 to 12 years old, 86% of the epileptics were detected by this procedure, whereas only 70% had an abnormal EEG. Using both procedures as complementary, the accuracy obtained was 96%. By symmetry analysis, 17% false positives were observed when the whole sample of 110 normal children and 150 children with some neurological disease (of which 93 were epileptic) were compared.

B. Averaged Evoked Responses

1. VERs

VERs to flashes are of higher amplitude in photosensitive epileptics. Amplitude and peak latency asymmetries have been reported by Jonkman (1967) and Ricardo (1974). The visual excitability cycle in epileptic patients shows a short refractory period with great facilitation of the late components (Floris et al., 1969). Cigánek (1977) described abnormal driving responses to 10 and 15 Hz in epileptic patients with generalized discharges. Lower amplitude of VERs to a checkerboard pattern, as well as great waveshape asymmetry of occipital responses, has been reported (Fernández et al., 1975).

a. Symmetry Analysis of VERs to Flashes. Ricardo et al. (1975), by the application of a discriminant equation obtained between a group of neurological patients and a control group, classified 64% of epileptic patients as abnormals. In this group, 85% had an abnormal EEG. Using both methods as complementary, an accuracy of 89% is reached. Discrimination based on the equation of VER measures yielded 23% false positives, when the whole sample of 92 normal subjects and 197 patients were compared. Therefore, the procedure is not accurate enough for the detection of epileptic patients.

b. Step-Wise Principal Component Analysis of VERs to Flashes. This procedure also yields a lower accuracy than the EEG for the identification of epileptic patients (John et al., 1977).

c. Driving Curves. By the analysis of the driving curves, 48% of the epileptics showed waveform asymmetries of the VERs; in 39%, no dominant response in the alpha range was observed. This results in an overall accuracy of 67% (Harmony et al., 1975).

2. AERs

In patients with temporal epilepsy, changes of the cortical AERs to clicks have been related to the degree of alterations of the EEG. According to Polujanova et al. (1977), when only localized spike activity was observed, without general EEG discharges, the response had higher amplitude and lower latency values. When the EEG alterations were generalized, there was a general reduction of amplitude of the AERs.

3. SSERs

Higher amplitude of SSERs in epileptic patients than in normal subjects has been a general finding (Broughton et al., 1967; Dawson, 1947a, 1947b; Fernández et al., 1975; A. M. Halliday, 1965, 1967).

4. Evoked-Response Battery

In a comparative study of 20 patients with temporal epilepsy and 20 normal subjects matched by age and sex, Fernández & Harmony (1978b) detected 95% of epileptic patients with no false positives. The analysis performed was a step-wise nonlinear discriminant analysis, based on the amplitude and the correlation coefficient of ERs in frontal, central, temporal, and occipital monopolar derivations, to a flash, to a checkerboard pattern, to three different tones, and to bilateral median nerve stimulation. Independent replication of the discriminant equations previously obtained, in a new group of 25 epileptic subjects, showed that 100% of temporal epileptics were correctly classified, whereas patients with generalized epilepsy were randomly discriminated. Such results suggest that there are differential characteristics of the averaged evoked responses according to the different types of epilepsy.

In a more recent study, the comparison of larger groups of temporal epileptics and normal subjects showed that with 10 variables, 75% of the epileptics and 94% of the normal subjects were adequately classified. The replication of this analysis yielded 68% correct classification in epileptic patients and 86% in normal subjects. The accuracy is still lower than the one obtained by visual assessment of the EEG.

C. Conclusions

Visual interpretation of the EEG has been, until now, the most efficient procedure for the diagnosis of epilepsy. It also permits identification of different electrophysiological patterns and localization of the abnormality in a high percentage of cases. But, as paroxysmal activity may not occur for long periods of time, the probability of its detection decreases with short time recordings. Thus, continuous monitoring of the EEG activity has been an extremely valuable tool in the study of epilepsy. Visual evaluation of these long-term recordings is obviously laborious and time consuming. Automatic spike detection is a solution for this problem. Another type of solution for the diagnosis of epileptic patients might be the study of some steady, not paroxysmal, electrophysiological characteristics. For example, the evoked responses are frequently altered in the epileptic patients. Neurometric procedures based on the analysis of the evoked responses have mainly been focused on amplitude and symmetry measurements. More intense research is needed in this direction in order to define the real value that they may have in the diagnosis of epilepsy.

IV. MULTIPLE SCLEROSIS (see Table 14.4)

A. EEG

1. Visual Assessment

The EEG in this disease does not show characteristic features, and whether it is abnormal or not appears to depend on the acuteness of the disease at the time of recording or the location of the lesion. Abnormal EEGs have been reported in 88% of cases during the acute phase and in only 36% during remissions (Cobb, 1963b). The abnormalities may be slight and diffuse or they may be focal, sometimes including epileptogenic activity.

B. Averaged Evoked Responses

1. VERs

a. Delayed VERs to a Pattern-Reversal Checkerboard. As has been mentioned in Chapter 3, Halliday's discovery of a characteristic delay of the major positive component of the VER to a pattern-reversal checkerboard in patients suffering or having suffered from photic neuritis and/or optic atrophy, in MS patients with a negative ophthalmological examination, opened a new field in the diagnosis of this disease. The incidence of delayed VERs in MS with previous episodes of optic neuritis is in the range of 87–100% according to different authors (see Table 14.6). In those patients with no previous opthalmologic antecedents, the accuracy obtained is in the range of 33–92%. The overall accuracy in all cases of MS is from 57–96%.

b. Steady-State VERs. Driving curves were abnormal in 47% of MS patients (Fernández et al., 1977). Using the apparent latency and the interocular latency difference as criteria in steady-state VERs to flicker and to pattern reversal, a total accuracy of 92% has been reported (Regan et al., 1976). Using similar criteria, Duwaer and Spekreijse (1978) have reported 67% detections, using steady-state responses to pattern reversal.

2. AERs

On the basis of amplitude and latency values of wave V, 65% of MS patients were detected. If middle auditory components were also considered, 77% of the patients had abnormal AERs (Robinson & Rudge, 1977a).

3. SSERs

Peak latency differences of the SSER far-field potentials that deviated from control values by at least 2.5 SD, absence of P_1, P_3, or N_1, and differences in the amplitude of the P_3 and N_1 potentials to left versus right median nerve stimulation that deviate from control values more than 2.5 SD, were the criteria used by Anziska et al. (1978) in the detection of MS patients. Abnormal results were obtained in 96% of the patients with definite MS.

Application of a discriminant equation obtained between a group of MS

TABLE 14.4
Accuracy of EEG and Different Neurometric Procedures in the Assessment of Multiple Sclerosis

Procedure	*Finding*	*Accuracy*	*Observations*	*Reference*
EEG Visual Interpretation	Slight diffuse or focal abnormalities	88% Acute phase 36% Remissions	Subjective component in interpretation	Cobb (1963b)
VERs to Pattern-Reversal Checkerboard	Characteristic delay of the major positive component	57% 96%	Accuracy dependent on previous episodes of optic neuritis	Shahrokhi et al. (1978) Halliday et al. (1973a)
Steady-State VERs to Pattern Reversal	Increased apparent latency and/or interocular latency difference	67% 54%		Duwaer and Spekreijse (1978) Regan et al. (1976)
Steady-state VERs to flicker	Increased apparent latency and/or interocular latency difference	62%		Regan et al. (1976)
Steady-State VERs to Flicker and to Pattern Reversal	Increased apparent latency and/or interocular latency difference	92%		Regan et al. (1976)

BAERs	Lower amplitude and higher latency values of wave V	65%		Robinson and Rudge (1977a)
BAERs and Middle AERs	Lower amplitude or higher latencies	77%		Robinson and Rudge (1977a)
Far-Field SSERs	Absence, increased latencies, differences of P_1, P_3, N_1	96% (Definite MS)		Anziska et al. (1978)
SSERT	Discrimination based on amplitude values of the single-cycle average evoked response to trains of electrical pulses.	100%		Sclabassi et al. (1974)
VERs to Pattern Reversal and SCERs	Delayed VERs, lower amplitude, and increased latencies of SCERs	59% (Possible MS)		Mastaglia et al. (1976)
ER Battery	Discrimination based on amplitude and waveform symmetry of VERs, AERs, and SSERs.	100%	15% false positives	Fernández et al. (1977)

patients and a control group, using the amplitude values of the single-cycle average evoked response obtained by trains of electrical pulses of different frequencies applied to the median nerve (SSERT), demonstrated 100% discrimination. The technique is highly specific: Demyelination must be present in the pathway under study for the observation of abnormal responses (Sclabassi et al., 1974).

4. Complementary Use of Pattern-Reversal VERs and Spinal-Cord Evoked Responses (SCERs)

Delayed VERs were observed in 83% of the group of definite MS and 33% of the probable and possible MS groups. Increased latency and reduced amplitude of SCERs were observed in 94% of the definite group, 50% of the probable, and 37% of the possible MS. Of the 27 cases in which both VERs and SCERs were recorded, 16 patients (59%) gave an abnormal result with one or the other or both techniques; six patients with normal VERs had abnormal SCERs, and four with normal SCERs had abnormal VERs. Thus, VERs and SCERs have a complementary role in investigating suspected MS (Mastaglia et al., 1976).

5. Evoked-Response Battery

Application of a discriminant equation, based on the amplitude and correlation coefficients of ERs to flash, to a checkerboard pattern, to three different tones, and to bilateral median nerve stimulation, between a control group and a group of nine probable and six possible MS patients, showed 100% detection of MS patients with 15% false positives (Fernández et al., 1977).

C. Conclusions

Application of ERs to the study of MS patients has shown that they are an extremely valuable tool in the diagnosis of this disease. The detection of abnormalities of the ERs in the absence of clinical symptoms related to the sensory modality studied unequivocally demonstrates the presence of various lesions. It is obvious that the combination of various types of ERs will improve the efficiency of the procedure.

15 Conclusions. Strategies for the Use of Neurometrics

In this volume, we have reviewed the major effects produced by different types of neurological diseases on the EEG and on the averaged evoked responses. This evidence, gathered by scientists devoted to the identification of functional correlates and quantitative evaluation of the brain's electrical activity, make possible the development of the neurometric methodology.

Evidence has been presented that demonstrates that neurometric procedures, either based on the analysis of the EEG or of the averaged evoked responses, surpass the accuracy of the conventional EEG examination in the identification of brain dysfunction caused by different neurological diseases. Using the neurometric methodology it is also possible to detect abnormalities that are clinically silent, and even to localize accurately lesions in the nervous system, which obviously increases its values as a diagnostic tool.

The objective, automatic nature of the methodology makes its adoption in large populations where there are not enough specialized personnel, both useful and economical. This is especially true in developing countries. Application of neurometrics will improve the efficiency of medical care in the whole population: in urban areas, where specialists in diverse neurological techniques are concentrated, it will provide a powerful adjunct to the neurologist. In rural or many urban areas, where a lack of specialists exists, it will make possible the detection, diagnosis and treatment of many patients by the general physician. Other patients, who need specialized examinations and treatments, will be detected and referred to the specialists. Thus, the specialized personnel will be primarily dedicated to examine and treat cases of the latter sort, who cannot be optimally treated by general physicians.

Therefore, in relation to the organization of a public health service for the application of neurometric procedures, two main approaches may be adopted, according to the economical and technical possibilities of a given region. The more economical solutions will utilize two different levels of examination. In the first level, rapid automatic primary screening for the detection of possible positive cases is performed. Subjects that should be submitted to this examination are those at risk for brain damage, and those who present some neurological symptoms. Those considered at risk are, for example, infants with prenatal and perinatal risk factors, childhood diseases, cranial traumas, chronic intoxication of workers in polluted environments, patients with peripheral signs of atherosclerosis, but asymptomatic from the neurological point of view, and so on. Subjects who are negative in the first examination, unless they continue presenting symptoms, will be considered as normal. Cases that are either positive in the primary screening or who continue to present symptoms, will be sent to a second level of examination. This will be a more detailed neurometric diagnostic examination, where the type of electrophysiological dysfunction and the probable location of damage will be identified. Results from the second examination may be sent to a general physician in those places where specialists are not available. The general physician should be able to take care of a large number of these patients, and will send other cases who require more specialized examinations to a place where specialists are concentrated. *In this way, the time of the scarce highly trained specialists will be used more efficiently*. Even in those areas that have enough specialists, it is more efficient to send the patients to them after a neurometric examination of the second type.

The primary screening procedure and the neurometric diagnostic examination may be performed by special purpose computers, operated by well-trained technicians. They provide automatic assessments that do not require skilled personnel to evaluate the results. The primary screening device, which may be based only on the examination of the EEG background activity or on the averaged evoked responses, depending on their relative utility and economy may yield an accuracy of approximately 80%. A high proportion of false negatives on the primary screening examination, who continue to present symptoms, can be detected by referral for the neurometric diagnostic examination, thus reducing the probability of ignoring the cases that have brain damage. The detailed neurometric diagnostic examination will provide information about the EEG background activity, the presence of spikes, the sensory pathway affected through the analysis of the ERs, the possible location of the lesion, and the type of diseases in which such abnormalities are more frequently seen.

The second approach is the creation of computer centers, based on general purpose computers, with data banks that may be fed by several terminals in order to perform a detailed neurometric study of both patients at risk or those with some definite neurological symptoms. The evaluation of the neurometric examination of the positive cases will be sent to neurological specialists, who will be able to analyze the reliability and utility of the neurometric procedures in the diagnosis of the patients, and communicate to the neurometricians the important failures or drawbacks of the procedure in order to improve it. Such centers will need many more experienced personnel and will be more expensive, but they will produce a progressive improvement of the neurometric methodology.

At present, the main emphasis of neurometrics has been in the development of diagnostic procedures; however, neurometrics is also very useful in the assessment of brain dysfunction in the follow-up of patients, in the evaluation of different treatments, and for the prognosis of the patients. From the clinical point of view, neurometrics may also be used for monitoring the brain state during anesthesia, surgical interventions, hemodialysis, and intensive care. Particularly important is the evaluation of newborns who have been submitted to risk factors during pregnancy and/or delivery, because earlier interventions will be much more effective for the remediation and compensation of central nervous system injuries. These studies should also improve preventive actions, identifying the electrophysiological correlates of the dysfunction produced by a specific risk factor in the newborn.

The sensitivity of the neurometric procedure to more subtle disorders than those that arise from neurological diseases, as has been demonstrated in the study of learning disabled children and behavioral problems, leads us to expect rapid expansion of applications of this technique to functional disorders and other clinical problems more directly related to the fields of psychiatry, psychology, and pedagogy.

References

Abraham, P., & McCallum, W. C. A permanent change in the EEG (CNV) of schizophrenics. *Electroenceph. Clin Neurophysiol.*, 1977, *43*, 533.

Abraham, P., McCallum, W. C., Docherty, T., Fox, A., & Newton, P. The CNV in schizophrenia. *Electroenceph. Clin Neurophysiol.*, 1974, *36*, 217-218.

Abraham, F. A., Melamed, E., & Lavy, S. Prognostic value of visual evoked potentials in occipital blindness following basilar artery occlusion. *Applied Neurophysiology*, 1975, *38*, 126-135.

Abrakov, L. V., Vedenskaya, I. V., & Dilman, V. M. The mechanism of the gross changes of the bioelectrical activity of the brain associated with metastatic cerebral tumors. *Vop. Neirokhir.*, 1962, *5*, 35-40. (Russian)

Adams, A. Studies on flat electroencephalogram in man. *Electroenceph. Clin. Neurophysiol.*, 1959, *11*, 34-41.

Adey, W. R. On-line analysis and pattern recognition techniques for the electroencephalogram. In G. F. Inbar (Ed.); *Signal analysis and pattern recognition in biomedical engineering*. New York; Wiley, 1974.

Adey, W. R. The influence of impressed electrical fields at EEG frequencies. In N. Burch & L. Altschuler (Eds.); *Behavior and brain electrical activity*. New York; Plenum Press, 1975, 363-390.

Adey, W. R., Dunlop, C. W., & Hendrix, C. E. Hippocampal slow waves; distribution and phase relationships in the course of approach learning. *Arch. Neurol.* (Chicago), 1960, *3*, 74-90.

Adey, W. R., Kado, R. T., & Walter, D. O. Computer analysis of EEG data from Gemini flight G7-7. *Aerospace Med.*, 1967, *38*, 345-359.

Adrian, E. D., & Matthews, B. H. C. The Berger rhythm: Potential changes from the occipital lobes in man. *Brain*, 1934, *57*, 355-385.

Agnew, H. W., Parker, J. C., Webb, W. B., & Williams, R. L. Amplitude measurement of the sleep electroencephalogram. *Electroenceph. Clin. Neurophysiol.*, 1967, *22*, 84-86.

Aird, R. B., & Gastaut, Y. Occipital and posterior electroencephalographic rhythms. *Electroenceph. Clin. Neurophysiol.*, 1959, *11*, 637-656.

Aitchinson, J., Habbema, J. D. F., & Kay, J. W. A critical comparison of two methods of statistical discrimination. *Appl. Statist.*, 1977, *26*, 15-25.

Albrecht, V., & Radil-Weiss, T. Some comments on the derivation of the Wiener filter for average evoked potentials. *Biol. Cybernetics*, 1976, *24*, 43-46.

Alferova, V. V. Visual evoked potentials in the EEG of children of different ages. *Zh. Vyssh. Nerv. Dyat.*, 1970, *20*, 1198-1203. (Russian)

Allen, A. R., & Starr, A. Sensory evoked potentials in the operating room. *Neurology*, 1977, *27*, 358.

Allison, T., Matsumiya, Y., Goff, G. D., & Goff, W. R. The scalp topography of human visual evoked potentials. *Electroenceph. Clin. Neurophysiol.*, 1977, *42*, 185-197.

Anderberg, M. R. *Cluster analysis for applications*. New York: Academic Press, 1973.

Alvarez, A., & Harmony, T. *Visual, auditory and somatosensory evoked responses in patients with intracranial tumors*. Unpublished results, 1978.

Anderson, T. W. *Introduction to multivariate statistical analysis*. New York: Wiley, 1958.

Anderson, T. W. Time series analysis. New York: Wiley, 1970.

Andrews, D. F., Granadesikan, R., & Warner, J. L. Transformations of multivariate data. *Biometrics*, 1971, *27*, 825-840.

Andrews, D. F., Granadesikan, R., & Warner, J. L. Methods for assessing multivariate normality. In P. R. Kishanaiah (Ed.), *Multivariate analysis* (Vol. 3), New York: Academic Press, 1973.

Anziska, B., Cracco, R. Q., Cook, A. W., & Feld, E. W. Somatosensory far field potentials: Studies in normal subjects and patients with multiple sclerosis. *Electroenceph. Clin. Neurophysiol.*, 1978, *45*, 602–610.

Aoki, Y. A clinical electroencephalographic study on photosensitive epilepsy, with special reference to visual evoked potential. *Folia Psychiat. Neurol. Jap.*, 1969, *23*, 103-120.

Arezzo, J., & Vaughan, H. G. Cortical potentials associated with voluntary movement in the monkey. *Brain Research*, 1975, *88*, 99-104.

Arlinger, S. D. N_1 latencies of the slow auditory evoked potential. *Audiology*, 1976, *15*, 370-375.

Arnal, D., Gerin, P., Salmon, D., Nakache, J. P., Maynard, P., Peronnet, F., & Hugonnier, R. Analyse statistique multivariée des potentiels évoqués moyens visuels dans l'amblyopie fonctionelle. *Electroenceph. Clin. Neurophysiol.*, 1971, *31*, 365-376.

Arnal, D., Gerin, P., Salmon, D., Ravault, M. P., Nakachi, J. P., & Peronnet, F. Les diverses composantes des potentiels évoqués moyen visuel chez l'homme. *Electroenceph. Clin. Neurophysiol.*, 1972, *32*, 499-511.

Artsenlova, O. K., & Ivanitsky, A. M. Relationships between the components of the evoked potential and background EEG in man. *Zh. Vyssh. Nerv. Deyat. Pavlov.*, 1967, *17*, 677-680. (Russian)

Arvidsson, A., Friberg, S., Matousek, M., & Petersén, I. Automatic selection of data in quantitative EEG analysis. *Electroenceph. Clin. Neurophysiol.*, 1977, *43*, 508.

Asselman, P., Chadwick, D. W., & Marsden, C. D. Visual evoked responses in the diagnosis and management of patients suspected of multiple sclerosis. *Brain*, 1975, *98*, 1261-1282.

Aunon, J. I., & Cantor, F. K. VEP and AEP variability: Interlaboratory vs. intralaboratory and intersession vs. intrasession variability. *Electroenceph. Clin. Neurophysiol.*, 1977, *42*, 705–708.

Aunon, J. I., & McGillem, C. D. *Techniques for processing single evoked potentials.* San Diego Biomedical Symposium, 1975, 211–218.

Aunon, J. I., & McGillem, C. D. High frequency components in the spectrum of the visual evoked potential. *Journal of Bioengineering*, 1977, *1*, 157–164.

Austin, G. M., & McCouch, G. P. Presynaptic components of intermediary cord potential. *Journal of Neurophysiology*, 1955, *18*, 441–451.

Baba, G., Asano, T., Nakamura, S., & Orimoto, T. Readiness potential recorded from the scalp and depth leads. *Applied Neurophysiology*, 1976/77, *39*, 268–271.

Babb, T. L., Manani, E., & Crandall, P. H. An electronic circuit for detection of EEG seizures recorded with implanted electrodes. *Electroenceph. Clin. Neurophysiol.*, 1974, *37*, 305-308.

Bach-y-Rita, G., Lion, G., Reynolds, J., & Ervin, F. An improved nasopharyngeal lead. *Electroenceph. Clin. Neurophysiol.*, 1969, *26*, 220-221.

Bacia, T., & Reid, K. Visual and somatosensory evoked potentials in man particularly in patients with focal epilepsy. *Electroenceph. Clin. Neurophysiol.*, 1965, *18*, 718.

Bacsy, Z., Szirtes, G., Auguszt, A., & Virat, A. Alteration of some components of visual evoked potentials in patients with homonymous hemianopsia. *Electroenceph. Clin. Neurophysiol.*, 1977, *43*, 531.

Baer, E. de, Machiels, M. B., & Kruidenier, C. Low level frequency following response. *Audiology*, 1977, *16*, 229-240.

Baker, J. B., Larson, S. J., Sances, A., & White, P. J. Evoked potentials as an aid to the diagnosis of multiple sclerosis. *Neurology* (Minn.), 1968, *18*, 286.

Barat, M., Paty, J., & Arné, L. Etude des potentiels évoqués auditifs et visuels dans différents types d'aphasie. *Rev. Neurol.*, 1974, *130*, 456-459.

Barlow, J. S. Rhythmic activity induced by photic stimulation in relation to intrinsic alpha activity of the brain in man. *Electroenceph. Clin. Neurophysiol.*, 1960, *12*, 317-326.

Barlow, J. S. Autocorrelation and crosscorrelation. In *Handbook of electroencephalography and clinical neurophysiology* (Vol. 5A) Amsterdam: Elsevier, 1973, 79-96.

Barlow, J. S. Some programs for the processing of EEG data on a small general purpose digital computer. In G. Dolce, & H. Künkel (Eds.), *CEAN*. Stuttgart: Gustav Fischer Verlag, 1975, 172-179.

Barlow, J. S., & Brazier, M. A. B. The pacing of EEG potentials of alpha frequency by low rates of repetitive flash. *Electroenceph. Clin. Neurophysiol.*, 1957, *9*, 161-162.

Barlow, J. S., & Cigánek, L. Lambda responses in relation to visual evoked responses in man. *Electroenceph. Clin. Neurophysiol.*, 1969, *26*, 183-192.

Barlow, J. S., & Freeman, M. Z. *Comparison of EEG activity recorded from homologous locations on the scalp by means of autocorrelation and crosscorrelation analysis* (Quarterly Progress Report No. 54). Cambridge, Mass.: Res. Lab. of Electronics, MIT, 1959, 173-181.

Barnet, A. B., & Goodwin, R. S. Averaged evoked electroencephalographic responses to clicks in the human newborn. *Electroenceph. Clin. Neurophysiol.*, 1965, *18*, 441-450.

Barnet, A. B., & Lodge, A. Click evoked EEG responses in normal and developmentally retarded infants. *Nature*, 1967, *214*, 252-255.

Barnet, A. B., Manson, J. I., & Wilner, E. Acute cerebral blindness in childhood. *Neurology*, 1970, *20*, 1147-1156.

Barnet, A. B., & Ohlrich, E. S. Evoked response decrement during auditory stimulation in normal and mongoloid infants. *Electroenceph. Clin. Neurophysiol.* 1971, *31*, 290-291.

Barnet, A. B., Ohlrich, E. S., Weiss, I. P., & Shanks, B. L. Auditory evoked potentials during sleep in normal children from ten days to three years of age. *Electroenceph. Clin. Neurophysiol.*, 1975, *39*, 29-41.

Barnet, A. B., Weiss, I. P., Sotillo, M. V., Ohlrich, E. S., Shkurovich, M. Z., & Cravioto, J. Abnormal auditory evoked potentials in early infancy malnutrition. *Science*, 1978, *201*, 450-452.

Barret, G., Blumhardt, L. D., Halliday, A. M., Halliday, E., & Kriss, A. A paradox in the lateralisation of the visual evoked response. *Nature* (London), 1976, *261*, 253-255.

Barret, G., Halliday, A. M., & Halliday, E. Asymmetries of the late components of the somatosensory evoked potential and P300 associated with handedness and side of stimulus delivery in a signal detection task. *Electroenceph. Clin. Neurophysiol.*, 1977, *43*, 538.

Baust, W., & Jörg, J. A neurophysiological method for the localization of transverse lesions of the spinal cord, using cortical evoked potentials. *Electroenceph. Clin. Neurophysiol.*, 1974, *36*, 441.

Baust, W., & Jörg, J. Clinical value of somatosensory cortical evoked potentials for the localization and diagnosis of spinal transverse regions. *Electroenceph. Clin. Neurophysiol.*, 1977, *43*, 513.

Bechtereva, N. P. *Biopotentiale der Grosshirnhemispheren bei supratentoriellen Tumoren.* Moscow: Medlis, 1960.

Beck, E. C., Doty, R. W., & Kodi, K. A. Electrocortical reactions associated with conditioned flexion reflexes. *Electroenceph. Clin. Neurophysiol.*, 1958, *10*, 279-289.

Becker, W., Hoehne, O., Iwase, K., & Kornhuber, H. H. Bereitschaftspotential, pramotorische Positievierung und andere Hirnpotentiale bei sakkadischen Augenwegungen. *Vision Res.*, 1972, *12*, 421-436.

Bergamasco, B. Excitability cycle of the visual cortex in normal subjects during psychosensory rest and cardiazolic activation. *Brain Res.*, 1966, *2*, 51-60.

Bergamasco, B., Benna, P., Covacich, A., & Gilli, M. Correlations between contingent negative variation and intellectual deficit: A study of adult subjects. *Electroenceph. Clin. Neurophysiol.*, 1977, *42*, 424.

Bergamasco, B., Bergamini, L., Mombelli, A. M., & Mutani, R. Longitudinal study of visual evoked potentials in subjects in post-traumatic coma. *Schweiz. Arch. Neurol. Neurochirurg. Psychiat.*, 1966, *97*, 1-10.

Bergamini, L., & Bergamasco, B. *Cortical evoked potentials in man*. Springfield: Charles C. Thomas, 1967. (a)

Bergamini, L., & Bergamasco, B. Possibility of the clinical use of sensory evoked potentials transcranially recorded in man. *Electroenceph. Clin. Neurophysiol.*, 1967, Suppl. *26*, 114-122. (b)

Bergamini, L., Bergamasco, B., Fra, L., Gandiglio, G., Mombelli, A. M., & Mutani, R. Somatosensory evoked cortical potentials in subjects with peripheral nervous lesions. *Electromyography*, 1965, *5*, 121-130.

Bergamini, L., Bergamasco, B., Fra, L., Gandiglio, G., Mombelli, A. M., & Mutani, R. Reponses corticales et peripheriques évoquées par stimulation du nerf dans la pathologie des cordons posterieurs. *Rev. Neurol.* (Paris), 1966, *155*, 99-112. (a)

Bergamini, L., Bergamasco, B., Mombelli, A. M., & Mutani, R. Autocorrelation analysis of EEG in coma. *Schweiz. Arch. Neurol. Psychiat.*, 1966, *97*, 11-20. (b)

Bickford, R. G. Automatic electroencephalographic control of general anesthesia. *Electroenceph. Clin. Neurophysiol.*, 1950, *2*, 93-96.

Bickford, R. G. An automatic recognition for spike-and-wave with simultaneous testing of motor response. *Electroenceph. Clin. Neurophysiol.*, 1959, *11*, 397-398.

Bickford, R. G. Computer analysis of background activity. In A. Rémond (Ed.), *EEG informatics. A didactic review of methods and applications of EEG data processing.* Amsterdam: Elsevier, 1977, 215-232.

Bickford, R. G., Brimm, J. E. Berger, L., & Aung, M. Application of compressed spectral array in clinical EEG. In P. Kellaway & I. Petersén (Eds.), *Automation of clinical electroencephalography.* New York: Raven Press, 1973, 55-64.

Bickford, R. G., Jacobson, J. L., & Cody, D. T. Nature of average evoked potentials to sound and other stimuli in man. *Ann. N.Y. Acad. Sci.*, 1964, *112*, 204-223.

Bigum, H. B., Dustman, R. E., & Beck, E. C. Visual and somatosensory evoked responses from mongoloid and normal children. *Electroenceph. Clin. Neurophysiol.*, 1970, *28*, 576-585.

Binnie, C. D., Batchelor, B. G., Bowring, P. A., Darby, C. E., Herbert, L., Lloyd, D. S. L., Smith, D. N., Smith, G. F., & Smith, M. A. Computer-assisted interpretation of clinical EEGs. *Electrenceph. Clin. Neurophysiol.*, 1978, *44*, 575-585.

Birchfield, R. I., Wilson, W. P., & Heyman, A. An evaluation of electroencephalography in cerebral infarction and ischemia due to arterioesclerosis. *Neurology* (Minn.), 1959, *9*, 859-870.

Birkemeier, W. P., Fontaine, A. B., Celesia, G. G., & Ma, K. M. Pattern recognition techniques for the detection of epileptic transients in EEG. *IEEE Transactions on Bio. Eng.*, 1978, *BME-25*, 213-217.

Blackman, R. B., & Tukey, J. W. *The measurement of power spectra from the point of view of communication engineering.* New York: Dover, 1958.

Blom, J. L., Barth, P. G., & Visier, S. L. Development of the visual evoked responses in children from 0 to 6 years. *Electroenceph. Clin. Neurophysiol.*, 1976, *41*, 435.

Blume, W. T., & Vera, S. A new computerized spike recognition programme: Its use at electrocorticography. *Electroenceph. Clin. Neurophysiol.*, 1977, *43*, 474.

Blumhardt, L. D., Barret, G., Halliday, A. M., & Kriss, A. The effect of experimental "scotomata" on the ipsilateral and contralateral responses to pattern reversal in one half field. *Electroenceph. Clin. Neurophysiol.*, 1978, *45*, 376-392.

Bodenstein, G., & Praetorius, H. M. Feature extraction from the electroencephalogram by adaptive segmentation. *Proc. of the IEEE*, 1977, *65*, 642-652.

Bodis-Wollner, I. Recovery from cerebral blindness: Evoked potential and psychophysical measurements. *Electroenceph. Clin. Neurophysiol.*, 1977, *42*, 178-184.

Bodis-Wollner, I., Atkin, A., Raab, E., & Wolkstein, M. Visual association cortex and vision in man: Pattern-evoked occipital potentials in a blind boy. *Science*, 1977, *198*, 629-631.

Bodis-Wollner, I., & Yahr, M. D. Latency of the pattern evoked potential in Parkinson's disease. Paper presented at the 11th World Congress of Neurology, Amsterdam, 1977.

Bohlin, T. Analysis of EEG signals with changing spectra using a short word Kalman estimator. *Mathematical Biosciences*, 1977, *35*, 221-259.

Böhm, M., & Droppa, J. Changes in visual cerebral evoked responses in man after brain strokes. *Electroenceph. Clin. Neurophysiol.*, 1969, *26*, 232.

Borda, R. P., & Frost, J. D. Error reduction in small sample averaging through use of the median rather than the mean. *Electroenceph. Clin. Neurophysiol.*, 1968, *25*, 391-392.

Bosaeus, E., Matousek, M., & Petersén, I. Correlation between paedopsychiatric findings and EEG variables in well functioning children of ages 5 to 16 years. *Scand. J. Psychol.*, 1977, *18*, 140-147.

Bostem, F. Postprocessing techniques. In A. Rémond (Ed.), *EEG informatics. A didactic review of methods and applications of EEG data processsing.* Amsterdam: Elsevier, 1977, 171-192.

Bostem, F., Rousseau, J. C., Degossely, M., & Dongier, M. Psychopathological correlations of the non-specific portion of visual and auditory evoked potentials and the associated contingent negative variation. *Electroenceph. Clin. Neurophysiol.*, 1967, Suppl. *26*, 131-138.

Box, G. E. P., & Jenkins, G. M. Time series analysis, forecasting and control. San Francisco: Holden-Day, 1970.

Branston, M. N., & Symon, L. Depression of the cortical evoked potential with reduction of local blood flow in baboons. *Journal of Physiology*, 1974, *24*, 98-99.

Brazier, M. A. B., & Barlow, J. S. Some applications of correlation analysis to clinical problems in electroencephalography. *Electroenceph. Clin. Neurophysiol.*, 1956, *8*, 325-331.

Brazier, M. A. B., & Casby, J. U. An application of the MIT digital electronic correlator to a problem in EEG: The EEG during mental calculation. *Electroenceph. Clin. Neurophysiol.*, 1951, *3*, 375.

Brezny, I. Visual evoked responses in myoclonic epilepsy. *Electroenceph. Clin. Neurophysiol.*, 1974, *36*, 78.

Brezny, I., & Gaziová, M. Late high voltage EEG responses to slowly repeated flashes. *Electroenceph. Clin. Neurophysiol.*, 1964, *16*, 383-387.

Bricolo, A., Turazzi, S., Faccioli, F., Odorizzi, F., Sciarretta, G., & Erculiani, P. Clinical application of compressed spectral array in long term EEG monitoring of comatose patients. *Electroenceph. Clin. Neurophysiol.*, 1978, *45*, 211-225.

Brillinger, D. R. *Time series, data analysis and theory.* New York: Holt, Rinehart and Winston, 1975.

Brinkman, R., & Ebner, A. Clinical value of the brain stem evoked response in coma. *Electroenceph. Clin. Neurophysiol.*, 1977, *43*, 525.

Brix, R. Grundlagen und klinische Anwendung der "Contingent Negative Variation" im Rahmen der "Evoked Response Audiometry." *Wiener Klinische Wochenschrift.*, 1975, *87* ,28-33.

Broughton, R. In E. Donchin & D. B. Lindsley (Eds.), *Averaged evoked potentials.* Washington, DC: NASA, 1969, 79-84.

Broughton, R. Acquisition of bioelectrical data: Collection and amplification. In *Handbook of electroencephalography and clincial neurophysiology.* (Vol. 3A). Amsterdam: Elsevier, 1976.

Broughton, R., Healey, T., Maru, J., Green, D. M., & Pagurek, B. A phase locked loop device for automatic detection of sleep spindles and stage 2. *Electroenceph. Clin. Neurophysiol.*, 1978, *44*, 677-680.

Broughton, R., Meier-Ewert, K. H., & Ebe, M. Visual and somatosensory evoked potentials of photosensitive epileptic subjects during wakefulness, sleep and following i.v. diazepam (Valium). *Electroenceph. Clin. Neurophysiol.*, 1966, *21*, 622.

Broughton, R, Meier-Ewert, K. H., & Ebe, M. Evoked visual, somatosensory, miogenic, oculogenic and electroretinographic potentials of photosensitive epileptic patients and normal control subjects. *Electroenceph. Clin. Neurophysiol.*, 1967, *23*, 492.

Broughton, R., Meier-Ewert, K. H., & Ebe, M. Evoked visual, somatosensory and retinal potentials in photosensitive epilepsy. *Elecroenceph. Clin. Neurophysiol.*, 1969, *27*, 373-386.

Brown, W. S., & Lehmann, D. Different lateralization for noun and verb evoked EEG scalp potential fields. *Electroenceph. Clin. Neurophysiol.*, 1977, *43*, 469.

Brown, W. S., Marsh, J. T., & Smith, J. C. Evoked potential waveform differences produced by the perception of different meanings of an ambiguous phrase. *Electroenceph. Clin. Neurophysiol.*, 1976, *41*, 113-123.

Buchsbaum, M. S. Average evoked response and stimulus intensity in identical and fraternal twins. *Physiological Psychology*, 1974, *2*, 365-370.

Buchsbaum, M. S., Henkin, R. I., & Christiansen, R. L. Age and sex differences in averaged evoked responses in a normal population, with observation on patients with gonadal dysgenesis. *Electroenceph. Clin. Neurophysiol.*, 1974, *37*, 137-144.

Buchsbaum, M. S., Van Kammen, D. P., & Murphy, D. L. Individual differences in average evoked responses to d- and l-amphetamine with and without lithium carbonate in depressed patients. *Psychopharmacology*, 1977, *51*, 129-135.

Buchwald, J. S., & Huang, C. M. Far-field acoustic response: Origins in the cat. *Science*, 1975, *189*, 382-384.

Burch, N. R. Period analysis of the EEG on a general purpose digital computer. *Ann. N.Y. Acad. Sci.*, 1964, *115*, 827-843.

Burch, N. R., Greiner, T., & Correl, E. Automatic analysis of EEG as an index of minimal changes in human consciousness. *Fed. Proc.*, 1955, *14*, 23.

Bures, J., Petrán, M., & Zachar, J. *Electrophysiological methods in biological research.* Prague: Academia Publishing House of the Czechoslovak Academy of Sciences, 1967.

Bynke, H., Olsson, J. E., & Rosén, I. Diagnostic value of visual evoked response, clinical eye examination and CFS analysis in chronic myelopathy. *Acta Neurol. Scand.*, 1977, *56*, 55-69.

Caccia, M. R., Ubialli, E., & Andreussi, L. Spinal evoked responses recorded from the epidural space in normal and diseased humans. *J. Neurol. Neurosurg. Psychiat.*, 1976, *39*, 962-972.

Callaway, E. Average Evoked Responses in Psychiatry. *J. Nerv. Ment. Dis.*, 1966, *143*, 80-94.

Callaway, E., & Harris, P. R. Coupling between cortical potentials from different areas. *Science*, 1974, *183*, 873-875.

Callaway, E., Jones, R. T., & Donchin, E. Auditory evoked potential variability in schizophrenia. *Electroenceph. Clin. Neurophysiol.*, 1970, *29*, 421-428.

Callaway, E., Tueting, P., & Koslow, S. H. (Eds.). *Event-related brain potentials in man.* New York: Academic Press, 1978.

Callaway, E., & Layne, R. S. Interaction between the visual evoked response and two spontaneous biological rhythms: The EEG alpha cycle and the cardiac arousal cycle. *Ann. N.Y. Acad. Sci.*, 1964, *112*, 421-431.

Calmes, R. L., & Cracco, R. Q. Comparison of somatosensory and somatomotor evoked responses to median nerve and digital nerve stimulation. *Electroenceph. Clin. Neurophysiol.*, 1971, *31*, 547-562.

Campbell, F. W., Atkinson, J., Francis, M. R., & Green, D. M. Estimation of auditory thresholds using evoked potentials. A clinical screening test. In J. E. Desmedt (Ed.), *Progress in clinical neurophysiology* (Vol. 2). Basel: Karger, 1977, 68-78.

Campbell, J., Bower, E., Dwyer, S. M., & Lodo, G. V. On the sufficiency of autocorrelation functions as EEG descriptors. *IEEE Trans. Biomed. Eng. BME*, 1967, *14*, 49-52.

Canali, G., & Carpitella, A. Rilievi statistici sul ritmo "en arceau." *Sist. nerv.*, 1956, *8*, 8-12.

Cant, B. R., Gronwell, D., & Burges, R. Auditory evoked responses after closed head injuries. *Electroenceph. Clin. Neurophysiol.*, 1974, *36*, 551-553.

Cantor, F. K., Young, R. R., & Wolpow, E. R. Enhanced ipsilateral photic responses in patients with unilateral cerebral pathology. *Electroenceph. Clin. Neurophysiol.*, 1974, *37*, 202.

Carmon, A., Lavy, S., & Schwartz, A. Correlation between electroencephalography and angiography in cerebrovascular accidents. *Electroenceph. Clin. Neurophysiol.*, 1966, *21*, 71-76.

Carmon, A., Mor, J., & Goldberg, J. Evoked cerebral responses to noxious thermal stimuli in humans. *Exp. Brain. Res.*, 1976, *25*, 103-107.

Carrie, J. R. G. The detection and quantification of transient and paroxysmal EEG abnormalities. In P. Kellaway & I. Petersen (Eds.), *Automation of clinical Electroencephalography,* New York: Raven Press, 1973, 217-226.

Carrie, J. R. G. Computer-assisted EEG sharp transient detection and quantification during overnight recordings in an epileptic patient. In P. Kellaway & I. Petersén (Eds.), *Quantitative analytic studies in epilepsy.* New York: Raven Press, 1976, 225-235.

Celesia, G. G. Visual evoked potentials in neurological disorders. *Am. J. EEG Technol.*, 1978, *18*, 47-59.

Celesia, G. G., & Chen, R. C. Parameters of spikes in human epilepsy. *Diseases of the Nervous System*, May, 1976, 277-281.

Celesia, G. G., & Daly, R. F. Effects of aging on visual evoked responses. *Arch. Neurol.*, 1977, *44*, 403-407. (a)

Celesia, G. G., & Daly, R. F. Visual electroencephalographic computer analysis (VECA): A new electrophysiological test for the diagnosis of optic nerve lesions. *Neurology* (Minn.), 1977, *27*, 637-641. (b)

Chatrian, G. E. Characteristics of unusual EEG patterns: Incidence, significance. *Electroenceph. Clin. Neurophysiol.*, 1964, *17*, 471-472.

Chatrian, G. E. The kappa rhythm. In *Handbook of electroencephalography and clinical neurophysiology* (Vol. 6A). Amsterdam: Elsevier, 1976.(a), 104-113.

Chatrian, G. E. Paroxysmal patterns in "normal" subjects. In *Handbook of electroencephalography and clinical neurophysiology* (Vol. 6A). Amsterdam: Elsevier, 1976. (b), 114-122.

Chatrian, G. E., Bergamini, L., Dandey, M., Klass, D. W., Lennox-Buchtal, M., & Petersén, I. A glossary of terms most commonly used by clinical electroencephalographers. Report of Committee on Terminology, IFSECN. *Electroenceph. Clin. Neurophysiol.*, 1974, *37*, 538-548.

Chatrian, G. E., Canfield, R. C., Knauss, T. A., & Lettich, E. Cerebral responses to electrical tooth pulp stimulation in man. *Neurology* (Minn.), 1975, *25*, 745-757.

Chatrian, G. E., & Lairy, G. C. (Eds.). The EEG of the waking adult. In *Handbook of electroencephalography and clinical neurophysiology* (Vol. 6A). Amsterdam: Elsevier, 1976.

Chatrian, G. E., Petersén, I., & Lazarte, J. A. The blocking of the rolandic wicket rhythm and some central changes related to movement. *Electroenceph. Clin. Neurophysiol.*, 1959, *11*, 497-510.

Chatrian, M. G. Etude électroencephalographique et electrocorticographique du rythme theta local dans les epilepsies temporales. *Rev. Neurol.*, 1953, *88*, 384-386.

Chiappa, K. H., Brimm, J. E., Allen, B. A., Leibig, B. E., Rossiter, V. S., Stockard, J. J., Burchiel, K. S., & Bickford, R. G. Computing in EEG and epilepsy. Evolution of a comprehensive EEG analysis and reporting system. In P. Kellaway & I. Petersén (Eds.), *Quantitative analytic studies in epilepsy*. New York: Raven Press, 1976, 329-342.

Chiappa, K. H., & Norwood, A. E. Brainstem auditory evoked responses in clinical neurology: Utility and neuropathological correlates. *Electroenceph. Clin. Neurophysiol.*, 1977, *43*, 518.

Chiappa, K. H., & Young, R. R. Carotid endarterectomy monitoring with a dedicated minicomputer. *Electroenceph. Clin. Neurophysiol.*, 1977, *43*, 518.

Chik, L., Sokol, R. J., & Rosen, M. G. Computer interpreted fetal electroencephalogram: Sharp wave detection and classification of infants for one year neurological outcome. *Electroenceph. Clin. Neurophysiol.*, 1977, *42*, 745-753.

Childers, D. G. Automated visual evoked response system. *Med. Biol. Eng. and Comput.*, 1977, *15*, 374-380.

Chiofalo, N., Fuentes, A., Rodriguez, R., Villavicencio, C., & Méndez, J. Etude statistique des correlations électroencephalographiques avec les données cliniques et anatomiques. A propos de 100 abces cérebraux. *Rev. EEG. Neurophysiol.*, 1976, *6*, 527-531.

Cigánek, L. The EEG response (evoked potential) to light stimulus in man. *Electroenceph. Clin. Neurophysiol.*, 1961, *13*, 165-172.

Cigánek, L. Excitability cycle of the visual cortex in man. *Ann. N.Y. Acad. Sci.*, 1964, *112*, 241-253.

Cigánek, L. Variability of the human visual evoked potential: Normative data. *Electroenceph. Clin. Neurophysiol.*, 1969, *27*, 35-42.

Cigánek, L. Visual evoked responses. In *Handbook of electroencephalography and clinical neurophysiology* (Vol. 8A). Amsterdam: Elsevier, 1975, 33-41.

Cigánek, L. Visual evoked potentials and the mechanisms of the generalized (centrencephalic) epileptic discharges. *Electroenceph. Clin. Neurophysiol.*, 1977, *43*, 466.

Cigánek, L., & Ingvar, D. H. Colour specific features of visual cortical responses in man evoked by monochromatic flashes. *Acta physiol. Scand.*, 1969, *76*, 82-92.

Cinca, I., Apostol, V., Pestroiu, D., Serbanescu, A., & Florescu, D. Automatic analysis of the EEG. A pattern recognition method. *Electroenceph. Clin. Neurophysiol.*, 1977, *43*, 551. (a)

Cinca, I., Florescu, D., Pestroiu, D., Serbanescu, A., & Apostol, V. Combined pattern recognition and time and frequency domain analysis in petit mal epilepsy. *Electroenceph. Clin. Neurophysiol.*, 1977, *43*, 551. (b)

Ciurea, E., & Crighel, E. The evoked bio-electric activity in cerebral circulatory insufficiency. Comparative research in patients with arteriosclerosis. *Revue Roumanie de Neurologie*, 1967, *4*, 129-137.

Clynes, M. In E. Donchin & D. B. Lindsley (Eds.), *Averaged evoked potentials*. Washington D.C., NASA, 1969, 86-91.

Coats, A. C., & Martin, J. L. Human auditory nerve action potentials and brain stem responses. *Archives of Otolaryngology*, 1977, *103*, 605-622.

Cobb, W. A. The normal adult EEG. In D. Hill & G. Parr (Eds.), *Electroencephalography*. London: MacDonald, 1963, 232–249. (a)

Cobb, W. A. The EEG of specific lesions. In D. Hill & G. Parr (Eds.), *electroencephalography*. London: MacDonald, 1963, 317–367. (b)

Cobb, W. A., & Dawson, G. D. The latency and form in man of the occipital potentials evoked by light flashes. *J. Physiol.*, 1960, *152*, 108-121.

Cobb, W. A., & Morocutti, C. (Eds.). The evoked potentials. *Electroenceph. Clin. Neurophysiol.*, 1967, Suppl. 26.

Cobb, W. A., & Morton, H. B. Harmonics in visual evoked responses. *Electroenceph. Clin. Neurophysiol.*, 1969, *26*, 538.

Coben, L. A. The effect of aging and of dimming the stimulus upon the visual evoked response to reversing checks in man. *Electroenceph. Clin. Neurophysiol.* 1977, *43*, 559.

Coger, R. W., Dymond, A. M., & Serafetinides, E. A. Classification of psychiatric patients with factor analytic EEG variables. *Proc. San Diego Biomedical Symposium*, 1976, *15*, 279-284.

Cohen, A. B. Stationarity of the human electroencephalogram. *Med. and Biol. Eng. and Comput.*, 1977, *15*, 513-518.

Cohen, A. B., Bravo-Fernández, E. J., & Sances, A. Quantification of computer analyzed serial EEGs from stroke patients. *Electroenceph. Clin. Neurophysiol.* 1976, *41*, 379-386.

Cohen, J. Very slow brain potentials relating to expectancy: The CNV. In E. Donchin & D. B. Lindsley (Eds.), *Averaged Evoked Responses.* Washington, D.C.: NASA, 1969, 143-163.

Cohen, J. The CNV in cases of hemispheric vascular lesions. *Electroenceph. Clin. Neurophysiol.*, 1975, *38*, 542.

Cohen, J., & Walter, W. G. The interaction of responses in the brain to semantic stimuli. *Psychophysiology*, 1966, *2*, 187-196.

Cohen, S. I., Silverman, A. J., & Shmavonian, B. M. Psychological studies in altered sensory environments. *J. Psychosom. Res.*, 1963, *6*, 259-281.

Cohn, R. Evoked visual cortical responses in homonymous hemianopic defects in man. *Electroenceph. Clin. Neurophysiol.*, 1963, *15*, 992.

Cohn, R. *Clinical electroencephalography*. New York: McGraw-Hill, 1949.

Cohn, R. Rhythmic after-activity in visual evoked responses. *Ann. N.Y. Acad. Sci.*, 1964, *112*, 281-291.

Cohn, R. Visual evoked responses in the brain injured monkey. *Arch. Neurol.*, 1969, *21*, 321-329.

Colon, E. J., Veer N . van der & de Weerd, J. P. C. A clinical study of the effect of different provocation tests on the power density spectra of the EEG. *Electroenceph. Clin. Neurophysiol.*, 1977, *43*, 502.

Conners, C., K. Cortical visual evoked responses in children with learning disorders. *Psychophysiology*, 1971, *7*, 418-428.

Cooley, J. W., & Tukey, J. W. An algorithm for the machine calculation of complex Fourier series. *Mathematics of Computation*, 1965, *19*, 297-301.

Cooper, R. Direct computer processing. In *Handbook of electroencephalography and clinical neurophysiology* (Vol. 4B). Amsterdam, Elsevier, 1972, 15-18.

Cooper, R., Scarratt, D., Tallis, R., & Van't Hoff, W. Some neurophysiological and psychometric measurements in mixoedema. *Electroenceph. Clin. Neurophysiol.*, 1977, *43*, 464.

Cooper, R., Winter, A. L., & Walter, W. G. Comparison of subcortical and scalp activity using chronically indwelling electrodes in man. *Electroenceph. Clin. Neurophysiol.*, 1965, *18*, 217-228.

Copenhaver, R. M., & Perry, N. M. Factors affecting visually evoked cortical potentials such as impaired vision of varying etiology. *Invest. Ophthal.*, 1964, *3*, 665-675.

Corletto, F., Gentilomo, A., Rosadini, G., Rossig, F., & Zattoni, J. Visual evoked potentials as recorded from the scalp and from the visual cortex before and after surgical removement of the occipital pole in man. *Electroenceph. Clin. Neurophysiol.*, 1967, *22*, 378-380.

Cracco, R. Q. Spinal evoked response: Peripheral nerve stimulation in man. *Electroenceph. Clin. Neurophysiol.*, 1973, *35*, 379-386.

Cracco, R. Q., & Cracco, J. B. Somatosensory evoked potential in man: Far field potentials. *Electroenceph. Clin. Neurophysiol.*, 1976, *41*, 460-466.

Creutzfeldt, O. D. The neuronal generation of the EEG. In *Handbook of electroencephalography and clinical neurophysiology* (Vol. 2C). Amsterdam: Elsevier, 1974.

Creutzfeldt, O. D., Kugler, J., Morocutti, C., & Sommer-Smith, J. A. Visual evoked potentials in normal human subjects and neurological patients. *Electroenceph. Clin. Neurophysiol.*, 1966, *20*, 98-106.

Creutzfeldt, O. D., & Kuhnt, U. The visual evoked potential: Physiological, developmental and clinical aspects. *Electroenceph. Clin. Neurophysiol.*, 1967, Suppl. *26*, 29-41.

Creutzfeldt, O. D., Watanabe, S., & Lux, H. D. Relations between EEG phenomena and potentials of single cortical cells. I:Evoked responses after thalamic and epicortical stimulation. *Electroenceph. Clin. Neurophysiol.*, 1966, *20*, 1-18.

Crevoisier, A. de, Peronnet, F., Girod, J., Challet, E., & Reval, M. Topography of auditory evoked potentials in children. *Electroenceph. Clin. Neurophysiol.*, 1976, *40*, 551.

Crighel, E., & Botez, M. I. Photic evoked potentials in man in lesions of the occipital lobes. *Brain*, 1966, *89*, 311-316.

Crighel, E., & Poilici, I. Photic evoked responses in patients with thalamic and brain stem lesions. *Confin. Neurol.*, 1968, *30*, 301-312.

Crighel, E., Sterman, C., & Marinchescu, C. Flash evoked responses in acute cerebrovascular diseases. The correlation with the clinical, electroencephalographic and rheoencephalographic course. *Revue Roumaine de Neurologie*, 1971, *8*, 275-284.

Crowell, D. H., Jones, R. H., Kapuniai, L. E., & Leung, P. Autoregressive representation of infant EEG for the purpose of hypothesis testing and classification. *Electroenceph. Clin. Neurophysiol.*, 1977, *43*, 317-324.

Czopf, J., Hegedüs, K., Kiss-Antal, M. Kellényi, L., & Karmos, G. Statistical analysis of EEG and clinical data in multiple sclerosis. Significance of the visual evoked response in the diagnosis of MS. *Electroenceph. Clin. Neurophysiol.*, 1976, *41*, 210.

Daly, D. M., Roeser, R. J., Aung, M. H., & Daly, D. D. Early evoked potentials in patients with acoustic neuroma. *Electroenceph. Clin. Neurophysiol.*, 1977, *43*, 151-159.

Daly, D. M., Roeser, R. J., & Moushegian, G. The frequency-following response in subjects with profound unilateral loss. *Electroenceph. Clin. Neurophysiol.*, 1976, *40*, 132-142.

Davis, A. E. Power spectral analysis of flash and click evoked responses. *Electroenceph. Clin. Neurophysiol.*, 1973, *35*, 287-291.

Davis, A. E., & Wada, J. A. Hemispheric asymmetry: Frequency analysis of visual and auditory evoked responses to non-verbal stimuli. *Electroenceph. Clin. Neurophysiol.*, 1974, *37*, 1-9.

Davis, A. E., & Wada, J. A. Hemispheric asymmetries in human infants: Spectral analysis of flash and click evoked potentials. *Brain and Language*, 1977, *4*, 23-31.

Davis, H. Principles of electric response audiometry. *Am. Otol. Rhinol. Lar.*, 1976, 85, Suppl. *28*.

Davis, H., Davis, P. A., Loomis, A. L., Harvey, N., & Hobart, G. A. Electrical reactions of the brain to auditory stimulation during sleep. *J. Neurophysiol.*, 1939, *2*, 500-514.

Davis, H., & Hirsh, S. K. Brain stem electric response audiometry (BSERA). *Acta Otolaryngol.*, 1977, *83*, 136-139.

Davis, H., Hirsh, S. K., Shelnutt, J., & Bowers, C. Further validation of evoked response audiometry (ERA). *Journal of Speech and Hearing Research*, 1967, *10*, 717-732.

Davis, H., & Onishi, S. Maturation of the auditory evoked potentials. Int. Aud., 1969, *8*: 24-33.

Davis, H., & Zerlin, S. Acoustic relations of the human vertex potential. *J. Acoust. Soc. Am.*, 1966, *39*, 109-116.

Dawson, G. D. Cerebral responses to electrical stimulation of peripheral nerve in man. *J. Neurol. Neurosurg. Psychiat., 1947, 10*, 134-140. (a)

Dawson, G. D. Investigations on a patient subject to myoclonic seizures. *J. Neurol. Neurosurg. Psychiat.*, 1947, *10*, 141-162. (b)

Dawson, G. D. The relative excitability and conduction velocity of sensory and motor nerve fibres in man. *J. Physiol.* (London), 1956, *131*, 436-451.

Debecker, J., & Carmeliet, J. Automatic supression of eye movements and muscle artifacts when averaging tape recorded cerebral evoked potentials. *Electroenceph. Clin. Neurophysiol.*, 1974, *37*, 513-515.

Debecker, J., & Desmedt, J. E. Les potentiels évoqués cerebraux et les potentiels de nerf sensible chez l'homme. *Acta Neurologica et Psychiatrica Belgica*, 1964, *64*, 1212-1248.

Deecke, L. Scheid, P., & Kornhuber, H. H. Distribution of readiness potential, premotion positivity and motor potential of the human cerebral cortex preceding voluntary finger movements. *Exp. Brain. Res.*, 1968, *7*, 158-168.

Defayolle, M., & Dinand, J. P. Application de l'analyse factorielle a l'étude de la structure de l'EEG. *Electroenceph. Clin. Neurophysiol.*, 1974, *36*, 319-322.

Delavnoy, J., Gerono, A., & Rousseau, J. C. Behavioral correlates of the motor potential. *Electroenceph. Clin. Neurophysiol.*, 1977, *43*, 510.

Delbeke, J., McComas, A. J., & Kopec, S. J. Analysis of evoked lumbosacral potentials in man. *J. Neurol. Neurosurg. Psychiat.*, 1978, *41*, 293-302.

DeMarco, P., & Tassinari, C. A. Extreme somatosensory evoked potentials (ESEP): An EEG sign forecasting the possible occurrence of seizures in children. *Electroenceph. Clin. Neurophysiol.*, 1977, *43*, 560.

Demetrescu, M. A new method for analysis of cerebral biopotentials. *Fisiol. Norm. Si Pat.*, 1957, *4*, 564-569.

Denoth, F. Some general remarks on Hjorth's parameters used in EEG analysis. In G. Dolce & H. Künkel (Eds.), *CEAN*, Stuttgart: Gustav Fischer Verlag, 1975, 9-18.

Desmedt, J. E. Somatosensory cerebral evoked potentials in man. In *Handbook of Electroencephalography and clinical neurophysiology* (Vol. 9). Amsterdam: Elsevier, 1971, 55-82.

Desmedt, J. E. (Ed.). Attention, voluntary contraction and event-related potentials. *Progress in clinical neurophysiology* (Vol. 1). Basel: Karger, 1977. (a)

Desmedt, J. E. (Ed.). Auditory evoked potentials in man. Psychopharmacology correlates of evoked potentials. *Progress in clinical neurophysiology* (Vol. 2). Basel: Karger, 1977. (b)

Desmedt, J. E., Brunko, E., & Debecker, J. Maturation of the somatosensory evoked potentials in normal infants and children, with special reference to the early N_1 component. *Electroenceph. Clin. Neurophysiol.*, 1976, *40*, 43-58.

Desmedt, J. E., Franken, L., Borenstein, S., Debecker, J., Lambert, C., & Manil, J. Le diagnostic des ralentissements de la conduction afferente dans les affections des nerfs peripheriques: Interet de l'extraction du potential évoqué cérébral. *Rev. Neurol.*, 1966, *115*, 255-262.

De Weerd, J. P. C., Martens, W. L. J., & Colon, E. J. Estimation of evoked potentials using time varying Wiener filtering. *Electroenceph. Clin. Neurophysiol.*, 1977, *43*, 476.

Diamond, A. L. Latency of the steady state visual evoked potential. *Electroenceph. Clin. Neurophysiol.*, 1977, *42*, 125-127.

Dietsch. G. Fourier-analyse von Elektroenzephalogrammen des Menschen. *Pflügers Arch. Ges.* Physiol., 1932, *230*, 106–112.

Dimitrijevic, M. R., Larssen, L. E., Lehmkuhl, D., & Sherwood, A. Evoked spinal cord and nerve root potentials in humans using a non-invasive recording technique. *Electroenceph. Clin. Neurophysiol.*, 1978, *45*, 331–340.

Dimov, S., Brefeith, J. L., Menini, C., & Naquet, R. A study of visual evoked potentials in twins with photosensitive epilepsy. *Electroenceph. Clin. Neurophysiol.*, 1974, *36*, 81–86.

Dinges, D., & Tepas, D. I. Luminance effects on visual evoked brain responses to flash onset and offset. *Bulletin of the Psychonom. Society.*, 1976, *8*, 105-108.

Dixon, W. F. *BMD computer programs.* Los Angeles: University of California, 1968.

Dobronravova, I. S., Grindel, O. M., & Bragina, N. N. Significance of EEG rhythms for the evaluation of the functional state of human brain in coma. *Electroenceph. Clin. Neurophysiol.*, 1977, *43*, 483.

Dobson, V. Spectral sensitivity of the 2 month infant as measured by the visually evoked cortical potential. *Vision Res.*, 1976, *16*, 367-374.

Dolce, G., & Künkel, H. (Eds.). *CEAN. Computerizea EEG analysis.* Stuttgart: Gustav Fischer Verlag, 1975.

Domino, E. F., Matsuoka, S., Waltz, J., & Cooper, I. S. Effects of cryogenic thalamic lesions on the somesthetic evoked response in man. *Electroenceph. Clin. Neurophysiol.*, 1965, *19*, 127-138.

Don, M., Allen, A. R., & Starr, A. Effect of click rate on the latency of auditory brain stem responses in humans. *The Annals of Otology, Rhinology and Laryngology*, 1977, *86*, 186-193.

Donchin, E. A multivariate approach to the analysis of the average evoked potentials. *IEEE Trans. Biomed. Eng.*, 1966, *BME-13*, 131-139.

Donchin, E. Data analysis techniques in average evoked potential research. In E. Donchin & D. B. Lindsley (Eds.), *Average evoked potentials.* Washington, D.C.: NASA, 1969, 199-217.

Donchin, E., Callaway, E., Cooper, R., Desmedt, J. E., Goff, W. R., Hillyard, S. A., & Sutton, S. Publication criteria for studies of evoked potentials. In J. E. Desmedt (Ed.), *Progress in clinical neurophysiology* (Vol. 1). Basel: Karger, 1977, 1-11.

Donchin, E., & Cohen, L. Averaged evoked potentials and intramodality selective attention. *Electroenceph. Clin. Neurophysiol.*, 1967, *22*, 537-546.

Donchin, E., & Lindsley, D. B. (Eds.). *Average evoked potentials*. Washington, D.C.: NASA, 1969.

Donker, D. N. J. Harmonic composition and topographic distribution of responses to sine wave modulated light (SML), their reproducibility and their interhemispheric relationships. *Electroenceph. Clin. Neurophysiol.*, 1975, *39*, 561-574.

Donker, D. N. J., Njio, L., Storm van Leeuwen, W., & Wieneke, G. H. Interhemispheric relationships of responses to sine wave modulated light in normal subjects and patients. *Electroenceph. Clin. Neurophysiol.*, 1978, *44*, 479-489.

Dorfman, L. J. Indirect estimation of spinal cord conduction velocity in man. *Electroenceph. Clin. Neurophysiol.*, 1977, *42*, 26-34.

Dorfman, L. J., Bosley, T. M., & Cummins, K. L. Electrophysiological localization of central somatosensory lesions in patients with multiple sclerosis. *Electroenceph. Clin. Neurophysiol.*, 1978, *44*; 742-753.

Doyle, D. J. Some comments of the use of Wiener filtering for the estimation of evoked potentials. *Electroenceph. Clin. Neurophysiol.*, 1975, *38*, 533-534.

Doyle, D. J. A proposed methodology for evaluation of the Wiener filtering method of evoked potential estimation. *Electroenceph. Clin. Neurophysiol.*, 1977, *43*, 749-751.

Drechsler, F., Wickboldt, J., Neuhanser, B., & Miltner, F. Somatosensory trigeminal evoked potentials in normal subjects and in patients with trigeminal neuralgia before and after thermocoagulation of the ganglion Gasseri. *Électroenceph. Clin. Neurophysiol.*, 1977, *43*, 496.

Dreyfus-Brisac, C. Sleep ontogenesis in early prematurity from 24 to 27 weeks of conceptional age. *Dev. Psychobiol.*, 1968, *1*, 162-169.

Dreyfus-Brisac, C. Ontogenesis of sleep in human prematures after 32 weeks of conceptional age. *Dev. Psychobiol.*, 1970, *3*, 91-121.

Dreyfus-Brisac, C., & Monod, N. Sleep of premature and full-term neonates: A polygraphic study. *Proc. R. Soc. Med.*, 1965, *58*, 67.

Dreyfus-Brisac, C., & Monod, N. Neonatal status epilepticus. In *Handbook of electroencephalography and clinical neurophysiology* (Vol. 15). Amsterdam: Elsevier, 1972, 38-51.

Drohocki, Z. L'intégrateur de l'electroproduction cérébrale pour l'ëlectroencéphalographie quantitative. *Rev. Neurol.*, 1948, *80*, 619.

Drohocki, Z. L'utilisation d'un analyseur statistique d'amplitudes, ASA, en électroencephalographie quantitative. *J. Physiol.* (Paris), 1969, *61*, Suppl. *2*, 275.

Duchowny, M. S., Weiss, I. P., Majlessi, H., & Barnet, A. B. Visual evoked responses in childhood cortical blindness after head trauma and meningitis. *Neurology*, 1974, *24*, 933-940.

Dumermuth, G. Electronic data processing in pediatric EEG research. *Neuropädiatrie*, 1971, *4*, 349-374.

Dumermuth, G. Sampling and data reduction. In *Handbook of electroencephalography and clinical neurophysiology* (Vol. 4A). Amsterdam: Elsevier, 1976, 22-30.

Dumermuth, G., Gasser, T., Hecker, A., Herdan, M., & Lange, B. Exploration of EEG components in the beta frequency range. In P. Kellaway & I. Petersén (Eds.), *Quantitative analytic studies in epilepsy,* New York: Raven Press, 1976, 533-558.

Dumermuth, G., Gasser, T., & Lange, B. Aspects of EEG analysis in the frequency domain. In G. Dolce, & H. Künkel (Eds.). *CEAN,* Stuttgart: Gustav Fischer Verlag, 1975.

Dumermuth, G., Huber, P. J., Kleiner, B., & Gasser, T. Analysis of the interelations between frequency bands of the EEG by means of the bispectrum. A preliminary study. *Electroenceph. Clin. Neurophysiol.*, 1971, *31*, 137-148.

Dumermuth, G., Walz, W., Scollo-Lavizzari, G., & Kleiner, B. Spectral analysis of EEG activity in different sleep stages in normal adults. *Europ. Neurol.*, 1972, *7*, 265-296.

Düsseldorf, J. J. Cortical somatosensoric evoked potentials to localize the focus of symptomatic epilepsy. *Proceedings of the 7th International Symposium on Epilepsy*, Berlin (West), June, 1975.

Dustman, R. E., & Beck, E. C. Long term stability of visually evoked potentials in man. *Science*, 1963, *142*, 1480-1481.

Dustman, R. E., & Beck, E. C. The visually evoked potentials in twins. *Electroenceph. Clin. Neurophysiol.*, 1965, *19*, 570-575. (a)

Dustman, R. E., & Beck, E. C. Phase of alpha brain waves, reaction time and visually evoked potentials. *Electroenceph. Clin. Neurophysiol.*, 1965, *18*, 433-440. (b)

Dustman, R. E., & Beck, E. C. Visually evoked potentials: Amplitude changes with age. *Science*, 1966, *151*, 1013-1015.

Dustman, R. E., & Beck, E. C. The effects of maturation and aging on the waveform of visually evoked potentials. *Electroenceph. Clin. Neurophysiol.*, 1969, *26*, 2-11.

Dustman, R. E., Schenkenberg, T., Lewis, E. G., & Beck, E. C. The cerebral evoked potential: Life span changes and twin studies. In J. E. Desmedt (Ed.), *Visual Evoked Potentials in man.* Oxford: Clarendon Press, 1977, 363-377.

Dutertre, F. Catalogue of the main EEG patterns. In *Handbook of electroencephalography and clinical neurophysiology,* Vol. 11. Amsterdam: Elsevier, 1977, 40-78.

Duwaer, A. L., & Spekreijse, H. Latency of luminance and contrast evoked potentials in multiple sclerosis patients. *Electroenceph. Clin. Neurophysiol.*, 1978, *45*, 244–258.

Eason, R. G., Oden, B. A., & White, C. T. Visually evoked cortical potentials and reaction time in relation to site of retinal stimulation. *Electroenceph. Clin. Neurophysiol.*, 1967, *22*, 313-324.

Eason, R. G., White, C. T., & Bartlett, N. Effects of checkerboard pattern stimulations on evoked cortical responses in relation to check size and visual field. *Psychon. Sci.*, 1970, *2*, 113-115.

Ebe, M., Meier-Ewert, K. H., & Broughton, R. Effects of intravenous diazepam (Valium) upon evoked potentials of photosensitive epileptic and normal subjects. *Electroenceph. Clin. Neurophysiol.*, 1969, *27*, 429-435.

Ebe, M., Mikami, I., & Ito, H. Clinical evaluation of electrical responses of retina and visual cortex in photic stimulation in opthalmic diseases. *Tonoku J. Exp. Med.*, 1964, *84*, 92-103.

Eccles, J. C., Kostyuk, P. G., & Schmidt, R. F. Central pathways responsible for depolarization of primary afferent fibres. *Journal of Physiology*, 1962, *161*, 237-257.

Eeg-Olofsson, O. The development of the electroencephalogram in normal adolescents from the age of 16 through 21 years. *Neuropädiatrie*, 1971, *3*, 11-45.

Eggermont, J. J. Detection of acoustic neurinoma on the basis of brain stem electrical responses. *Electroenceph. Clin. Neurophysiol.*, 1977, *43*, 582.

Ehle, A., & Sklar, F. Alterations of visual evoked responses in patients with hydrocephalus. *Electroenceph. Clin. Neurophysiol.*, 1977, *43*, 504.

Ehrenberg, B. L., & Penry, J. K. Computer recognition of generalized spike-wave discharges. *Electroenceph. Clin. Neurophysiol.*, 1976, *41*, 25-36.

Ellenberg, C., Dennis, J. P., & Ziegler, S. B. The visually evoked potential in Huntington disease. *Neurology*, 1978, *28*, 95-97.

Ellenberg, C., & Ziegler, S. B. Visual evoked potentials and quantitative perimetry in multiple sclerosis. *Ann. Neurol.*, 1977, *1*, 561-564.

Ellingson, R. J. The incidence of EEG abnormality among patients with mental disorders of apparently non-organic origin: A critical review. *Am. J. Psychol.* 1955, *3*, 263-275.

Ellingson, R. J. Variability of visual evoked responses in the human newborn. *Electroenceph. Clin. Neurophysiol.*, 1970, *29*, 10-19.

Ellingson, R. J., Danahy, T., Nelson, B., & Lahtrop, G. H. Variability of auditory evoked potentials in human newborns. *Electroenceph. Clin. Neurophysiol.*, 1974, *36*, 155-162.

Ellingson, R. J., Lahtrop, G. H., Nelson, B., & Danahy, T. Visual evoked potentials in infants: Further observations. *Electroenceph. Clin. Neurophysiol.*, 1974, *36*, 87.

Elmgren, J., & Löwenhard, P. Un análisis factorial del EEG humano. *Rev. de Psicología General y Aplicada* (Madrid), 1973, *28*, 255-271.

Elmquist, D. Automatic EEG analysis according to the method of "normalized slope descriptors." Experience in a clinical routine material. *Electroenceph. Clin. Neurophysiol.*, 1974, *37*, 215.

Elul, R. Gaussian behavior of the electroencephalogram: Changes during performance of mental tasks. *Science*, 1969, *164*, 328-331.

Enslein, K., Ralston, A., & Wilf, H. S. (Eds.) *Statistical methods for digital computers* (Vol. 3). New York: Wiley, 1977.

Ertekin, C. Studies on the human evoked electrospinogram. I: The origin of the segmental evoked potentials. *Acta Neurol. Scand.*, 1976, *53*, 3–20.

Ertekin, C. *Human evoked electrospinogram in patients with diseases of the spinal cord and roots.* Paper presented at the 11th World Congress of Neurology, Amsterdam, 1977.

Ertekin, C. Comparison of the human evoked electrospinogram recorded from the intrathecal, epidural and cutaneous levels. *Electroenceph. Clin. Neurophysiol.*, 1978, *44*, 683-690.

Ertl, J., & Schafer, E. W. Cortical activity preceding speech. *Life Sci.*, 1967, *6*, 473-479.

Estévez, O., & Spekreijse, H. Relationship between pattern appearance-disappearance and pattern-reversal responses. *Exp. Brain. Res.*, 1974, *19*, 233-238.

Etévenon, P., & Pidoux, B. From biparametric to multidimensional analysis of EEG. In A. Rémond (Ed.), *EEG informatics. A didactic review of methods and applications of EEG data processing.* Amsterdam: Elsevier, 1977, 193-214.

Etévenon, P., Rioux, P., Pidoux, B., & Verdeaux, G. Microprogrammed Fast Fourier analysis of EEG. On-line statistical spectral analysis and off-line spike detection. In P. Kellaway & I. Petersén (Eds.), *Quantitative analytic studies in epilepsy.* New York: Raven Press, 1976, 355-374.

Everitt, B. S. *Graphical techniques for multivariate data.* London: Heinemann Educational Books, 1978.

Feinsod, M., & Hoyt, W. F. Subclinical optic neuropathy in multiple sclerosis. *J. Neurol. Neurosurg. Psychiat.*, 1975, *38*, 1109-1114.

Feller, W. An introduction to probability theory and its applications (Vol. 2). Havana: Instituto del Libro, 1965.

Feller, W. An introduction to probability theory and its applications (Vol. 1). Havana: Instituto del Libro, 1967.

Fenton, G. W., Fenwick, P., Dollimore, J., Hirsch, S. R., & Dunn, L. Power spectral analysis of the EEG in schizophrenia. *Electroenceph. Clin. Neurophysiol.*, 1977, *43*, 561.

Fenwick, P. Mathematico-statistical modelling of the EEG. *Electroenceph. Clin. Neurophysiol.*, 1975, *36*, 564-565.

Fenwick, P. Mitchie, P., Dollimore, J., & Fenton, G. W. Mathematical simulation of the electroencephalogram using autoregressive series. *Biomed. Comput.*, 1971, *2*, 281.

Fernández, G., & Harmony, T. Symmetry of visual evoked responses to patterned stimuli. Normative data. *Activitás Nervosa Superior* (Praha), 1977, *19*, 169-172. (a)

Fernández, G., & Harmony, T. Symmetry of auditory evoked responses. Normative data. *Activitás Nervosa Superior* (Praha), 1977, *19*, 172-175. (b)

Fernández, G., & Harmony, T. Efecto del tratamiento anticonvulsivo sobre los potenciales evocados en pacientes epilépticos. *Cenic*, 1978, *9*, 153–161.

Fernández, G., & Harmony, T. *Neurometric assessment in temporal epilepsy*. In J. Majkowski (Ed.), *Epilepsy. A clinical and experimental research*. Warsaw: International League against epilepsy, the Polish Chapter, 1980, 56–62.

Fernández, G., Harmony, T., & Rodríguez, R. L. Evoked responses in epilepsy. In B. Holmgren & T. Harmony (Eds.), *Applications of computers to the study of the nervous system*. Havana: CENIC, 1975.

Fernández, G., Otero, G., Ricardo, J., & Harmony, T. Estudio de los potenciales evocados visuales y de la correlación de la actividad electroencefalográfica entire distintas áreas de pacientes neurológicos. *Cenic*, 1970, *2*, 37-49.

Fernández, G., Pérez, N. L., & Harmony, T. *Visual, auditory and somatosensory evoked responses in multiple sclerosis*. Paper presented at the 11th World Congress of Neurology, Amsterdam, 1977.

Fernández-Bouzas, A., Ballesteros, A., Harmony, T., Mellado, E., & Gallardo, M. *Transcatheter embolization of brain arteriovenous malformations and meningiomas: Anatomofunctional correlation of effects*. Paper presented at the 11th World Congress of Neurology, Amsterdam, 1977.

Fernández-Bouzas, A., & Harmony, T. *Evoked responses in atherosclerotic patients*. Unpublished results, 1979.

Fernández-Bouzas, A., Harmony, T., Nápoles, E., & Szava, S. *EDTA treatment of patients with occlusive cerebrovascular disease*. Presented at the Ninth World Congress of Neurological Sciences, New York, 1969.

Ferris, G. S., Davis, G. D., Dorsen, M., & Hackett, E. R. Changes in latency and form of the photically induced average evoked responses in human infants. *Electroenceph. Clin. Neurophysiol.*, 1967, *22*, 305-312.

Figueredo, P., Pascual, J., Pozo, D., & Harmony, T. *Análisis de la simetría electroencefalográfica en el niño*. Unpublished results, 1978.

Findji, F., Renault, B., Baillon, J. F., & Rémond, A. Preliminary results of an original method of statistical analysis of EEG signals considered as a succesion of half-waves. *Rev. Electroenceph. Neurophysiol. Clin.*, 1973, *3*, 304-309.

Fink, M. Cerebral electrometry. Quantitative EEG applied to human psychopharmacology. In G. Dolce & H. Künkel (Eds.), *CEAN*, Stuttgart: Gustav Fischer Verlag, 1975, 270-288.

Fink, M., Itil, T. M., & Shapiro, D. Digital computer analysis of the human EEG in psychiatric research. *Comprehen. Psychiat.*, 1967, *8*, 521-538.

Fiorentini, A., & Maffei, L. Evoked potentials in astigmatic subjects. *Vision Res.*, 1973, *13*, 1781-1783.

Floris, V., Morocutti, C., Amabile, G., Bernardi, G., & Rizzo, P. A. Cerebral reactivity in psychiatric and epileptic patients. *Electroenceph. Clin. Neurophysiol.*, 1969, *27*, 680.

Floris, V., Morocutti, C., Amabile, G., Bernardi, G., Rizzo, P. A., & Vasconetto, C. Recovery cycle of visual evoked potentials in normal and schizophrenic subjects. *Electroenceph. Clin. Neurophysiol.*, 1967, Suppl. *26*, 74-81.

Foit, A., & Cigánek, L. Possibilities of the diagnostic use of somatosensory evoked potentials. *Electroenceph. Clin. Neurophysiol.*, 1975, *39*, 547.

Forssman, H., & Frey, T. Electroencephalograms of boys with behavior disorders. *Acta psychiat. et neurol. Scand.*, 1953, *28*, 61-73.

Frankel, H., El-Negamy, E., & Sedgwick, E. M. Spinal somatosensory evoked responses in normal subjects and in patients with paraplegia. *Electroenceph. Clin. Neurophysiol.*, 1978, *44*, 130.

Frantzen, E., Harvald, B., & Haugsted, H. The arteriographic and electroencephalographic findings in cerebral apoplexy. *Danish Med. Bulletin*, 1959, *6*, 12-19.

Freeman, R. D. & Thibos, L. N. Visual evoked response in humans with abnormal visual experience. J. Physiol. (London), 1975, *247*, 711-724.

Friberg, S. Automatic EEG diagnosis presented as speech or printed-out. *Electroenceph. Clin. Neurophysiol.*, 1977, *43*, 508.

Friberg, S., Magnusson, R. I., Matousek, M., & Petersén, I. Automatic EEG diagnosis by means of digital processing. In P. Kellaway & I. Petersén (Eds.), *Quantitative analytic studies in epilepsy*. New York: Raven Press, 1976.

Frost, J. D. The promise technology holds for the future of electroencephalography. *Amer. J. EEG Technol.*, 1972, *12*, 65-75.

Fukushima, T., Mayanagi, Y., & Bonchard, G. Thalamic evoked potentials to somatosensory stimulation in man. *Electroenceph. Clin. Neurophysiol.*, 1976, *40*, 481-490.

Gaillard, A. W. K., & Perdok, J. The two components of the CNV. *Electroenceph. Clin. Neurophysiol.*, 1977, *43*, 485.

Galambos, R., & Hecox, K. Clinical applications of the brain stem auditory evoked potentials. In J. E. Desmedt (Ed.), *Progress in clinical neurophysiology* (Vol. 2). Basel: Karger, 1977, 1-19.

Gallais, P., Collomb, H., Milletto, G., Cardaire, G., & Blanc-Garin, J. Confrontation entre les données de l'électroencephalogramme et des examens psychologiques chez 522 sujets repartis en trois groupes differents. II. Confrontations des données de l'électroencephalogramme et de l'examen psychologique chez 113 jeunes soldats. In H. Fischgold & H. Gastaut (Eds.), Conditionnement et réactivité en électroencephalographie. *Electroenceph. Clin. Neurophysiol.*, 1957, Suppl. *6*, 294-303.

Gantchev, G., & Yankov, I. Somatosensory evoked potential elicited with the stretch reflex. *Electroenceph. Clin. Neurophysiol.*, 1974, *37*, 321-324.

Gasser, T. Goodness of fit tests for correlated data. *Biometrika*, 1975, *62*, 563-570.

Gasser, T. General characteristics of the EEG as a signal. In A. Rémond (Ed.), *EEG informatics. A didactic review of methods and applications of EEG data processing.* Amsterdam: Elsevier, 1977, 37-56.

Gastaut, H. Effets des stimulations physiques sur l'EEG de l'homme. *Electroenceph. Clin. Neurophysiol.*, 1949, Suppl. *2*, 69-82.

Gastaut, H., Franck, G., Krolikowska, W., Naquet, R., Régis, H., & Roger, J. Etude des potentiels évoqués visuels chez des hemianopsique présentant des crises épileptiques visuelles dans leur champ aveugle. *Rev. Neurol.*, 1963, *108*, 316-322.

Gastaut, H., Gastaut, Y., Roger, A., Corriol, J., & Naquet, R. Etude electroencephalographique du cycle de excitabilité cortical. *Electroenceph. Clin. Neurophysiol.*, 1951, *3*, 401-428.

Gastaut, H., Lee, M. C., & Laboureur, P. Comparative EEG and psychometric data for 825 French naval pilots and 511 control subjects of the same age. *Aerospace Med.*, 1960, *31*, 547-552.

Gastaut, H., & Tassinari, C. A. Epilepsies. In *Handbook of electroencephalography and clinical neurophysiology* (Vol. 13A). Amsterdam: Elsevier, 1975.

Gastaut, H., Terzian, H. and Gastaut, Y. Etude d'une activité électroencephalographique meconnue: Le rythme rolandique en arceau. *Marseille med.* 1952, *89*, 296-310.

Gauthier, P., & Gottesmann, C. Etude de la variation contingente negative et de l'onde postimperative en presence d'interferences. *Electroenceph. Clin. Neurophysiol.*, 1976, *40*, 143-152.

Gerin, P., Artru, F., Fischer, G., Reval, M., Courjon, J., & Munier, F. Reflections on the diagnostic value of average evoked potentials in deep coma. *Electroenceph. Clin. Neurophysiol.*, 1970, *29*, 100.

Gerin, P., Pernier, J., & Peronnet, F. Amplitude des potentiels évoqués moyens auditifs du vertex et intensité des stimuli. *Brain Res. Osaka*, 1972, *36*, 89-100.

Gerin, P., Ravault, M. P., David, C., Munier, F., & Parmeland, D. Occipital average responses and lesions of optic nerve. *C. R. Soc. Biol.* (Paris), 1966, *160*, 1445-1453.

Gerken, G. M., Moushegian, G., Stillman, R. D., & Rupert, A. L. Human frequency following response to monaural and binaural stimuli. *Electroenceph. Clin. Neurophysiol.*, 1975, *38*, 379-386.

Gersch, W., Yonemoto, J., & Naitoh, P. Automatic classification of multivariate EEGs using an amount of information measure and the eigenvalues of parametric time series model features. *Computers and Biomedical Research*, 1977, *10*, 297–318.

Gevins, A. S., Yeager, C. L., Diamond, S. L., Spire, J. P., Zeitlin, G. M., & Gevins, A. H. *Automated analysis of the electrical activity of the human brain (EEG): A progress report* (Proc. of the IEEE). 1975, *63*, 1382-1399.

Gevins, A. S., Yeager, C. L., Diamond, S. L., Zeitlin, G. M., Spire, J. P., & Gevins, A. H. Sharp transient analysis and thresholded linear coherence spectra of paroxysmal EEGs. In P. Kellaway & I. Petersén (Eds.), *Quantitative analytic studies in epilepsy.* New York: Raven Press, 1976, 463-482.

Gevins, A. S., Yeager, C. L., Zeitlin, G. M., Ancoli, S., & Dedon, M. F. On-line computer rejection of EEG artifact. *Electroenceph. Clin. Neurophysiol.*, 1977, *42*, 267-274. (a)

Gevins, A. S., Zeitlin, G. M., Ancoli, S., & Yeager, C. L. Computer rejection of EEG artifact. II:Contamination by drowsiness. *Electroenceph. Clin. Neurophysiol.*, 1977, *42*, 31-42. (b)

Giannitrapani, D. Developing concepts of lateralization of cerebral functions. *Cortex*, 1967, *3*, 353-370.

Giannitrapani, D. EEG changes under differing auditory stimulation. *Arch. Gen. Psychiat.*, 1970, *23*, 445-453.

Giannitrapani, D., & Kayton, L. Schizophrenia and EEG spectral analysis. *Electroenceph. Clin. Neurophysiol.*, 1974, *36*, 377-386.

Gibbs, E. L., & Gibbs, F. A. Electroencephalographic evidence of thalamic and hypothalamic epilepsy. *Neurology* (Minn.), 1951, *1*, 136-144. (a)

Gibbs, F. A., & Gibbs, E. L. *Atlas of electroencephalography, Vol. 1: Methodology and control*. Cambridge, Mass.: Addison-Wesley, 1951. (b)

Gibbs, F. A., & Gibbs, E. L. *Atlas of electroencephalography, Vol. 2: Epilepsy*. Cambridge, Mass.: Addison-Wesley, 1952.

Gibbs, F. A., & Gibbs, E. L. Fourteen and six per second positive spikes. *Electroenceph. Clin. Neurophysiol.*, 1963, *15*, 553-558.

Gibbs, F. A., & Gibbs, E. L. *Atlas of electroencephalography, Vol. 3: Neurological and psychiatric disorders*. Cambridge, Mass.: Addison-Wesley, 1964.

Gibbs, F. A., Gibbs, E. L., & Lennox, W. G. Electroencephalographic classification of epileptic patients and control subjects. *Arch Neurol. Psychiat.*, 1943, *50*, 111-128.

Giblin, D. R. Somatosensory evoked potentials in healthy subjects and in patients with lesions of the Nervous System. *Ann. N.Y. Acad. Sci.*, 1964, *112*, 93-142.

Gilden, L., Vaughan, H. G., & Costa, L. D. Summated human electroencephalographic potentials associated with voluntary movement. *Electroenceph. Clin. Neurophysiol.*, 1966, *20*, 433-438.

Gilroy, J., Lynn, G. E., Ristow, G. E., & Pellerin, R. J. Auditory evoked brain stem potentials in a case of "locked in" syndrome. *Archives of Neurology*, 1977, *34*, 492-495.

Glaser, E. M., Suter, C. M., Dasheiff, R., & Goldberg, A. The human frequency-following response: Its behavior during continuous tone and tone burst stimulation. *Electroenceph. Clin. Neurophysiol.*, 1976, *40*, 25-32.

Glass, J. O., Crowder, J. V., Kennerdeel, J. S., & Merikangos, J. R. Visually evoked potentials from occipital and precentral cortex in visually deprived humans. *Electroenceph. Clin. Neurophysiol.*, 1977, *43*, 207-217.

Gloor, P. The EEG and differential diagnosis of epilepsy. In H. Van Duijn, D. N. J. Donker, & A. C. Van Huffelen (Eds.), *Current concepts in clinical neurophysiology*. The Hague: N. V. Drukkerij, Trio, 1977, 9-22.

Gloor, P., Ball, G., & Schaul, N. Brain lesions that produce delta waves in the EEG. *Neurology*, 1977, *27*, 326-333.

Gloor, P., Kalaby, O., & Giard, N. The electroencephalogram in diffuse encephalopathies. Electroencephalographic correlates of grey and white matter lesions. *Brain*, 1968, *91*, 779-802.

Goff, G. D., Matsumiya, Y., Allison, T., & Goff, W. R. The scalp topography of human somatosensory and auditory evoked potentials. *Electroenceph. Clin. Neurophysiol.*, 1977, *42*, 57-76.

Goff, W. R., Allison, T., Lyons, W., Fisher, T. C., & Conte, R. Origins of short latency auditory evoked potentials in man. In J. E. Desmedt (Ed.), *Progress in clinical neurophysiology* (Vol. 2). Basel: Karger, 1977, 30-40.

Goff, W. R., Matsumiya, Y., Allison, T., & Goff, G. D. Cross-modality comparisons of averaged evoked potentials. In E. Donchin and D. B. Lindsley (Eds.), *Average evoked potentials*, Washington, D.C.: NASA, 1969.

Goff, W. R., Rosner, B. S., & Allison, T. Distribution of cerebral somatosensory evoked responses in normal man. *Electroenceph. Clin Neurophysiol.*, 1962, *14*, 697-713.

Goldberg, P., & Samson-Dollfus, D. A time domain analysis method applied to recognition of EEG rhythms. In G. Dolce & H. Künkel (Eds.), *CEAN*, Stuttgart: Gustav Fischer Verlag, 1975, 19-26.

Golberg, P., Samson-Dollfus, D., & Grémy, F. An approach to an automatic pattern recognition of the electroencephalogram: Background rhythm and paroxysmal events. *Meth. Inform. Med.*, 1973, *12*, 155-163.

Goldie, L., & VanVelzer, C. Innate sleep rhythms. *Brain*, 1965, *88*, 1043-1056.

Goldstein, L. Time domain analysis of the EEG. The integrative method. In G. Dolce & H. Künkel (Eds.), *CEAN*, Stuttgart: Gustav Fischer Verlag, 1975, 251-270.

Goldstein, L., Murphree, H., Sugerman, A. A., Pfeiffer, C. C., & Jenney, E. H. Quantitative EEG analysis of naturally occurring and drug-induced psychiatric states in human males. *Clin. Pharmacol. Ther.*, 1963, *4*, 10-21.

Goldstein, L., Sugerman, A. A., Stolberg, H., Murphree, H., & Pfeiffer, C. C. Electrocerebral activity in schizophrenic and non-psychiatric subjects. Quantitative EEG amplitude analysis. *Electroenceph. Clin. Neurophysiol.*, 1965, *19*, 350-361.

Goldstein, R., McRandle, C. C., & Smith, M. A. Early and late AERs to clicks in neonates. *Electroenceph. Clin. Neurophysiol.*, 1974, *37*, 207.

Goodin, D. S., Squires, K. C., Henderson, B. H., & Starr, A. Age-related variations in evoked potentials to auditory stimuli in normal human subjects. *Electroenceph. Clin. Neurophysiol.*, 1978, *44*, 447-458.

Goodwin, G. E. The significance of alpha variants in the EEG, and their relationships to an epileptiform syndrome. *Amer. J. Psychiat.*, 1947, *104*, 369-379.

Gotman, J., & Gloor, P. Automatic recognition and quantification of interictal epileptic activity in the human scalp EEG. *Electroenceph. Clin. Neurophysiol.*, 1976, *41*, 513-529.

Gotman, J., Gloor, P. & Ray, W. F. A quantitative comparison of traditional reading of the EEG and interpretation of computer extracted features in patients with supratentorial brain lesions. *Electroenceph. Clin. Neurophysiol.*, 1975, *38*, 623-639.

Gotman, J., Gloor, P., & Schaul, N. Comparison of traditional reading of the EEG and automatic recognition of interictal epileptic activity. *Electroenceph. Clin. Neurophysiol.*, 1978, *44*, 48-60.

Gotman, J., Skuce, D. R., Thompson, C. J., Gloor, P., Ives, J. R., & Ray, W. F. Clinical applications of spectral analysis and extraction of features from electroencephalograms with slow waves in adult patients. *Electroenceph. Clin. Neurophysiol.*, 1973, *35*, 225-235.

Grall, Y., Rigaudiere, F., Delthil, S., Legargassen, J. F., & Sourdille, J. Potentiels évoqués et acuite visuelle. *Vision. Res.*, 1976, *16*, 1007-1012.

Grass, A. M., & Gibbs, F. A. A Fourier transform of the electroencephalogram. *J. Neurophysiol.*, 1938, *1*, 521-526.

Grigorieva, L. P. The visual evoked potential and colour discrimination of the normal colour defective subjets. *Electroenceph. Clin. Neurophysiol.*, 1977, *43*, 457.

Grindel, O. D., Boldyreva, G. N., Burashnikov, E. N., & Andrevski, V. M. On the possibility of application of correlation analysis of the human electroencephalogram. *Zn. Vyssh. Nerv. Deyat. Pavlova*, 1964, *14*, 745-754. (Russian)

Groll-Knapp, E., Ganglberger, J. A., & Maider, M. Voluntary movement-related slow potentials in cortex and thalamus in man. In J. E. Desmedt (Ed.), *Progress in clinical neurophysiology* (Vol. 1). Basel: Karger, 1977, 164-173.

Grosveld. F., & De Rijke, W. Individual differences in the amplitude-histogram of the parieto-occipital EEG. *Electroenceph. Clin. Neurophysiol.*, 1977, *43*, 481.

Grünewald, G., Grünewald-Zuberbier, E., & Netz, J. Late components of average evoked potentials in children with different abilities to concentrate. *Electroenceph. Clin. Neurophysiol.*, 1978, *44*, 617-625.

Grünewald, G., Grünewald-Zuberbier, E., Netz, J., Sander, G., & Hömberg, V. Relationships between the late component of the contingent negative variation and the bereitschaftspotential. *Electroenceph. Clin. Neurophysiol.*, 1977, *43*, 517.

Grünewald-Zuberbier, E., Grünewald, G., Netz, J., & Klenkler-Wehler, A. EEG alpha attenuation responses, contingent negative variation (CNV) and vertex potentials in reaction time tasks in children with different ability to concentrate. *Electroenceph. Clin. Neurophysiol.*, 1977, *43*, 517.

Hagne, I., Persson, J., Magnusson, R., & Petersén, I. Spectral analysis via Fast Fourier Transform of waking EEG in normal infants. In P. Kellaway & I. Petersén (Eds.), *Automation of clinical EEG*, New York: Raven Press, 1973, 103-143.

Hall, R. A., Griffin, R. B., Mayer, D. L., Hopkins, K. H., & Rappaport, M. Evoked potential, stimulus intensity and drug treatment in hyperkinesis. *Psychophysiology*, 1976, *13*, 405-418.

Halliday, A. M. The incidence of large cerebral evoked responses in myoclonic epilepsy. *Electroenceph. Clin. Neurophysiol.*, 1965, *19*, 102.

Halliday, A. M. Changes in the form of cerebral evoked responses in man associated with various lesions of the nervous system. In Recent advances in clinical neurophysiology. *Electroenceph. Clin. Neurophysiol.*, 1967, Suppl. *25*, 178-192.

Halliday, A. M. The effect of lesions of the visual pathway and cerebrum on the visual evoked response. In *Handbook of electroencephalography and clinical neurophysiology* (Vol. 8A), Amsterdam: Elsevier, 1975, 119-128. (a)

Halliday, A. M. Somatosensory evoked responses. In *Handbook of electroencephalography and clinical neurophysiology* (Vol. 8A). Amsterdam: Elsevier, 1975, 60-67. (b)

Halliday, A. M. The effect of lesions of the afferent pathways and cerebrum on the somatosensory response. In *Handbook of electroencephalography and clinical neurophysiology* (Vol. 8A). Amsterdam: Elsevier, 1975, 129–137. (c)

Halliday, A. M. Cortical evoked potentials in man: Clinical observations. In H. Spekreijse & L. H. Van der Tweel (Eds.), *Spatial contrast. Report of a workshop*. Amsterdam: North Holland, 1977, 84-89.

Halliday, A. M., Barret, G., Blumhardt, L. D., Halliday, E., & Kriss, A. The pattern evoked response in hemianopia. *Electroenceph. Clin. Neurophysiol.*, 1977, *43*, 537.

Halliday, A. M., & Halliday, E. Cortical evoked potentials in patients with benign essential myoclonus and progressive myoclonic epilepsy. *Electroenceph. Clin. Neurophysiol.*, 1970, *29*, 106.

Halliday, A. M., Halliday, E., Kriss, A., McDonald, W. I., & Mushin, J. The pattern evoked potential in compression of the anterior visual pathways. *Brain*, 1976, *99*, 357-374.

Halliday, A. M., & Mason, A. A. The effect of hypnotic anaesthesia on cortical responses. *J. Neurol. Neurosurg. Psychiat.*, 1964, *27*, 300-312.

Halliday, A. M., McDonald, W. I., & Mushin, J. Delayed pattern-evoked responses in optic neuritis. *Lancet*, 1972, *1*, 982-985.

Halliday, A. M., McDonald, W. I., & Mushin, J. Delayed pattern evoked responses in optic neuritis in relation to visual acuity. *Trans. Ophthalmol. Soc. U.K.*, 1973, *93*, 315-324. (a)

Halliday, A. M., McDonald, W. I., & Mushin, J. Visual evoked response in the diagnosis of multiple sclerosis. *Brit. Med. J.*, 1973, *4*, 661-664. (b)

Halliday, A. M., McDonald, W. I., & Mushin, J. The dissociation of amplitude and latency changes in the pattern-evoked response following optic neuritis. *Electroenceph. Clin. Neurophysiol.*, 1974, *36*, 218. (a)

Halliday, A. M., McDonald, W. I., & Mushin, J. The value of the patterned-evoked response in the diagnosis of multiple sclerosis. *Electroenceph. Clin. Neurophysiol.*, 1974, 36, 551-553. (b)

Halliday, A. M., McDonald, W. I., & Mushin, J. Delayed visual evoked responses in progressive spastic paraplegia. *Electroenceph. Clin. Neurophysiol.*, 1974, *37*, 328. (c)

Halliday, A. M., & Wakefield, G. S. Cerebral evoked potentials in patients with dissociated sensory loss. *J. Neurol. Neurosurg. Psychiat.*, 1963, *26*, 211-219.

Halliday, R., Rosenthal, J. H., Naylor, H., & Callaway, E. Averaged evoked potential predictors of clinical improvement in hyperactive children treated with methylphenidate: An initial study and replication. *Psychophysiology*, 1976, *13*, 429-439.

Hamel, B., Bourne, J. R., Ward, J. W., & Teschan, P. Transient and steady state visually evoked cortical potentials in renal disease. *Electroenceph. Clin. Neurophysiol.*, 1976, *40*, 316.

Hamel, B., Bourne, J. R., Ward, J. W., & Teschan, P. Visually evoked cortical potentials in renal failure: Transient potentials. *Electroenceph. Clin. Neurophysiol.*, 1978, *44*, 606-616.

Hanley, J., Rickless, W. R., Crandall, P. H., & Walter, R. D. Automatic recognition of EEG correlates of behavior in a chronic schizophrenic patient. *Amer. J. Psychiat.*, 1972, *128*, 1524-1528.

Hannan, E. J. Multiple time series. New York: Wiley, 1970.

Harding, G. F. A. The use of visual evoked responses to flash stimuli in assessment of visual defect. *Electroenceph. Clin. Neurophysiol.*, 1974, *36*, 551-553.

Harker, L. A., Hosick, E. C., Voots, R. J., & Mendel, M. I. Influence of succinylcholine on middle component auditory evoked potentials. *Arch. of Otolaryngology*, 1977, *103*, 133–137.

Harman, H. H. *Modern factor analysis.* Chicago: University of Chicago Press, 1960.

Harmony, T. EEG and VER symmetry. Unpublished results, 1977.

Harmony, T. Driving activity. A quantitative study. *Activitas Nervosa Superior* (Praha), 1975, *17*, 116–119.

Harmony, T., & Fernández, G. Application of a non linear discriminant analysis for the differentiation of normal, epileptic and multiple sclerosis subjects on the basis of some evoked response parameters. In *First international symposium on data analysis and informatics* (Vol. 1). Colloques IRIA: Versailles, 1977, 281–290.

Harmony, T., & Alvarez, A. Evoked responses after head trauma. *Activitas Nervosa Superior* (Praha), 1981, *23*, 303–310.

Harmony, T., Fernández, G., Alvarez, A., & Roche, M. A. Visual, auditory and somatosensory evoked responses in cerebrovascular diseased patients. *Activitas Nervosa Superior* (Praha), 1978, *20*, 161-177. (a)

Harmony, T., Fernández, G., & Ricardo, J. "Driving curve" for the evaluation of brain damage. In B. Holmgren & T. Harmony (Eds.), *Applications of computers to the study of the nervous system*, Havana: CENIC, 1975.

Harmony, T., Fernández-Bouzas, A., Fernández, G., & Alvarez, A. Utilización de las respuestas evocadas en la evaluación del tratamiento a pacientes neurológicos. *Revista Hospital Psiquiátrico de La Habana*, 1978, *19*, 405–412. (b)

Harmony, T., Otero, G., Ricardo, J., & Fernández, G. Polarity coincidence correlation coefficient and signal energy ratio of the ongoing EEG activity. I:Normative data. *Brain. Res.*, 1973, *61*, 133-140. (a)

Harmony, T., Ricardo, J., Otero, G., Fernández, G., & Valdés, P. Symmetry of the visual evoked potentials in normal subjects. *Electroenceph. Clin. Neurophysiol.*, 1973, *35*, 237-240. (b)

Harmony, T., Valdés, P., Fernández, G., Alvarez, A., & Solis, M. Neurometric assessment of different groups of neurological patients on the basis of some evoked response parameters. Unpublished results, 1978. (c)

Harner, R. N. Computer analysis and clinical EEG interpretation: Perspective and application. In G. Dolce & H. Künkel (Eds.), *CEAN*, Stuttgart: Gustav Fischer Verlag, 1975, 337-343.

Harner, R. N. EEG analysis in the time domain. In A. Rémond, (Ed.), *EEG informatics. A didactic review of methods and application of EEG data processing*. Amsterdam: Elsevier, 1977, 57-82.

Harner, R. N., & Ostergren K. A. Sequential analysis of quasistable and paroxysmal activity. In P. Kellaway & I. Petersén (Eds.), *Quantitative analytic studies in epilepsy*. New York: Raven Press, 1976, 343-353.

Harner, R. N., & Ostergren, K. A. Clinical application of computerized EEG topography (CET). *Electroenceph. Clin. Neurophysiol.*, 1977, *42*, 721-722.

Harter, M. R., & White, C. T. Effects of contour sharpness and check size on visually evoked cortical potentials. *Vision Res.*, 1968, *8*, 701-711.

Harter, M. R., & White, C. T. Evoked cortical responses to checkerboard patterns: Effect of check size as a function of visual acuity. *Electroenceph. Clin. Neurophysiol.*, 1970, *28*, 48-54.

Hartwell, J. W., & Erwin, C. W. Evoked potential analysis: On-line signal optimization using a minicomputer. *Electroenceph. Clin. Neurophysiol.*, 1976, *41*, 416-421.

Harvold, V., & Skinhoj, E. EEG in cerebral apoplexy. *Acta Psychiatrica and Neurol. Scand.*, 1956, *31*, 181-185.

Hashimoto, I., Ishiyama, Y., & Tozuka, G. Alterations in brain stem auditory evoked responses and their relationships to lesions of the brain stem. *Electroenceph. Clin. Neurophysiol.*, 1977, *43*, 472.

Havlicek, V., Childiaeva, R., & Chernik, V. Ontogeny of the EEG power characteristics of quiet sleep periodic cerebral rhythm in preterm infants. *Neuropädiatrie*, 1975, *6*, 151-161.

Hazemann, P., Oliver, L., & Fischgold, H. Potentiel évoqué somestesique ipsilateral enregistré au niveau du scalp, chez l'homme hémispherectomisé. *C. R. Acad. Sc. Paris*, 1969, *268*, 195-198.

Hecox, K., & Galambos, R. Brain stem auditory evoked responses in human infants and adults. *Arch. Otolaryngol.*, 1974, *99*, 30-33.

Hecox, K., Squires, N., & Galambos, R. The dependence of human brainstem evoked potentials on signal duration and rise-fall time. *J. Acoust. Soc. Am.* 1974, *56*, 563.

Hecox, K., Squires, N., & Galambos, R. Brainstem auditory evoked response in man. I:Effect of stimulus rise-fall and duration. *J. Acoust. Soc. Am.*, 1976, *60*, 1187-1192.

Hennerici, M., Wenzel, D., & Freund, H. J. The comparison of small-size rectangle and checkerboard stimulation for the evaluation of delayed visual evoked responses in patients suspected of multiple sclerosis. *Brain*, 1977, *100*, 119-136.

Hill, D. EEG in episodic psychotic and psychopathic behaviour. *Electroenceph. Clin. Neurophysiol.*, 1952, *4*, 419-442.

Hill, D. Epilepsy: clinical aspects. In D. Hill & G. Parr (Eds.), *Electroencephalography*. London: MacDonald, 1963, 250-294.

Hill, D., & Parr, G. (Eds.) *Electroencephalography*. London: MacDonald, 1963.

Hillyard, S. A. The CNV and the vertex evoked potential during signal detection: A preliminary report. In E. Donchin & D. B. Lindsley, (Eds.), *Average evoked responses*. Washington, D.C.: NASA, 1969, 349-353.

Hirose, N., & Hishikawa, Y. An electrophysiological study on dystonic seizures induced by movement. *Electroenceph. Clin. Neurophysiol.*, 1977, *43*, 462.

Hjorth, B. EEG analysis based on time domain properties. *Electroenceph. Clin. Neurophysiol.*, 1970, *29*, 306-310.

Hjorth, B. The physical significance of time domain descriptors in EEG analysis. *Electroenceph. Clin. Neurophysiol.*, 1973, *34*, 321-325.

Hoeppner, T. J., & Lolas, F. Visual evoked responses and visual symptoms in multiple sclerosis. *Electroenceph. Clin. Neurophysiol.*, 1977, *43*, 569.

Holder, G. E. The effects of chiasmal compression on the pattern visual evoked potential. *Electroenceph. Clin. Neurophysiol.*, 1978, *45*, 278-280.

Horwitz, S., Larson, S., & Sances, A. Evoked potentials as an adjunct to the auditory evaluation of patients. *Proc. Symp. Biomed. Eng.*, 1966, *1*, 49-52.

Horyd, W., Myga, W., & Kulczycki, J. Visual evoked responses in patients with subacute sclerosing panencephalitis. *Electroenceph. Clin. Neurophysiol.*, 1977, *43*, 553.

Hrbek, A., Hrbkova, M., & Lenard, H. G. Somatosensory evoked responses in newborn infants. *Electroenceph. Clin. Neurophysiol.*, 1968, *25*, 443-448.

Hrbek, A., Hrbkova, M., & Lenard, H. G. Somatosensory, auditory and visual evoked responses in newborn infants during sleep and wakefulness. *Electroenceph. Clin. Neurophysiol.*, 1969, *26*, 597-603.

Hrbek, A., Karlberg, P., & Olsson, T. Development of visual and somatosensory evoked responses in pre-term newborn infants. *Electroenceph. Clin. Neurophysiol.*, 1973, *34*, 225-232.

Hrbek, A., Karlberg, P., Kjellmer, I., Olsson, T., & Riha, M. Clinical application of evoked electroencephalographic responses in newborn infants. I:Perinatal asphyxia. *Develop. Med. Child. Neurol.*, 1977, *19*, 34-44.

Hrbek, A., & Mares, P. Cortical evoked responses to visual stimulation in full-term and premature newborns. *Electroenceph. Clin. Neurophysiol.*, 1964, *16*, 577-581.

Hrbek, A., Vitová, Z., & Mares, P. The development of cortical evoked responses to visual stimulation during childhood. *Activitas Nervosa Superior* (Praha), 1966, *8*, 39-46.

Hrbkova, M. Somatosensory responses evoked by tendon taps in normal adults and neurological patients. *Electroenceph. Clin. Neurophysiol.*, 1969, *27*, 669.

Hughes, J. R. Usefulness of photic stimulation in routine electroencephalography. *Neurology* (Minn.), 1960, *10*, 777-782.

Hume, A. L., & Cant, B. R. Conduction time in central somatosensory pathways in man. *Electroenceph. Clin. Neurophysiol.*, 1978, *45*, 361-375.

Ilyanok, V. A. Effect of intensity and depth of pulsation of flickering light on the electrical activity of the human brain. *Biophysics*, 1961, *6*, 72-82.

Ilyanok, V. A. Spatial distribution of assimilated rhythm over the cerebral cortex in man. *Zh. Vyssh. Nerv. Deyat. Pavlova*, 1964, *14*, 763-770. (Russian)

Imahori, K., & Suhara, K. On the statistical method in the brain-wave study. *Folia Psychiat. Neurol. Jap.*, 1949, *3*, 137-155.

Irwin, D. A., Knott, J. R., McAdam, D. W., & Rebert, C. S. Motivational determinants of the contingent negative variation. *Electroenceph. Clin. Neurophysiol.* 1966, *21*, 538-543.

Isaksson, A. On time variable properties of EEG signals examined by means of Kalman filter method (Tech. Report No. 95). Stockholm: Dept. of Telecommunication Theory, Royal Institute of Technology, 1975.

Isaksson, A., & Wennberg, A. Visual evaluation and computer analysis of the EEG. A comparison. *Electroenceph. Clin. Neurophysiol.*, 1975, *38*, 79-86. (a)

Isaksson, A., & Wennberg, A. An EEG simulator—a means of objective clinical interpretation of the EEG. *Electroenceph. Clin. Neurophysiol.*, 1975, *39*, 313-320. (b)

Isaksson, A., & Wennberg, A. Spectral properties of non-stationary EEG signals evaluated by means of Kalman filtering: Application examples from a vigilance test. In P. Kellaway & I. Petersén (Eds.), *Quantitative analytic studies in epilepsy,* New York: Raven Press, 1976, 389-402.

Ishikawa, K. Studies on the visual evoked responses to paired light flashes in schizophrenics. *Kurume med. J.*, 1968, *15*, 153-167.

Itil, T. M., Marasa, J., Saletu, B., Davis, S., & Mucciardi, A. N. Computerized EEG: Predictor of outcome in schizophrenia. *The Journal of Nervous and Mental Diseases*, 1975, *160*, 188-203.

Ivanitsky, A. M. Evoked responses and analysis of stimuli in human cerebral cortex. *Zh. Vyssh. Nerv. Deyat. Pavlova*, 1969, *19*, 1020. (Russian)

Ives, J. R., & Gloor, P. Update: chronic sphenoidal electrodes. *Electroenceph. Clin. Neurophysiol.*, 1978, *44*, 789-790.

Ives, J. R., Thompson, C. J., & Woods, J. K. Acquisition by telemetry and computer analysis of 4 channel long term EEG recording from patients subject to "petit mal" absense attacks. *Electroenceph. Clin. Neurophysiol.*, 1973, *34*, 665-668.

Jacob, H. *Ein beitrag zur automatischen in echtzeit ablaufenden analyse von kontinui erlichen und intermittiereden aktivitaten im elektroenzephalogramm.* Thesis, Hannover, 1976.

Jacobson, J. H., Hirose, T., & Suzuki, T. A. Simultaneous EEG and VER in lesions of the optic pathway. *Investigative Ophthal.*, 1968, *6*, 279-292.

Jardine, C. J., Jardine, N., & Sibson, C. The structure and construction of taxonomic hierarchies. *Math Biosc.*, 1967, *1*, 173-179.

Jasper, H. H. The ten-twenty electrode system of the International Federation. *Electroenceph. Clin. Neurophysiol.*, 1958, *10*, 371-375.

Jasper, H. H., & Andrews, H. L. Human brain rhythms. I:Recording techniques and preliminary results. *J. Gen. Psychol.*, 1936, *14*, 98-126.

Jasper, H. H., & Andrews, H. L. Electroencephalography. III: Normal differentiation of occipital and precentral regions in man. *Arch. Neurol. Psychiat.* (Chic.), 1938, *39*, 96-115.

Jasper, H. H., & Kershman, J. Classification of the EEG in epilepsy. *Electroenceph. Clin. Neurophysiol.*, 1949, *1*, 123-131.

Jeffreys, D. A. Cortical source locations of pattern-related visual evoked potentials recorded from the human scalp. *Nature*, 1971, *229*, 502-504.

Jeffreys, D. A., & Axford, J. G. Source location of pattern specific components of human visual evoked potentials. I:Components of striate cortical origin. *Exp. Brain Res.*, 1972, *16*, 1-21. (a)

Jeffreys, D. A., & Axford, J. G. Source location of pattern specific components of human visual evoked potentials. II:Components of extrastriate cortical origin. *Exp. Brain Res.*, 1972, *16*, 22-40. (b)

Jewett, D. L., Romano, M. N., & Williston, J. S. Human auditory evoked potentials: Possible brain stem components detected on the scalp. *Science*, 1970, *167*, 1517-1518.

Jewett, D. L., & Williston, J. S. Auditory evoked far fields averaged from the scalp of humans. *Brain*, 1971, *94*, 681-696.

John, E. R. *Neurometric assessment of learning disabled children*. Unpublished results, 1979.

John, E. R. *Functional neuroscience, Vol. II. Neurometrics: Clinical applications of quantitative electrophysiology*. Hillsdale, New Jersey: Lawrence Erlbaum Associated, 1977.

John, E. R., Bartlett, F., Shimokochi, M., & Kleinman, D. Neural readout from memory. *Journal of Neurophysiology*, 1973, *36*, 898-924.

John, E. R., Karmel, B. Z., Corning, W. C., Easton, P., Brown, D., Ahn, H., John, M., Harmony, t., Prichep, L., Toro, A., Gerson, I., Bartlett, F., Thatcher, R. W., Kaye, H., Valdés, P., & Schwartz, E. Neurometrics. *Science*, 1977, *196*, 1393-1410.

John, E. R., & Laupheimer, R. *A method for the analysis of symmetry of brain wave activity*. U. S. Patent No. 3696808, 1972.

John, E. R., Ruchkin, D. S., & Vidal, J. S. Measurement of Event-Related Potentials. In E. Callaway, P. Tueting, & S. H. Koslow (Eds.), *Event-related brain potentials in man*. New York: Academic Press, 1978.

John, E. R., Ruchkin, D. S., & Villegas, J. Signal analysis and behavioral correlates of evoked potential configurations in cats. *Ann. N.Y. Acad. Sci.*, 1964, *112*, 362-420.

Johnson, L., Lubin, A., Naitoh, P., Nute, C., & Austin, M. Spectral analysis of the EEG of dominant and non-dominant alpha subjects during waking and sleeping. *Electroenceph. Clin. Neurophysiol.*, 1969, *26*, 361-370.

Jones, D. P., Binnie, C. D., Bown, R. L., Lloyd, D. S. L., & Watson, B. W. The contingent negative variation and psychological findings in chronic hepatic encephalopathy. *Electroenceph. Clin. Neurophysiol.*, 1976, *40*, 661-665.

Jones, R. T., Blacker, K. H., Callaway, E., & Layne, R. S. The auditory evoked response as a diagnostic and prognostic measure in schizophrenia. *The American J. of Psychiatry*, 1965, *122*, 33-41.

Jones, S. J. Short latency potentials from the neck and scalp following median nerve stimulation. *Electroenceph. Clin. Neurophysiol.*, 1977, *43*, 853-863.

Jones, S. J., & Small, D. G. The dipolar distribution of subcortical somatosensory evoked potentials in man. *Electroenceph. Clin. Neurophysiol.*, 1977, *43*, 537.

Jones, S. J., & Small, D. G. Spinal and subcortical evoked potentials following stimulation of the posterior tibial nerve in man. *Electroenceph. Clin. Neurophysiol.*, 1978, *44*, 299-306.

Jones, T. A., Schorn, V., Siu, G., Stockard, J. J., Rossiter, V. S., Bickford, R. G., & Sharbrough, F. W. Effects of local and systemic cooling on brain-stem auditory evoked responses. *Electroenceph. Clin. Neurophysiol.*, 1977, *43*, 469.

Jonkman, E. J. *The average cortical response to photic stimulation.* Thesis, University of Amsterdam, 1967.

Joseph, J. P., Lesèvre, N., & Dreyfus-Brisac, C. Spatio-temporal organization of EEG in premature infants and full-term newborns. *Electroenceph. Clin. Neurophysiol.*, 1976, *40*, 153–168.

Kaiser, E. Telemetry and video recording on magnetic tape cassettes in long term EEG. In P. Kellaway & I. Petersén (Eds.), *Quantitative analytic studies in epilepsy.* New York: Raven Press, 1976, 279–288.

Kaiser, E., Magnusson, R. I., & Petersén, I. Reverse correlation. In *Handbook of electroencephalography and clinical neurophysiology* (Vol. 5A). Amsterdam: Elsevier, 1973, 100–108.

Kaiser, E., & Petersén, I. Reverse correlation of 14 and 6 per second positive spikes. In P. Kellaway & I. Petersén (Eds.), *Clinical electroencephalography of children.* Stockholm: Almquist and Wiksell, 1968, 153-166.

Kaiser, E., & Sem-Jacobsen, C. W. "Yes-no" data reduction in EEG automatic pattern recognition. *Electroenceph. Clin. Neurophysiol.*, 1962, *14*, 953-956.

Kalman, R. E. A new approach to linear filtering and prediction problems. *Trans. ASME J. Basic. Eng. Ser. D82*, 1960.

Kamp, A., & Vliegenthart, W. E. Spectral changes of the EEG in human frontal cortex related to stimulus-response tasks. *Electroenceph. Clin. Neurophysiol.*, 1977, *43*, 566.

Kamphuisen, H. C. Average EEG responses to sinusoidally modulated light in normal subjects and patients. *Electroenceph. Clin. Neurophysiol.*, 1969, *27*, 674.

Kaplan, P. E. Blink reflex studies and somatosensory cerebral evoked potentials in patients with stroke and aphasia. *Electromyograph. Clin. Neurophysiol.*, 1978, *18*, 107-112.

Kardel, T., & Stigby, B. Period-amplitude analysis of the electroencephalogram correlated with liver function in patients with cirrhosis of the liver. *Electroenceph. Clin. Neurophysiol.*, 1975, *38*, 605-609.

Kato, M., Lüders, H., Miyoshi, S., & Kuroiwa, Y. Clinical study of evoked cortical potentials. I:Somatosensory evoked potentials. *Clin. Neurol.* (Tokyo), 1970, *10*, 539-547.

Katz, S., Blackburn, J. G., Perot, P. L., & Lam, C. F. The effects of low spinal injury on somatosensory evoked potentials from forelimb stimulation. *Electroenceph. Clin. Neurophysiol.*, 1978, *44*, 236-238.

Kavanagh, R. N., Darcey, T. M., & Fender, D. H. The dimensionality of the human visual evoked potential. *Electroenceph. Clin. Neurophysiol.*, 1976, *40*, 633–640.

Kellaway, P. Automation of clinical electroencephalography: The nature and scope of the problem. In P. Kellaway, & I. Petersén (Eds.), *Automation of clinical electroencephalography,* New York: Raven Press, 1973, 1-24.

Kellaway, P., & Maulsby, R. *The normative electroencephalographic data reference library.* (Final Report, Contractor Report NASA 1200). Washington, D.C.: National Aeronautics and Space Administration, 1967.

Kellaway, P., & Petersén, I. (Eds.). *Automation of clinical electroencephalography,* New York: Raven Press, 1973.

Kellaway, P., & Petersén, I. (Eds.). *Quantitative analytic studies in epilepsy.* New York: Raven Press, 1976.

Kelly, D. L., Goldring, S., & O'Leary, J. Averaged evoked somatosensory responses from exposed cortex in man. *Arch. Neurol.*, 1965, *13*, 1-9.

Kitasato, H. The relation between the photic driving of EEG and the response evoked by photic stimulation in man. *Jap. J. Physiol.*, 1966, *16*, 238-253.

Kitasato, H., & Hatsuda, T. The cortical responses evoked by double photic stimuli in various states of man. *Jap. J. Physiol.*, 1966, *16*, 227-237.

Kjellman, A., Larsson, L. E., & Prevec, T. S. Potentials evoked by tapping recorded from the human scalp over the cortical somatosensory region. *Electroenceph. Clin. Neurophysiol.*, 1967, *23*, 396.

Klein, F. F. A waveform analyzer applied to the human EEG. *IEEE Trans. Biomed. Eng.*, 1976, *BME-23*, 246-252.

Knoll, O. Continuous spectral analysis of the EEG during hemodialysis for monitoring CNS functions. *Electroenceph. Clin. Neurophysiol.*, 1977, *43*, 492.

Knott, J. R. The theta rhythm. In *Handbook of electroencephalography and clinical neurophysiology* (Vol. 6A). Amsterdam: Elsevier, 1976, 69-76.

Kodera, K., Yamane, H., Yamada, O., & Suzuki, J. Brain stem response audiometry at speech frequencies. *Audiology*, 1977, *16*, 469-479.

Kohn, M., & Lifshitz, K. A nonparametric statistical evaluation of changes in evoked potentials to different stimuli. *Psychophysiology*, 1976, *13*, 392-398.

Kohn, M., Lifshitz, K., & Litchfield, D. Average evoked potentials and frequency modulation. *Electroenceph. Clin. Neurophysiol.*, 1978, *45*, 236-243.

Kondo, N. Clinical study of somatosensory evoked potentials in orthopaedic surgery. *International Orthopaedics* (Sicot), 1977, *1*, 9-15.

Kooi, K. A. Voltage-time characteristics of spikes and other rapid electroencephalographic transients: Semantic and morphological considerations. *Neurology* (Minnesota), 1966, *16*, 59-66.

Kooi, K. A. *Fundamentals of electroencephalography*. New York: Harper and Row, 1971.

Kooi, K. A., & Bagchi, B. K. Visual evoked responses in man: Normative data. Ann. N.Y. Acad. Sci., 1964, *112*, 254-269. (a)

Kooi, K. A., & Bagchi, B. K. Observations on early components of visual evoked responses and occipital rhythms. *Electroenceph. Clin. Neurophysiol.*, 1964, *17*, 638-643. (b)

Kooi, K. A., Güvener, A. M., & Bagchi, B. K. Visual evoked responses in lesions of the higher optic pathways. *Neurology*, 1965, *15*, 841-848.

Kooi, K. A., & Thomas, M. H. Electronic analysis of cerebral responses to repetitive photic stimulation in patients with brain damage. *Electroenceph. Clin. Neurophysiol.*, 1958, *10*, 417-424.

Kooi, K. A., Tipton, A. C., & Marshall, R. E. Polarities and field configurations of the vertex components of the human auditory evoked response: A reinterpretation. *Electroenceph. Clin. Neurophysiol.*, 1971, *31*, 166-169.

Kopec, S. J., & Edelwejn, Z. *Evoked cerebral and sensory nerve potential.* Paper presented at the Conference of Electroencephalography and Clinical Neurophysiology, Kolobrzeg, Poland, 1978.

Korol, S., & Stangos, N. Les potentiels visuels évoqués moyennés dans la compression du nerf optique et leur comportement aprés décompression. *Arch. Opht.* (Paris), 1974, *34*, 209-214.

Kornhuber, H. H., & Deecke, L. Hirnpotentialänderungen beim Menschen vor and nach Willkürbewegungen, dargestellt mit Magnetband Speicherung und Rückwärtsanalyse. *Pflügers. Arch. ges. Physiol.*, 1964, *281*, 52.

Kornhuber, H. H., & Deecke, L. Hirnpotentialänderungen bei Willkürbewegungen und passiven Bewegungen des Menschen: Bereitschaftspotential und reafferente Potentiale. *Pflügers. Arch. ges. Physiol.*, 1965, *284*, 1-17.

Koshevnikov, V. A. Basis of a method for analysis of cerebral biopotentials as a complex oscillatory process. *Probl. Fiziol. Akust.*, 1955, *3*, 102-116. (Russian)

Koshevnikov, V. A. Some methods of automatic measurements of the electroencephalogram. *Electroenceph. Clin. Neurophysiol.*, 1958, *10*, 269-278.

Koshino, K., Kuroch, R., & Mogami, H. Flashing diode evoked potentials and optic nerve function during surgery. *Electroenceph. Clin. Neurophysiol.*, 1977, *43*, 449.

Krekule, I., & Radil-Weiss, T. Crosscorrelation and crosspectral analysis in relation to changes in vigilance level. *Activitas Nervosa Superior* (Praha), 1966, *8*, 193-194. (Czechoslovakian)

Kress, G. Area luminance effects and the visual evoked brain response. *Perception and Psychophysics*, 1975, *17*, 37-42.

Kruskal, J. B. Multidimensional scaling by optimizing goodness of fit to a non-metric hypothesis. *Psychometrika*, 1964, *29*, 1-27.

Kuhlo, W. The beta rhythms. In *Handbook of electroencephalography and clinical neurophysiology* (Vol. 6A). Amsterdam: Elsevier, 1976, 29-45. (a)

Kuhlo, W. Slow posterior rhythms. In *Handbook of electroencephalography and clinical neurophysiology* (Vol. 6A). Amsterdam: Elsevier, 1976, 89-103. (b)

Kuhlo, W., Heintel, H., & Vogel, F. The 4-5 c/sec rhythm. *Electroenceph. Clin. Neurophysiol.*, 1969, *26*, 613-618.

Künkel, H. Historical review of principal methods. In A. Rémond (Ed.), *EEG informatics. A didactic review of methods and applications of EEG data processing*. Amsterdam: Elsevier, 1977, 9-25.

Künkel, H., & EEG project group. Hybrid computing system for EEG analysis. In G. Dolce & H. Künkel (Eds.), *CEAN*, Stuttgart: Gustav Fischer Verlag, 1975, 365-383.

Kuroiwa, Y., Kato, M. and Umezaki, H. Computer analysis of cortical evoked potentials. Applications to agnostic syndrome study. *Proc. Austr. Ass. Neurol.*, 1968, *5*, 497-500.

Kutas, M., & Donchin, E. The effect of handedness, of responding hand, and of response form on the contralateral dominance of the readiness potential. In J. E. Desmedt (Ed.), *Progress in clinical neurophysiology* (Vol. 1). Basel: Karger, 1977, 189-210.

Laget, P., Flores-Guevara, R., D'Allest, A. M., Ostre, C., Raimbault, J., & Mariani, J. La maturation des potentiels évoqués visuels chez l'enfant normal. *Electroenceph. Clin. Neurophysiol.*, 1977, *43*, 732-734.

Laget, P., Mano, H., & Houdart, R. De l'interet des potentiels évoqués somesthesiques dans l'étude des lesions du lobe parietal de l'homme. *Neurochirurgie* (Paris), 1967, *13*, 841-853.

Laget, P., & Salbreux, R. *Atlas d'electorencephalographie infantile*. Paris: Masson, 1967.

Laget, P., Salbreux, R., Raimbault, J., D'Allest, A. M., & Mariani, J. Relationships between changes in somesthesic evoked responses and electroencephalographic findings in the child with hemiplegia. *Developmental Medicine and Child Neurology*, 1976, *18*, 620-631.

Lansing, R. W., & Barlow, J. S. Rhythmic after activity to flashes in relation to the background alpha which precedes and follows the photic stimuli. *Electroenceph. Clin. Neurophysiol.*, 1972, *32*, 149-160.

Lansing, R. W., & Thomas, H. The laterality of photic driving in normal adults. *Electroenceph. Clin. Neurophysiol.*, 1964, *16*, 290-294.

Larsen, L. E., & Walter, D. O. On automatic methods of sleep staging by spectra of electroencephalogram. *Agressologie*, 1969, *10*, 611-624.

Larsen, L. E., & Walter, D. O. On automatic methods of sleep staging by EEG spectra. *Electroenceph. Clin. Neurophysiol.*, 1970, *28*, 459-467.

Larson, S. J., Sances, A., & Baker, J. B. Evoked cortical potentials in patients with stroke. *Circulation*, 1966, *33* Suppl. *2*, 15-19. (b)

Larson, S. J., Sances, A., & Christenson, P. C. Evoked somatosensory potentials in man. *Arch. Neurol.* (Chicago), 1966, *15*, 88-93. (a)

Larsson, L. E., & Prevec, T. S. Somatosensory response to mechanical stimulation as recorded in the human EEG. *Electroenceph. Clin. Neurophysiol.*, 1970, *28*, 162-172.

Lavy, S., Carmon, A., & Schwartz, A. Depression of electrical cortical activity in acute cerebrovascular accidents. *Confinia Neurologica* (Basel), 1964, *24*, 182-188.

Lee, R. G., & Blair, R. D. G. Evolution of EEG and visual evoked response changes in Jacob-Creutzfeldt disease. *Electroenceph. Clin. Neurophysiol.*, 1973, *35*, 133-142.

Lee, R. G., & White, D. G. Modification of the human somatosensory evoked response during voluntary movement. *Electroenceph. Clin. Neurophysiol.*, 1974, *36*, 56-62.

Legewie, H., & Probst, W. On-line analysis of EEG with a small computer. *Electroenceph. Clin. Neurophysol.*, 1969, *27*, 533-535.

Lehmann, D. Multichannel topography of human alpha EEG fields. *Electroenceph. Clin. Neurophysiol.*, 1971, *31*, 439-449.

Lehmann, D., & Fender, D. H. Average visual evoked potentials in humans: Mechanism of dichoptic interaction studied in a subject with a split chiasma. *Electroenceph. Clin. Neurophysiol.*, 1969, *27*, 142.

Lehmann, D., Kavanagh, R. N., & Fender, D. H. Field studies of averaged visually evoked EEG potentials in a patient with a split chiasma. *Electroenceph. Clin. Neurophysiol.*, 1969, *26*, 193-199.

Lehtinen, L., & Bërgstrom, L. Naso-ethmoidal electrode for recording the electrical activity of the inferior surface of the frontal lobe. *Electroenceph. Clin. Neurophysiol.*, 1970, *29*, 303-305.

Lehtonen, J. B., & Koivikko, M. J. The use of a non-cephalic reference electrode in recording cerebral evoked potentials in man. *Electroenceph. Clin. Neurophysiol.*, 1971, *31*, 154-156.

Lehtonen, J. B., & Lehtinen, L. Alpha rhythm and uniform visual field in man. *Electroenceph. Clin. Neurophysiol.*, 1972, *32*, 139-147.

Lenard, H. G., Von Bernuth, H., & Hutt, S. J. Acoustic evoked responses in newborn infants: The influence of pitch and complexity of the stimulus. *Electroenceph. Clin. Neurophysiol.*, 1969, *27*, 121-127.

Lesèvre, N. Etude des réponses moyennes recuilles sur la région postérieure du scalp chez l'homme au cours de l'exploration visuelle ("complexe lambda"). *Psychol. franc.*, 1967, *12*, 26-36.

Lesèvre, N., & Joseph, J. P. Topographical organization of the visual evoked potential recorded on the scalp: Individualization of different spatial components occurring at the same moment. *Electroenceph. Clin. Neurophysiol.*, 1977, *43*, 504.

Lesèvre, N., & Rémond, A. Potentiels évoqués pour l'apparition de patterns: Effets de la dimension du pattern et de la densité des contrastes. *Electroenceph. Clin. Neurophysiol.*, 1972, *32*, 593-604.

Levillain, D., Pouliquen, A., Rogler, M. & Samson-Dollfus, D. Electro-clinical study of visual evoked potentials in 16 cases of lateral homonymous hemianopia. *Electroenceph. Clin. Neurophysiol.*, 1974, *36*, 83.

Levy, L. L., Segerberg, L. H., Schmidt, R. P., Turrell, R. C., & Roseman, E. The electroencephalogram in subdural hematoma. *J. Neurosurg.*, 1952, *9*, 588.

Lewis, E. G., Dustman, R. E., & Beck, E. C. Evoked response similarity in monozygotic and unrelated individuals: A comparative study. *Electroenceph. Clin. Neurophysiol.*, 1972, *23*, 309-316.

Lewis, E. G., Dustman, R. E., & Beck, E. C. Visual and somatosensory evoked potential characteristics of patients undergoing hemodialysis and kidney transplantation. *Electroenceph. Clin. Neurophysiol.*, 1978, *44*, 223-231.

Liberson, W. T. Study of evoked potentials in aphasics. *Am. J. Phys. Med.*, 1966, *45*, 135-142.

Lieb, J. P., Woods, S. C., Siccardi, A., Crandall, P. H., Walter, D. O., & Leake, B. Quantitative analysis of depth spiking in relation to seizure foci in patients with temporal lobe epilepsy. *Electroenceph. Clin. Neurophysiol.*, 1978, *44*, 641-663.

Lifshitz, K., & Gradijan, J. Differentiation of schizophrenic and other groups by auditory evoked characteristics. *Electroenceph. Clin. Neurophysiol.*, 1974, *37*, 211.

Lilliefords, H. W. On the Kolmogorov-Smirnov test for normality with mean and variance unknown. *J. Amer. Stat. Ass.*, 1967, *62*, 399-402.

Lin, T., & Standley, C. C. Importancia de los métodos epidemiológicos en psiquiatría. Cuadernos de Salud Pública, *16*, Ginebra: Organización Mundial de la Salud, 1964.

Lindgren, A. *Statistical theory*. New York: Macmillan, 1962.

Lindsley, D. B. Brain potentials in children and adults. *Science*, 1936, *84*, 354.

Lion, K. S., & Winter, D. F. A method for discrimination between signal and random noise of electrobiological potentials. *Electroenceph. Clin. Neurophysiol.*, 1953, *5*, 109-111.

Livanov, M. N., & Ananiev, W. M. Electrophysiological study of the spread of activity in the rabbit cerebral cortex. *Fiziol. Zh. SSSR.*, 1955, *41*, 461-469.

Livanov, M. N., Gavrilova, N. A., & Aslanov, A. S. Intercorrelations between different cortical regions of human brain during mental activity. *Neuropsychologia*, 1964, *2*, 281-289.

Livanov, M. N., & Rusinov, V. S. *Mathematical analysis of the electrical activity of the brain*. Cambridge, Mass.: Harvard University Press, 1968.

Lombroso, C. T., Duffy, F. H., & Robb, R. M. Selective suppression of cerebral evoked potentials to patterned light in amblyopia exanopsia. *Electroenceph. Clin. Neurophysiol.*, 1969, *27*, 238-247.

Loomis, A. L., Harvey, N., & Hobart, G. A. Distribution of disturbance-patterns in the human electroencephalogram, with special reference to sleep. *J. Neurophysiol.*, 1938, *1*, 413-430.

Lopes da Silva, F. H., Dijk, A., & Smits, H. Detection of nonstationarities in EEGs using the autoregressive model- An application to EEGs of epileptics. In G. Dolce & H. Künkel (Eds.), *CEAN*, Stuttgart: Gustav Fischer Verlag, 1975, 180-199.

Lopes da Silva, F. H., Ten Broeke, W., Van Hulten, K., & Lommen, J. G. EEG nonstationarities detected by inverse filtering in scalp and cortical recordings of epileptics; statistical analysis and spatial display. In P. Kellaway & I. Petersén (Eds.), *Quantitative analytic studies in epilepsy. New York: Raven Press, 1976.*

Lopes da Silva, F. H., Van Hulten, K., Lommen, J. G., Storm van Leeuwen, W., Van Vellen, C. W. M., & Viegenthart, W. Automatic detection and localization of epileptic foci. *Electroenceph. Clin. Neurophysiol.*, 1977, *43*, 1-13.

Lorente de No, R. Analysis of the activity of the chains of internuncial neurons. *J. Neurophysiology*, 1938, *1*, 207-244.

Low, M. D. Event-related potentials and the CNV. In A. Rémond (Ed.), *EEG informatics. A didactic review of methods and applications of EEG data processing*. Amsterdam: Elsevier, 1977, 347-362.

Low, M. D., Borda, R. P., Frost, J. D., & Kellaway, P. Surface negative slow potential shift associated with conditioning in man. *Neurology*, 1966, *16*, 771-782.

Low, M. D., Coats, A. C., Rettig, G. M., & McSherry, J. W. Anxiety, attentiveness-alertness: A phenomenological study of the CNV. *Neuropsychologia*, 1967, *5*, 379-384.

Low, M. D., & Purves, S. J. Sensory evoked potentials, CNV and the EEG in patients with proven brain lesion. *Electroenceph. Clin. Neurophysiol.*, 1975, *39*, 208.

Lowitzch, K., Kuhnt, U., Sakmann, C. Maurer, K., Hopf, H. C., Schott, D., & Thäter, K. Visual pattern evoked responses and blink responses in assessment of MS diagnosis. *J. Neurol.*, 1976, *213*, 17-32.

Loynes, R. M. On the concept of the spectrum for non-stationary processes. *J. R. statis. Soc. B.*, 1968, *30*, 1-30.

Lucioni, R., & Penati, G. Sulla frequenza e sul significate in psichiatria dei tracciati cosidetti piatti. *Riv. Neurol.*, 1966, *36*, 200-208.

Lücking, C. H. Variability of visual evoked responses in epileptic patients. *Electroenceph. Clin. Neurophysiol.*, 1969, *27*, 702.

Lücking, C. H., Creutzfeldt, O. D., & Heinemann, U. Visual evoked potentials of patients with epilepsy and of a control group. *Electroenceph. Clin. Neurophysiol.*, 1970, *29*, 557-566.

Lüders, H. The effect of aging on the waveform of the somatosensory cortical evoked potential. *Electroenceph. Clin. Neurophysiol.*, 1970, *29*, 450-460.

Lüders, H., Daube, J. R., Taylor, W. F., & Klass, D. W. A computer system for statistical analysis of EEG transients. In P. Kellaway & I. Petersén, (Eds.), *Quantitative analytic studies in epilepsy*. New York: Raven Press, 1976, 403–430.

Lüders, H., Kato, M., & Kuroiwa, Y. Cortical evoked potentials in hepatolenticular degeneration. *Electroenceph. Clin. Neurophysiol.*, 1969, *27*, 425.

Lüders, H., Miyoshi, S., & Kuroiwa, Y. Electrophysiological studies on cerebral evoked potentials in myoclonus epilepsy. *Electroenceph. Clin. Neurophysiol.*, 1972, *32*, 203.

Lugaresi, E., & Pazzaglia, P. Interictal electroencephalogram. In *Handbook of electroencephalography and clinical neurophysiology*, (Vol. 13). Amsterdam: Elsevier, 1975, 7-10.

Lundervold, A. EEG in patients with coma due to localized brain lesions. In *Handbook of electroencephalography and clinical neurophysiology*, (Vol. 12). Amsterdam: Elsevier, 1975, 37-46.

Lütcke, A., Meitins, L., & Masach, A. The presentation of background activity, focal findings, follow up studies and paroxysmal events by means of the "normalized slope descriptors" of Hjorth. *Electroenceph. Clin. Neurophysiol.*, 1974, *37*, 215.

Lynn, G. E., Gilroy, J., & Maulsby, R. Auditory brainstem potential in vertebral basilar artery disease. *Electroenceph. Clin. Neurophysiol.*, 1977, *43*, 465.

Maccolini, E., Meduri, R., Cavicchi, S., & Cristini, G. Multivariate analysis of visual evoked response. *Albrecht. v. Graefes. Arch. Klin. Exp. Ophthal.*, 1977, *202*, 275-283.

MacGillivray, B. B. Traditional methods of examination in clinical EEG. In *Handbook of electroencephalography and clinical neurophysiology*, (Vol. 3C). Amsterdam: Elsevier, 1974.

MacGillivray, B. B. The application of automated EEG analysis to the diagnosis of epilepsy. In A. Rémond (Ed.), *EEG informatics. A didactic review of methods and applications of EEG data processing*. Amsterdam: Elsevier, 1977, 243-262.

MacGillivray, B. B., & Wadbrook, D. G. A system for extracting a diagnosis from the clinical EEG. In G. Dolce & H. Künkel (Eds.), *CEAN*. Stuttgart, Gustav Fischer Verlag, 1975, 344-364.

MacGillivray, B. B., & Wadbrook, D. G. Automated clinical EEG reporting by small computer. *Electroenceph. Cln. Neurophysiol.*, 1977, *43*, 539.

MacLean, C., Cordaro, T., Appenzeller, O, & Rhodes, J. M. Flash evoked potentials in migraine. *Electroenceph. Clin. Neurophysiol.*, 1975, *38*, 544-545.

Madkour, O., & Abdel Hamid, T. Somatosensory evoked cortical potentials in man. *Electroenceph. Clin. Neurophysiol.*, 1967, *22*, 392.

Magnus, O, & Ponsen, L. The influence of the phase of the alpha rhythm on the cortical evoked response to photic stimulation. *Electroenceph. Clin. Neurophysiol.*, 1965, *18*, 427-428.

Magnus, O., Van der Wulp, C. J. M., Van der Holst, M. J. C., Van Huffelen, A. C., & Heimans, J. Application of computer analysis to EEG interpretation. *Electroenceph. Clin. Neurophysiol.*, 1977, *43*, 547.

Majkowski, J., Horyd, W., Kicinska, M., Narebski, J., Goscinski, I., & Darwaj, B. Reliability of electroencephalography. *Polish Medical Journal*, 1971, *10*, 1223-1230.

Malkovich, J. F., & Afifi, A. A. On tests for multivariate normality. *J. Amer. Stat. Ass.*, 1973, *63*, 176-179.

Marciano, F., Monod, N., & Nalfe, G. Computer classification of newborn sleep states. *Electroenceph. Clin. Neurophysiol.*, 1977, *43*, 475.

Marchesi, G. F., Tascini, G., Angeleri, F., Quattrini, A., & Scarpino, O. Automatic quantification and computerized statistical analysis of interictal discharges in epilepsies with asynchronous and alternating foci. *Acta med. Rom.*, 1976, *14*, 312-332.

Marcus, M. M. , & Zuercher, E. Auditory evoked response from specific and nonspecific cortex in schizophrenia. *Electroenceph. Clin. Neurophysiol.*, 1977, *43*, 564.

Mardia, K. V. Measures of multivariate skewness and kurtosis with applications. *Biometrika*, 1970, *57*, 519-530.

Marko, H., & Petsche, H. Ein Gerät zur gleichzeitigen Frequenz und Amplitudenanalyze von EEG-kurven bei trei Wählbasis. *Arch. Psychiat. Nervenkr.* 1957, *196*, 191-195.

Marsh, J. T., Brown, W. S., & Smith, J. C. Differential brainstem pathways for the conduction of auditory frequency-following responses. *Electroenceph. Clin. Neurophysiol.*, 1974, *36*, 415-424.

Marsh, J. T., Brown, W. S., & Smith, J. C. Far-field recorded frequency-following responses: Correlates of low pitch auditory perception in humans. *Electroenceph. Clin. Neurophysiol.*, 1975, *38*, 113-119.

Martin, P. Trois aspects EEG des hematomes intracérebraux. *Electroenceph. Clin. Neurophysiol.*, 1953, *5*, 133-136.

Martin, W. B., Johnson, L. C., Viglione, S. S., Naitoh, P., Joseph, R. D., & Moses, J. D. Pattern recognition of EEG-EOG as a technique for all-night sleep stage scoring. *Electroenceph. Clin. Neurophysiol.*, 1972, *32*, 417-427.

Masland, W. S., & Goldensohn, E. S. Asymmetric response to photic stimulation. *Electroenceph. Clin. Neurophysiol.*, 1967, *23*, 77-97.

Massone, C., Gasparetto, B., & Rodriguez, G. A computer based system for human EEG sleep analysis. *Electroenceph. Clin. Neurophysiol.*, 1977, *43*, 543.

Mastaglia, F. L., Black, J. L., & Collins, D. W. K. Visual and spinal evoked potentials in diagnosis of multiple sclerosis. *Br. Med. J.*, 1976, *2*, 732-733.

Matejcek, M., & Devos, J. E. Selected methods of quantitative EEG analysis and their applications in psychotropic drug research. In P. Kellaway & I. Petersén (Eds.), *Quantitative analytic studies in epilepsy.* New York: Raven Press, 1976, 183-206.

Matejcek, M., & Schenk, G. K. Quantitative analysis of the EEG by means of iterative interval analysis. *Electroenceph. Clin. Neurophysiol.*, 1973, *34*, 775.

Matousek, M. *Automatic analysis in clinical electroencephalography.* (Research Report No. 9). Prague: Psychiatric Research Institute, 1967.

Matousek, M. Frequency analysis in routine electroencephalography. *Electroenceph. Clin. Neurophysiol.*, 1968, *24*, 365-373.

Matousek, M. (Ed.). Frequency and correlation analysis. In *Handbook of electroencephalography and clinical neurophysiology.* Amsterdam: Elsevier (Vol. 5A). 1973.

Matousek, M. Clinical application of EEG analysis: Presentation of EEG results and dialogue with the clinician. In A. Rémond (Ed.), *EEG informatics. A didactic review of methods and applications of EEG data processing.* Amsterdam: Elsevier, 1977, 233-242.

Matousek, M., & Petersén, I. Objective measurement of maturation defects and other EEG abnormalities by means of frequency analysis. *Proceedings of the V World Congress of Psychiatry*, Mexico, 1971.

Matousek, M., & Petersén, I. Frequency analysis of the EEG in normal children and adolescents. In P. Kellaway, & I. Petersén (Eds.), *Automation of clinical electroencephalography.* New York: Raven Press, 1973, 75–102. (a)

Matousek, M., & Petersén, I. Automatic evaluation of the EEG background activity by means of age dependent EEG quotients. *Electroenceph. Clin. Neurophysiol.*, 1973, *35*, 603-612. (b)

Matousek, M., Petersén, I., & Friberg, S. Automatic assessment of randomly selected routine EEG records. In G. Dolce, & H. Künkel (Eds.), *CEAN*, Stuttgart: Gustav Fischer Verlag, 1975.

Matsumiya, Y., Gennarelli, T. A., & Lombroso, C. T. Somatosensory evoked responses in the hemispherectomised man. *Electroenceph. Clin. Neurophysiol.*, 1971, *31*, 289.

Matthews, W. B., Beauchamp, M., & Small, D. G. Cervical somatosensory evoked responses in man. *Nature*, 1974, *252*, 230-232.

Maynard, D. E. The cerebral function analyser monitor (CFAM). *Electroenceph. Clin. Neurophysiol.*, 1977, *43*, 479.

McAdam, D. W. Increases in CNS excitability during negative cortical slow potentials in man. *Electroenceph. Clin. Neurophysiol.*, 1969, *26*, 216-219.

McAdam, D. W., Irwin, D. A., Rebert, C. S., & Knott, J. R. Conative control of the Contingent Negative Variation. *Electroenceph. Clin. Neurophysiol.*, 1966, *21*, 194-195.

McAdam, D. W., & Seales, D. M. Bereitschaftspotential enhancement with increased level of motivation. *Electroenceph. Clin. Neurophysiol.*, 1969, *27*, 73–75.

McCallum, W. C., & Cummins, B. The effects of brain lesions on the Contingent Negative Variation in neurosurgical patients. *Electroenceph. Clin. Neurophysiol.*, 1973, *35*, 449–456.

McCallum, W. C., & Walter, W. G. The effects of attention and distraction on the Contingent Negative Variation in normal and neurotic subjects. *Electroenceph. Clin. Neurophysiol.*, 1968, *25*, 319–329.

McGillem, C. D., & Aunon, J. I. *Measured characteristics of single visual evoked brain potentials.* Paper presented at San Diego Biomedical Symposium, 1976.

McGillem, D., & Aunon, J. I. Measurments of signal components on single visually evoked brain potentials. *IEEE Trans. Biomed. Eng.*, 1977, *BME-24*, 232-241.

McInnes, A. The spinal evoked responses in multiple sclerosis. *Electroenceph. Clin. Neurophysiol.*, 1978, *44*, 131.

McQueen, J. B. *Some methods for classification and analysis of multivariate observations.* (Proc. Symp. Math. Statist. and Probability). Berkeley: University of California Press, 1967, 281-289.

Meienberg, P., & Gerster, F. A computer program on-line processing of polygraphic sleep records. *Electroenceph. Clin. Neurophysiol.*, 1977, *43*, 467.

Meijes, P. Some characteristics of the early components of the somatosensory evoked responses to mechanical stimuli in man. *Psychiat. Neurol. Neurosurg.*, 1969, *72*, 263-268.

Mendel, M. I. Influence of stimulus level and sleep stage on the early components of the averaged electroencephalographic response to clicks during all-night sleep. *J. of Speech and Hearing Research*, 1974, *17*, 5-15.

Mendel, M. I., Adkinson, C. D., & Harker, L. A. Middle components of the auditory potentials in infants. *Ann. Otol. Rhinol. Laryngol.*, 1977, *86*, 293-299.

Mendel, M. I., & Hosick, E. C. Effects of secobarbital on the early components of the auditory evoked potentials. *Revue de Laringologie*, 1975, *96*, 178-184.

Mezan, I. The human averaged response to trains of photic stimuli. *Electroenceph. Clin. Neurophysiol.*, 1974, *37*, 323.

Michael, W. F., & Halliday, A. M. Differences between the occipital distribution of upper and lower field pattern evoked responses in man. *Brain Res.*, 1971, *32*, 311-324.

Michel, F., & Peronnet, F. Extinction gauche au test dichotique: Lésion hémisphérique ou lésion commisurale? In F. Michel & B. Schott (Eds.), *Les syndromes de disconnexion calleuse chez l'homme.* Actes du Coll. Int. de Lyon, 1974, 85–117.

Mol, J. M. F. Cerebral response to sinusoidally modulated light in man. *Electroenceph. Clin. Neurophysiol.*, 1969, *26*, 536.

Monod, N., & Dreyfus-Brisac, C. Prognostic value of the neonatal EEG in full-term newborns. In O. Magnus (Ed.), *Handbook of electroencephalography and clinical neurophysiology* (Vol. 15). Amsterdam: Elsevier, 1972.

Montagu, J. D. The relationship between the intensity of repetitive photic stimulation and the cerebral response. *Electroenceph. Clin. Neurophysiol.*, 1967, *23*, 152-161.

Morgan, A., Gerin, P., & Charachon, D. L'audiometrie electroencephalographique. *Acta Oto-Rhino-Laryngologica Belgica*, 1970, *24*, 4.

Morley, G., & Liedtke, C. E. Averaged evoked potentials as a localizing technique in aphasia. Paper presented at *San Diego Biomedical Symposium*, 1976, *15*, 217–223.

Morley, G., & Liedtke, C. E. Automated evoked potential analysis using peak and latency discrimination. Paper presented at the *San Diego Biomedical Symposium*, 1977, 291-298.

Morocutti, C., Amabile, G., & Bernardi, G. Study of the visual evoked response in epileptics. *Neopsichiatria*, 1968, *34*, 585-593.

Morocutti, C., Sommer-Smith, J. A., & Creutzfeldt, O. D. Das visuelle reaktionspotential bei normalen Versuchspersonen und charakteristische Veränderungen bei Epileptikern. *Arch. Psychiat. Nervenkr.*, 1966, *208*, 234–254.

Morrell, F. Electrophysiological analysis of the auditory evoked potential in a patient with a left hemispherectomy. *Electroenceph. Clin. Neurophysiol.*, 1974, *36*, 223.

Morrison, D. F. *Multivariate statistical methods*. New York: McGraw Hill, 1976.

Moushegian, G. The frequency-following response in man. In J. E. Desmedt (Ed.), *Progress in clinical neurophysiology* (Vol. 2). Basel: Karger, 1977, 20-29.

Moushegian, G., Rupert, A. L., & Stillman, R. D. Scalp recorded early responses in man to frequencies in the speech range. *Electroenceph. Clin. Neurophysiol.*, 1973, *35*, 665-667.

Mundy-Castle, A. C. An analysis of central responses to photic stimulation in normal adults. *Electroenceph. Clin. Neurophysiol.*, 1953, *5*, 1-22.

Nagao, H. On some test criteria for covariance matrix. *The Annals of Statistics*, 1973, *1*, 700-709.

Nagypol, T., Tomka, I., & Bodó, M. Pattern recognitioin and analyzer system for the evaluation of correlations between epileptic spike and background EEG activities. *Electroenceph. Clin. Neurophysiol.*, 1976, *41*, 213.

Naitoh, P., Johnson, C. L., & Lubin, A. Modification of surface negative slow potential (CNV) in the human brain after total sleep loss. *Electroenceph. Clin. Neurophysiol.*, 1971, *30*, 17-22.

Nakanishi, T., Shimada, Y., Sakuta, M., & Toyokura, Y. The initial positive component of the scalp-recorded somatosensory evoked potential in normal subjects and in patients with neurological disorders. *Electroenceph. Clin. Neurophysiol.*, 1978, *45*, 26-34.

Nakanishi, T., Shimada, Y., & Toyokura, Y. Somatosensory evoked responses to mechanical stimulation in normal subjects and in patients with neurological disorders. *J. of the Neurological Sciences*, 1974, *21*, 289-298.

Namerow, N. S. Somatosensory evoked responses in multiple sclerosis patients with varying sensory loss. *Neurology*, 1968, *18*, 1197-1204.

Namerow, N. S., & Enns, N. Visual evoked responses in patients with multiple sclerosis. *J. Neurol. Neurosurg. Psychiat.*, 1972, *35*, 829-833.

Namerow, N. S., Sclabassi, R. J., & Enns, N. F. Somatosensory responses to stimulus trains: Normative data. *Electroenceph. Clin. Neurophysiol.*, 1974, *37*, 11-21.

Needham, W. E., Dustman, R. E., Bray, P. F., & Beck, E. C. Intelligence, EEG and visual evoked potentials in centrencephalic epilepsy. *Electroenceph. Clin. Neurophysiol.*, 1971, *30*, 94.

Netchine, S., Harrison, S., Berges, J., & Lairy, G. C. Contribution a l'étude de la signification des rythmes mu. *Rev. Neurol.*, 1964, *11*, 339-341.

NINCDS. *Neurological and sensory disabilities: Estimated numbers and costs*. National Institute of Health Publication, USA, 1973, 73-152.

Nishitani, H., & Kooi, K. A. Cerebral evoked responses in hypothyroidism. *Electroenceph. Clin. Neurophysiol.*, 1968, *24*, 554-560.

Njiokiktjien, C. J., Visser, S. L, & Rijke, W. EEG and visual evoked responses in children with learning disorders. *Neuropädiatrie*, 1977, *8*, 134–147.

Noel, P., & Desmedt, J. E. Somatosensory cerebral evoked potentials after vascular lesions of the brain stem and diencephalon. *Brain*, 1975, *98*, 113-128.

Nogawa, E., Katayama, K., Tabata, Y., Kawahara, T., & Ohshio, T. Visual evoked potentials estimated by Wiener filtering. *Electroenceph. Clin. Neurophysiol.*, 1973, *35*, 375-378.

Nogawa, T., Katayama, K., Tabata, Y., Ohshio, T., & Kawahara, T. Digital methods for amplitude and phase analysis of the EEG. *Journal of the Kansai Medical University*, 1976, Suppl. *28*, 1-20.

Novikova, L. A., & Filchikova, L. I. Influence of defocussing an optic stimulus on human evoked potential. *J. Higher. Nerv. Activity.*, 1977, *27*, 98-106.

Novikova, L. A., & Tolstova, V. A. Investigation of neurophysiological mechanisms of visual deprivation in man. *Electroenceph. Clin. Neurophysiol.*, 1977, *43*, 482.

Obrist, W. D. Problems of aging. In *Handbook of electroencephalography and clinical neurophysiology* (Vol. 6A). Amsterdam: Elsevier, 1976, 275-292.

Obrist, W. D., & Busse, E. W. The electroencephalogram in old age. In W. P. Wilson (Ed.), *Applications of electroencephalography in psychiatry*. Durham, N.C.: Duke University Press, 1965, 185-205.

Obrist, W. D., & Henry, C. E. Electroencephalographic findings in aged psychiatric patients. *J. Nerv. Ment. Dis.*, 1958, *126*, 254-267.

Obrist, W. D., Henry C. E., & Justiss, W. A. Longitudinal changes in the senescent EEG: A 15 year study. In *Proceedings of the Seventh International Congress of Gerontology*, Vienna, 1966, 35-38.

O'Connor, K. P. Contingent Negative Variation differences between elderly normal and demented subjects. *Electroenceph. Clin. Neurophysiol.*, 1977, *43*, 471.

O'Connor, K. P., Shaw, J. C., & Ongley, C. O. The EEG and differential diagnosis in psychiatric disorders of the senium. *Electroenceph. Clin. Neurophysiol.*, 1977, *43*, 506.

Ohlrich, E. S., & Barnet, A. B. Auditory evoked responses during the first year of life. *Electroenceph. Clin. Neurophysiol.*, 1972, *32*, 161-169.

Ohlrich, E.S., Barnet, A. B., Weiss, I. P., & Shanks, B. L. Auditory evoked potential in early childhood: A longitudinal study. *Electroenceph. Clin. Neurophysiol.*, 1978, *44*, 411-423.

Ojemann, G. A., & Henkin, R. I. Steroid dependent changes in human visual evoked potentials. *Life Sciences*, 1967, *6*, 327-334.

Olson, C. L. Comparative robustness of six tests in multivariate analysis of variance. *J. of the Amer. Statist. Ass.*, 1974, *69*, 894-908.

Oosterhuis, H. G., Ponsen, L., Jonkman, E. J., & Magnus, O. The average visual evoked response in patients with cerebrovascular disease. *Electroenceph. Clin. Neurophysiol.*, 1969, *27*, 23-24.

Ornitz, E. M., Forsythe, A. B., Tanguay, P. E., Ritvo, E. R., de la Pena, A., & Ghahremani, J. The recovery cycle of the averaged auditory evoked response during sleep in autistic children. *Electroenceph. Clin. Neurophysiol.*, 1974, *37*, 173-174. (b)

Ornitz, E. M., Ritvo, E. R., Panman, L. M., Lee, Y. H., Carr, E. M., & Walter, R. D. The auditory evoked response in normal and autistic children during sleep. *Electroenceph. Clin. Neurophysiol.*, 1968, *25*, 221.

Ornitz, E. M., Tanguay, P. E., Forsythe, A. B., de la Peña, A., & Ghahremani, J. The recovery cycle of the averaged auditory evoked response during sleep in normal children. *Electroenceph. Clin. Neurophysiol.*, 1974, *37*, 113-122. (a)

Ostow, M. Flickered light as a provocative test in electroencephalography. *Electroenceph. Clin. Neurophysiol.*, 1949, *1*, 245.

Otero, G., Harmony, T., & Ricardo, J. Polarity coincidence correlation coefficient and signal energy ratio of the ongoing EEG activity. II: Brain tumors. *Activitas Nervosa Superior* (Praha), 1975, *17*, 120-126. (a)

Otero, G., Harmony, T., & Ricardo, J. Polarity coincidence correlation coefficient and signal energy ratio of the ongoing EEG activity. III:Cerebrovascular lesions. *Activitas Nervosa Superior* (Praha), 1975, *17*, 127-133. (b)

Otero, G., Harmony, T., & Ricardo, J. Polarity coincidence correlation coefficient and signal energy ratio of the ongoing EEG activity in brain damaged patients. In B. Holmgren & T. Harmony (Eds.), *Applications of computers to the study of the nervous system.* Havana: CENIC, 1975. (c)

Otero, G., Harmony, T., Ricardo, J., Llorente, S., Peñalver, J. C., Estévez, M., & Roche, M. A. Coeficiente de correlación de polaridad y relación de energía de la actividad electroencefalográfica. IV Epilepsias. *Cenic*, 1974, *5*, 67-72.

Otto, D. A., & Benignus, A. *Slow positive shifts during sustained motor activity in humans.* Paper presented at the 28th Annual Meeting of the American EEG Society, Seattle, Washington, 1974.

Otto, D. A., & Leifer, L. J. The effects of modifying response and performance feedback parameters on the CNV in humans. *Electroenceph. Clin. Neurophysiol.*, 1973, Suppl. *33*, 29-37.

Padmos, P., Haaijman Joost, J., & Spekreijse, H. Visually evoked cortical potentials to patterned stimuli in monkey and man. *Electroenceph. Clin. Neurophysiol.*, 1973, *35*, 153-163.

Pagni, C. A. Somatosensory evoked potentials in thalamus and cortex of man. *Electroenceph. Clin. Neurophysiol.*, 1967, Suppl. *26*, 147-155.

Palestini, M., Pisano, M., Rosadini, G., & Rossi, G. F. Excitability cycle of the visual cortex during sleep and wakefulness. *Electroenceph. Clin. Neurophysiol.*, 1965, *19*, 267-283.

Pampiglione, G., & Kerridge, J. EEG abnormalities from the temporal lobe studied with sphenoidal electrodes. *J. Neurol. Neurosurg. Psychiat.*, 1956, *19*, 117-129.

Papakostopoulos, D. Sustained macropotentials preceding selfspaced movements in left and right handed subjects. *Electroenceph. Clin. Neurophysiol.*, 1978, *44*, 791.

Papakostopoulos, D., Cooper, R., & Crow, H. J. Inhibition of cortical evoked potentials and sensation by self-initiated movements in man. *Nature*, 1975, *258*, 321-324.

Papakostopoulos, D., Winter, A. L., & Newton, P. New technique for the control of eye potential artifacts in multichannel CNV recordings. *Electroenceph. Clin. Neurophysiol.*, 1973, *34*, 651-653.

Papatheophilov, R., & Turland, D. N. The electroencephalogram of normal adolescent males: visual assessment and relationship with other variables. *Develop. Med. Child Neurol.*, 1976, *18*, 603-619.

Papp, N., & Ktonas, P. Critical evaluation of complex demodulation techniques for the quantification of bioelectrical activity. Paper presented at *San Diego Biomedical Symposium*, 1976.

Parmelee, A. H., Schulz, H. R., & Disbrow, M. A. Sleep patterns of the newborn. *J. Pediat.*, 1961, *58*, 241-250.

Parzen, E. *Stochastic processes*. San Francisco: Holden-Day, 1962.

Pastrnákova, I., Peregrin, J., & Sverak, J. Visual evoked responses to blank and checkerboard patterned flashes and visual acuity. *Physiol. Bohemoslov.*, 1975, *24*, 459.

Peacock, S. M. Averaged "after-activity" and the alpha regeneration cycle. *Electroenceph. Clin. Neurophysiol.*, 1970, *28*, 278-295.

Peacock, S. M., & Conroy, R. C. Further considerations of the regional responses to photic stimulation as shown by epoch averaging. *Electroenceph. Clin. Neurophysiol.*, 1974, *36*, 163-170.

Peronnet, F., & Michel, F. The asymmetry of the auditory evoked potentials in normal man and in patients with brain lesions. In J. E. Desmedt (Ed.), *Progress in clinical neurophysiology*. Basel: Karger, 1977, 120-141.

Peronnet, F., Michel, F., Echallier, J. F., & Girod, J. Coronal topography of human auditory evoked responses. *Electroenceph. Clin. Neurophysiol.*, 1974, *37*, 225-230.

Persson, J. Comments on estimations and tests of EEG amplitude distributions. *Electroenceph. Clin. Neurophysiol.*, 1974, *37*, 309-313.

Petersén, I., & Eeg-Olofsson, O. The development of the electroencephalogram in normal children from the age of one through 15 years. Non paroxysmal activity. *Neuropädiatrie*, 1970, *2*, 247.

Petersén, I., Eeg-Olofsson, O., Hagne, I., & Selldén, U. EEG of selected healthy children. *Electroenceph. Clin. Neurophysiol.*, 1965, *19*, 613-620.

Petersén, I., Kaiser, E., & Magnusson, R. I. Need and implementation of centers for automatic analysis and automatic interpretation of clinical EEG. In P. Kellaway & I. Petersén (Eds.), *Automation of clinical electroencephalography*. New York: Raven Press, 1973, 25-30.

Petersén, I., & Matousek, M. Automatic analysis and interpretation of EEG. In B. Holmgren & T. Harmony (Eds.), *Application of computers to the study of the nervous system*. Havana: CENIC, 1975.

Petersén, I., & Sörbye, R. Slow posterior rhythms in adults. *Electroenceph. Clin. Neurophysiol.*, 1962, *14*, 161-170.

Petsche, H. Das Vektor-EEG, ein neuer Weg zur Klärung hirnelektrischer Vorgänge. *Wien. Z. Nervenheilk.*, 1952, *5*, 304–320.

Petsche, H. EEG topography. In *Handbook of electroencephalography and clinical neurophysiology*. (Vol. 5A). Amsterdam: Elsevier, 1972.

Pfefferbaum, A. Handedness and cortical hemisphere effects in sine wave stimulated evoked responses. *Neuropsychol.*, 1971, *9*, 237-240.

Pfurtscheller, G., & Fischer, G. A new approach to spike detection using a combination of inverse and matched filter techniques. *Electroenceph. Clin. Neurophysiol.*, 1978, *44*, 243-247.

Picard, P., Navarranne, P., Labourer, P., Grousset, G., & Jest, C. Confrontations des données de l'electroencephalogramme et des examens psychologiques chez 522 sujets repartis en trois groupes différents. III:Confrontations des données de l'electroencephalogramme et de l'examen psychologique chez 309 candidats pilotes a l'aéronautique.

In H. Fischgold & H. Gastaut (Eds.), *Conditionement et reactivité en electroencephalographie. Electroenceph. Clin. Neurophysiol.*, 1957, *Suppl.*, *6*, 304–314.

Picton, T. W., & Hillyard, S. A. Human auditory evoked potentials. II: Effects of attention. *Electroenceph. Clin. Neurophysiol.*, 1974, *36*, 191-200.

Picton, T. W., Hillyard, S. A., Krausz, H. I., & Galambos, R. Human auditory evoked potentials. I:Evaluation of components. *Electroenceph. Clin. Neurophysiol.*, 1974, *36*, 179-190.

Picton, T. W., Woods, D. L., & Proulx, G. B. Human auditory sustained potentials. I:The nature of the response. *Electroenceph. Clin. Neurophysiol.*, 1978, *45*, 186-197.

Pitot, M., & Gastaut, Y. Aspects électroencephalographiques inhabituels des séquelles des traumatismes craniens II:Le rythmes pósterieurs a 4 cycles-seconde. *Rev. Neurol.*, 1956, *94*, 189-191.

Polujanova, L., Vasilieva, V., & Kamaskaja, V. Functional meaning of the late waves of the evoked potentials to significant auditory stimuli in patients with temporal epilepsy. *Electroenceph. Clin. Neurophysiol.*, 1977, *43*, 456.

Popivanov, D. Analysis of the evoked potential in relation to a preceding epoch of background activity. *Electroenceph. Clin. Neurophysiol.*, 1974, *37*, 323.

Popivanov, D. Classification of evoked potentials before averaging. *Electroenceph. Clin. Neurophysiol.*, 1977, *43*, 671.

Popov, G. A. *Principios de la planificacíon sanitaria en la USSR*. Cuadernos de Salud Pública, *43*, Ginebra: Organización Mundial de la Salud, 1972.

Popov, S. Influence of semantic and acoustic parameters of verbal stimuli on brain activity. *Electroenceph. Clin. Neurophysiol.*, 1977, *43*, 562.

Popov, S., Ovtcharova, P., Raitchev, R., & Tzicalova, R. Evoked activity with verbal stimulation in aphasia. *Electroenceph. Clin. Neurophysiol.*, 1977, *43*, 561.

Praetorius, H. M., Bodenstein, G., & Creutzfeldt, O. D. Adaptive segmentation of EEG records: A new approach to automatic EEG analysis. *Electroenceph. Clin. Neurophysiol.*, 1977, *42*, 89-94.

Preston, M. J., Guthrie, J. T., Kirsch, I., Gertman, D., & Childs, B. VERs in normal and disabled adult readers. *Psychophysiology*, 1977, *14*, 8-14.

Prevec, T. S., & Butinar, D. Changes in somatosensory evoked potentials in multiple sclerosis patients. *Electroenceph. Clin. Neurophysiol.*, 1977, *43*, 574.

Prevec, T. S., Lokar, J., & Cernelc, S. The use of CNV in audiometry. *Audiology*, 1974, *13*, 447-457.

Priestley, M. B. Evolutionary spectra and non-stationary processes. *J. R. Statist, B.* 1965, *27*, 204-237.

Priestley, M. B. Design relation for non-stationary processes. *J. R. Statist. Soc. B.*, 1966, *28*, 228-240.

Priestley, M. B., & Rao, T. S. A test for non-stationarity of time series. *J. R. Statist. Soc. B.*, 1969, *31*, 140-149.

Prior, P. F., Maynard, D. E., & Brierley, J. B. Use of the cerebral function analyzer monitor (CFAM) in: 1) Intravenous infusion anaesthesia and 2) Hypoxia and ischaemia. *Electroenceph. Clin. Neurophysiol.*, 1977, *43*, 530.

Prior, P. F., Maynard, D. E., & Scott, D. F. A new device for continuous monitoring of cerebral activity: Its use following cerebral anoxia. *Electroenceph. Clin. Neurophysiol.*, 1970, *28*, 423-424.

Procházka, M. Some factors affecting the amplitude of averaged evoked potentials in man. *Electroenceph. Clin. Neurophysiol.*, 1971, *30*, 276.

Pronk, R. A. F., Simons, A. J. R., & de Boer, S. J. EEG as a monitoring parameter during open heart surgery. Technical aspects. *Electroenceph. Clin. Neurophysiol.*, 1977, *43*, 542.

Pruell, G. Spectral estimators of EEG (alpha band) and circadian rhythm. *Electroenceph. Clin. Neurophysiol.*, 1977, *43*, 580. (a)

Pruell, G. Clinical, electroencephalographic and biochemical follow-up studies of acute brain infarction in man and dog. *Electroenceph. Clin. Neurophysiol.*, 1977, *43*, 557. (b)

Puri, M. L. Non parametric techniques in statistical inference. Cambridge: Cambridge University Press, 1970.

Puri, M. L., & Sen, P. K. Non parametric methods in multivariate analysis. New York: Wiley, 1971.

Purpura, D. P., Scharff, T., & McMurtry, J. G. Intracellular study of internuclear inhibition in ventrolateral thalamic neurons. *Journal of Neurophysiology*, 1965, *28*, 487-496.

Purves, S. J., & Low, M. D. Visual evoked potentials to reversing pattern light emitting diode stimulation in normal subjects and patients with demyelinating disease. *Electroenceph. Clin. Neurophysiol.*, 1976, *41*, 651.

Quilter, P. M., Wadbrook, D. G., & MacGillivray, B. B. Automatic elimination of eye movement artifacts in EEG signal processing. *Electroenceph. Clin. Neurophysiol.*, 1977, *43*, 539.

Ragot, R. A., & Rémond, A. EEG field mapping. *Electroenceph. Clin. Neurophysiol.*, 1978, *45*, 417-421.

Ramos, A., Schwartz, E., & John, E. R. *Unit activity and evoked potentials during readout from memory.* Paper presented at the XXIV International Congress of Physiological Sciences, New Delhi, 1974.

Rao, T. S., & Tong, H. A. A test for time-dependence of linear open-loop systems. *J. R. Statist. Soc. B.*, 1972, *34*, 235-240.

Rapin, I., & Bergman, M. Auditory evoked responses in uncertain diagnosis. *Arch Otolaryngol.*, 1969, *90*, 307-314.

Rapin, I., & Graziani, J. Auditory evoked responses in normal, brain damaged, and deaf infants. *Neurology*, 1967, *17*, 881-894.

Rapin, I., & Schimmel, H. Assessment of auditory sensitivity in infants and in uncooperative handicapped children by using the late components of the average auditory evoked potential. In J. E. Desmedt (Ed), *Progress in clinical neurophysiology* (Vol. 2). Basel: Karger, 1977.

Rapin, I., Schimmel, H., Tourk, L. M., Krasnegor, N. A., & Pollak, C. Evoked responses to clicks and tones oV varying intensity in waking adults. *Electroenceph. Clin. Neurophysiol.*, 1966, *21*, 335-344.

Rappaport, M., Hall, K., Hopkins, K. H., Belleza, T., Berrol, S., & Reynolds, G. Evoked brain potentials and disability in brain damaged patients. *Arch. of Physiol. Med. and Rehabilitation*, 1977, *58*, 333-338.

Ravault, M. P., Gerin, P., David, C., & Munier, F. Optic nerve function and occipital evoked responses. *Arch Ophtal.* (Paris), 1966, *26*, 641-660.

Rayport, M., Vaughan, H. G., & Rosengart, C. L. Simultaneous recording of visual averaged evoked response to flash from scalp and calcarine cortex in man. *Electroenceph. Clin. Neurophysiol.*, 1964, *17*, 610.

Regan, D. Chromatic adaptation and steady state evoked potentials. *Vision Res.*, 1968, *8*, 149-158.

Regan, D. *Evoked potentials in psychology, Sensory physiology and clinical medicine.* New York: Wiley Interscience, 1972.

Regan, D. Evoked potentials in basic and clinical research. In A. Rémond (Ed.), *EEG informatics. A didactic review of methods and applications of EEG data processing.* Amsterdam: Elsevier, 1977, 319-346. (a)

Regan, D. Clinical applications of steady state evoked potentials: Speedy methods of refracting the eye and assessing visual acuity in amblyopia. In J. E. Desmedt (Ed.), *Cerebral evoked potentials in man.* London: Oxford University, 1977. (b)

Regan, D., & Heron, J. R. Clinical investigation of lesions of the visual pathway: A new objective technique. *J. Neurol. Neurosurg. Psychiat.*, 1969, *32*, 479-483.

Regan, D., & Milner, B. A. Objective perimetry by evoked potential recordings: Limitations. *Electroenceph. Clin. Neurophysiol.*, 1978, *44*, 393-397.

Regan, D., Milner, B. A., & Heron, J. R. Delayed visual perception and delayed visual evoked potentials in the spinal form of multiple sclerosis and in retrobulbar neuritis. *Brain*, 1976, *99*, 43-66.

Regan, D., & Richards, W. Brightness and contrast evoked potentials. *J. Opt. Soc. Amer.*, 1973, *63*, 606-611.

Regan, D., & Spekreijse, H. Evoked potential indications of color blindness. *Vision Res.*, 1974, *14*, 89-95.

Rémond, A. Integrated and topological analysis of the EEG. *Electroenceph. Clin. Neurophysiol.*, 1961, Suppl. *20*, 64-67.

Rémond, A. Level of organization of evoked responses in man. *Ann. N.Y. Acad. Sci.*, 1964, *112*, 143-159.

Rémond, A. The importance of topographic data in EEG phenomena and an electric model to reproduce them. *Electroenceph. Clin. Neurophysiol.*, 1968, Suppl. *27*, 29-49.

Rémond, A. An EEGer's approach to automatic data processing. In G. Dolce & H. Künkel (Eds.), *CEAN*, Stuttgart: Gustav Fischer Verlag, 1975, 128-136.

Rémond, A. (Ed.). *EEG informatics. A didactic review of methods and applications of EEG data processing.* Amsterdam: Elsevier, 1977.

Rémond, A. (Ed.). *Handbook of electroencephalography and clinical neurophysiology*, Amsterdam: Elsevier.

Rémond, A., & Conte, C. Organisation spatio-temporelle des responses EEG a la S. L. I. á la fréquence de 10 c/s. *Rev. Neurol.* (Paris), 1962, *107*, 250-257.

Rémond, A., & Lesèvre, N. Distribution topographique des potentiels évoqués occipitaux chez l'homme normal. *Rev. Neurol.*, 1965, *112*, 317-330.

Rémond, A., & Lesèvre, N. Variations in average evoked potentials as a function of the alpha rhythm phases. *Electroenceph. Clin. Neurophysiol.*, 1967, Suppl. *26*, 45-52.

Rémond, A., & Renault, B. La théorie des objects électrographiques. *Rev. EEG Neurophysiol.*, 1972, *23*, 241-256.

Rémond, A., Renault, B., Baillou, J. F., & Bienenfeld, G. Automatic time domain analysis of EEG waves. In M. Matejcek & G. K. Schenk, *Quantitative analysis in EEG.* Basel: Sandoz, 1975, 321-323.

Rémond, A., & Storm van Leeuwen, W. Why analyze, quantify or process routine clinical EEG. In A. Rémond (Ed.), *EEG informatics. A didactic review of methods and applications of EEG data processing.* Amsterdam: Elsevier, 1977.

Rémond, A., & Torres, F. A method of electrode placement with a view to topographical research. *Electroenceph. Clin. Neurophysiol.*, 1964, *17*, 577-578.

Rêmond, A., Torres, F., Lesèvre, N., & Conte, C. Quelques considerations au sujet de la distribution topographique des ondes lambda. *Rev. Neurol.*, 1964, *111*, 344.

Renault, B., Joseph, J. P., Lagarce, M., Baillon, J. F., & Rémond, A. Etudes des criteres électroencephalographiques de classification automatique des individus d'une population. *Rev. EEG Neurophysiol.*, 1975, *5*, 313-316.

Reneaw, J., & Hnatiow, G. *Evoked response audiometry: A topical and historical review.* Baltimore: University Park Press, 1975.

Rentscheller, I., & Spinelli, D. Accuracy of evoked potential refractometry using bar gratings. *Acta ophthalmologica*, 1978, *56*, 67-74.

Rey, J. H., Pond, D. A., & Evans, C. C. Clinical and electroencephalographic studies of temporal lobe function. *Proc. R. Soc. Med.*, 1949, *42*, 891-904.

Rhee, R. S., Goldensohn, E. S., & Kini, R. C. EEG characteristics of solitary intracranial lesions in relationship to anatomical location. *Electroenceph. Clin. Neurophysiol.*, 1975, *38*, 553.

Ricardo, J. Simetría de los potenciales evocados visuales en el hombre. Thesis, Havana, Havana University, 1974.

Ricardo, J., Harmony, T., & Otero, G. Symmetry of visual evoked potentials in neurological patients. In B. Holmgren & T. Harmony (Eds.), *Applications of computers to the study of the nervous system*. Havana: CENIC, 1975.

Ricardo, J., Harmony, T., Otero, G., & Llorente, S. Estudio de la respuesta de seguimiento por medio de la actividad evocada filtrada. *CENIC*, 1974, *5*, 57-66.

Richey, E. T., Kooi, K. A., & Tourtelotte, W. W. Visually evoked responses in multiple sclerosis. *J. Neurol. Neurosurg. Psychiat.*, 1971, *34*, 275-280.

Rietveld, W. J. Contributions of various retinal areas to the visual evoked potential in the human cortex. *Acta Physiol. Pharmacol. Neerl.*, 1965, *13*, 160-170.

Rietveld, W. J., Tordoir, W. E. M., Hagenoow, J. R. B., Lubbers, J. A., & Spoor, T. A. Visual evoked responses to blank and to checkerboard patterned flashes. *Acta Physiol. Pharmacol. Neerl.*, 1967, *14*, 259-284.

Rizzo, P. A., Amabile, G., Caporali, M., Spadero, M., Zanasi, M., & Morocutti, C. A CNV study in a group of patients with traumatic head injuries. *Electroenceph. Clin. Neurophysiol.*, 1978, *45*, 281-285.

Robinson, K., & Rudge, P. Abnormalities of the auditory evoked potentials in patients with multiple sclerosis. *Brain*, 1977, *100*, 19-40. (a)

Robinson, K., & Rudge, P. The early components of the auditory evoked potentials in multiple sclerosis. In J. E. Desmedt (Ed.), *Progress in clinical neurophysiology* (Vol. 2). Basel: Karger, 1977, Vol. 2, 58-67. (b)

Rodin, E. A., Grisell, J. L., Gudobba, R. D., & Zachary, G. Relationship of EEG background rhythms to photic evoked responses. *Electroenceph. Clin. Neurophysiol.*, 1965 , *19*, 301-304.

Rodríguez, V., Garriga, E., Valdés, P., & Harmony, T. *Métodos de clasificación automática.* Paper presented at the VI Seminario Cientifico CENIC, Havana, 1977.

Roger, A., & Bert, J. Etudes des corrélations entre les differentes variables EEG. *Rev. Neurol.*, 1959, *101*, 334-360.

Rohrbaugh, J. W., Syndulko, K., & Lindsley, D. B. Brain wave components of the Contingent Negative Variation in humans. *Science*, 1976, *191*, 1055-1057.

Rohuer, F., Plane, C., & Solé, P. Intéret des potentiels évoqués visuels dans les affectations du nerf optique. *Arch. Ophtal.* (Paris), 1969, *29*, 555–564.

Rose, F. C. *Visual evoked potentials in migraine patients.* Paper presented at the 11th World Congress of Neurology, Amsterdam, 1977.

Rossini, P. M., Torrioli, M. G., Sollazzo, D., Albertini, G., & Gambi, D. VER and EEG recording in the assessment of pre-term newborn infants. *Electroenceph. Clin. Neurophysiol.*, 1977, *43*, 481.

Roth, W. T., Krainz, P. L., Ford, J. M., Tinklenberg, J. R., Rothbart, R. M., & Kopell, B. S. Parameters of temporal recovery of the human auditory evoked potential. *Electroenceph. Clin. Neurophysiol.*, 1976, *40*, 623-632.

Rowe, M. J. The brain stem auditory evoked response in post concussion vertigo. *Electroenceph. Clin. Neurophysiol.*, 1977, *43*, 454.

Rowe, M. J. Normal variability of the brain-stem auditory evoked response in young and old subjects. *Electroenceph. Clin. Neurophysiol.*, 1978, *44*, 459-470.

Ruchkin, D. S. Error of correlation coefficient estimates from polarity coincidences. *IEEE Trans. Inf. Theory*, 1965, *IT-11*, 296-297. (a)

Ruchkin, D. S. An analysis of average response computation based upon aperiodic stimuli. *IEEE Trans. Biomed. Eng.*, 1965, *BME-12*, 87-94. (b)

Ruchkin, D. S. Sorting of non homogeneous sets of evoked potentials. *Communications in Behavioral Biology*, 1971, *5*, 383-396.

Ruchkin, D. S., & Walter, D. O. A shortcoming of the median evoked response. *IEEE Trans. Biomed. Eng.*, 1975, *BME-23*, 245.

Ruhm, H. B., Walter, E., & Flanigin, H. Acoustically evoked potentials in man: Mediation of early components. *Laryngoscope*, 1967, *77*, 806-822.

Rust, J. Genetic effects in the cortical auditory evoked potential: A twin study. *Electroenceph. Clin. Neurophysiol.*, 1975, *39*, 321-327.

Sainio, K., Kaste, M., & Stenberg, D. *Quantitative EEG and rcBF in ischaemic brain infarction. Value in early diagnosis.* Paper presented at the 11th World Congress of Neurology, Amsterdam, 1977.

Salamy, A., & McKean, C. M. Postnatal development of human brain stem potentials during the first year of life. *Electroenceph. Clin. Neurophysiol.*, 1976, *40*, 418-426.

Salamy, A., McKean, C. M., & Buda, F. Maturational changes in auditory transmission as reflected in human brain stem potentials. *Brain Res.*, 1975, *96*, 361-366.

Saletu, B., Itil, T. M., & Saletu, M. Auditory evoked response, EEG and thought process in schizophrenics. *American Journal of Psychiatry*, 1971, *128*, 336-344.

Saletu, B., Saletu, M., & Itil, T. M. The relationships between psychopathology and evoked responses before, during and after psychotropic drug treatment. *Biological Psychiatry*, 1973, *6*, 46-74.

Saletu, B., Saletu, M., Simeon, J., Viamontes, G., & Itil, T. M. Comparative symptomatological and evoked potential studies with d-amphetamine, thioridazine and placebo in hyperkinetic children. *Biological Psychiatry*, 1975, *10*, 253-275.

Saltzberg, B. Period analysis. In *Handbook of electroencephalography and clinical neurophysiology* (Vol. 5A). Amsterdam: Elsevier, 1973, 67-75.

Saltzberg, B., & Burch, N. R. A new approach to signal analysis in electroencephalography. *IRE Trans. Med. Electron.*, 1957, *8*, 24-30.

Saltzberg, B., & Burch, N. R. Period analytic estimates of moments of the power spectrum: A simplified EEG time domain procedure. *Electroenceph. Clin. Neurophysiol.*, 1971, *30*, 568-570.

Saltzberg, B., Heath, R. G., & Edwards, R. J. EEG spike detection in schizophrenia research. Digest of the 7th Int. Conf. Med. Biol. Eng. Stockholm, 1967.

Saltzberg, B., Lustick, L. S., & Heath, R. G. A non-parametric method of determining general EEG changes due to administration of drugs. *Electroenceph. Clin. Neurophysiol.*, 1970, *28*, 102.

Saltzberg, B., Lustick, L. S., & Heath, R. G. Detection of focal depth spiking in the scalp EEG of monkeys. *Electroenceph. Clin. Neurophysiol.*, 1971, *31*, 327-333.

Samland, O., Przuntek, H., & Dommasch, D. Cortical evoked potentials in hepatolenticular degeneration. *Electroenceph. Clin. Neurophysiol.*, 1976, *41*, 665.

Sammon, J. W. A non linear mapping for data structure analysis. *IEEE Trans. Comput.*, 1969, *C-18*, 401-409.

Samson-Dollfus, D. *L'EEG du prémature jusqu'á l'age de 3 mois et du noveau-né á terme*. Thesis, University of Paris, 1955.

Samson-Dollfus, D., & Pouliquen, A. Visual evoked potentials applied to the study of lateral homonymous hemianopia. *Electroenceph. Clin. Neurophysiol.*, 1977, *42*, 859.

Sato, K., Keiich, M., Sata, H., Ochi, N., & Ishino, T. On random fluctuations in EEG and evoked potentials. *The Japanese Journal of Physiology*, 1970, *21*, 167-185.

Sato, K., Kitajima, H., Mimura, K., Hirota, N., Tagawa, Y., & Ochi, N. Cerebral visual evoked potentials in relation to EEG. *Electroenceph. Clin. Neurophysiol.*, 1971, *30*, 123-138.

Sato, K., Ono, K., Chiba, G., & Fukata, K. On some methods for EEG pattern discrimination. *Intern. J. Neuroscience.*, 1977, *7*, 201-206.

Satterfield, J. H., & Braley, B. W. Evoked potentials and brain maturation in hyperactive and normal children. *Electroenceph. Clin. Neurophysiol.*, 1977, *43*, 43-51.

Saunders, M. G. Amplitude probability density studies on alpha-like patterns. *Electroenceph. Clin. Neurophysiol.*, 1963, *15*, 761-767.

Saunders, M. G. Averaging photic driving responses. *Electroenceph. Clin. Neurophysiol.*, 1976, *40*, 214.

Schafer, E. W. P. Cortical activity preceding speech: Semantic specificity. *Nature* (London), 1967, *216*, 1338-1339.

Schenk, G. K. Vektorielle zero-crossing-technik. *EEG-EMG*, 1972, *3*, 198.

Schenk, G. K. The pattern-oriented aspect of EEG quantification. Model and clinical basis of the Iterative Time Domain Approach. In P. Kellaway & I. Petersén (Eds.), *Quantitative analytic studies in epilepsy*. New York: Raven Press, 1976, 431-462.

Schenkenberg, T., Dustman, R. E., & Beck, E. C. Changes in evoked responses related to age, hemisphere and sex. *Electroenceph. Clin. Neurophysiol.*, 1971, *30*, 163.

Scherrer, J., Verley, R., & Garma, L. A review of French studies in the ontogenical field. In W. Himwich (Ed.), *Developmental neurobiology* (Vol. 16). Springfield: Charles C. Thomas, 1970, 528-549.

Schneider, J. Cerebral tumours and evoked potentials. *Electroenceph. Clin. Neurophysiol.*, 1968, *25*, 586.

Schwartz, E., & John, E. R. Unpublished observations, 1976. See John, 1977.

Schwartz, M., & Shagass, C. Recovery functions of human somatosensory and visual evoked potentials. *Ann. N.Y. Acad. Sci.*, 1964, *112*, 510-525.

Schwartzova, K., & Synek, V. The significance of diffuse slow activity in the EEG in cerebral arterioesclerosis. *Electroenceph. Clin. Neurophysiol.*, 1969, *26*, 230.

Schweitzer, P. K., & Tepas, D. I. Intensity effect of the auditory evoked brain response to stimulus onset and cessation. *Perception and Psychophysics*, 1974, *16*, 396-400.

Schwent, V. L., Hillyard, S. A., & Galambos, R. Selective attention and the auditory vertex potential. Effects of stimulus delivery rate. *Electroenceph. Clin. Neurophysiol.*, 1976, *40*, 604-614. (a)

Schwent, V. L., Hillyard, S. A., & Galambos, R. Selective attention and the auditory vertex potential. II:Effects of signal intensity and masking noise. *Electroenceph. Clin. Neurophysiol.*, 1976, *40*, 615-622. (b)

Sclabassi, R. J., Namerow, N. S., & Enns, N. F. Somatosensory response to stimulus trains in patients with multiple sclerosis. *Electroenceph. Clin. Neurophysiol.*, 1974, *37*, 23-33.

Shagass, C. *Evoked brain potentials in psychiatry*. New York: Plenum, 1972.

Shagass, C., Amadeo, M., & Roemer, R. A. Spatial distribution of potentials evoked by half-field pattern reversal and pattern-onset stimuli. *Electroenceph. Clin. Neurophysiol.*, 1976, *41*, 609-622.

Shagass, C., Schwartz, M., & Straumanis, J. J. Subject factors related to variability of averaged evoked responses. *Electroenceph. Clin. Neurophysiol.*, 1966, *20*, 97.

Shagass, C., Straumanis, J. J., Roemer, R. A., & Amadeo, M. Evoked potentials of schizophrenics in several sensory modalities. *Biological Psychiatry*, 1977, *12*, 221-235.

Shahrokhi, F., Chiappa, K. H., & Young, R. Y. Pattern shift visual evoked responses. *Arch. of Neurology*, 1978, *35*, 65-71.

Shannon, C. E., & Weaver, W. *The mathematical theory of communication*. University of Illinois Press, 1949.

Shapiro, S. S., & Wilk, M. S. An analysis of variance test for normality. *Biometrika*, 1965, *52*, 591-611.

Shapiro, S. S., Wilk, M. S., & Chen, S. J. A. A comparative study of tests of normality. *J. Amer. Stat. Ass.*, 1968, *63*, 1343-1372.

Sheridan, F. P., Yeager, C. L., Oliver, W. A., & Simon, A. Electroencephalography as a diagnostic and prognostic aid in studying the senescent individual: A preliminary report. *J. Geront.*, 1955, *10*, 53-59.

Sheuler, W., & Ulrich, G. Event related potentials and EEG in a case of auditory agnosia. *Electroenceph. Clin. Neurophysiol.*, 1977, *43*, 480.

Shibasaki, H. Movement-associated cortical potentials in unilateral cerebral lesions. *J. Neurol.*, 1975, *209*, 189-198.

Shibasaki, H., & Kato, M. Movement associated cortical potentials with unilateral and bilateral simultaneous hand movement. *J. Neurol.*, 1975, *208*, 191-199.

Shibasaki, H., & Kuroiwa, Y. *Clinical studies of the movement-related cortical potentials*. Paper presented at the 11th World Congress of Neurology, Amsterdam, 1977.

Shibasaki, H., Tamashita, Y., & Kuroiwa, Y. Electroencephalographic studies of myoclonus. *Electroenceph. Clin. Neurophysiol.*, 1977, *43*, 455. (b)

Shibasaki, H., Tamashita, Y., & Tsuji, S. Somatosensory evoked potentials. *J. of Neurol. Sciences*, 1977, *34*, 427-439. (a)

Shimizu, H. Evoked response in VIIIth nerve lesions. *Laryngoscope*, 1968, *78*, 2140-2152.

Shimoji, K., Higashi, T., & Kano, T. Epidural recordings of spinal electrogram in man. *Electroenceph. Clin. Neurophysiol.*, 1971, *30*, 236-239.

Shimoji, K., Kano, T., Morioka, T., & Ikezono, E. Evoked spinal electrogram in a quadriplegic patient. *Electroenceph. Clin. Neurophysiol.*, 1973, *35*, 659-662.

Shimoji, K., Matsuki, M., & Shimizu, H. Waveform characteristics and spatial distribution of evoked spinal electrogram in man. *J. Neurosurg.*, 1977, *46*, 304-314.

Shipley, T., Jones, R. W., & Fry, A. Evoked visual potentials and human color vision. *Science*, 1965, *150*, 1162-1164.

Shipton, H. W. A new frequency-selective toposcope for electroencephalography. *Med. Biol. Eng.*, 1963, *1*, 403-495.

Short, M. J., Musella, L., & Wilson, W. P. Correlation of affect and EEG in senile psychoses. *J. Geront.*, 1968, *23*, 324-327.

Siegel, S. *Diseño experimental no paramétrico*. Havana: Instituto del Libro, 1970.

Simonova, O., Foth, B., & Stein, J. EEG studies of healthy population—normal rhythms of resting recording. *Act. Univ. Carol. Med* (Praha), 1967, *13*, 543-551.

Simson, R., Vaughan, H. G., & Ritter, W. The scalp topography of potentials associated with missing visual or auditory stimuli. *Electroenceph. Clin. Neurophysiol.*, 1976, *40*, 33-42.

Simson, R., Vaughan, H. G., & Ritter, W. The scalp topography of potentials in auditory and visual go/no go tasks. *Electroenceph. Clin. Neurophysiol.*, 1977, *43*, 864-875.

Sklar, B., Hanley, J., & Simmons, W. W. A computer analysis of EEG spectral signatures from normal and dyslexic children. *Trans. Biomed. Eng..*, 1973, *20*, 20-26.

Small, D. G., Beauchamp, M., & Matthews, W. B. Spinal evoked potentials in multiple sclerosis. *Electroenceph. Clin. Neurophysiol.*, 1977, *42*, 141-145.

Small, D. G., & Jones, S. J. Subcortical somatosensory evoked potentials following stimulation at the wrist or the ankle in normal subjects. *Electroenceph. Clin. Neurophysiol.*, 1977, *43*, 536.

Smith, J. C., Marsh, J. T., & Brown, W. S. Far-field recorded frequency-following responses: Evidence for the locus of brainstem sources. *Electroenceph. Clin. Neurophysiol.*, 1975, *39*, 465-472.

Smith, J. R. Automatic analysis and detection of EEG spikes. *IEEE Trans. Biomed. Eng.*, 1974, *BME-21*, 1-7.

Sohmer, H., Feinmesser, M., Bauberger-Tell, L., & Edelstein, E. Cochlear, brain stem and cortical evoked responses in nonorganic hearing loss. *Ann. Otol.*, 1977, *86*, 227-234. (a)

Sohmer, H., Pratt, H., & Kinarti, R. Sources of frequence following responses (FFR) in man. *Electroenceph. Clin. Neurophysiol.*, 1977, *42*, 656-664. (b)

Sohmer, H., & Student, M. Auditory nerve and brain-stem evoked responses in normal, autistic, minimal brain dysfunction and psychomotor retarded children. *Electroenceph. Clin. Neurophysiol.*, 1978, *44*, 380-388.

Sokol., S. Measurement of infant visual acuity from pattern reversal evoked potentials. *Vision Res.*, 1978, *18*, 33-39.

Spehlman, R. The averaged electrical responses to diffuse and to patterned light in the human. *Electroenceph. Clin. Neurophysiol.*, 1965, *19*, 560-569.

Spehr, W., Sartorius, H., Beiglund, K., Hjorth, B., Kablitz, C., Plog, U., Wiedemann, P. H., & Zapf, K. EEG and haemodialysis. A structural survey EEG spectral analysis,

Hjorth's EEG descriptors, blood variables and psychological data. *Electroenceph. Clin. Neurophysiol.*, 1977, *43*, 787-797.

Spekreijse, H., de Vries-Khoe, L. H., & van den Berg, T. J. T. P. The development of luminance and pattern EP's in infants. *Electroenceph. Clin. Neurophysiol.*, 1977, *43*, 576.

Spekreijse, H., & Van der Tweel, L. H. *Flicker and noise. Clnical electroretinography.* Supplement of Vision Research, Proceedings of the third International Symposium held in October, 1964. Oxford: Pergamon Press, 1966, 275-280.

Spekreijse, H., Van der Tweel, L. H., & Zuidema, T. Contrast evoked potentials in man. *Vision Res.*, 1973, *13*, 1577-1601.

Spilker, B., & Callaway, E. Augmenting and reducing in averaged visual evoked responses to sine wave light. *Psychophysiology*, 1969, *6*, 49-57.

Spilker, B., Kamiya, J., Callaway, E., & Yeager, C. L. Visual evoked responses in subjects trained to control alpha rhythms. *Psychphysiology*, 1969, *5/6*, 683-695.

Spoelstra, P. J., Wieneke, G. H., & Storm Van Leeuwen, W. A system for the EEG power spectra in clinical situation. *Electroenceph. Clin. Neurophysiol.*, 1977, *43*, 564.

Spunda, J., & Radil-Weiss, T. A simple instrument suitable for measuring the instantaneous frequency of the dominant activity. *Electroenceph. Clin. Neurophysiol.*, 1972, *32*, 434-437.

Squires, K. C., & Donchin, E. Beyond averaging: The use of discriminant function to recognize event related potentials elicited by single auditory stimuli. *Electroenceph. Clin. Neurophysiol.*, 1976, *41*, 449-459.

Starr, A. Auditory brain stem responses in brain death. *Brain*, 1976, *99*, 543-554.

Starr, A. Clinical relevance of brain stem auditory evoked potentials in brain stem disorders in man. In J. E. Desmedt (Ed.), *Progress in clinical neurophysiology* (Vol. 2). Basel: Karger, 1977.

Starr, A. Sensory evoked potentials in clinical disorders of the nervous system. *Ann. Rev. Neurosci.*, 1978, *1*, 103-127.

Starr, A., & Achor, L. J. Auditory brain stem responses in neurological disease. *Arch. Neurol.*, 1975, *32*, 761-768.

Starr, A., & Hamilton, H. E. Correlation between confirmed sites of neurological lesions and abnormalities of far-field auditory brain stem responses. *Electroenceph. Clin. Neurophysiol.*, 1976, *41*, 595-608.

Stenberg, D., Sainio, K., & Kaste, M. EEG frequency descriptors in cerebral infarction. *Electroenceph. Clin. Neurophysiol.*, 1977, *43*, 524.

Sterman, M. B., Harper, R. M., Havens, B., Hoppenbrouwers, T., McGinty, D. J., & Hodgman, J. E. Quantitative analysis of infant EEG development during quiet sleep. *Electroenceph. Clin. Neurophysiol.*, 1977, *43*, 371-385.

Stevens, J. R., Kodamo, H., Lonsbury, B., & Mills, L. Ultradian characteristics of spontaneous seizures discharges recorded by radio telemetry in man. *Electroenceph. Clin. Neurophysiol.*, 1971, *31*, 313-325.

Stillman, R. D., Crow, G., & Moushegian, G. Components of the frequency-following potential in man. *Electroenceph. Clin. Neurophysiol.*, 1978, *44*, 438-446.

Stockard, J. J., & Rossiter, V. S. Clinical and pathologic correlates of brain stem auditory response abnormalities. *Neurology*, 1977, *27*, 316-325.

Stockard, J. J., Rossiter, V. S., Jones, T. A., & Sharbrough, F. W. Effects of centrally acting drugs on brainstem auditory responses. *Electroenceph. Clin. Neurophysiol.*, 1977, *43*, 550.

Stockard, J. J., Rossiter, V. S., & Wiederholt, W. C. Brainstem auditory evoked responses in suspected central pontine myelinolysis. *Arch. Neurol.*, 1976, *33*, 726-728.

Stohr, P. E., & Goldring, S. Origin of somatosensory evoked scalp responses in man. *J. Neurosurg.*, 1969, *31*, 117-121.

Storm van Leeuwen, W., Bickford, R. G., Brazier, M., Cobb, W. A., Dondey, M., Gastaut, use of spectral analysis in clinical EEG. *Electroenceph. Clin. Neurophysiol.*, 1977, *43*, 566.

Storm van Leeuwen, W., Bickford, R., Brazier, M., Cobb, W. A., Dondey, M., Gastaut, H., Gloor, P., Henry, C. E., Hess, R., Knott, J. R., Kugler, J., Lairy, G. C., Loeb, C., Magnus, O., Oller-Daurella, L., Petsche, H., Schwab, R., Walter, W. G., & Widen L. Proposal for an EEG terminology by the terminology committee of the international federation for electroencephalography and clinical neurophysiology. *Electroenceph. Clin. Neurophysiol.*, 1966, *20*, 306-310.

Storm van Leeuwen, W., Lopes da Silva, F. H., & Kamp, H. (Eds.) Evoked responses. In *Handbook of electroencephalography and clinical neurophysiology* (Vol. 8A). Amsterdam: Elsevier, 1975.

Strackee, J., & Cerri, S. A. Some statistical aspects of digital Wiener filtering and detection of prescribed frequency components in time averaging of biological signals. *Biological Cybernetics*, 1977, *28*, 55-61.

Straumanis, J. J., Shagass, C., & Schwartz, M. Visually evoked cerebral response changes associated with chronic brain syndromes and aging. *J. Gerontol.*, 1965, *20*, 498-505.

Streletz, L. J., Katz, L., Hohenberger, M., & Cracco, R. Q. Scalp recorded auditory evoked potentials and sonomotor responses: An evaluation of components and recording techniques. *Electroenceph. Clin. Neurophysiol.*, 1977, *43*, 192-206.

Sugerman, A. A., Goldstein, L., Murphee, H. B., Pfeiffer, C. C., & Jenney, E. H. EEG and behavioral changes in schizophrenia. *Arch gen Psychiat.*, 1964, *10*, 340-344.

Sulg, I., Hokkanen, E., Saarela, E., Arranto, J., Sotaniemi, K., Reunanen, M., & Hollmen, A. *Computerized quantitative EEG and blood pressure monitoring during high risk surgery*. Paper presented at the 11th World Congress of Neurology, Amsterdam, 1977.

Surwillo, W. W. Cortical evoked response recovery functions: Physiological manifestations of the psychological refractory period? *Psychophysiology*, 1977, *14*, 32-39. (a)

Surwillo, W. W. Changes in the electroencephalogram accompanying the use of stimulant drugs (methylphenidate and dextroamphetamine) in hyperactive children. *Biological Psychiatry*, 1977, *12*, 787-799. (b)

Suzuki, H. Phase relationships of alpha rhythm in man. *Jap. J. Physiol.*, 1974, *24*, 569-586.

Suzuki, T. A., & Taguchi, K. Cerebral evoked responses to auditory stimuli in waking man. *Ann. Otolaryngol.*, 1965, *74*, 128–139.

Suzuki, T. A., Taguchi, K. Cerebral evoked responses to auditory stimuli in young children during sleep. *Ann. Otol. Rhinol. Laryngol.*, 1968, *77*, 102-110.

Symann-Lovett, N., Gascon, G. G., Matsumiya, Y., & Lombroso, C. T. Waveform difference in visual evoked responses between normal and reading disabled children. *Neurology*, 1977, *27*, 156-159.

Syndulko, K., & Lindsley, D. B. Motor and sensory determinants of cortical slow potential shifts in man. In J. E. Desmedt (Ed.), *Progress in clinical neurophysiology* (Vol. 1). Basel: Karger, 1977, 97–131.

Szirtes, J., Rothenberger, A., & Jürgens, R. Averaged evoked potentials to verbal stimuli in normal, aphasic and right hemisphere damaged subjects. *Electroenceph. Clin. Neurophysiol.*, 1977, *43*, 467.

Taghavy, A. Somatosensory evoked potentials in tumours of the corpus callosum. *Electroenceph. Clin. Neurophysiol.*, 1977, *42*, 436.

Takahashi, K. Frequency analysis of clinical EEG with a digital computer. Comparative study with Fourier analysis. *Electroenceph. Clin. Neurophysiol.*, 1977, *43*, 483.

Takahashi, K., & Fujitani, Y. Somatosensory and visual evoked potentials in hyperthyroidism. *Electroenceph. Clin. Neurophysiol.*, 1970, *29*, 551-556.

Tamura, K. Ipsilateral somatosensory evoked response in man. *Folia Psychiat. Neurol. Jap.*, 1972, *26*, 83-94.

Tamura, K., Lüders, H., & Kuroiwa, Y. Further observations on the effect of aging on the wave form of the somatosensory cortical evoked potential. *Electroenceph. Clin. Neurophysiol.*, 1972, *33*, 325-327.

Tanguay, P. E., Lee, J. C. M., & Ornitz, E. M. A detailed analysis of the auditory evoked response wave form in children during REM and stage 2 sleep. *Electroenceph. Clin. Neurophysiol.*, 1973, *35*, 241-248.

Tatsuno, J., Marsoner, H. J., & Wageneder, F. M. Topography of acoustically evoked potentials triggered by alpha activity. *Acta Biol. Med. German*, 1970, *25*, 441-446.

Tchavdarov, D., & Matveev, M. Value and application of simultaneous amplitude period analysis. *Electroenceph. Clin. Neurophysiol.*, 1977, *43*, 532.

Tepas, D. I., Boxerman, L. A., & Anch, A. M. Auditory evoked brain responses: Intensity functions from bipolar human scalp recordings. *Percep. Psychophys.*, 1972, *11*, 217-221.

Thatcher, R. W., & John, E. R. *Functional neuroscience, Vol. I. Foundations of cognitive processes*. Hillsdale, New Jersey: Lawrence Erlbaum Associateds, 1977.

Thomsen, J., Terkildsen, K., & Osterhammel, P. Auditory brain stem responses in patients with acoustic neuromas. *Scand. Audiol.*, 1978, *7*, 1-5.

Thornton, A. R., Bilaterally recorded early acoustic responses. *Scand. Audiol.*, 1975, *41*, 173-181.

Thornton, A. R., Mendel, M. I., & Anderson, C. V. Effects of stimulus frequency and intensity on the middle components of the averaged auditory electroencephalographic response. *Journal of Speech and Hearing Res.*, 1977, *20*, 81-94.

Timsit, Koninckx, N., Dargent, J., Fontaine, O., & Dougier, M. Etude de la durée des VCN chez un groupe de sujets normaux, un groupe de néurosés et un groupe de psychotiques. In J. Dangent & M. Dougier, (Eds.), *Variations contingentes négatives*. Belgium: University of Liege, 1969, 206-214.

Timsit-Berthier, M., Gerono, A., & Rousseau, J. CNV variations of amplitude and duration during low level of arousal: The "distraction-arousal" hypothesis reconsidered. *Electroenceph. Clin. Neurophysiol.*, 1977, *43*, 471.

Toman, J. Flicker potentials and alpha rhythm in man. *J. Neurophysiol.*, 1941, *4*, 51-61.

Townsend, R. E., Lubin, A., & Naitoh, P. Stabilization of alpha frequency by sinusoidally modulated light. *Electroenceph. Clin. Neurophysiol.*, 1975, *39*, 515-518.

Tukey, J. W. Commentary, a data analyst's comments on a variety of points and issues. In E. Callaway, P. Tueting, & S. H. Koslow (Eds.), *Event-related potentials in man*. New York: Academic Press, 1978.

Tyner, F. S., & Knott, J. R. Amplitude asymmetries when using subdermal electrodes: Is accurate head marking sufficient? *Electroenceph. Clin. Neurophysiol.*, 1977, *43*, 767.

Ulett, G. Electroencephalograms of dogs with experimental space-occupying intracranial lesions. *Arch. Neurol. Psychiat.*, 1945, *54*, 141-149.

Umezaki, H., & Morrell, F. Developmental study of photic responses evoked in premature infants. *Electroenceph. Clin. Neurophysiol.*, 1970, *28*, 55-63.

Ungan, P., & Basar, E. Comparison of Wiener filtering and selective averaging of evoked potentials. *Electroenceph. Clin. Neurophysiol.*, 1976, *40*, 516-520.

Ungher, J., Ciurea, E., & Volanski, D. Influence of brain lesions on the electrical response to rhythmic photic stimulation. *Fiziol. Z.*, 1961, *47*, 704-710. (Russian)

Valdés, P. Principal component analysis of visual evoked responses. Unpublished results, 1974.

Valdés, P. Propiedades estocásticas de los potenciales evocados visuales. Thesis, Havana University, 1978.

Valdés, P., & Baez, O. *Utilizacíon del análisis discriminante no lineal paso a paso en la selección de variables.* Paper presented at the VI Seminario CENIC, 1977.

Valdés, P., Harmony, T., & Ricardo, J. Clasificación de los potenciales evocados visuales del hombre. *CENIC*, 1974, *5*, 73-80.

Valdés, P., Ricardo, J., & Harmony, T. Automatic classification of visual evoked potentials. In B. Holmgren & T. Harmony (Eds.), *Application of computers to the study of the nervous system.* Havana: CENIC, 1975.

Valdés, P., Valdés, M., & Baez, O. Método de extraccion de components relacionados a eventos en los respuestas. Unpublished results, 1979.

Van der Sandt, W. Clinical application of Evoked Response Audiometry. *South African Medical Journal.*, 1969, *43*, 33-35.

Van der Tweel, L. H., Sem-Jacobsen, C. W., Kamp, A., Storm van Leeuwen, W., & Veringa, F. T. H. Objective determination of response to modulated light. *Acta Physiol. Pharmacol. Neerl.*, 1958, *7*, 528.

Van der Tweel, L. H., & Verduyn-Lunel, H. F. E. Human visual responses to sinusoidally modulated light. *Electroenceph. Clin. Neurophysiol.*, 1965, *18*, 587-598.

Van Dis, H., Corner, M., Dapper, R., & Hanewald, G. Consistency of individual differences in the human EEG during quiet wakefulness. *Electroenceph. Clin. Neurophysiol.*, 1977, *43*, 574.

Van Hoek, L. O., & Thijssen, J. M. Contributions of luminosity and color contrast to the steady state evoked respons. *Ophthal. Res.*, 1977, *9*, 54-61.

Van Huffelen, A. C., Van der Wulp, C. J. M., Poortvliet, M. J. C., Van der Holst, M. J. C., & Magnus, O. Computerized EEG analysis in patients with ischemic cerebrovascular disease. A- Spontaneous activity. *Electroenceph. Clin. Neurophysiol.*, 1977, *43*, 545.

Varner, J. L., Ellingson, R. J., Danahy, T., & Nelson, B. Interhemispheric amplitude symmetry in the EEGs of full-term newborns. *Electroenceph. Clin. Neurophysiol.*, 1977, *43*, 846-852.

Vaughan, H. G. The relationship of brain activity to scalp recordings of event related potentials. In E. Donchin & D. B. Lindsley (Eds.), *Average evoked potentials.* Washington, D.C.: NASA, 1969, 45-75.

Vaughan, H. G. The motor potentials. In *Handbook of electroencephalography and clinical neurophysiology* (Vol. 8A). Amsterdam: Elsevier, 1975, 86-91.

Vaughan, H. G., Arezzo, J., & Pickoff, A. S. The intracranial sources of the averaged auditory evoked response in the monkey. *Electroenceph. Clin. Neurophysiol.*, 1974, *37*, 199-213.

Vaughan, H. G., Costa, L. D., Gilden, L., & Schimmel, H. Identification of sensory and motor components of cerebral activity in simple reaction tasks. *Proceedings of the 73rd Convention of the American Psychological Association*, 1965, *1*, 179-180.

Vaughan, H. G., & Gross, E. G. Cortical responses to light in unaesthetized monkeys and their alteration by visual system lesions. *Exp. Brain Res.*, 1969, *8*, 19-36.

Vaughan, H. G., & Katzman, R. Evoked responses in visual disorders. *Ann. N.Y. Acad. Sci.*, 1964, *112*, 305-319.

Vaughan, H. G., Katzman, R., & Taylor, J. Alterations of visual evoked response in the presence of homonymous visual defects. *Electroencehp. Clin. Neurophysiol.*, 1963, *15*, 737-746.

Vaughan, H. G., & Ritter, W. The sources of auditory evoked responses recorded from the human scalp. *Electroenceph. Clin. Neurophysiol.*, 1970, *28*, 360-367.

Velasco, M., López, M., Zenteno-Alanís, G., & Velasco, F. Signos electroencefalográficos de las neoplasias intracraneales. Valoración crítica de 136 casos con diagnóstico histopatológico. *Arch. Invest. Med.*, 1970, *1*, 93-108.

Velasco, M., & Velasco, F. Differential effect of selective attention on early and late components of cortical and subcortical somatic evoked responses in man. *Electroenceph. Clin. Neurophysiol.*, 1975, *39*, 157-163.

Velasco, M., Velasco, F., Lombardo, P. C., & Lombardo, L. Somatosensory evoked potentials in patients with cerebrovascular lesions verified by computerized axial tomography. *Electroenceph. Clin. Neurophysiol.*, 1977, *43*, 488.

Velasco, M., Velasco, F., Maldonado, H., & Machado, J. P. Differential effect of thalamic and subthalamic lesions on early and late components of the somatic evoked potentials in man. *Electroenceph. Clin. Neurophysiol.*, 1975, *39*, 163-171.

Verzeano, M. Pacemarkers, synchronization and epilepsy. In H. Petsche & M. A. B. Brazier (Eds.), *Synchronization of EEG activities in epilepsies*. New York: Springer Verlag, 1972, 154-188.

Victor, N. A non linear discriminant analysis. *Computer Programs in Biomedicine*, 1971, *2*, 36-50.

Vidal, J. J. *Neurocybernetics and man-machine* (Proceeding of International Conference on Cybernetics). San Francisco, 1975.

Viglione, S. S. *Final report: Validation of the epileptic seizure warning system*. Huntington Beach, California, McDonnel Douglas Astronautics Company, 1975.

Viglione, S. S., Ordon, V. A., & Risch, F. A methodology for detecting ongoing changes in the EEG prior to clinical seizures. MDAC Paper WD 1399 A. Huntington Beach, California, McDonnel Douglas Astronautics Company, 1970.

Viglione, S. S., Ordon, V. A., & Risch, F. Device for prediction of onset of seizures. *Electroenceph. Clin. Neurophysiol.*, 1974, *36*, 215-216.

Viglione, S. S., & Walsh, G. O. Epileptic seizure prediction. *Electroenceph. Clin. Neurophysiol.*, 1976, *41*, 649.

Visser, S. L., Stam, F. C., Van Tilburg, W., Op den Velde, W., Blom, J. L., & De Rijke, W. Visual evoked response in senile and presenile dementia. *Electroenceph. Clin. Neurophysiol.*, 1976, *40*, 385-392.

Vitová, Z. Cerebral responses to flickering light in clinical research. *Activitas Nervosa Superior* (Praha), 1973, *15*, 63-69.

Vitová, Z., & Faladová, L. Visual evoked responses and cerebral disorders in children. *Electroenceph. Clin. Neurophysiol.*, 1975, *39*, 439. (a)

Vitová, Z., & Faladová, L. Somatosensory responses in clinical research. *Activitas Nervosa Superior* (Praha), 1975, *17*, 1-6. (b)

Vitová, Z., & Hrbek, A. Ontogeny of cerebral responses to flickering light in human infants during wakefulness and sleep. *Electroenceph. Clin. Neurophysiol.*, 1970, *28*, 391.

Vivion, M. C., Goldstein, R., Wolf, K. E., & McFarland, W. H. Middle components of human auditory averaged electroencephalographic response: Waveform variations during averaging. *Audiology*, 1977, *16*, 21-37.

Vogel, F. The genetic basis of the normal human electroencephalogram. *Hum. Genet.*, 1970, *10*, 91-114.

Vogel, F., & Fujiya, Y. The incidence of some inherited EEG variants in normal Japanese and German males. *Human Genet.*, 1969, *7*, 38-42.

Vogel, F., & Götze, W. Statistische Betrachtungen über die ß-wellen im EEG des Menschen. *Dtsch. Z. Nervenheilk.*, 1962, *184*, 112-136.

Vogel, W., Broverman, D. M., Klaiber, E. L., & Kobayashi, Y. EEG driving responses as a function of monoamine oxidase. *Electroenceph. Clin. Neurophysiol.*, 1974, *36*, 205-207. (a)

Vogel, W., Broverman, D. M., Klaiber, E. L., & Kobayashi, Y. The effect of MAO inhibitors on the EEG driving response to light in normal subjects. *Electroenceph. Clin. Neurophysiol.*, 1974, *37*, 202. (b)

Vogel, W., Broverman, D. M., Klaiber, E. L., & Kun, K. J. EEG response to photic stimulation as a function of cognitive style. *Electroenceph. Clin. Neurophysiol.*, 1969, *27*, 186.

Voitinsky, E., Livshitz, M. E., & Romm, B. I. Study of differential law of amplitude distribution of brain potentials. *Biofisika*, 1972, *17*, 922-924.

Volavka, J., Feldstein, S., Abrams, R., Dombush, R., & Fink, M. EEG and clinical change after bilateral and unilateral electroconvulsive therapy. *Electroenceph. Clin. Neurophysiol.*, 1972, *32*, 631-639.

Volavka, J., Last, S. L., & Maynard, D. E. EEG frequency analysis during light sleep. *Activitas Nervosa Superior* (Praha), 1969, *11*, 234-237.

Volavka, J., Matousek, M., & Roubicek, J. EEG frequency analysis in schizophrenia. An attempt to reconsider the role of age. *Acta psychiat. Scand.*, 1966, *42*, 237-245.

Volavka, J., Matousek, M., Roubicek, J., Feldstein, S., Brezinova, N., Prior, P. I., Scott, D. F., & Synek, V. The reliability of visual EEG assessment. *Electroenceph. Clin. Neurophysiol.*, 1971, *31*, 294.

Von Albert, H. H. Automated analysis of prolonged EEG recordings in epileptic patients. In J. K. Penry (Ed.), *Epilepsy, the eighth international symposium*. New York: Raven Press, 1977.

Vos, J. E. Between EEG machine and computer: Data storage and data conversion. In A. Rémond (Ed.), *EEG informatics. A didactic review of methods and applications of EEG data processing*. Amsterdam: Elsevier, 1977, 143-155.

Wagle, B. Multivariate beta distribution and a test for multivariate normality. *J. R. Statist. Soc.*, 1968, *30*, 511-516.

Walter, D. O. Spectral analysis for electroencephalogram: Mathematical determination of neurophysiological relationships from records of limited duration. *Exp. Neurol.*, 1963, *8*, 155-181.

Walter, D. O. The method of complex demodulation. In Advances in EEG analysis, *Electroenceph. Clin. Neurophysiol.*, 1968, Suppl. *27*, 53-57. (a)

Walter, D. O. A posteriori "Wiener filtering" of average evoked responses. In Advances in EEG analysis. *Electroenceph. Clin. Neurophysiol.*, 1968, Suppl. *27*, 61-70. (b)

Walter, D. O. Digital processing of bioelectrical phenomena. In *Handbook of electroencephalography and clinical neurophysiology* (Vol. 4B). Amsterdam: Elsevier, 1972.

Walter, D. O., & Adey, W. R. Spectral analysis of electroencephalograms recorded during learning in the cat. *Exp. Neurol.*, 1963, *8*, 155-181.

Walter, D. O., & Brazier, M. A. B. (Eds.). Advances in EEG analysis. *Electroenceph. Clin. Neurophysiol.*, 1968, Suppl. *27*.

Walter, D. O., Rhodes, J. M., & Adey, W. R. Discriminating among states of consciousness by EEG measurements. A study of four subjects. *Electroenceph. Clin. Neurophysiol.*, 1967, *22*, 22-29.

Walter, D. O., Rhodes, J. M., Brown, D., & Adey, W. R. Comprehensive spectral analysis of human EEG generators in posteriori cerebral regions. *Electroenceph. Clin. Neurophysiol.*, 1966, *20*, 224-237.

Walter, S. T., & Arfel, G. Responses aux stimulations visuelles dans les états de coma aigu et de coma chronique. *Electroenceph. Clin. Neurophysiol.*, 1972, *32*, 27-41.

Walter, V. J., & Walter, W. G. The central effects of rhythmic sensory stimulation. *Electroenceph. Clin. Neurophysiol.*, 1949, *1*, 57.

Walter, W. G. The location of cerebral tumors by electroencephalography. *Lancet*, 1936, *2*, 305-308.

Walter, W. G. An automatic low frequency analyzer. *Electron. Eng.*, 1943, *16*, 3-13.

Walter, W. G. Normal rhythms. Their development, distribution and significance. In D. Hill & G. Parr (Eds.), *Electroencephalography*. London: MacDonald, 1950, 203-277.

Walter, W. G., Cooper, R., Aldridge, V. J., Mc Callum, W. C., and Winter, A. L. Contingent negative variation: an electric sign of sensorimotor association and expectancy in human brain. Nature 1964, *203*, 380-384. (a)

Walter, W. G. The convergence and interaction of visual, auditory and tactile responses in human nonspecific cortex. *Ann. N.Y. Acad. Sci.*, 1964, *112*, 320-361. (b)

Walter, W. G. Brain responses to semantic stimuli. *J. Psychosom. Res.*, 1965, *9*, 51-61.

Walter, W. G. The Contingent Negative Variation as an aid to psychiatric diagnosis. In M. Kletzman & J. Zubin (Eds.), *Objective indication of psychopathology*. New York: Academic Press, 1970.

Walter, W. G. Evoked response general. In *Handbook of electroencephalography and clinical neurophysiology* (Vol. 8A). Amsterdam: Elsevier, 1975, 20-32.

Walter, W. G., & Dovey, V. J. Electroencephalography in cases of subcortical tumour. *J. Neurol. Neurosurg. Psychiat.*, 1944, *7*, 57-65.

Walter, W. G., Dovey, V. J., & Shipton, H. W. Analysis of the electrical response of the human cortex to photic stimulation. *Nature*, 1946, *19*, 540-541.

Walter, W. G., & Shipton, H. W. A new toposcopic display system. *Electroenceph. Clin. Neurophysiol.*, 1951, *3*, 281-292.

Ward, W. D. The Contingent Negative Variation in hyperkinetic children. *Electroenceph. Clin. Neurophysiol.*, 1976, *41*, 645.

Wastell, D. G. Statistical detection of individual evoked responses: An evaluation of Woody's adaptive filter. *Electroenceph. Clin. Neurophysiol.*, 1977, *42*, 835-839.

Wegner, J. T., & Struve, F. A. Incidence of the 14 and 6 per second positive spike pattern in adult clinical population: An empirical note. *J. Nervous and Mental Diseases*, 1977, *164*, 340-345.

Weinberg, H., Michalewski, H., & Koopman, R. The influence of discriminations on the form of the Contingent Negative Variation. *Neuropsychologia*, 1976, *14*, 87-95.

Weinberg, H., & Papakostopoulos, D. The frontal CNV: Its dissimilarity to CNVs recorded from other sites. *Electroenceph. Clin. Neurophysiol.*, 1975, *39*, 21-28.

Weinberg, H., Walter, W. G., & Crow, H. J. Intracerebral events in humans related to real and imaginary stimuli. *Electroenceph. Clin. Neurophysiol.*, 1970, *29*, 1-9.

Weiss, M. S. Non Gaussian properties of the EEG during sleep. *Electroenceph. Clin. Neurophysiol.*, 1973, *34*, 200-202.

Weitzman, E. D., & Graziani, L. J. Maturation and topography of the auditory evoked response of the prematurely born infant. *Developmental Psychobiology*, 1968, *1*, 79-89.

Weitzman, E. D., Graziani, L. J., & Duhamel, L. Maturation and topography of the auditory evoked response of the prematurely born infant. *Electroenceph. Clin. Neurophysiol.*, 1967, *23*, 82.

Wennberg, A. *Spectral parameter analysis (SPA) of the EEG. Clinical application*. Thesis, Karolinska Institute, Stockholm, 1975.

Wennberg, A., & Isaksson, A. Simulation of nonstationary EEG signals as a means of objective interpretation of the EEG. In P. Kellaway & I. Petersén (Eds.), *Quantitative analytic studies in epilepsy*. New York: Raven Press, 1976, 493-508.

Wennberg, A., & Zetterberg, L. H. Application of a computer-based model for EEG analysis. *Electroenceph. Clin. Neurophysiol.*, 1971, *31*, 457-468.

Werre, P. F., & Smith, C. J. Variability of responses evoked by flashes in man. *Electroenceph. Clin. Neurophysiol.*, 1964, *17*, 644-652.

Whitton, J. L., Lue, F., & Moldofsky, H. A spectral method for removing eye movement artifacts from the EEG. *Electroenceph. Clin. Neurophysiol.*, 1978, *44*, 735-741.

Wicke, J. D., Donchin, E., & Lindsley, D. B. Visual evoked potentials as a function of flash luminance and duration. *Science*, 1964, *146*, 83-85.

Wicke, J. D., Goff, W. R., Wallace, J. D., & Allison, T. On-line statistical detection of average evoked potentials: Applications to evoked response audiometry. *Electroenceph. Clin. Neurophysiol.*, 1978, *44*, 328-343.

Wiederholt, W. C., & Kritchevsky, M. Early components of the human averaged somatosensory evoked potential. Paper presented at the 11th World Congress of Neurology, Amsterdam, 1977.

Wiener, N. *Extrapolation, interpolation and smoothing of stationary time series*. New York: Wiley, 1949.

Wildberger, H. G. H., Van Lith, G. H. M., Winjgaarde, R., & Mak, G. T. M. Visually evoked cortical potentials in the evaluation of homonymous and bitemporal visual field defects. *Brit. J. Ophthal.*, 1976, *60*, 273-278.

Williams, R. L., Karakan, I., & Hursch, C. J. *Electroencephalography of human sleep: Clinical applications*. New York: Wiley, 1974.

Williamson, P. D., Goff, W. R., & Allison, T. Somatosensory evoked responses in patients with unilateral cerebral lesions. *Electroenceph. Clin. Neurophysiol.*, 1970, *28* 566-575.

Wishart, D. An algorithm for hierarchical classification. *Biometrics*, 1969, *22*, 165-170.

Wolpaw, J. R., & Penry, J. K. A temporal component of the auditory evoked response. *Electroenceph. Clin. Neurophysiol.*, 1975, *39*, 609-620.

Wolpaw, J. R., & Penry, J. K. Hemispheric differences in the auditory evoked response. *Electroenceph. Clin. Neurophysiol.*, 1977, *43*, 99-102.

Woody, C. D. Characterization of an adaptive filter for the analysis of variable latency neuroelectric signals. *Medical and Biological Engineering*, 1967, *5*, 539-553.

Yagi, A., Ball, L., & Callaway, E. Optimum parameters for the measurement of cortical coupling. *Physiological Psychology*, 1976, *4*, 33-38.

Yamada, T., Kimura, J., Young, S., & Powers, M. Somatosensory evoked potentials elicited by bilateral stimulation of the median nerve and its clinical applications. *Neurology*, 1978, *28*, 218-224.

Yamada, O., Yamane, H., & Kodera, K. Simultaneous recordings of the brain stem response and the frequency-following response to low frequency tone. *Electroenceph. Clin. Neurophysiol.*, 1977, *43*, 362–370.

Yamamoto, K., Shimazono, Y., & Miyasaka, M. Automatic EEG analysis in normal subjects. *Electroenceph. Clin. Neurophysiol.*, 1977, *43*, 468.

Yeager, C. L., Gevins, A. S., & Henderson, J. H. A concise method of EEG classification for compiling a clinical EEG data base. *Electroenceph. Clin. Neurophysiol.*, 1977, *43*, 459.

Yingling, C. D. Lateralization of cortical coupling during complex verbal and spatial behavior. In J. E. Desmedt (Ed.), *Progress in clinical neurophysiology* (Vol. 3). Basel: Karger, 1977.

Zappoli, R., Papini, M., Briani, S., Benvenutti, P., & Pasquinelli, A. CNV in patients with known frontal lobe lesion. *Electroenceph. Clin. Neurophysiol.*, 1975, *39*, 216.

Zeese, J. A. Pattern evoked responses in multiple sclerosis. *Electroenceph. Clin. Neurophysiol.*, 1976, *40*, 315.

Zetterberg, L. H. Estimation of parameters for a linear difference equation with application to EEG analysis. *Math. Biosci.*, 1969, *5*, 227-275.

Zetterberg, L. H. Experience with analysis and simulation of EEG signals with parametric descriptors of spectra. In P. Kellaway & I. Petersén (Eds.), *Automation of clinical electroencephalography*. New York: Raven Press, 1973, 161-202. (b)

Zetterberg, L. H. Spike detection by computer and by analog equipment. In P. Kellaway & I. Petersén (Eds.), *Automation of clinical electroencephalography*. New York: Raven Press, 1973, 227-234. (a)

Zetterberg, L. H. *Means and methods for processing of physiological signals with emphasis on EEG analysis*. Technical Report No. 84. Telecommunication Theory Electrical Engineering. Stockholm: Royal Institute of Technology, 1974.

Zhirmynskaya, E. A., Voitenko, G. A., & Konyukhova, G. P. Changes of correlational functions in different types of alterations of bioelectrical activity of the brain. *Zh. Nevropat. Psikhiat.*, 1970, *70*, 376-382. (Russian)

Zimmermann, G. N., & Knott, J. R. Slow potentials of the brain related to speech processing in normal speakers and stutterers. *Electroenceph. Clin. Neurophysiol.*, 1974, *37*, 599-607.

Author Index

A

D

G

L

M

Q

R

S

Subject Index

A

B

T

V

X,Y,Z